BIOMETALS IN NEURODEGENERATIVE DISEASES

BIOMETALS IN NEURODEGENERATIVE DISEASES

Mechanisms and Therapeutics

Edited by

ANTHONY R. WHITE
Cell and Molecular Biology
QIMR Berghofer Medical Research Institute,
Herston, QLD, Australia

MICHAEL ASCHNER
Department of Molecular Pharmacology
Albert Einstein College of Medicine
Bronx, NY, United States

LUCIO G. COSTA
Department of Environmental and Occupational
Health Sciences University of Washington
Seattle, WA, United States

ASHLEY I. BUSH
Florey Institute of Neuroscience and Mental Health
University of Melbourne
Parkville, VIC, Australia

ELSEVIER

ACADEMIC PRESS
An imprint of Elsevier

Academic Press is an imprint of Elsevier
125 London Wall, London EC2Y 5AS, United Kingdom
525 B Street, Suite 1800, San Diego, CA 92101-4495, United States
50 Hampshire Street, 5th Floor, Cambridge, MA 02139, United States
The Boulevard, Langford Lane, Kidlington, Oxford OX5 1GB, United Kingdom

Library of Congress Cataloging-in-Publication Data
A catalog record for this book is available from the Library of Congress

British Library Cataloguing-in-Publication Data
A catalogue record for this book is available from the British Library

ISBN: 978-0-12-804562-6

For information on all Academic Press publications visit our website at
https://www.elsevier.com/books-and-journals

Publisher: Mara Conner
Acquisition Editor: Melanie Tucker
Editorial Project Manager: Kristi Anderson
Production Project Manager: Karen East and Kirsty Halterman
Designer: Victoria Pearson

Typeset by Thomson Digital

Contents

7. Metals and Prions: Twenty Years of Mining the Awe

DAVID R. BROWN

8. Manganese and Neurodegeneration

DINAMENE MARQUES DOS SANTOS, MICHAEL ASCHNER, ANA P. MARREILHA DOS SANTOS

9. Zinc in Autism

STEFANIE GRABRUCKER, ANDREAS M. GRABRUCKER

10. Metals and Motor Neuron Disease

PER M. ROOS

11. Metals and Lysosomal Storage Disorders

HENNA KONTTINEN, KATARÍNA LEJAVOVÁ, TARJA MALM, KATJA M. KANNINEN

12. Developmental Exposure to Metals and its Contribution to Age-Related Neurodegeneration

LUCIO G. COSTA

13. Metal Biology Associated with Huntington's Disease

TERRY JO V. BICHELL, TIMOTHY C. HALBESMA, K. GRACE TIPPS, AARON B. BOWMAN

19. Metals and Autophagy in Neurotoxicity

PENG SU, MICHAEL ASCHNER, JINGYUAN CHEN, WENJING LUO

20. An Overview of Multifunctional Metal Chelators as Potential Treatments for Neurodegenerative Diseases

FRANK W. LEWIS, DAVID TÉTARD

21. Abnormal Function of Metalloproteins Underlies Most Neurodegenerative Diseases

KATJA M. KANNINEN, ANTHONY R. WHITE

Contributors

Alessandro Alimonti National Institute of Health, Rome, Italy

Michael Aschner Albert Einstein College of Medicine, Bronx, NY, United States

Terry Jo V. Bichell Vanderbilt Brain Institute; Vanderbilt University Medical Center, Nashville, TN, United States

Stephen C. Bondy Center for Occupational and Environmental Health, University of California, Irvine, CA, United States

Valentina Borghesani CNRS, LCC (Laboratory of Chemical Coordination); University of Toulouse, Toulouse, France

Aaron B. Bowman Vanderbilt Brain Institute; Vanderbilt University Medical Center, Nashville, TN, United States

Sonia Brescianini Center for Epidemiology, Surveillance and Health Promotion, National Institute of Health, Rome, Italy

David R. Brown University of Bath, Bath, United Kingdom

Maria C. Buscarinu Center for Experimental Neurological Therapies, S. Andrea Hospital, "Sapienza" University of Rome, Rome, Italy

Ashley I. Bush The Florey Institute of Neuroscience and Mental Health, The University of Melbourne, Parkville, VIC, Australia

Bárbara R. Cardoso The Florey Institute of Neuroscience and Mental Health, The University of Melbourne, Parkville, VIC, Australia; University of São Paulo, São Paulo, Brazil

Benedetta Cerasoli Center for Experimental Neurological Therapies, S. Andrea Hospital, "Sapienza" University of Rome, Rome, Italy

Jingyuan Chen Fourth Military Medical University, Xi'an, China

James R. Connor The Pennsylvania State University College of Medicine, Hershey, PA, United States

Lucio G. Costa University of Washington, Seattle, WA, United States; University of Parma, Parma, Italy

Peter J. Crouch University of Melbourne, Melbourne, VIC, Australia

Melisa del Barrio CNRS, LCC (Laboratory of Chemical Coordination); University of Toulouse, Toulouse, France

David C. Dorman North Carolina State University, Raleigh, NC, United States

Peter Faller Biometals and Biological Chemistry, Institute of Chemistry, UMR 7177, University of Strasbourg, Strasbourg, France

Michela Ferraldeschi Center for Experimental Neurological Therapies, S. Andrea Hospital, "Sapienza" University of Rome, Rome, Italy

Arianna Fornasiero Center for Experimental Neurological Therapies, S. Andrea Hospital, "Sapienza" University of Rome, Rome, Italy

Andreas M. Grabrucker Institute for Anatomy and Cell Biology; WG molecular Analysis of Synaptopathies, Ulm University, Ulm, Germany

Stefanie Grabrucker Institute for Anatomy and Cell Biology, Ulm University, Ulm, Germany

Mark A. Greenough The Florey Institute of Neuroscience and Mental Health, The University of Melbourne, Melbourne, VIC, Australia

Timothy C. Halbesma Vanderbilt University Medical Center, Nashville, TN, United States

Dominic J. Hare The Florey Institute of Neuroscience and Mental Health, The University of Melbourne, Parkville, VIC; University of Technology Sydney, Broadway, NSW, Australia

Christelle Hureau CNRS, LCC (Laboratory of Chemical Coordination); University of Toulouse, Toulouse, France

Hong Jiang Medical College of Qingdao University; Shandong Provincial Collaborative Innovation Center for Neurodegenerative Disorders, Qingdao University, Qingdao, China

Katja M. Kanninen A.I. Virtanen Institute for Molecular Sciences, University of Eastern Finland, Kuopio, Finland

Henna Konttinen A.I. Virtanen Institute for Molecular Sciences, University of Eastern Finland, Kuopio, Finland

Katarína Lejavová A.I. Virtanen Institute for Molecular Sciences, University of Eastern Finland, Kuopio, Finland

Frank W. Lewis Northumbria University Newcastle, Newcastle, United Kingdom

Wenjing Luo Fourth Military Medical University, Xi'an, China

Tarja Malm A.I. Virtanen Institute for Molecular Sciences, University of Eastern Finland, Kuopio, Finland

Dinamene Marques dos Santos University of Lisbon, Lisboa, Portugal

Ana P. Marreilha dos Santos University of Lisbon, Lisboa, Portugal

Carlo Mattei Center for Experimental Neurological Therapies, S. Andrea Hospital, "Sapienza" University of Rome, Rome, Italy

Rosella Mechelli Center for Experimental Neurological Therapies, S. Andrea Hospital, "Sapienza" University of Rome, Rome, Italy

Alexandra I. Mot University of Melbourne, Melbourne, VIC, Australia

Anne M. Nixon The Pennsylvania State University College of Medicine, Hershey, PA, United States

Carlos M. Opazo The Florey Institute of Neuroscience and Mental Health, The University of Melbourne, Melbourne, VIC, Australia

George Perry The University of Texas at San Antonio (UTSA), San Antonio, TX, United States

Anna Pino National Institute of Health, Rome, Italy

Germán Plascencia-Villa The University of Texas at San Antonio (UTSA), San Antonio, TX, United States

Alejandra Ramírez Muñoz The Florey Institute of Neuroscience and Mental Health, The University of Melbourne, Melbourne, VIC, Australia

Giovanni Ristori Center for Experimental Neurological Therapies, S. Andrea Hospital, "Sapienza" University of Rome, Rome, Italy

Silvia Romano Center for Experimental Neurological Therapies, S. Andrea Hospital, "Sapienza" University of Rome, Rome, Italy

Per M. Roos Karolinska Institutet, Institute of Environmental Medicine, Stockholm, Sweden

Carlo Salustri Institute of Cognitive Sciences and Technologies (CNR), Fatebenefratelli Hospital, Rome, Italy

Marco Salvetti Center for Experimental Neurological Therapies, S. Andrea Hospital, "Sapienza" University of Rome, Rome, Italy

Mariacristina Siotto Don Carlo Gnocchi Foundation ONLUS, Italy

Rosanna Squitti IRCCS, Institute Center St. John of God Fatebenefratelli, Brescia, Italy

Maria A. Stazi National Institute of Health, Rome, Italy

Peng Su Fourth Military Medical University, Xi'an, China

David Tétard Northumbria University Newcastle, Newcastle, United Kingdom

K. Grace Tipps Vanderbilt University Medical Center, Nashville, TN, United States

Mariacarla Ventriglia Institute of Cognitive Sciences and Technologies (CNR), Fatebenefratelli Hospital, Rome, Italy

Anthony R. White QIMR Berghofer Medical Research Institute, Herston, QLD, Australia

Miguel José-Yacamán The University of Texas at San Antonio (UTSA), San Antonio, TX, United States

Preface

Biological metals (biometals) have key functions in the brain but can also induce degenerative changes due to abnormalities in homeostatic mechanisms. The scientific literature in this field is advancing rapidly with approximately 300 publications per year adding to our knowledge of how biometals contribute to neurodegenerative diseases, such as Alzheimer's disease, Parkinson's disease, motor neuron disease, and others. Despite this rapid increase in our understanding of biometals in brain disease, the fields of biomedicine and neuroscience have often overlooked this information. The need to bring the research on biometals in neurodegeneration to the forefront of biomedical research is essential if we are to understand neurodegenerative disease processes and develop effective therapeutics. There are currently few sources of consolidated research on biometals and neurodegeneration that are available to biomedical researchers, clinicians, students, and others. This book on biometals in neurodegeneration provides an authoritative and timely resource to bring together the major findings in the field for ease of access to those working in neuroscience or biomedicine, or with an interest in metals and their role in the brain function, disease, and as therapeutic targets.

Overview of chapters included in *Biometals in Neurodegenerative Diseases: Mechanisms and Therapeutics.*

Alzheimer's disease is the leading form of neurodegeneration contributing to the majority of an estimated 36 million cases of dementia worldwide. With an ageing world population, estimates for global Alzheimer's disease prevalence are in the order of 115 million patients by 2050. It is therefore fitting that the opening chapter of this book covers biometals in Alzheimer's disease. Mot and Crouch (Chapter 1, pp. 1–18) provide a comprehensive insight into the contribution of biometals including copper, zinc, and iron in several major pathological features of Alzheimer's disease including amyloid peptide aggregation and tau phosphorylation. The chapter finishes with an insight into where therapeutic approaches to biometal modulation in Alzheimer's disease may progress in the future. Staying with the role of biometals in Alzheimer's disease, Squitti et al. (Chapter 2, pp. 19–34) provides a deeper insight into the role of copper in this disorder, describing the pathways of copper metabolism and brain copper handling as well as interesting aspects of copper toxicity and the role of ceruloplasmin and nonceruloplasmin copper in Alzheimer's disease. This is followed by a very interesting insight into a biometal that receives less coverage than it should, selenium and its role in neurodegeneration. This biometal forms a critical inorganic component of the amino acid selenocysteine, which is involved in at least 25 different proteins. Abnormal selenium stasis is found in many forms of leading neurodegenerative diseases, and selenium-based therapeutics have the potential to make significant impacts in these disorders as discussed by Cardoso et al. (Chapter 3, pp. 35–50).

The subsequent three chapters by Nixon and Connor (Chapter 4, pp. 51–66), Ferraldeschi et al. (Chapter 5, pp. 67–82) and Stephen Bondy (Chapter 6, pp. 83–94) cover important aspects of biometals in inflammation and how this modulates outcomes in neurodegeneration. Nixon and Connor et al. describe how the high iron (Fe) gene, HFE genotype, affects macrophage phenotype in disease. Mutations in HFE appear to alter macrophage (and microglial) iron distribution with potentially important outcomes for neurodegeneration. Ferraldeschi et al. follow this with an expanded insight into the role of biometals in oxidative-mediated neuroinflammatory processes, with a more detailed focus on biometal effects in multiple sclerosis. Bondy then provides a valuable account of the various mechanisms leading to biometal-mediated neuroinflammation, including the formation of haptens, the production of reactive oxygen and nitrogen species, the sequestering of reducing capacity and the formation of inflammation-provoking colloids.

David Brown (Chapter 7, pp. 95–116) brings us a very informative and insightful account of 20 years of metals research in prion diseases, dispelling some common myths and providing a comprehensive account of where we have come to in this field. Iron, zinc, copper, and manganese all have key roles to play in prion protein stasis in diseases, such as Creutzfeld–Jakob disease. Staying with the biometal, manganese, Marques dos Santos et al. (Chapter 8, pp. 117–152) provide an in-depth coverage of this element in neurodegeneration, providing valuable information on the role of manganese in neurobiology, environmental exposure in humans, and subsequent pathways to neurotoxicity and neurodegeneration.

Although autism spectrum disorder (ASD) is not classically categorized as a neurodegenerative disorder, there are shared comorbidities between ASD and neurodegenerative disorders including altered biometal stasis in the brain. Grabrucker and Grabrucker (Chapter 9, pp. 153–174) delve into the role of these biometal changes in ASDs, providing an interesting account of how biometals can affect neuro-synaptic functions resulting in the features that characterize ASD. Although a rare disorder, motor neuron disease (MND) has been the center of recent major international funding efforts. The disease is rapid with most cases fatal in 2–5 years after onset, and no long-term effective treatment exists. Although the cause in most cases remains unknown, Per Roos (Chapter 10, pp. 175–194) describes a key role for possible environmental exposure to biometals including lead, manganese, and mercury in disease etiology, and how these metals may contribute to neuropathological changes. In the last of the chapters covering the general role of biometals in neurodegeneration, Konttinen et al. (Chapter 11, pp. 195–216) cover important aspects of biometals in another group of rare disorders, the lysosomal storage diseases (LSDs). Lysosomes are key sites of biometal homeostasis, and abnormalities in lysosomal function as occurs in LSDs, leads to significant biometal abnormalities with potentially major impacts leading to neurodegeneration in these disorders.

The second half of this volume covers molecular and cellular aspects of metals in brain health, dysfunction, and neurotoxicity. Lucio G. Costa (Chapter 12, pp. 217–230) starts this section with a review of how environmental exposure to metals, such as lead and arsenic in early life can affect outcomes in later life neurodegeneration including Alzheimer's disease. The mechanism of this predisposition is unclear but could be related to epigenetic changes induced by biometals. Bichell et al. (Chapter 13, pp. 231–264) follow this with an account of metal biology in Huntington's disease including potential iron, copper, and manganese interactions with a range of homeostatic enzymes and proteins in the brain. Del Barrio et al. (Chapter 14, pp. 265–282) return us to Alzheimer's disease again with a critical insight into the fundamental copper coordination by amyloid peptide, the major protein form deposited in Alzheimer's brains. The review describes how copper drives aggregation and reactive oxygen species generation through interaction with the amyloid peptide.

Delving deeper into the cells of the brain, Plascencia-Villa et al. (Chapter 15, pp. 283–312) explore the role of biometals in mitochondrial function and how this contributes to a range of neurodegenerative disorders. Abnormalities in biometal handling in the cell powerhouse leads to major outcomes including reactive oxygen species formation, abnormal cell signaling, and altered energy production with important consequences for highly metabolic neurons. Another important aspect of biometal involvement in neurodegeneration is biometal transportation. Changes to key biometal transporters in the brain can have profound effects on the handling and action of copper, zinc, iron, manganese etc. And conversely, altered metal levels can affect transporter expression and localization. Hong Jiang (Chapter 16, pp. 313–348) provides a comprehensive coverage of metal transporters for the main neuro-metals and how changes to these transporters can underlie neurodegenerative outcomes.

One of the most important techniques used to understand how biometals contribute to neurodegeneration is metal imaging. David Dorman (Chapter 17, pp. 349–362) describes one of the central biometal imaging techniques applied to neurodegenerative disease, magnetic resonance imaging (MRI), and how it can be used to understand and differentiate the roles of iron, manganese, and copper in brain disorders. Brain protein accumulation is a major feature of most neurodegenerative diseases and is often associated with impaired mechanisms for clearance of aggregated or abnormally folded proteins. Ramírez Muñoz et al. (Chapter 18, pp. 363–376) describe how metals play a fundamental role in protein clearance and how this can be affected by abnormal metal homeostasis, contributing further to neurodegenerative disease pathology. Related to this, Su et al. (Chapter 19, pp. 377–398) contribute a key insight to the role of metals in autophagic processes. A key cellular mechanism for clearance of unwanted cell material, autophagy is a complex process involving many proteins and subcellular compartments. Studies have found major impairments to autophagy in neurodegenerative diseases and this is now a common putative therapeutic target. Su et al., explore the role of metals in autophagy and how abnormalities to metal homeostasis can contribute to pathological autophagic changes.

Of course, one of the major reasons for increasing our understanding of biometals in neurodegeneration is to develop therapeutic approaches for these disorders. In the penultimate chapter, Lewis and Tétard (Chapter 20, pp. 399–414) provide us with a comprehensive overview of metal chelators as potential new treatments for neurodegeneration. The future of these therapeutics appears to be in development of multifunctional agents that target metals and additional pathological features of neurodegeneration, such as oxidative stress. Time will tell if this approach provides much needed advances in neurodegenerative disease therapeutics. The final chapter by Kanninen and White (Chapter 21, pp. 415–438) then takes an overarching view of biometals in neurodegeneration and provides a review of the role for metalloproteins in many forms of neurodegenerative disease, leading us to consider whether neurodegenerative diseases should be categorized as metallopathies.

Whether student, clinician, or specialized biometals researcher, we hope that the reader will be able to gain exciting new insights into biometals and neurodegeneration. We believe that this volume will have an important place in the medical literature and provide a valuable reference source for many years in this major field of neurodegenerative disease research.

Anthony R. White
Michael Aschner
Lucio G. Costa
Ashley I. Bush

CHAPTER

1

Biometals and Alzheimer's Disease

Alexandra I. Mot, Peter J. Crouch

University of Melbourne, Melbourne, VIC, Australia

OUTLINE

INTRODUCTION

Alzheimer's disease (AD) was first described in 1906 by Dr. Alois Alzheimer, and is now the third leading cause of death in industrial countries.[1] The disease is clinically characterized by the progressive loss of memory and other cognitive domains including language, attention, orientation, and problem solving abilities.[2] The biggest risk factor for AD is age,[3] and given the ageing population demographic of our society the incidence of AD is likely to increase in the future. This highlights the urgent need for the development of effective disease-modifying therapies to halt or slow disease progression. Although the aetiology of sporadic AD remains largely unknown, the disease is associated with distinct pathological abnormalities which distinguish the condition from other forms of dementia.[4] Macroscopically, AD is characterized by progressive cortical atrophy particularly of the frontal, parietal, and temporal lobes.[5] Microscopically, the disease is characterized by neuronal and synaptic loss, extracellular senile plaques composed of aggregated amyloid beta (Aβ) peptides, and intracellular neurofibrillary tangles (NFTs) composed of hyperphosphorylated forms of the protein tau.[6,7]

According to the amyloid cascade hypothesis which was first suggested in 1992, the Aβ peptide plays a central role in AD pathogenesis.[8] The amyloid precursor protein (APP) is cleaved through one of two pathways by the metalloproteinases α-secretase, γ-secretase, or

Biometals in Neurodegenerative Diseases. http://dx.doi.org/10.1016/B978-0-12-804562-6.00001-4

the beta-site amyloid precursor protein-cleaving enzyme 1 (BACE 1) which is a β-secretase.[9] The nonamyloidogenic pathway involves cleavage of the extracellular APP domain by α-secretase followed by cleavage of the intramembranous domain by γ-secretase. By contrast, in the amyloidogenic pathway the initial cleavage of the extracellular APP domain is mediated by BACE 1 resulting in the production of the Aβ peptide.[10] Although Aβ is generated in all brain regions and is ubiquitously expressed throughout the body, not all brain regions are affected.[11,12] This indicates that Aβ expression alone is not sufficient to cause disease, and it is therefore likely that other factors in the affected brain regions are able to either induce Aβ toxicity or to make these brain regions in other ways vulnerable to disease. Consistent with this is the fact that phase three clinical trials performed on drugs that inhibit Aβ production or lower Aβ levels through immunotherapy have failed to alter disease progression.[13–16] Alternative therapeutic approaches are therefore urgently needed.

Biologically functional metal ions (also known as biometals) are tightly regulated in the heathy brain and a breakdown in the homeostasis mechanisms that compartmentalize and regulate these metals can substantially affect brain function.[17] The following sections will examine how copper, zinc, and iron play a role in AD pathogenesis through interactions with disease-associated proteins. Lastly, therapeutic attempts to restore biometal homeostasis in AD will be reviewed.

THE ROLE OF COPPER IN AD

Copper is a redox-active metal and exists in either oxidized (Cu^{2+}) or reduced (Cu^{+}) valence states.[18] Many enzymes utilize this change in copper oxidation state, in the presence of oxygen, to catalyze redox chemistry for a wide range of important biochemical reactions. Some important copper-containing enzymes are: Cu/Zn-superoxide dismutase (SOD1), which converts the superoxide free radical into hydrogen peroxide,[19] cytochrome *c* oxidase (COX) which plays a key role in the mitochondrial electron transport chain,[20] and ceruloplasmin (Cp) which functions as a ferroxidase to facilitate iron export from cells.[21] All of these proteins require copper binding to perform their function, and low copper levels could therefore lead to oxidative stress, mitochondrial dysfunction, and intracellular iron accumulation, all of which are observed in AD.[22–24] The same chemistry which makes copper useful in biology also allows free copper to catalyze the formation of the hydroxyl radical via the Fenton reaction.[25] Therefore, because the free form of the metal is potentially damaging, absorption and excretion of copper are tightly regulated in the body. Copper transport across cellular membranes occurs predominantly via the transporters high affinity copper uptake protein 1 (Ctr1) and ATPase copper-transporting alpha and beta polypeptides (ATP7a and ATP7b).[26] Neurodegeneration is a feature of both Menkes disease, which is caused by mutations in the gene encoding ATP7a[27,28] and Wilson disease, which is caused by mutations in the gene encoding ATP7b.[29,30] This demonstrates that copper dysregulation is detrimental to brain health.

In the AD brain overall copper levels are decreased within affected regions[31,32] but are enriched within plaques and neurofibrillary tangles.[33] From this a complex picture emerges where abnormal copper distribution in AD leads to copper deficiency within affected brain regions. In the healthy brain, postsynaptic N-methyl-D-aspartic acid (NMDA) neurites release ionic copper into the synaptic cleft, facilitated by ATP7a, at a concentration of around

15 μM.[34,35] Within the synaptic cleft copper causes S-nitrosylation of NMDA receptors, which inhibits their activation.[36] The sequestration of copper within amyloid plaques has been proposed as a mechanism by which the pool of free copper within the synaptic cleft is depleted leading to increased activation of NMDA receptors.[37] In contrast with decreased brain copper levels in AD, the serum and cerebrospinal fluid (CSF) levels of copper are significantly elevated in AD patients when compared to age-matched controls.[38,39] This may correlate with increased expression of ceruloplasmin (a major copper-binding protein in serum) in AD, although excess copper is not bound to this carrier protein.[40] Furthermore, increased serum copper was reported to correlate well with higher levels of serum peroxides in AD patients.[41] Taken together these studies indicate that altered copper distribution in AD brain, serum, and CSF contributes to disease pathogenesis.

Copper binds to APP in the amino-terminal ectodomain (between residues 142 and 166)[42] and catalytically reduces copper (II) to copper (I).[43] The structure of the APP copper binding domain consist of four ligands (His-147, His-151, Tyr-168, and Met-170),[42] which show structural homology to other copper chaperones. As a ubiquitously expressed protein, APP may play a role in regulating metal ion homeostasis. This is supported by studies which have shown that chronic copper overload or copper deficiency can both up- and downregulate APP mRNA expression in mouse fibroblasts.[44,45] Furthermore, another study found that a low copper diet in healthy individuals was associated with decreased APP protein expression in platelets.[46] Conversely, both in vivo and in vitro studies in APP-knockout mice have shown that copper levels are significantly increased in brain and liver tissues as well as in cortical neuron and fibroblast primary cultures derived from these animals.[47,48] One of these studies also found that APP-knockout primary cortical neurons are susceptible to copper-induced toxicity through copper (I) production which caused localized oxidative stress.[47] Moreover, the overexpression of mutant APP in various transgenic mouse lines decreased copper levels in both in vivo and in vitro contexts.[49–51] Additionally, copper promotes an increase in cell surface APP by increasing its exocytosis and reducing its endocytosis, respectively.[52] Collectively these studies indicate that the interaction between copper and APP may contribute to AD pathogenesis.

Copper binds to the Aβ peptide in a pH-dependent manner and $A\beta_{1-16}$ has been shown to be the minimal sequence required for copper binding.[53] Between pH 6 and 7, Aβ binds to copper at Asp1, His6, and His13/14; while at pH 8, the binding sites shift to His6, His13, and His14.[54] At pH 10 or higher, Asp1, Ala2, Glu3, and Phe4 can also form a complex with copper.[55,56] Of particular interest is the fact that Aβ purified from human brain plaques contains fewer histidine residues, which has been explained by copper-mediated oxidation.[57] Copper modifies Aβ by promoting dityrosine crosslinking of the peptide, which may act as a seed to accelerate Aβ aggregation and induce oligomer formation.[58,59] Aβ toxicity is partially dependant on copper and can be attenuated in cell culture by copper chelation.[60,61] The mechanism of copper-Aβ induced cytotoxicity might involve oxidative stress, as the complex catalytically generates hydrogen peroxide.[62] Furthermore, another study found that the copper-Aβ complex could inhibit COX function thereby impairing mitochondrial energy production.[63]

Copper also binds to the tau protein and certain fragments in the four-repeat microtubule-binding domain of tau (residues 256–273, 287–304, and 306–336) were shown to aggregate in the presence of copper in vitro.[64,65] Furthermore, copper binding to tau induces hydrogen peroxide production,[66] which recapitulates what is observed in AD brains where copper-containing NFTs are a source of oxidative stress.[67] Chronic copper exposure accelerates tau hyperphosphorylation via abnormal cyclin-dependent kinase 5 (Cdk5) activation, resulting in dissociation of tau from microtubules in an AD mouse model.[68] However, copper delivery drugs have been shown to decrease glycogen synthase kinase 3 beta (GSK-3β)-dependent tau phosphorylation.[69] These studies indicate that copper alters tau phosphorylation through diverse mechanisms.

THE ROLE OF ZINC IN AD

Zinc is another transition metal which plays an important role in diverse cellular functions. With the possible exception of pancreatic β islets, the brain contains the highest concentration of zinc within the body.[70] Within the healthy brain, the majority of zinc is compartmentalized in membrane-bound metalloproteins (particularly metallothioneins MT-I, II, and III).[71] Diverse classes of proteins require bound zinc for normal function, including metalloenzymes (e.g., SOD1), transcription factors, and signaling kinases.[72,73] In its free ionic form, zinc in the brain is highly enriched in glutamatergic nerve terminals where it is released (at concentrations of 1–100 μM) upon neuronal activation.[74] Synaptic zinc has a functional role in signal transmission and acts as an antagonist to NMDA receptors.[75] Intracellular zinc uptake is facilitated by a number of zinc-importing proteins (ZIPs), particularly ZIPs 1–5 and 7–15.[76] Zinc uptake can also be mediated by NMDA receptor-dependent voltage-gated L-type Ca^{2+}, Ca^{2+}-permeable AMPA/kainate channels, and Na^{+}/Zn^{+} exchangers.[77–79] Approximately 50% of zinc uptake requires the AD-linked presenilin protein, however, the mechanism by which presenilin contributes to zinc uptake is unknown.[80] Intracellular zinc sequestration or export occurs via the zinc transport (ZnT) protein family. ZnT-2, 5, 7, and 8 are expressed at low levels within the brain, while ZnT-3 is found in granule, pyramidal, and interneuron cells of the hippocampus and plays a role in transporting zinc into glutamatergic vesicles.[81] Indeed, a loss of synaptic zinc in ZnT-3-knockout mice causes age-depend cognitive decline,[82] demonstrating the importance of synaptic zinc in brain function.

Bulk tissue analyses of postmortem AD brains have yielded inconsistent results. Earlier work showed no difference in brain zinc levels between AD and controls,[83,84] while latter studies showed a decrease in zinc levels in several AD brain regions including the neocortex, superior frontal and parietal gyri, medial temporal gyrus and thalamus, and the hippocampus.[85,86] Conflicting reports have, however, also shown elevated zinc levels in multiple AD brain regions including the amygdala, hippocampus, cerebellum, olfactory areas, and superior temporal gyrus.[31,87] These discrepancies could be a result of the examination of different brain regions and/or the utilization of different sample preparations (e.g., tissue fixation affects zinc measurement).[88] Moreover, bulk tissue analyses are unlikely to reveal changes in zinc compartmentalization. Indeed, studies have shown that in AD there is a redistribution of zinc into extracellular plaques and surrounding neuropil.[33,89] While the cause of zinc dysregulation in AD remains unknown, changes to several proteins involved in zinc homeostasis including MT-I, MT-II, MT-III, ZnT-1, ZnT-3, ZnT4, and ZnT-6 in AD[90–93] are likely to contribute to the aberrant compartmentalization of zinc within the brain. Interestingly, estrogen can also modulate levels of ZnT-3 which is of particular significance given that sex is another major risk factor for AD.[94] The serum and CSF levels of zinc are decreased in AD patients when compared to age-matched controls,[38,95] which could in part be explained by nutritional deficiency associated with advanced age.[17]

Zinc binds to APP in a conserved region of amino acids between residues 170 and 188 and this domain consists of two key cysteine ligands at position 186 and 187, which are crucial for binding as well as other potential ligands (e.g., Cys174, Met170, Asp177, and Glu184).[96,97] Zinc interferes with APP processing by altering the function of key secretases involved in APP cleavage. A disintegrin and metalloproteinase domain-containing protein 10 (ADAM 10), the α-secretase involved in the nonamyloidogenic processing of APP, is a zinc-dependent enzyme and thus zinc increases APP proteolysis.[98] Zinc also increases presenilin 1 expression which facilities cellular zinc uptake,[80] although the activity of the γ-secretase complex is inhibited by zinc.[99] Furthermore, the binding of zinc to Aβ within the APP protein sequence can mask the proteolytic cleavage site,[100] thus inhibiting degradation of Aβ by matrix metalloproteases.[101]

Zinc binds to Aβ between residues 6 and 28 with up to three zinc ions bound to histidines 6, 13, and 14.[96,97,100] Zinc binding rapidly induces the aggregation of Aβ into insoluble precipitates, which typify AD pathology.[102] Zinc-induced plaque formation in AD is also supported by the anatomical distribution of plaque and zinc in the brain. Although Aβ is ubiquitously expressed, plaque formation only occurs in neocortical regions of AD-affected brains which closely align with the expression of ZnT3.[103] APP transgenic mice crossed with ZnT3-knockout mice exhibited decreased Aβ burden,[103] which demonstrates the contribution of endogenous zinc to amyloid burden in AD. Furthermore, zinc sequestration into amyloid deposits induces loss of functional zinc in the synapse.[102] Synaptic zinc deficiency is further exacerbated in AD by concomitant loss of ZnT3 expression.[33] Therefore, by two mechanisms labile zinc is made deficient in the brain neuropil in AD.

Zinc can directly bind to tau monomers with moderate affinity, altering its confirmation, and can induce both the fibrillization and the aggregation of the protein.[104,105] Zinc also modulates the translation and phosphorylation of tau by affecting the activities of GSK-3β, protein kinase B, ERK1/2, and c-Jun N-terminal kinase.[106,107] Furthermore, zinc is elevated in neurons with neurofibrillary tangle pathology.[89]

THE ROLE OF IRON IN AD

Iron is a transition metal which can exist in oxidation states from −2 to +8, but in biological systems only ferrous (Fe^{2+}) and ferric (Fe^{3+}) states exist. The cycling between Fe^{2+} and Fe^{3+} is utilized in biology for various electron transfer (redox) reactions essential to life.[108,109] Furthermore, iron is required for other essential biological processes including: the transport of oxygen (where iron is bound to haemoglobin),[110] regulation of protein expression,[111,112] cell growth[113] and cell differentiation,[114] as well as brain development,[115] neurotransmitter synthesis,[116] and myelin production.[117] Although essential to biological processes, when in excess, iron is toxic because it can react with oxygen through the Fenton reaction to generate superoxide anions and hydroxyl radicals,[118] which are a source of oxidative stress.[119] For these reasons iron levels are tightly regulated within the body and disruption of these homeostatic processes can cause either iron-deficient anemia or iron overload disorders.[120] Iron homeostasis is maintained via the coordinated action of several proteins including the iron carrier protein transferrin, the transferrin receptor for iron import, the ferroportin channel for iron export, the iron storage protein ferritin, ferrireductases which reduce iron to its ferrous state, and ferroxidases which oxidize iron to its ferric state. Circulation iron, once oxidized to its ferric state using the ferroxidase ceruloplasmin, cannot cross the blood brain barrier (BBB), but requires an iron complexed to transferrin to bind the transferrin receptor on the lumen side of endothelial cells.[121,122] The transferrin complex then enters the cell via endocytosis where iron assimilates with a labile iron pool within the cytosol and is available for incorporation into iron-binding proteins, such as ferritin.[123] This process is highly regulated by the abundance or the deficiency in both transferrin (with or without iron incorporated) and its receptor.[124,125]

In the AD brain iron levels are elevated[126,127] and especially enriched within neurofibrillary tangles[24] and amyloid plaques,[128] the latter of which has an iron concentration three times higher than that which is found in the surrounding normal neuropil.[33] Iron accumulation occurs in the AD cortex, but not the cerebellum, which is consistent with the anatomical profile of neurodegeneration in AD.[129,130] The iron storage protein ferritin binds most iron within the brain,[127] and this protein increases with age and in AD.[131] Neuronal iron deposition causes oxidative stress which likely contributes to elevated oxidative stress observed in the AD brain.[132] Furthermore, iron-induced oxidative stress has been shown to initiate several apoptotic pathways in neurons and damage lipids and proteins (including the NMDA receptor) resulting in synaptic dysfunction and neuronal cell death.[133–135] A number of iron-associated proteins have an altered expression profile in AD, which could partly explain the cause of iron accumulation in AD. Ferritin has been reported to be elevated in AD and colocalizes with amyloid plaques.[126] Transferrin, which is normally expressed solely by oligodendrocytes, is also expressed in astrocytes in the AD brain[126] and was found to be increased in frontal cortex of AD.[136] Lower ceruloplasmin expression was found in AD brains,[137] as well as its ferroxidase activity in plasma.[138] Taken together, it is likely that the iron accumulation observed in AD is a result of multiple failures in its regulatory proteins. Reports of iron levels in serum and CSF have yet to show a consistent change in AD.[38,139] While serum iron levels may be unchanged, a recent study has shown that CSF ferritin levels can predict AD outcomes.[140]

Iron binds to APP via the iron-responsive element type II located within the 5′ untranslated region of its mRNA sequence.[141] Under conditions of high iron levels, such as are seen in the AD brain, restricted translation of APP by iron-responsive proteins is diminished, leading to increased translation of the transcript.[111] Conversely, the same study also found that iron chelation decreased translation of the transcript. Iron may also alter APP cleavage by modulating furin, a proconvertase involved in the regulation of α-secretase-dependent processing.[142] Since ferrous iron has a low affinity for transferrin, it requires oxidation by a ferroxidase before it can be removed from the cell.[143] Ceruloplasmin is the classic ferroxidase[144,145]; however, this protein is not expressed in neurons.[146] In one recent study APP was proposed as the analogous neuronal ferroxidase.[129] This study found that APP-knockout mice exhibit iron accumulation in brain and peripheral tissues, and loss of APP ferroxidases activity in the AD brain is coincident with iron retention in the tissue.

Iron in both Fe^{2+} and Fe^{3+} states binds to the Aβ peptide at residues Asp1, Glu3, His6, His13, and His14.[147,148] Iron promotes the aggregation of Aβ in vitro,[149] which can be prevented by iron chelation.[150] The iron-aggregated Aβ is also toxic to cultured cells,[151,152] which has been suggested to be mediated by reactive oxygen species,[153] by Fenton chemistry,[154] or by the activation of the Bcl-2-related apoptosis pathway.[155] Taken together, these studies suggest a role for iron-mediated Aβ toxicity in AD.

Iron also binds to the tau protein, and the binding of Fe^{3+}, but not Fe^{2+}, causes aggregation of hyperphosphorylated tau that can be reversed by reducing Fe^{3+} to Fe^{2+} or by iron chelation.[156,157] Within the AD brain, iron enrichment colocalizes with NFTs and is a source of reactive oxygen species.[24,67] Iron also affects the phosphorylation status of tau: Fe^{3+} decreases tau phosphorylation[158] while Fe^{2+} increases tau phosphorylation.[159,160] Furthermore, a recent study has shown that the iron-export capability of APP requires the binding of tau to APP.[161,162] In tau-knockout primary cortical neurons, APP was inappropriately trafficked and not presented on the extracellular surface where it acts as a ferroxidase.[161] Total tau levels are decreased in the AD cortex,[163,164] and loss of tau expression causes iron- and age-dependent cognitive loss and cortical atrophy in mice.[161] These studies demonstrate the apparent interconnection between iron overload, tau, and APP in the pathogenesis of AD.

THERAPEUTIC TARGETING OF BIOMETALS IN AD

Given that targeting Aβ in multiple ways has so far failed to confer clinical benefits,[13–16] there is a need to target other pathways in AD. Targeting biometals by restoring metal ion homeostasis represents an alternative potential therapeutic avenue. To achieve this, sophisticated compounds are needed which can correct metal miscompartmentalization in AD by redistributing metal ions from extracellular plaques (preventing Aβ aggregation) into metal ion-deficient neurons (to restore normal function). Several potential metal-based AD therapeutics are discussed later.

5-Chloro-7-iodo-quinolin-8-ol (clioquinol) is a derivative of 8-hydroxyquinoline that was widely used as an antiparasitic agent before it was withdrawn from clinical use owing to a speculated severe side effect, subacute myelo-optic-neuropathy (SMON). This side effect was only observed in Japan,[165] and the association between SMON and clioquinol has since been questioned.[166] Although it was initially considered a moderate chelator of iron, copper, and zinc,[167] clioquinol has more recently been characterized as a copper/zinc ionophore, which functions to redistribute these metals into cells.[168,169] In addition, clioquinol is believed to confer neuroprotection by iron chelation, as iron binds to clioquinol,[170] and a number of the reported beneficial effects of clioquinol are iron dependent.[154,171] Preclinical studies have shown promising outcomes, including deceased Aβ brain burden,[166] inhibition of Aβ oligomer formation,[172,173] and rescue of memory impairment in clioquinol treated animals.[166] Furthermore, a phase two clinical trial[174] and a case study[175] reported improvement in cognitive outcomes for patients with AD. However, complications with large-scale manufacturing of the compound have hindered further exploration for its use in AD.

A second-generation 8-hydroxyquinoline derivative, PBT2, has shown even greater therapeutic efficiency in an AD mouse model[176] as well as in a phase two clinical trial.[177,178] However, in another more recent phase two clinical trial, PBT2 did not show an improved Pittsburgh compound B-PET scan when compared to placebo patients.[179] While patients on PBT2 had a lower Pittsburgh compound B-PET signal, the result was confounded by an inexplicable reduction in the placebo group. The proposed mechanism for neuroprotection of this drug is by acting as a copper-zinc ionophore, redistributing copper and zinc inside the cell, which induces inhibitory phosphorylation of the α- and β-isoforms of GSK-3 and subsequently lowers Aβ levels.[180] More comprehensive clinical studies are needed to further investigate the utility of this compound as an AD therapeutic.

Given that the mechanisms of action for both clioquinol and PBT2 probably involve their copper ionophore activity, copper-containing bis(thiosemicarbazone) compounds have been explored for their potential to treat AD. One compound, Cu^{II}(gtsm), delivers copper to neurons and has been shown to lower Aβ levels, GSK3β activity, and tau phosphorylation levels in cell culture and AD model mice, which was accompanied by improved cognition in these mice.[69,181] Another compound, Cu^{II}(atsm), delivers copper selectively to cells with an impaired electron transport chain[182] and has not been shown to be beneficial in the APP/PS1 mouse model of AD.[69] Further studies are needed to examine the utility of these copper-containing bis(thiosemicarbazone) ligands for the treatment of AD.

Given the role for iron in regulating APP translation,[111] decreasing iron overload in AD via iron chelators has shown promise in both preclinical and clinical trials. The iron chelators epigallocatechin-3-gallate (EGCG) and M-30 have been shown to reduce APP expression in cultured cells.[183,184] Furthermore, the iron chelator deferoxamine inhibits amyloidogenic APP processing in cultured cells and in AD model mice, which also attenuated Aβ burden within the brain and reversed spatial memory impairment.[185,186] Intramuscular injection of deferoxamine was tested in a single-blind clinical trial of 48 AD patients over a 24-month period and deferoxamine treatment reduced the rate of cognitive decline by half.[187] Despite this encouraging trial outcome obtained in 1991, further clinical developments of compounds that target iron in AD have not occurred.

CONCLUSIONS

Through interactions with disease-associated proteins, including APP, Aβ, and tau, the biometals copper, zinc, and iron appear to play an important role in AD pathogenesis (Table 1.1). Altered biometal homeostasis in AD has opened up new opportunities for the development of disease-modifying therapeutics. Preclinical and clinical data indicate that targeting biometals by restoring metal ion homeostasis remains a promising prospect for the treatment of AD.

TABLE 1.1 Biometal Interactions With Disease-Associated Proteins in Alzheimer's Disease

	Amyloid precursor protein (APP)	**Amyloid beta (Aβ)**	**Tau**
Copper	• Alters APP expression • Increases cell surface APP	• Causes Aβ aggregation • Causes reactive oxygen species formation • Causes mitochondrial dysfunction	• Causes tau aggregation • Alters tau phosphorylation • Causes reactive oxygen species formation
Zinc	• Inhibits degradation of Aβ • Alters APP cleavage	• Causes Aβ aggregation	• Causes tau aggregation • Alters tau phosphorylation • Alters tau expression
Iron	• Alters APP expression • Alters APP cleavage	• Causes Aβ aggregation • Causes reactive oxygen species formation	• Causes tau aggregation • Alters tau phosphorylation • Causes reactive oxygen species formation

References

1. Mattson MP. Pathways towards and away from Alzheimer's disease. *Nature*. 2004;430(7000):631–639.
2. Jalbert JJ, Daiello LA, Lapane KL. Dementia of the Alzheimer type. *Epidemiol Rev*. 2008;30:15–34.
3. Ferri CP, Prince M, Brayne C, Brodaty H, Fratiglioni L, Ganguli M, Hall K, Hasegawa K, Hendrie H, Huang Y, Jorm A, Mathers C, Menezes PR, Rimmer E, Scazufca M. Global prevalence of dementia: a Delphi consensus study. *Lancet*. 2005;366(9503):2112–2117.
4. Selkoe DJ. Alzheimer's disease: genes, proteins, and therapy. *Physiol Rev*. 2001;81(2):741–766.
5. McDonald CR, McEvoy LK, Gharapetian L, Fennema-Notestine C, Hagler Jr DJ, Holland D, Koyama A, Brewer JB, Dale AM. Regional rates of neocortical atrophy from normal aging to early Alzheimer disease. *Neurology*. 2009;73(6):457–465.
6. Grundke-Iqbal I, Iqbal K, Tung YC, Quinlan M, Wisniewski HM, Binder LI. Abnormal phosphorylation of the microtubule-associated protein tau (tau) in Alzheimer cytoskeletal pathology. *Proc Natl Acad Sci USA*. 1986;83(13):4913–4917.
7. Masters CL, Simms G, Weinman NA, Multhaup G, McDonald BL, Beyreuther K. Amyloid plaque core protein in Alzheimer disease and Down syndrome. *Proc Natl Acad Sci USA*. 1985;82(12):4245–4249.
8. Hardy JA, Higgins GA. Alzheimer's disease: the amyloid cascade hypothesis. *Science*. 1992;256(5054):184–185.
9. Tanzi RE, Gusella JF, Watkins PC, Bruns GA, St George-Hyslop P, Van Keuren ML, Patterson D, Pagan S, Kurnit DM, Neve RL. Amyloid beta protein gene: cDNA, mRNA distribution, and genetic linkage near the Alzheimer locus. *Science*. 1987;235(4791):880–884.
10. Vassar R, Bennett BD, Babu-Khan S, Kahn S, Mendiaz EA, Denis P, Teplow DB, Ross S, Amarante P, Loeloff R, Luo Y, Fisher S, Fuller J, Edenson S, Lile J, Jarosinski MA, Biere AL, Curran E, Burgess T, Louis JC, Collins F, Treanor J, Rogers G, Citron M. Beta-secretase cleavage of Alzheimer's amyloid precursor protein by the transmembrane aspartic protease BACE. *Science*. 1999;286(5440):735–741.
11. Spillantini MG, Hunt SP, Ulrich J, Goedert M. Expression and cellular localization of amyloid beta-protein precursor transcripts in normal human brain and in Alzheimer's disease. *Brain Res Mol Brain Res*. 1989;6(2-3):143–150.
12. Arai H, Lee VM, Messinger ML, Greenberg BD, Lowery DE, Trojanowski JQ. Expression patterns of beta-amyloid precursor protein (beta-APP) in neural and nonneural human tissues from Alzheimer's disease and control subjects. *Ann Neurol*. 1991;30(5):686–693.
13. Green RC, Schneider LS, Amato DA, Beelen AP, Wilcock G, Swabb EA, Zavitz KH. Effect of tarenflurbil on cognitive decline and activities of daily living in patients with mild Alzheimer disease: a randomized controlled trial. *JAMA*. 2009;302(23):2557–2564.
14. Doody RS, Raman R, Farlow M, Iwatsubo T, Vellas B, Joffe S, Kieburtz K, He F, Sun X, Thomas RG, Aisen PS, Siemers E, Sethuraman G, Mohs R. A phase 3 trial of semagacestat for treatment of Alzheimer's disease. *N Engl J Med*. 2013;369(4):341–350.
15. Doody RS, Thomas RG, Farlow M, Iwatsubo T, Vellas B, Joffe S, Kieburtz K, Raman R, Sun X, Aisen PS, Siemers E, Liu-Seifert H, Mohs R. Phase 3 trials of solanezumab for mild-to-moderate Alzheimer's disease. *N Engl J Med*. 2014;370(4):311–321.
16. Salloway S, Sperling R, Fox NC, Blennow K, Klunk W, Raskind M, Sabbagh M, Honig LS, Porsteinsson AP, Ferris S, Reichert M, Ketter N, Nejadnik B, Guenzler V, Miloslavsky M, Wang D, Lu Y, Lull J, Tudor IC, Liu E, Grundman M, Yuen E, Black R, Brashear HR. Two phase 3 trials of bapineuzumab in mild-to-moderate Alzheimer's disease. *N Engl J Med*. 2014;370(4):322–333.
17. Duce JA, Bush AI. Biological metals and Alzheimer's disease: implications for therapeutics and diagnostics. *Prog Neurobiol*. 2010;92(1):1–18.
18. Ridge PG, Zhang Y, Gladyshev VN. Comparative genomic analyses of copper transporters and cuproproteomes reveal evolutionary dynamics of copper utilization and its link to oxygen. *PLoS One*. 2008;3(1):e1378.
19. Robinson NJ, Winge DR. Copper metallochaperones. *Annu Rev Biochem*. 2010;79:537–562.
20. Horn D, Barrientos A. Mitochondrial copper metabolism and delivery to cytochrome c oxidase. *IUBMB Life*. 2008;60(7):421–429.
21. Wong BX, Ayton S, Lam LQ, Lei P, Adlard PA, Bush AI, Duce JA. A comparison of ceruloplasmin to biological polyanions in promoting the oxidation of Fe(2+) under physiologically relevant conditions. *Biochim Biophys Acta*. 2014;1840(12):3299–3310.
22. Perry G, Cash AD, Smith MA. Alzheimer disease and oxidative stress. *J Biomed Biotechnol*. 2002;2(3):120–123.

23. Moreira PI, Carvalho C, Zhu X, Smith MA, Perry G. Mitochondrial dysfunction is a trigger of Alzheimer's disease pathophysiology. *Biochim Biophys Acta*. 2010;1802(1):2–10.
24. Smith MA, Harris PL, Sayre LM, Perry G. Iron accumulation in Alzheimer disease is a source of redox-generated free radicals. *Proc Natl Acad Sci USA*. 1997;94(18):9866–9868.
25. Madsen E, Gitlin JD. Copper and iron disorders of the brain. *Annu Rev Neurosci*. 2007;30:317–337.
26. Ip V, Liu JJ, Mercer JF, McKeage MJ. Differential expression of ATP7A, ATP7B and CTR1 in adult rat dorsal root ganglion tissue. *Mol Pain*. 2010;6:53.
27. Vulpe C, Levinson B, Whitney S, Packman S, Gitschier J. Isolation of a candidate gene for Menkes disease and evidence that it encodes a copper-transporting ATPase. *Nat Genet*. 1993;3(1):7–13.
28. Kodama H, Murata Y, Kobayashi M. Clinical manifestations and treatment of Menkes disease and its variants. *Pediatr Int*. 1999;41(4):423–429.
29. Bull PC, Thomas GR, Rommens JM, Forbes JR, Cox DW. The Wilson disease gene is a putative copper transporting P-type ATPase similar to the Menkes gene. *Nat Genet*. 1993;5(4):327–337.
30. Merle U, Stremmel W, Encke J. Perspectives for gene therapy of Wilson disease. *Curr Gene Ther*. 2007;7(3):217–220.
31. Deibel MA, Ehmann WD, Markesbery WR. Copper, iron, and zinc imbalances in severely degenerated brain regions in Alzheimer's disease: possible relation to oxidative stress. *J Neurol Sci*. 1996;143(1-2):137–142.
32. Magaki S, Raghavan R, Mueller C, Oberg KC, Vinters HV, Kirsch WM. Iron, copper, and iron regulatory protein 2 in Alzheimer's disease and related dementias. *Neurosci Lett*. 2007;418(1):72–76.
33. Lovell MA, Robertson JD, Teesdale WJ, Campbell JL, Markesbery WR. Copper, iron and zinc in Alzheimer's disease senile plaques. *J Neurol Sci*. 1998;158(1):47–52.
34. Hopt A, Korte S, Fink H, Panne U, Niessner R, Jahn R, Kretzschmar H, Herms J. Methods for studying synaptosomal copper release. *J Neurosci Methods*. 2003;128(1-2):159–172.
35. Hartter DE, Barnea A. Evidence for release of copper in the brain: depolarization-induced release of newly taken-up 67copper. *Synapse*. 1988;2(4):412–415.
36. Schlief ML, Craig AM, Gitlin JD. NMDA receptor activation mediates copper homeostasis in hippocampal neurons. *J Neurosci*. 2005;25(1):239–246.
37. Stys PK, You H, Zamponi GW. Copper-dependent regulation of NMDA receptors by cellular prion protein: implications for neurodegenerative disorders. *J Physiol*. 2012;590(6):1357–1368.
38. Basun H, Forssell LG, Wetterberg L, Winblad B. Metals and trace elements in plasma and cerebrospinal fluid in normal aging and Alzheimer's disease. *J Neural Transm Park Dis Dement Sect*. 1991;3(4):231–258.
39. Squitti R, Lupoi D, Pasqualetti P, Dal Forno G, Vernieri F, Chiovenda P, Rossi L, Cortesi M, Cassetta E, Rossini PM. Elevation of serum copper levels in Alzheimer's disease. *Neurology*. 2002;59(8):1153–1161.
40. Squitti R, Pasqualetti P, Dal Forno G, Moffa F, Cassetta E, Lupoi D, Vernieri F, Rossi L, Baldassini M, Rossini PM. Excess of serum copper not related to ceruloplasmin in Alzheimer disease. *Neurology*. 2005;64(6):1040–1046.
41. Squitti R, Rossini PM, Cassetta E, Moffa F, Pasqualetti P, Cortesi M, Colloca A, Rossi L, Finazzi-Agro A. d-penicillamine reduces serum oxidative stress in Alzheimer's disease patients. *Eur J Clin Invest*. 2002;32(1):51–59.
42. Barnham KJ, McKinstry WJ, Multhaup G, Galatis D, Morton CJ, Curtain CC, Williamson NA, White AR, Hinds MG, Norton RS, Beyreuther K, Masters CL, Parker MW, Cappai R. Structure of the Alzheimer's disease amyloid precursor protein copper binding domain. A regulator of neuronal copper homeostasis. *J Biol Chem*. 2003;278(19):17401–17407.
43. Multhaup G, Schlicksupp A, Hesse L, Beher D, Ruppert T, Masters CL, Beyreuther K. The amyloid precursor protein of Alzheimer's disease in the reduction of copper(II) to copper(I). *Science*. 1996;271(5254):1406–1409.
44. Armendariz AD, Gonzalez M, Loguinov AV, Vulpe CD. Gene expression profiling in chronic copper overload reveals upregulation of Prnp and App. *Physiol Genomics*. 2004;20(1):45–54.
45. Bellingham SA, Lahiri DK, Maloney B, La Fontaine S, Multhaup G, Camakaris J. Copper depletion down-regulates expression of the Alzheimer's disease amyloid-beta precursor protein gene. *J Biol Chem*. 2004;279(19):20378–20386.
46. Davis CD, Milne DB, Nielsen FH. Changes in dietary zinc and copper affect zinc-status indicators of postmenopausal women, notably, extracellular superoxide dismutase and amyloid precursor proteins. *Am J Clin Nutr*. 2000;71(3):781–788.
47. White AR, Multhaup G, Maher F, Bellingham S, Camakaris J, Zheng H, Bush AI, Beyreuther K, Masters CL, Cappai R. The Alzheimer's disease amyloid precursor protein modulates copper-induced toxicity and oxidative stress in primary neuronal cultures. *J Neurosci*. 1999;19(21):9170–9179.

48. Bellingham SA, Ciccotosto GD, Needham BE, Fodero LR, White AR, Masters CL, Cappai R, Camakaris J. Gene knockout of amyloid precursor protein and amyloid precursor-like protein-2 increases cellular copper levels in primary mouse cortical neurons and embryonic fibroblasts. *J Neurochem*. 2004;91(2):423–428.
49. Bayer TA, Schafer S, Simons A, Kemmling A, Kamer T, Tepest R, Eckert A, Schussel K, Eikenberg O, Sturchler-Pierrat C, Abramowski D, Staufenbiel M, Multhaup G. Dietary Cu stabilizes brain superoxide dismutase 1 activity and reduces amyloid Abeta production in APP23 transgenic mice. *Proc Natl Acad Sci USA*. 2003;100(24):14187–14192.
50. Maynard CJ, Cappai R, Volitakis I, Cherny RA, White AR, Beyreuther K, Masters CL, Bush AI, Li QX. Overexpression of Alzheimer's disease amyloid-beta opposes the age-dependent elevations of brain copper and iron. *J Biol Chem*. 2002;277(47):44670–44676.
51. Phinney AL, Drisaldi B, Schmidt SD, Lugowski S, Coronado V, Liang Y, Horne P, Yang J, Sekoulidis J, Coomaraswamy J, Chishti MA, Cox DW, Mathews PM, Nixon RA, Carlson GA, St George-Hyslop P, Westaway D. In vivo reduction of amyloid-beta by a mutant copper transporter. *Proc Natl Acad Sci USA*. 2003;100(24):14193–14198.
52. Acevedo KM, Hung YH, Dalziel AH, Li QX, Laughton K, Wikhe K, Rembach A, Roberts B, Masters CL, Bush AI, Camakaris J. Copper promotes the trafficking of the amyloid precursor protein. *J Biol Chem*. 2011;286(10):8252–8262.
53. Minicozzi V, Stellato F, Comai M, Dalla Serra M, Potrich C, Meyer-Klaucke W, Morante S. Identifying the minimal copper- and zinc-binding site sequence in amyloid-beta peptides. *J Biol Chem*. 2008;283(16):10784–10792.
54. Drew SC, Noble CJ, Masters CL, Hanson GR, Barnham KJ. Pleomorphic copper coordination by Alzheimer's disease amyloid-beta peptide. *J Am Chem Soc*. 2009;131(3):1195–1207.
55. Dorlet P, Gambarelli S, Faller P, Hureau C, Pulse EPR. spectroscopy reveals the coordination sphere of copper(II) ions in the 1-16 amyloid-beta peptide: a key role of the first two N-terminus residues. *Angew Chem Int Ed Engl*. 2009;48(49):9273–9276.
56. Karr JW, Szalai VA. Role of aspartate-1 in Cu(II) binding to the amyloid-beta peptide of Alzheimer's disease. *J Am Chem Soc*. 2007;129(13):3796–3797.
57. Atwood CS, Huang X, Khatri A, Scarpa RC, Kim YS, Moir RD, Tanzi RE, Roher AE, Bush AI. Copper catalyzed oxidation of Alzheimer Abeta. *Cell Mol Biol*. 2000;46(4):777–783.
58. Atwood CS, Perry G, Zeng H, Kato Y, Jones WD, Ling KQ, Huang X, Moir RD, Wang D, Sayre LM, Smith MA, Chen SG, Bush AI. Copper mediates dityrosine cross-linking of Alzheimer's amyloid-beta. *Biochemistry*. 2004;43(2):560–568.
59. Ali FE, Separovic F, Barrow CJ, Cherny RA, Fraser F, Bush AI, Masters CL, Barnham KJ. Methionine regulates copper/hydrogen peroxide oxidation products of Abeta. *J Pept Sci*. 2005;11(6):353–360.
60. You H, Tsutsui S, Hameed S, Kannanayakal TJ, Chen L, Xia P, Engbers JD, Lipton SA, Stys PK, Zamponi GW. Abeta neurotoxicity depends on interactions between copper ions, prion protein, and N-methyl-D-aspartate receptors. *Proc Natl Acad Sci USA*. 2012;109(5):1737–1742.
61. Wu WH, Lei P, Liu Q, Hu J, Gunn AP, Chen MS, Rui YF, Su XY, Xie ZP, Zhao YF, Bush AI, Li YM. Sequestration of copper from beta-amyloid promotes selective lysis by cyclen-hybrid cleavage agents. *J Biol Chem*. 2008;283(46):31657–31664.
62. Huang X, Atwood CS, Hartshorn MA, Multhaup G, Goldstein LE, Scarpa RC, Cuajungco MP, Gray DN, Lim J, Moir RD, Tanzi RE, Bush AI. The A beta peptide of Alzheimer's disease directly produces hydrogen peroxide through metal ion reduction. *Biochemistry*. 1999;38(24):7609–7616.
63. Crouch PJ, Blake R, Duce JA, Ciccotosto GD, Li QX, Barnham KJ, Curtain CC, Cherny RA, Cappai R, Dyrks T, Masters CL, Trounce IA. Copper-dependent inhibition of human cytochrome c oxidase by a dimeric conformer of amyloid-beta1-42. *J Neurosci*. 2005;25(3):672–679.
64. Ma QF, Li YM, Du JT, Kanazawa K, Nemoto T, Nakanishi H, Zhao YF. Binding of copper (II) ion to an Alzheimer's tau peptide as revealed by MALDI-TOF MS, CD, and NMR. *Biopolymers*. 2005;79(2):74–85.
65. Zhou LX, Du JT, Zeng ZY, Wu WH, Zhao YF, Kanazawa K, Ishizuka Y, Nemoto T, Nakanishi H, Li YM. Copper (II) modulates in vitro aggregation of a tau peptide. *Peptides*. 2007;28(11):2229–2234.
66. Su XY, Wu WH, Huang ZP, Hu J, Lei P, Yu CH, Zhao YF, Li YM. Hydrogen peroxide can be generated by tau in the presence of Cu(II). *Biochem Biophys Res Commun*. 2007;358(2):661–665.
67. Sayre LM, Perry G, Harris PL, Liu Y, Schubert KA, Smith MA. In situ oxidative catalysis by neurofibrillary tangles and senile plaques in Alzheimer's disease: a central role for bound transition metals. *J Neurochem*. 2000;74(1):270–279.

68. Kitazawa M, Cheng D, Laferla FM. Chronic copper exposure exacerbates both amyloid and tau pathology and selectively dysregulates cdk5 in a mouse model of AD. *J Neurochem*. 2009;108(6):1550–1560.
69. Crouch PJ, Hung LW, Adlard PA, Cortes M, Lal V, Filiz G, Perez KA, Nurjono M, Caragounis A, Du T, Laughton K, Volitakis I, Bush AI, Li QX, Masters CL, Cappai R, Cherny RA, Donnelly PS, White AR, Barnham KJ. Increasing Cu bioavailability inhibits Abeta oligomers and tau phosphorylation. *Proc Natl Acad Sci USA*. 2009;106(2):381–386.
70. Frederickson CJ. Neurobiology of zinc and zinc-containing neurons. *Int Rev Neurobiol*. 1989;31:145–238.
71. Ebadi M, Elsayed MA, Aly MH. The importance of zinc and metallothionein in brain. *Biol Signals*. 1994;3(3):123–126.
72. Vallee BL, Coleman JE, Auld DS. Zinc fingers, zinc clusters, and zinc twists in DNA-binding protein domains. *Proc Natl Acad Sci USA*. 1991;88(3):999–1003.
73. Szallasi Z, Bogi K, Gohari S, Biro T, Acs P, Blumberg PM. Non-equivalent roles for the first and second zinc fingers of protein kinase Cdelta. Effect of their mutation on phorbol ester-induced translocation in NIH 3T3 cells. *J Biol Chem*. 1996;271(31):18299–18301.
74. Sensi SL, Paoletti P, Bush AI, Sekler I. Zinc in the physiology and pathology of the CNS. *Nat Rev Neurosci*. 2009;10(11):780–791.
75. Paoletti P, Ascher P, Neyton J. High-affinity zinc inhibition of NMDA NR1-NR2A receptors. *J Neurosci*. 1997;17(15):5711–5725.
76. Lovell MA. A potential role for alterations of zinc and zinc transport proteins in the progression of Alzheimer's disease. *J Alzheimers Dis*. 2009;16(3):471–483.
77. Koh JY, Choi DW. Zinc toxicity on cultured cortical neurons: involvement of N-methyl-D-aspartate receptors. *Neuroscience*. 1994;60(4):1049–1057.
78. Jia Y, Jeng JM, Sensi SL, Weiss JH. Zn2+ currents are mediated by calcium-permeable AMPA/kainate channels in cultured murine hippocampal neurones. *J Physiol*. 2002;543(Pt 1):35–48.
79. Cheng C, Reynolds IJ. Calcium-sensitive fluorescent dyes can report increases in intracellular free zinc concentration in cultured forebrain neurons. *J Neurochem*. 1998;71(6):2401–2410.
80. Greenough MA, Volitakis I, Li QX, Laughton K, Evin G, Ho M, Dalziel AH, Camakaris J, Bush AI. Presenilins promote the cellular uptake of copper and zinc and maintain copper chaperone of SOD1-dependent copper/zinc superoxide dismutase activity. *J Biol Chem*. 2011;286(11):9776–9786.
81. Kelleher SL, Lonnerdal B. Zinc transporters in the rat mammary gland respond to marginal zinc and vitamin A intakes during lactation. *J Nutr*. 2002;132(11):3280–3285.
82. Adlard PA, Parncutt JM, Finkelstein DI, Bush AI. Cognitive loss in zinc transporter-3 knock-out mice: a phenocopy for the synaptic and memory deficits of Alzheimer's disease?. *J Neurosci*. 2010;30(5):1631–1636.
83. Ehmann WD, Markesbery WR, Alauddin M. Quantitation, localization and variations of brain zinc with aging by instrumental neutron activation analysis. In: Frederickson CJ, Howell GA, Kassarskis EJ, eds. *Neurobiology of Zinc. Part A. Physiochemistry, Anatomy, and Techniques*. New York: Alan R. Liss; 1984:329–342.
84. Hershey LA, Hershey CO, Varnes AW, Wongmongkolrit T, Strain WH. Zinc content in CSF, brain and other tissues in Alzheimer's Disease and aging. In: Frederickson CJ, Howell GA, Kassarskis EJ, eds. *The Neurobiology of Zinc. Part B. Deficiency, Toxicity and Pathology*. New York: Alan R. Liss; 1984:325–334.
85. Panayi AE, Spyrou NM, Iversen BS, White MA, Part P. Determination of cadmium and zinc in Alzheimer's brain tissue using inductively coupled plasma mass spectrometry. *J Neurol Sci*. 2002;195(1):1–10.
86. Corrigan FM, Reynolds GP, Ward NI. Hippocampal tin, aluminum and zinc in Alzheimer's disease. *Biometals*. 1993;6(3):149–154.
87. Danscher G, Jensen KB, Frederickson CJ, Kemp K, Andreasen A, Juhl S, Stoltenberg M, Ravid R. Increased amount of zinc in the hippocampus and amygdala of Alzheimer's diseased brains: a proton-induced X-ray emission spectroscopic analysis of cryostat sections from autopsy material. *J Neurosci Methods*. 1997;76(1):53–59.
88. Schrag M, Dickson A, Jiffry A, Kirsch D, Vinters HV, Kirsch W. The effect of formalin fixation on the levels of brain transition metals in archived samples. *Biometals*. 2010;23(6):1123–1127.
89. Suh SW, Jensen KB, Jensen MS, Silva DS, Kesslak PJ, Danscher G, Frederickson CJ. Histochemically-reactive zinc in amyloid plaques, angiopathy, and degenerating neurons of Alzheimer's diseased brains. *Brain Res*. 2000;852(2):274–278.
90. Yu WH, Lukiw WJ, Bergeron C, Niznik HB, Fraser PE. Metallothionein III is reduced in Alzheimer's disease. *Brain Res*. 2001;894(1):37–45.

91. Adlard PA, West AK, Vickers JC. Increased density of metallothionein I/II-immunopositive cortical glial cells in the early stages of Alzheimer's disease. *Neurobiol Dis*. 1998;5(5):349–356.
92. Lovell MA, Smith JL, Xiong S, Markesbery WR. Alterations in zinc transporter protein-1 (ZnT-1) in the brain of subjects with mild cognitive impairment, early, and late-stage Alzheimer's disease. *Neurotox Res*. 2005;7(4):265–271.
93. Beyer N, Coulson DT, Heggarty S, Ravid R, Irvine GB, Hellemans J, Johnston JA. ZnT3 mRNA levels are reduced in Alzheimer's disease post-mortem brain. *Mol Neurodegener*. 2009;4:53.
94. Lee JY, Kim JH, Hong SH, Cherny RA, Bush AI, Palmiter RD, Koh JY. Estrogen decreases zinc transporter 3 expression and synaptic vesicle zinc levels in mouse brain. *J Biol Chem*. 2004;279(10):8602–8607.
95. Baum L, Chan IH, Cheung SK, Goggins WB, Mok V, Lam L, Leung V, Hui E, Ng C, Woo J, Chiu HF, Zee BC, Cheng W, Chan MH, Szeto S, Lui V, Tsoh J, Bush AI, Lam CW, Kwok T. Serum zinc is decreased in Alzheimer's disease and serum arsenic correlates positively with cognitive ability. *Biometals*. 2010;23(1):173–179.
96. Bush AI, Multhaup G, Moir RD, Williamson TG, Small DH, Rumble B, Pollwein P, Beyreuther K, Masters CL. A novel zinc(II) binding site modulates the function of the beta A4 amyloid protein precursor of Alzheimer's disease. *J Biol Chem*. 1993;268(22):16109–16112.
97. Bush AI, Pettingell Jr WH, de Paradis M, Tanzi RE, Wasco W. The amyloid beta-protein precursor and its mammalian homologues. Evidence for a zinc-modulated heparin-binding superfamily. *J Biol Chem*. 1994;269(43):26618–26621.
98. Lammich S, Kojro E, Postina R, Gilbert S, Pfeiffer R, Jasionowski M, Haass C, Fahrenholz F. Constitutive and regulated alpha-secretase cleavage of Alzheimer's amyloid precursor protein by a disintegrin metalloprotease. *Proc Natl Acad Sci USA*. 1999;96(7):3922–3927.
99. Hoke DE, Tan JL, Ilaya NT, Culvenor JG, Smith SJ, White AR, Masters CL, Evin GM. In vitro gamma-secretase cleavage of the Alzheimer's amyloid precursor protein correlates to a subset of presenilin complexes and is inhibited by zinc. *FEBS J*. 2005;272(21):5544–5557.
100. Bush AI, Pettingell Jr WH, Paradis MD, Tanzi RE. Modulation of A beta adhesiveness and secretase site cleavage by zinc. *J Biol Chem*. 1994;269(16):12152–12158.
101. Crouch PJ, Tew DJ, Du T, Nguyen DN, Caragounis A, Filiz G, Blake RE, Trounce IA, Soon CP, Laughton K, Perez KA, Li QX, Cherny RA, Masters CL, Barnham KJ, White AR. Restored degradation of the Alzheimer's amyloid-beta peptide by targeting amyloid formation. *J Neurochem*. 2009;108(5):1198–1207.
102. Bush AI, Pettingell WH, Multhaup G, d Paradis M, Vonsattel JP, Gusella JF, Beyreuther K, Masters CL, Tanzi RE. Rapid induction of Alzheimer A beta amyloid formation by zinc. *Science*. 1994;265(5177):1464–1467.
103. Lee JY, Cole TB, Palmiter RD, Suh SW, Koh JY. Contribution by synaptic zinc to the gender-disparate plaque formation in human Swedish mutant APP transgenic mice. *Proc Natl Acad Sci USA*. 2002;99(11):7705–7710.
104. Boom A, Authelet M, Dedecker R, Frederick C, Van Heurck R, Daubie V, Leroy K, Pochet R, Brion JP. Bimodal modulation of tau protein phosphorylation and conformation by extracellular Zn2+ in human-tau transfected cells. *Biochim Biophys Acta*. 2009;1793(6):1058–1067.
105. Mo ZY, Zhu YZ, Zhu HL, Fan JB, Chen J, Liang Y. Low micromolar zinc accelerates the fibrillization of human tau via bridging of Cys-291 and Cys-322. *J Biol Chem*. 2009;284(50):34648–34657.
106. An WL, Bjorkdahl C, Liu R, Cowburn RF, Winblad B, Pei JJ. Mechanism of zinc-induced phosphorylation of p70 S6 kinase and glycogen synthase kinase 3beta in SH-SY5Y neuroblastoma cells. *J Neurochem*. 2005;92(5):1104–1115.
107. Pei JJ, An WL, Zhou XW, Nishimura T, Norberg J, Benedikz E, Gotz J, Winblad B. P70 S6 kinase mediates tau phosphorylation and synthesis. *FEBS Lett*. 2006;580(1):107–114.
108. Lenhoff HM, Nicholas DJ, Kaplan NO. Effects of oxygen, iron, and molybdenum on routes of electron transfer in Pseudomonas fluorescens. *J Biol Chem*. 1956;220(2):983–995.
109. Malkin R, Rabinowitz JC. Nonheme iron electron-transfer proteins. *Annu Rev Biochem*. 1967;36:113–148.
110. Sanders-Loehr J. Involvement of oxo-bridged binuclear iron centers in oxygen transport, oxygen reduction, and oxygenation. *Prog Clin Biol Res*. 1988;274:193–209.
111. Rogers JT, Randall JD, Cahill CM, Eder PS, Huang X, Gunshin H, Leiter L, McPhee J, Sarang SS, Utsuki T, Greig NH, Lahiri DK, Tanzi RE, Bush AI, Giordano T, Gullans SR. An iron-responsive element type II in the 5′-untranslated region of the Alzheimer's amyloid precursor protein transcript. *J Biol Chem*. 2002;277(47):45518–45528.
112. Friedlich AL, Tanzi RE, Rogers JT. The 5′-untranslated region of Parkinson's disease alpha-synuclein messengerRNA contains a predicted iron responsive element. *Mol Psychiatry*. 2007;12(3):222–223.

113. Verger C, Imbenotte J. Decreased heme content and cessation of cell growth in cultured chick embryo fibroblasts in the presence of horse serum: stimulation of heme synthesis and cell growth by iron. *J Cell Physiol.* 1982;113(2):193–196.
114. Landschulz W, Thesleff I, Ekblom P. A lipophilic iron chelator can replace transferrin as a stimulator of cell proliferation and differentiation. *J Cell Biol.* 1984;98(2):596–601.
115. Beard J. Iron deficiency alters brain development and functioning. *J Nutr.* 2003;133(5 Suppl 1):1468S–1472S.
116. Agarwal KN. Iron and the brain: neurotransmitter receptors and magnetic resonance spectroscopy. *Br J Nutr.* 2001;85(Suppl 2):S147–S150.
117. Schulz K, Kroner A, David S. Iron efflux from astrocytes plays a role in remyelination. *J Neurosci.* 2012;32(14):4841–4847.
118. Fenton JM, Pellin MJ, Govindjee, kaufmann KJ. Primary photochemistry of the reaction center of photosystem I. *FEBS Lett.* 1979;100(1):1–4.
119. Zigler Jr JS, Jernigan Jr HM, Garland D, Reddy VN. The effects of "oxygen radicals" generated in the medium on lenses in organ culture: inhibition of damage by chelated iron. *Arch Biochem Biophys.* 1985;241(1):163–172.
120. Zhang AS, Enns CA. Iron homeostasis: recently identified proteins provide insight into novel control mechanisms. *J Biol Chem.* 2009;284(2):711–715.
121. Morris CM, Keith AB, Edwardson JA, Pullen RG. Uptake and distribution of iron and transferrin in the adult rat brain. *J Neurochem.* 1992;59(1):300–306.
122. Aisen P. Entry of iron into cells: a new role for the transferrin receptor in modulating iron release from transferrin. *Ann Neurol.* 1992;32(Suppl):S62–S68.
123. Eckenroth BE, Steere AN, Chasteen ND, Everse SJ, Mason AB. How the binding of human transferrin primes the transferrin receptor potentiating iron release at endosomal pH. *Proc Natl Acad Sci USA.* 2011;108(32):13089–13094.
124. Caughman SW, Hentze MW, Rouault TA, Harford JB, Klausner RD. The iron-responsive element is the single element responsible for iron-dependent translational regulation of ferritin biosynthesis. Evidence for function as the binding site for a translational repressor. *J Biol Chem.* 1988;263(35):19048–19052.
125. Kikinis Z, Eisenstein RS, Bettany AJ, Munro HN. Role of RNA secondary structure of the iron-responsive element in translational regulation of ferritin synthesis. *Nucleic Acids Res.* 1995;23(20):4190–4195.
126. Connor JR, Menzies SL, St Martin SM, Mufson EJ. A histochemical study of iron, transferrin, and ferritin in Alzheimer's diseased brains. *J Neurosci Res.* 1992;31(1):75–83.
127. Collingwood JF, Mikhaylova A, Davidson M, Batich C, Streit WJ, Terry J, Dobson J. In situ characterization and mapping of iron compounds in Alzheimer's disease tissue. *J Alzheimers Dis.* 2005;7(4):267–272.
128. Goodman L. Alzheimer's disease; a clinico-pathologic analysis of twenty-three cases with a theory on pathogenesis. *J Nerv Ment Dis.* 1953;118(2):97–130.
129. Duce JA, Tsatsanis A, Cater MA, James SA, Robb E, Wikhe K, Leong SL, Perez K, Johanssen T, Greenough MA, Cho HH, Galatis D, Moir RD, Masters CL, McLean C, Tanzi RE, Cappai R, Barnham KJ, Ciccotosto GD, Rogers JT, Bush AI. Iron-export ferroxidase activity of beta-amyloid precursor protein is inhibited by zinc in Alzheimer's disease. *Cell.* 2010;142(6):857–867.
130. Andrasi E, Farkas E, Scheibler H, Reffy A, Bezur L. Al, Zn, Cu, Mn and Fe levels in brain in Alzheimer's disease. *Arch Gerontol Geriatr.* 1995;21(1):89–97.
131. Bartzokis G, Tishler TA. MRI evaluation of basal ganglia ferritin iron and neurotoxicity in Alzheimer's and Huntingon's disease. *Cell Mol Biol.* 2000;46(4):821–833.
132. Hare D, Ayton S, Bush A, Lei P. A delicate balance: iron metabolism and diseases of the brain. *Front Aging Neurosci.* 2013;5:34.
133. Salvador GA, Uranga RM, Giusto NM. Iron and mechanisms of neurotoxicity. *Int J Alzheimers Dis.* 2010;2011:720658.
134. Munoz P, Humeres A, Elgueta C, Kirkwood A, Hidalgo C, Nunez MT. Iron mediates N-methyl-D-aspartate receptor-dependent stimulation of calcium-induced pathways and hippocampal synaptic plasticity. *J Biol Chem.* 2011;286(15):13382–13392.
135. Mattson MP. Metal-catalyzed disruption of membrane protein and lipid signaling in the pathogenesis of neurodegenerative disorders. *Ann NY Acad Sci.* 2004;1012:37–50.
136. Loeffler DA, Connor JR, Juneau PL, Snyder BS, Kanaley L, DeMaggio AJ, Nguyen H, Brickman CM, LeWitt PA. Transferrin and iron in normal, Alzheimer's disease, and Parkinson's disease brain regions. *J Neurochem.* 1995;65(2):710–724.

137. Connor JR, Tucker P, Johnson M, Snyder B. Ceruloplasmin levels in the human superior temporal gyrus in aging and Alzheimer's disease. *Neurosci Lett.* 1993;159(1-2):88–90.
138. Torsdottir G, Kristinsson J, Snaedal J, Sveinbjornsdottir S, Gudmundsson G, Hreidarsson S, Johannesson T. Case-control studies on ceruloplasmin and superoxide dismutase (SOD1) in neurodegenerative diseases: a short review. *J Neurol Sci.* 2010;299(1-2):51–54.
139. Strozyk D, Launer LJ, Adlard PA, Cherny RA, Tsatsanis A, Volitakis I, Blennow K, Petrovitch H, White LR, Bush AI. Zinc and copper modulate Alzheimer Abeta levels in human cerebrospinal fluid. *Neurobiol Aging.* 2009;30(7):1069–1077.
140. Ayton S, Faux NG, Bush AI. Ferritin levels in the cerebrospinal fluid predict Alzheimer's disease outcomes and are regulated by APOE. *Nat Commun.* 2015;6:6760.
141. Venti A, Giordano T, Eder P, Bush AI, Lahiri DK, Greig NH, Rogers JT. The integrated role of desferrioxamine and phenserine targeted to an iron-responsive element in the APP-mRNA 5'-untranslated region. *Ann NY Acad Sci.* 2004;1035:34–48.
142. Silvestri L, Camaschella C. A potential pathogenetic role of iron in Alzheimer's disease. *J Cell Mol Med.* 2008;12(5A):1548–1550.
143. Ayton S, Lei P, Bush AI. Metallostasis in Alzheimer's disease. *Free Radic Biol Med.* 2013;62:76–89.
144. Osaki S. Kinetic studies of ferrous ion oxidation with crystalline human ferroxidase (ceruloplasmin). *J Biol Chem.* 1966;241(21):5053–5059.
145. Harris ZL, Takahashi Y, Miyajima H, Serizawa M, MacGillivray RT, Gitlin JD. Aceruloplasminemia: molecular characterization of this disorder of iron metabolism. *Proc Natl Acad Sci USA.* 1995;92(7):2539–2543.
146. Klomp LW, Farhangrazi ZS, Dugan LL, Gitlin JD. Ceruloplasmin gene expression in the murine central nervous system. *J Clin Invest.* 1996;98(1):207–215.
147. Bousejra-ElGarah F, Bijani C, Coppel Y, Faller P, Hureau C. Iron(II) binding to amyloid-beta, the Alzheimer's peptide. *Inorg Chem.* 2011;50(18):9024–9030.
148. Nair NG, Perry G, Smith MA, Reddy VP. NMR studies of zinc, copper, and iron binding to histidine, the principal metal ion complexing site of amyloid-beta peptide. *J Alzheimers Dis.* 2010;20(1):57–66.
149. Mantyh PW, Ghilardi JR, Rogers S, DeMaster E, Allen CJ, Stimson ER, Maggio JE. Aluminum, iron, and zinc ions promote aggregation of physiological concentrations of beta-amyloid peptide. *J Neurochem.* 1993;61(3):1171–1174.
150. Huang X, Atwood CS, Moir RD, Hartshorn MA, Tanzi RE, Bush AI. Trace metal contamination initiates the apparent auto-aggregation, amyloidosis, and oligomerization of Alzheimer's Abeta peptides. *J Biol Inorg Chem.* 2004;9(8):954–960.
151. Schubert D, Chevion M. The role of iron in beta amyloid toxicity. *Biochem Biophys Res Commun.* 1995;216(2):702–707.
152. Liu B, Moloney A, Meehan S, Morris K, Thomas SE, Serpell LC, Hider R, Marciniak SJ, Lomas DA, Crowther DC. Iron promotes the toxicity of amyloid beta peptide by impeding its ordered aggregation. *J Biol Chem.* 2011;286(6):4248–4256.
153. Rottkamp CA, Raina AK, Zhu X, Gaier E, Bush AI, Atwood CS, Chevion M, Perry G, Smith MA. Redox-active iron mediates amyloid-beta toxicity. *Free Radic Biol Med.* 2001;30(4):447–450.
154. Rival T, Page RM, Chandraratna DS, Sendall TJ, Ryder E, Liu B, Lewis H, Rosahl T, Hider R, Camargo LM, Shearman MS, Crowther DC, Lomas DA. Fenton chemistry and oxidative stress mediate the toxicity of the beta-amyloid peptide in a Drosophila model of Alzheimer's disease. *Eur J Neurosci.* 2009;29(7):1335–1347.
155. Kuperstein F, Yavin E. Pro-apoptotic signaling in neuronal cells following iron and amyloid beta peptide neurotoxicity. *J Neurochem.* 2003;86(1):114–125.
156. Yamamoto A, Shin RW, Hasegawa K, Naiki H, Sato H, Yoshimasu F, Kitamoto T. Iron (III) induces aggregation of hyperphosphorylated tau and its reduction to iron (II) reverses the aggregation: implications in the formation of neurofibrillary tangles of Alzheimer's disease. *J Neurochem.* 2002;82(5):1137–1147.
157. Amit T, Avramovich-Tirosh Y, Youdim MB, Mandel S. Targeting multiple Alzheimer's disease etiologies with multimodal neuroprotective and neurorestorative iron chelators. *FASEB J.* 2008;22(5):1296–1305.
158. Egana JT, Zambrano C, Nunez MT, Gonzalez-Billault C, Maccioni RB. Iron-induced oxidative stress modify tau phosphorylation patterns in hippocampal cell cultures. *Biometals.* 2003;16(1):215–223.
159. Lovell MA, Xiong S, Xie C, Davies P, Markesbery WR. Induction of hyperphosphorylated tau in primary rat cortical neuron cultures mediated by oxidative stress and glycogen synthase kinase-3. *J Alzheimers Dis.* 2004;6(6):659–671.

160. Chan A, Shea TB. Dietary and genetically-induced oxidative stress alter tau phosphorylation: influence of folate and apolipoprotein E deficiency. *J Alzheimers Dis*. 2006;9(4):399–405.
161. Lei P, Ayton S, Finkelstein DI, Spoerri L, Ciccotosto GD, Wright DK, Wong BX, Adlard PA, Cherny RA, Lam LQ, Roberts BR, Volitakis I, Egan GF, McLean CA, Cappai R, Duce JA, Bush AI. Tau deficiency induces parkinsonism with dementia by impairing APP-mediated iron export. *Nat Med*. 2012;18(2):291–295.
162. Islam K, Levy E. Carboxyl-terminal fragments of beta-amyloid precursor protein bind to microtubules and the associated protein tau. *Am J Pathol*. 1997;151(1):265–271.
163. Shin RW, Iwaki T, Kitamoto T, Sato Y, Tateishi J. Massive accumulation of modified tau and severe depletion of normal tau characterize the cerebral cortex and white matter of Alzheimer's disease. Demonstration using the hydrated autoclaving method. *Am J Pathol*. 1992;140(4):937–945.
164. Khatoon S, Grundke-Iqbal I, Iqbal K. Levels of normal and abnormally phosphorylated tau in different cellular and regional compartments of Alzheimer disease and control brains. *FEBS Lett*. 1994;351(1):80–84.
165. Tateishi J. Subacute myelo-optico-neuropathy: clioquinol intoxication in humans and animals. *Neuropathology*. 2000;20(Suppl):S20–S24.
166. Cherny RA, Atwood CS, Xilinas ME, Gray DN, Jones WD, McLean CA, Barnham KJ, Volitakis I, Fraser FW, Kim Y, Huang X, Goldstein LE, Moir RD, Lim JT, Beyreuther K, Zheng H, Tanzi RE, Masters CL, Bush AI. Treatment with a copper-zinc chelator markedly and rapidly inhibits beta-amyloid accumulation in Alzheimer's disease transgenic mice. *Neuron*. 2001;30(3):665–676.
167. Treiber C, Simons A, Strauss M, Hafner M, Cappai R, Bayer TA, Multhaup G. Clioquinol mediates copper uptake and counteracts copper efflux activities of the amyloid precursor protein of Alzheimer's disease. *J Biol Chem*. 2004;279(50):51958–51964.
168. Park MH, Lee SJ, Byun HR, Kim Y, Oh YJ, Koh JY, Hwang JJ. Clioquinol induces autophagy in cultured astrocytes and neurons by acting as a zinc ionophore. *Neurobiol Dis*. 2011;42(3):242–251.
169. Nitzan YB, Sekler I, Frederickson CJ, Coulter DA, Balaji RV, Liang SL, Margulis A, Hershfinkel M, Silverman WF. Clioquinol effects on tissue chelatable zinc in mice. *J Mol Med*. 2003;81(10):637–644.
170. Tamura Z, Yoshioka M, Imanari T, Fukaya J, Kusaka J. Identification of green pigment and analysis of clioquinol in specimens from patients with subacute myelo-optico-neuropathy. *Clin Chim Acta*. 1973;47(1):13–20.
171. Atamna H, Frey II WH. A role for heme in Alzheimer's disease: heme binds amyloid beta and has altered metabolism. *Proc Natl Acad Sci USA*. 2004;101(30):11153–11158.
172. LeVine 3rd H, Ding Q, Walker JA, Voss RS, Augelli-Szafran CE. Clioquinol and other hydroxyquinoline derivatives inhibit Abeta(1-42) oligomer assembly. *Neurosci Lett*. 2009;465(1):99–103.
173. Mancino AM, Hindo SS, Kochi A, Lim MH. Effects of clioquinol on metal-triggered amyloid-beta aggregation revisited. *Inorg Chem*. 2009;48(20):9596–9598.
174. Ritchie CW, Bush AI, Mackinnon A, Macfarlane S, Mastwyk M, MacGregor L, Kiers L, Cherny R, Li QX, Tammer A, Carrington D, Mavros C, Volitakis I, Xilinas M, Ames D, Davis S, Beyreuther K, Tanzi RE, Masters CL. Metal-protein attenuation with iodochlorhydroxyquin (clioquinol) targeting Abeta amyloid deposition and toxicity in Alzheimer disease: a pilot phase 2 clinical trial. *Arch Neurol*. 2003;60(12):1685–1691.
175. Ibach B, Haen E, Marienhagen J, Hajak G. Clioquinol treatment in familiar early onset of Alzheimer's disease: a case report. *Pharmacopsychiatry*. 2005;38(4):178–179.
176. Adlard PA, Cherny RA, Finkelstein DI, Gautier E, Robb E, Cortes M, Volitakis I, Liu X, Smith JP, Perez K, Laughton K, Li QX, Charman SA, Nicolazzo JA, Wilkins S, Deleva K, Lynch T, Kok G, Ritchie CW, Tanzi RE, Cappai R, Masters CL, Barnham KJ, Bush AI. Rapid restoration of cognition in Alzheimer's transgenic mice with 8-hydroxy quinoline analogs is associated with decreased interstitial Abeta. *Neuron*. 2008;59(1):43–55.
177. Lannfelt L, Blennow K, Zetterberg H, Batsman S, Ames D, Harrison J, Masters CL, Targum S, Bush AI, Murdoch R, Wilson J, Ritchie CW. Safety, efficacy, and biomarker findings of PBT2 in targeting Abeta as a modifying therapy for Alzheimer's disease: a phase IIa, double-blind, randomised, placebo-controlled trial. *Lancet Neurol*. 2008;7(9):779–786.
178. Faux NG, Ritchie CW, Gunn A, Rembach A, Tsatsanis A, Bedo J, Harrison J, Lannfelt L, Blennow K, Zetterberg H, Ingelsson M, Masters CL, Tanzi RE, Cummings JL, Herd CM, Bush AI. PBT2 rapidly improves cognition in Alzheimer's Disease: additional phase II analyses. *J Alzheimers Dis*. 2010;20(2):509–516.
179. Ayton S, Lei P, Bush AI. Biometals and their therapeutic implications in Alzheimer's disease. *Neurotherapeutics*. 2015;12(1):109–120.

180. Crouch PJ, Savva MS, Hung LW, Donnelly PS, Mot AI, Parker SJ, Greenough MA, Volitakis I, Adlard PA, Cherny RA, Masters CL, Bush AI, Barnham KJ, White AR. The Alzheimer's therapeutic PBT2 promotes amyloid-beta degradation and GSK3 phosphorylation via a metal chaperone activity. *J Neurochem*. 2011;119(1):220–230.
181. Donnelly PS, Caragounis A, Du T, Laughton KM, Volitakis I, Cherny RA, Sharples RA, Hill AF, Li QX, Masters CL, Barnham KJ, White AR. Selective intracellular release of copper and zinc ions from bis(thiosemicarbazonato) complexes reduces levels of Alzheimer disease amyloid-beta peptide. *J Biol Chem*. 2008;283(8):4568–4577.
182. Donnelly PS, Liddell JR, Lim S, Paterson BM, Cater MA, Savva MS, Mot AI, James JL, Trounce IA, White AR, Crouch PJ. An impaired mitochondrial electron transport chain increases retention of the hypoxia imaging agent diacetylbis(4-methylthiosemicarbazonato)copperII. *Proc Natl Acad Sci USA*. 2012;109(1):47–52.
183. Reznichenko L, Amit T, Zheng H, Avramovich-Tirosh Y, Youdim MB, Weinreb O, Mandel S. Reduction of iron-regulated amyloid precursor protein and beta-amyloid peptide by (-)-epigallocatechin-3-gallate in cell cultures: implications for iron chelation in Alzheimer's disease. *J Neurochem*. 2006;97(2):527–536.
184. Avramovich-Tirosh Y, Amit T, Bar-Am O, Zheng H, Fridkin M, Youdim MB. Therapeutic targets and potential of the novel brain- permeable multifunctional iron chelator-monoamine oxidase inhibitor drug, M-30, for the treatment of Alzheimer's disease. *J Neurochem*. 2007;100(2):490–502.
185. Hanson LR, Fine JM, Renner DB, Svitak AL, Burns RB, Nguyen TM, Tuttle NJ, Marti DL, Panter SS, Frey II WH. Intranasal delivery of deferoxamine reduces spatial memory loss in APP/PS1 mice. *Drug Deliv Transl Res*. 2012;2(3):160–168.
186. Guo C, Wang T, Zheng W, Shan ZY, Teng WP, Wang ZY. Intranasal deferoxamine reverses iron-induced memory deficits and inhibits amyloidogenic APP processing in a transgenic mouse model of Alzheimer's disease. *Neurobiol Aging*. 2013;34(2):562–575.
187. Crapper McLachlan DR, Dalton AJ, Kruck TP, Bell MY, Smith WL, Kalow W, Andrews DF. Intramuscular desferrioxamine in patients with Alzheimer's disease. *Lancet*. 1991;337(8753):1304–1308.

CHAPTER

2

Copper in Alzheimer's Disease

Rosanna Squitti, Mariacarla Ventriglia**, Mariacristina Siotto†, Carlo Salustri***

***IRCCS, Institute Center St. John of God Fatebenefratelli, Brescia, Italy**
****Institute of Cognitive Sciences and Technologies (CNR), Fatebenefratelli Hospital, Rome, Italy**
†Don Carlo Gnocchi Foundation ONLUS, Italy

OUTLINE

INTRODUCTION

Alzheimer's disease (AD) is the most common form of dementia in the elderly and represents one of the most socially costly diseases in all developed countries. Research has made tremendous progress in the last years but is still hindered by the fact that AD develops only in humans, while it is unfound in the animal world. Diagnosis is based on cognitive tests: Mini-mental state examination (MMSE)[1] is used to screen for cognitive impairment at the very early stage of cognitive decline. Diagnosis is always uncertain as other forms of dementia share symptoms. Thus, even the most confident diagnosis of a living patient is always delivered as "probable AD" according to [NINCDS-ADRDA] criteria.[2,3] Certainty comes only with a *postmortem* autopsy.

Biometals in Neurodegenerative Diseases. http://dx.doi.org/10.1016/B978-0-12-804562-6.00002-6

AD presents itself in two forms: "late onset" and "early onset." The name of the first one derives from the fact that it normally appears after age 65. It is the most common form of AD, affecting 90%–95% of all patients. It is also often called "sporadic" as it does not show Mendelian inheritance traits. Sporadic AD is the result of a complex interaction of genetic and nongenetic factors. No single culprit can be named and age remains the greatest recognized risk factor. However, recently researchers have discovered that the inheritance of some specific genes increases the chance of developing the disease. Due to the statistical nature of this observation, these genes have been named "susceptibility" genes as they have not been proven to directly cause AD but the presence of one or more of them makes an individual more susceptible to develop the disease. In particular, inheritance of the ε4 allele of the apolipoprotein E (*APOE*) gene has been established to be one of the major risk factors of AD.

Recently, researchers have also found that oxidative stress can cause major cellular damage and have uncovered the neurodegenerative effects of the breakdown of essential metals' homeostasis. Iron, copper, zinc, and manganese, which are all indispensable for our life (Box 2.1), can easily enter toxic biochemical reactions resulting in oxidative stress when they are not kept under control by specialized proteins or transporters.

Today, the involvement of iron, zinc, and copper in AD is extensively documented by several meta-analyses published in the last few years. Among these essential metals, though, copper appears to have a special role. In fact, a 2011 meta-analysis demonstrated that, while neurocortical iron and zinc levels do not change in the AD brain, copper decreases significantly.[4] At the same time, meta-analyses of iron, zinc, and copper in general circulation (plasma and serum) of AD patients have shown no change of systemic iron, decreased levels of systemic zinc, and increased levels of systemic copper.[5] In this scenario, we will see later in this chapter that it is fundamental to distinguish between two different "types" of copper: copper that circulates tightly bound to ceruloplasmin (often called copper "bound" to Cp) and copper that circulates loosely attached to and constantly exchanged among albumin and other low molecular compounds (we will call it "non-Cp-Cu" or sometimes "free" copper).[6]

THE PHYSIOLOGY OF COPPER

Copper Absorption and Distribution

Copper levels in our body are the result of how much copper is absorbed through the intestine and how much is excreted via the liver. Food is of course the main source of intake, but there is some preoccupation about the still widely used copper pipes which may expose us to a nonnegligible involuntary intake of copper from drinking water.[7] Following a modern "normal" diet, we ingest between 0.6 and 1.6 mg of copper per day (Fig. 2.2).

However, contrary to iron that almost entirely remains in our body, copper is excreted by several ways.

Altogether a healthy 70 kg human body contains no more than 110 mg[18] (Box 2.2). The biggest share of copper is in the skeleton (including the bone marrow) and in the skeletal muscles with about 46 mg and 26 mg, respectively. The liver contains about 10 mg. About 9 mg are found in the brain and 6 mg in the blood. Normal mean levels of serum copper are 11–24,4 μmol/L.[19]

BOX 2.1

BIOMETALS: HOW HAVE THEY BECOME SO IMPORTANT.

Iron, copper, zinc and manganese are all essential for life. Two-thirds of the proteins in our body use these metals. Thus, the biology of these metals has an important impact on our health and the breakdown of their homeostasis often leads to disease. Biometals are very useful when kept under control but become extremely dangerous when their levels become deregulated (Fig. 2.1).

Biometals have come a long way. Up to about 2.45 billion years ago, the Earth's atmosphere contained only small amounts of free oxygen, probably produced entirely by the reaction of sunlight with water vapor from volcanoes. Cyanobacteria living in the oceans produced the energy for their lives by photosynthesis, via *photosystems that utilized copper and iron to exchange electrons*. Oxygen was a by-product of this process and was normally captured by dissolved iron present in the environment. However, at the beginning of the Siderian, the first period of the Proterozoic, the photosynthesis-produced oxygen reached saturation levels and the atmosphere started being filled with dioxygen (O_2). As a result, about 2.45 billion years ago, all primitive forms of anaerobic life on the Earth rapidly ceased to exist. This Great Oxygenation Event, also known as Oxygen Catastrophe, Oxygen Crisis or Great Oxydation, changed forever Earth's life, which now depends on breathing oxygen.

As gaseous oxygen built up, the atmosphere began to change from one that was chemically reducing to an oxidizing (i.e., rust-forming) one. Iron, weathered from basaltic volcanoes, became oxidized before it reached the oceans. This resulted in the formation of red beds, whose red color comes from the particular variety of iron mineral precipitated on land, mostly hematite (Fe_2O_3) (Fig. 2.1).

Thus, the history of the Earth's early crust also tells us the story of its early atmosphere and explains the strict connection of essential metals in human metabolism. This is the reason why they are essential for life and why concentrations of these metals in our body, and specifically in our brain, are enormously elevated (up to 300 times higher) with respect to those of environmental metal, such as aluminum.

Copper in the body appears in two oxidation states: Cu^{1+} and Cu^{2+}, which play an important role in how copper is managed throughout the life cycle. Food copper is mainly in a Cu^{2+} state but it must be first reduced to Cu^{1+} in order to be transported across the enterocytes' membrane. This process takes place via reductases, such as the cytochrome b558, Steap 2, and CYBRD1.[20] There is evidence that DMT1, which is known to regulate iron uptake, also participates in the uptake of copper.[21]

Cu^{1+} is then imported into the enterocyte[22] (Table 2.2). Inside the enterocyte, several chaperone proteins load copper onto specific enzymes: the main ones are the cytochrome C oxidase assembly homolog (COX17), which delivers copper to mitochondria, antioxidant protein 1 homolog (ATOX1), and ATP7A protein, which transport copper to the *trans*-Golgi

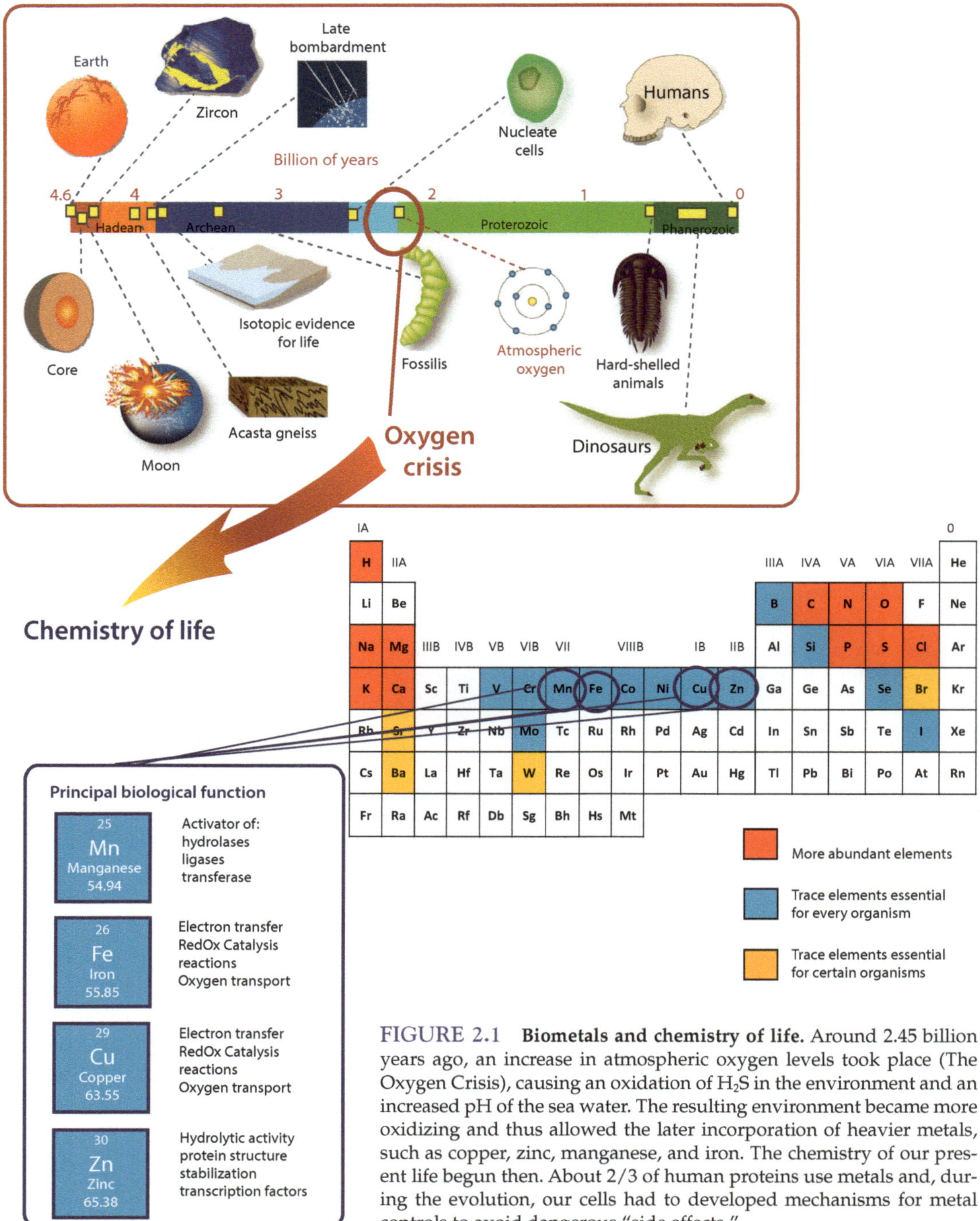

FIGURE 2.1 **Biometals and chemistry of life.** Around 2.45 billion years ago, an increase in atmospheric oxygen levels took place (The Oxygen Crisis), causing an oxidation of H_2S in the environment and an increased pH of the sea water. The resulting environment became more oxidizing and thus allowed the later incorporation of heavier metals, such as copper, zinc, manganese, and iron. The chemistry of our present life begun then. About 2/3 of human proteins use metals and, during the evolution, our cells had to developed mechanisms for metal controls to avoid dangerous "side effects."

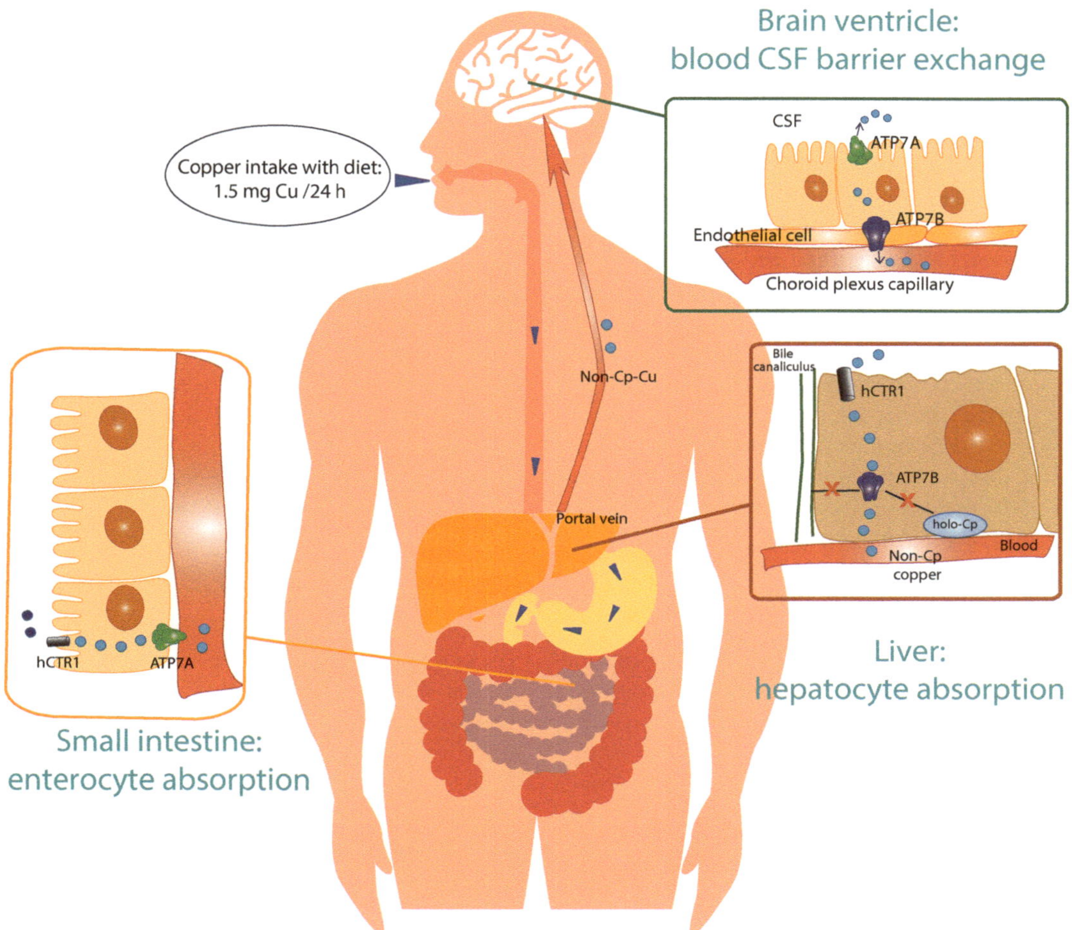

FIGURE 2.2 **Absorption of copper in conditions of altered homeostasis.** We normally ingest 1.5 mg/day of copper via food and water and the homeostasis of this metal is finely regulated. *Yellow box*: absorption of copper into the enterocyte: Cu^{2+} is reduced from reductases. The integral membrane protein hCTR-1 imports Cu^{1+} which is loaded onto copper-dependent enzymes, via several chaperone proteins (not shown). ATP7A transports copper to the *trans*-Golgi network and pumps out of the enterocyte's basolateral membrane (*via* vesicular compartment). Copper is then transported to the liver bound to albumin or α2 macroglobulin or amino acids via the portal vein. *Brown Box:* The liver is the main storage organ for copper. Copper intake in the hepatocytes resembles the one in the enterocytes, following the same mechanism of reduction by reductase, hCTR-1-mediated absorption, and delivery to chaperones. In the liver, ATP7B, the homolog of enterocytes' ATP7A, incorporates copper into ceruloplasmin. In normal conditions, about 85%–95% of copper tightly binds ceruloplasmin, whereas the remainder loosely binds to and is exchanged among albumin, α2 macroglobulin, amino acids, peptides, and several micronutrients. An excess of copper induces the translocation of ATP7B from the *trans*-Golgi network to the canalicular membrane (via vesicular compartment), where the metal is secreted in the bile. The figure shows an altered copper homeostasis characterized by a failure in the holoceruloplasmin biosynthesis and by a failure in copper excretion into the bile. The consequence is the production of an excess of copper not bound to ceruloplasmin into the blood system. *Green box*: Uptake of copper into brain cells requires the reduction from Cu^{2+} to Cu^{1+}. This reaction is performed by unidentified reductases probably analogous to those present in other organs. The secretion of copper is assigned principally to ATP7A, via vesicular compartment which secrete copper into the synapse, but there is also an ATP7B which acts near the choroid plexus capillary.

BOX 2.2

COPPER IN THE DIET

The World Health Organization (WHO) has classified copper as an essential element whose absence or deficiency from the diet produces functional or structural abnormalities, and reports that the minimal intake to prevent copper deficiency is 0.9 mg/day (WHO, 1996). Thus, the balance between copper absorption and excretion must be tightly regulated. In a normal individual, copper absorption reaches about 30% of the total intake[8–10] but decreases if dietary copper intake increases, varying from 56% under a low copper regimen to 12% under a high copper regimen.[9,10] Several factors, including age, sex, food type, oral contraceptives and more, can affect the absorption rate. Food, supplements, and water are the primary sources of copper exposure in developed countries. Taking vitamin or mineral supplements increases exposure by about 2 mg/day, while drinking-water contributes 0.1–1 mg/day in most countries. The most relevant sources of dietary copper and the foods with low copper content are listed in Table 2.1. It is important to consider that the content of copper in food varies with local conditions and practices, as copper compounds are widely used as bactericides or fungicides on many crops. Also copper emissions from smelting and casting industries can be particularly intense in certain areas. All these factors definitely affect the copper content in cereals, fruit and vegetables and, to a lesser extent, meat and animal products.[11–13] Cooking, food storage and food processing also affect the quantity of copper present in any given food. Reduced stomach acidity may also increase the risk for copper deficiency. The concomitance of high dietary copper intake and a diet high in saturated fats has been recognized to be associated with cognitive decline.[14,15] This hypothesis is supported by the evidence of accumulation of metal-transporting proteins and compounds in key sites of the attentional circuits.[16] Evidence-based medicine recommends both dietary and lifestyle guidelines for establishing an adequate intake of copper. Among other targets, these guidelines also intend to prevent or at least improve conditions associated with the risk of AD.[17]

TABLE 2.1 Foods with the Highest and with the Lowest Content of Bioavailable Copper

Food (100 g)	Copper (mg)	Food (100 g)	Copper (mg)
Animal liver (veal)	11.86	Egg	0.023
Oysters	5.71	Sole, codfish, grouper	0.019
Sesame seeds	4.08	Cauliflower, cabbage	0.017
Cocoa	3.79	Carrots	0.017
Nuts (cashew)	2.19	Peppers	0.017
Seafood (calamari)	2.11	Milk	0.011
Dried herbs (basil)	2.10	Sugar	0.007
Sunflower seeds	1.60	Turnips	0.005
Sun dried tomatoes	1.42	Oil	0
Pumpkin	1.34	Butter	0

TABLE 2.2 Copper Absorption and Distribution in the Intestine

Enterocyte	Protein involved	function
Apical surface	• cytochrome b558 ferric/cupric reductase • Steap2 • CYBRD1	Reduction of Cu^{2+} to Cu^{1+}
Membrane	• hCTR-1 • DMT-1?	Import of Cu^{1+}
Cytosol	• Copper chaperones • COX17 • ATOX1 • CCS • ATP7A • MT	Transport
Basolateral membrane	• ATP7A	Transmigration and export of copper into circulation
Circulation	• Albumin • α2-macroglobulin • Amino acids	Transport of copper

network, and CCS, the copper chaperone to SOD1 in the cytosol.[22] Copper is then pumped out of the enterocyte's basolateral membrane by ATP7A and transported to the liver by albumin or α2–macroglobulin via the portal vein (Table 2.2, Fig. 2.2). In the liver, copper is partly stored and partly redistributed to other organs.

Copper in the Liver

The liver plays a most fundamental role in initiating copper movement and usage by balancing duodenal absorption and biliary excretion. As in the enterocytes, copper intake in the hepatocytes follows the same mechanism of reduction, hCTR-1-mediated absorption, and transfer to chaperones (Table 2.3, Fig. 2.2). ATP7B, which is the homolog of enterocytes' ATP7A, incorporates copper into ceruloplasmin (Table 2.3, Fig. 2.2). In the liver, however, copper divides into two "types": a first type, about 85%–95% of the total, becomes tightly bound to the big protein ceruloplasmin, while the remainder binds loosely to albumin, α2 macroglobulin, amino acids, peptides and several micronutrients, and is constantly exchanged among all these low-molecular-weight compounds.

Within the hepatocytes, an excess of copper induces the translocation of ATP7B from the *trans*-Golgi network to the canalicular membrane, where the metal is secreted in the bile (Table 2.3, Fig. 2.2).

Copper's Path From General Circulation to the Brain

In order to regulate the transfer of substances from the blood to the different body systems, several "filters" are necessary: two are the most important: the "blood–cerebrospinal fluid" barrier (BCB) and the "blood–brain" barrier (BBB).

TABLE 2.3 Copper Absorption and Distribution in the Liver

Hepatocyte	Protein involved	function
Apical Membrane	• cytochrome b558 ferric/cupric reductase • Steap2 • hCTR-1 • DMT-1?	Reduction of Cu^{2+} to Cu^{1+} Import of Cu^{1+}
Cytosol	Copper chaperones: • COX17 • ATOX1 • CCS (for SOD) • APP • MT	Transport and delivery of copper into specific proteins
	• ATP7B (*trans* Golgi)	Copper loading into ceruloplasmin
Interface with Bile canaliculus	• ATP7B	Transmigration from *trans* Golgi and Export of excess copper into bile
Basolateral outer membrane	• ceruloplasmin	"transport" of copper structurally bound and not exchangeable (85:95% of serum copper)
Circulation	• Albumin • α2-macroglobulin • Amino acids	Transport of exchangeable non-Cp-Cu

The cerebrospinal fluid (CSF), which is produced by the choroid plexuses from arterial blood, plays an important role in the metabolism of the central nervous system (CNS) and is essential for its homeostasis. Like other elements and substances, copper must cross the BCB to reach the CSF. The mechanism of this passage is not fully understood and we still don't know whether copper is moved into the CSF by active transport or passive diffusion. However, normal CSF copper levels range between 0.5 and 2.5 μmol/L, reviewed in Ref. [23].

The highest copper accumulations are in BBB tissues (choroid plexus and cerebral capillaries) and brain parenchyma and to a lesser extent in CSF. The BBB is the principal gate of copper into the brain parenchyma, whereas the BCB appears more involved in the regulation of copper homeostasis in CSF.

Cu^{2+} is reduced to Cu^{1+} before uptake into brain cells (Table 2.4; Fig. 2.2), a process that is performed by still unidentified reductases. However, in comparison to other cell types, it seems that the brain presents an over control of metal uptake: beside hCTR1, two other proteins, the APP and the prion protein (PrP), are located on the surface of brain cells and appear to be involved in copper regulation.

After entering the brain, chaperones ATOX1 (or HAH1), CCS, COX17 or metallothioneins deliver Cu^{1+} to the intracellular compartments. ATP7A has a main role in pumping copper into synaptic vesicles at the glutamatergic synapse, where this metal acts as a modulator of neurotransmission.[24] ATP7B is instead expressed in some isolated regions of the brain.[25]

TABLE 2.4 Copper Absorption and Distribution in the Brain

Blood CSF Barrier	Protein involved	Function
Blood Brain Barrier	• Unidentified reductases	Reduction of Cu^{2+} to Cu^{1+}
Brain cells surface	• hCTR-1 • APP • PrP	Import of Cu^{1+}
Membrane	• hCTR-1 • APP • PrP • Copper chaperones • COX17 • ATOX1 • CCS • ATP7A/ATP7B • MT	Transport and delivery of copper into specific proteins

The Key Role of Ceruloplasmin

Ceruloplasmin is a big protein mainly synthesized in the liver but also expressed endogenously by the CNS. In the hepatocytes, ceruloplasmin uploads six copper atoms in its structure in a process mediated by the protein ATP7B. The copper-loaded ceruloplasmin, normally referred to as holo-ceruloplasmin, is immediately transferred to the blood.

Ceruloplasmin catalyzes the oxidation of Fe^{2+} to Fe^{3+} via the following chemical reaction

$$4\,Fe^{2+} + 4\,H^{+} + O_2 \rightarrow 4\,Fe^{3+} + 2\,H_2O$$

This is a key reaction as it permits iron to be bussed to various organs by the protein transferrin, which accepts only Fe^{3+}. It is also a "safe" reaction as its by-product is simply water.

At physiological pH, oxidation of Fe^{2+} may trigger dangerous Fenton or Haber-Weiss reactions. Fortunately, ceruloplasmin normally limits the production of oxygen radicals by scavenging H_2O_2.[26] In this scenario, copper plays an important role because the synthesis of holo-ceruloplasmin strictly depends on the amount of copper available in the liver.

A reduced availability of copper results in the production of apo-ceruloplasmin, which has no ferroxidase capability and is rapidly degraded in plasma. A reduction of ferroxidase activity due to a decreased presence of ceruloplasmin results in more Fe^{2+} available for Fenton reactions.

This is why aceruloplasminemia, which is an autosomal recessive trait causing a drop in ceruloplasmin activity, causes severe iron overload and is often misdiagnosed as hemochromatosis. Moreover, ceruloplasmin prevents lipid peroxidation. Patients with aceruloplasminemia show evidence of increased lipid peroxidation and impaired fatty acid oxidation. The rate of serum iron oxidation, which is required for iron mobilization and iron release from tissue storage[27] is also regulated by ceruloplasmin. In summary, ceruloplasmin is a protein essential for iron metabolism and for antioxidant defense and is implicated in the molecular mechanisms of hepatic disease and neurodegenerative disorders.[28] Also genetic mutations of the *ATP7B* gene, which produces the above mentioned intermediary protein ATP7B, may cause low holo-ceruloplasmin levels. This is what actually happens in Wilson's disease (WD), which is the paradigmatic disease of free copper toxicosis or accumulation in both liver and brain.[29]

COPPER TOXICITY

The Role of Copper in Alzheimer's Disease

It is well known that the presence of amyloid plaques and neurofibrillary tangles, respectively outside and inside the neuronal space is the hallmark of the AD brain. The major constituent of the plaques is amyloid-beta (Aβ), a 39–43 amino-acid peptide, generated from the cleavage of the transmembrane protein APP. APP, which has multiple selective copper-binding sites, appears to mediate redox activity, which causes the precipitation of Aβ, even at low concentrations (Box 2.3)

Enhanced concentrations of copper have been reported to colocalize within both amyloid plaques and neurofibrillary tangles.[30] The fact that Aβ deposition in plaques is an age-dependent phenomenon but Aβ production does not increase with age, suggests that changes in biometal homeostasis, which are age-dependent, may play a key role in the Aβ transformation and neurotoxicity. Biometal deposits have been found also in other brain areas known to be affected by AD, as for example, the basal ganglia,[31] even though the total content of copper in the brain appears decreased.[4] All the above considerations and findings have led to hypothesizing a synergic involvement of zinc, iron, copper and Aβ in AD. This notion, subsequently enriched by further findings, was eventually proposed as the *Metal Hypothesis*

BOX 2.3

METALS AND Aβ

The interaction between transition metals and Aβ can be described by the following reactions[33]:

$$(A\beta)^2 + Me^{n+} \rightarrow A\beta : A\beta^+ + Me^{(n-1)+}$$

where Me generically stands for metal. This reaction has two negative effects: the first is the production of an insoluble Aβ peptide, the second the production of a superoxide anion via the following reaction

$$Fe^{2+} + O_2 \rightarrow Fe^{3+} + O_2^-$$

The generated superoxide can now participate in a Haber-Weiss reaction with peroxide

$$O_2^- + H_2O_2 \rightarrow \bullet OH + OH^- + O_2$$

which produces reactive oxygen species (ROS). The only way the superoxide anion can be depleted is by a dismutation:

$$O^{2-} + O_2^- + 2H^+ \rightarrow H_2O_2 + O_2$$

which is generally, but not exclusively, accelerated by superoxide dismutases, as for example, SOD1, see Ref. [34] for a review of the biology of metals in AD.

of AD.[32] This hypothesis proposes that it is the interaction of Aβ with zinc, iron, and copper at glutamatergic synapses that promotes the aggregation of Aβ in insoluble plaques, short-circuiting the entire neuronal network to which those synapses belong, and thus driving AD pathogenesis.[32]

Beside the experimental and theoretical models of copper toxicity in AD, we can take advantage of meta-analyses to depict a possible role of essential metals and specifically of copper in this disease. Meta-analyses of both local brain and general systemic circulation demonstrated an imbalance of essential metals in AD. More specifically, while iron appears unchanged, zinc homeostasis appears disturbed[4] and copper imbalance is evident when considering as a whole the results from the different meta-analyses.[4–6] In fact, meta-analyses evaluating the differences in the levels of the fraction of non-Cp-Cu in serum[6] demonstrated increased levels of the metal in general circulation. This metal fraction is redox active, and makes up 5%–10% of total serum copper.[25,35] Because of its looser binding to albumin and micronutrient pools in the blood, non-Cp-Cu is available to meet tissue needs in the body. If the non-Cp-Cu pool becomes expanded, though, this copper becomes toxic, as exemplified by WD.[8] The results of the meta-analysis and of subsequent studies demonstrated an increase of this pool of copper in general circulation.[6] This increase in non-Cp-Cu can account for the increase of total serum copper found in AD.[5,23,36] Considered as a whole, these meta-analyses demonstrate the existence of a copper "failure" in AD, consisting in a copper decrease in the brain,[4] an increase in the blood,[5] and an increase of non-CP-Cu in the serum.[6] Increased non-Cp-Cu and decreased brain copper in AD is a condition biologically plausible on the basis on the Long Evans Cinnamon (LEC) rat model of WD. In fact, these rats exhibit inbred *ATP7B* mutation and as a consequence they have increased non-Cp-Cu in serum, decreased total copper in the brain and increased redox active labile copper in the brain.[37] James and colleagues,[38] in line with the result of the meta-analysis by Schrag et al,[4] demonstrated decreased levels of total copper in specific areas of the AD brain and increased levels of redox active labile copper in the same areas. LEC rats exhibit also decreased levels of ceruloplasmin-specific activity in general circulation, and decreased levels of ceruloplasmin specific activity have been found in AD.[39] More specifically, a recent study demonstrated decreased levels of ceruloplasmin specific activity in AD with respect to healthy controls, along with increased non-Cp-Cu.[40] According to Bradford Hill criteria (information available at: https://en.wikipedia.org/wiki/Bradford_Hill_criteria) all these findings are of relevance for causation of the metal with AD.

P-type ATPases, and in particular ATP7B, are copper efflux pumps that regulate the amount of copper released by the hepatocyte via bile canalicula, and copper loading into nascent ceruloplasmin during its biosynthesis. Defects in copper loading into ceruloplasmin increases the amount of non-Cp-Cu released into blood circulation. Increased apo-ceruloplasmin in the serum of AD patients have been demonstrated in AD[40] and signs of liver hypofunction ascribable to disturbing effects of non-Cp-Cu on hepatocytes.[41] Moreover, the non-Cp-Cu increase is tightly related to the AD clinical picture, revealing direct effects on brain functions.[11,42,43] This implies an increased non-Cp-Cu inside the brain.[38] In some of our previous studies we have found signs of non-Cp-Cu moving from serum to CSF through the BBB,[44] and of non-Cp-Cu correlations with CSF markers of AD.[44] It is well known from WD studies that ATP7B failure causes serum non-Cp-Cu to increase beyond the normal reference range (>1.6 μmol/L).

If on the one hand the correlative association between abnormally increased levels of non-Cp-Cu and cognitive decline has been extensively reported in the literature, recently reviewed in [45] on the other hand the causative connection relates to some genetic studies.[46–48] However, causation evidence is strongly provided by a bulk of studies carried out on in vitro and animal models and by "proof of concept" phase II clinical trials, demonstrating changing in the clinical history of patients in relative small size AD cohorts.[45,49,50]

Genetics of Copper and AD

Two recent genome wide association studies (GWAS) identified loci affecting metal metabolism.[51,52] These studies identified two regions on chromosome 1 as having significant association on concentrations in erythrocytes. A deeper analysis revealed that the genes in this region of chromosome 1 do not code for proteins with known functions, which have been associated with disease relevant to Cu metabolism. Among the 20 disease-associated loci, CLU, the gene that encodes clusterin, has been demonstrated to increase the risk of sporadic AD.[53] CLU is a molecular chaperone that has multiple roles in apoptosis but also aids protein folding and Aβ clearance. It has been reported that CLU directly interacts with ATP7A and ATP7B, facilitating their degradation *in vitro* and modulates their copper-export function.[54]

As expected, these GWAS did not find significant association between single nucleotide polymorphisms (SNPs) in the chromosomal region where *ATP7B* is located and AD. The GWAS outcome can be explained by the paradigm "common disease – common gene variants", which is currently the basis for GWAS, and by the complex structure of the *ATP7B* gene. In fact, GWAS hardly detects rare variants, which are instead supposed to account for the missing hereditability of complex diseases, especially if referred to the *ATP7B* gene, which is a high polymorphic gene, as previously described.[55]

With a perspective different from GWAS, thus using a hypothesis-driven approach,[56] we theorized that the mechanism for increased non-Cp-Cu in AD could be related to genetic defects interfering with the ATP7B function, causing altered loading of Cu into nascent ceruloplasmin. On this line, we started an extensive study on the *ATP7B* gene in AD patients, which is still in progress.

Analysis of the *ATP7B* gene is complex, since it is a highly polymorphic gene. The 1000-Genome project has identified more than 1300 variations of *ATP7B* in human populations.[56] Worldwide detection of *ATP7B* mutations is actually difficult since most mutations are rare, reported only within single families and often prevalent in specific ethnic groups. As a result, the database regarding both the gene's properties and the possible dysfunctions of the proteins they encode appears still unsatisfactory.[57]

Our hypothesis-driven approach was inspired by the study of Gupta et al.,[58] which presented a set of SNP markers. These SNPs were highly heterozygous across most of the world populations and could be used in combination with analyses of prevalent mutations as a comprehensive strategy for determining pre-symptomatic and carrier sibs of WD patients. We took advantage of this knowledge in WD to study in AD these four alleles of the *ATP7B* gene, which are informative of the *ATP7B* gene structure.[58] We focused our attention on this set of four SNPs, namely: rs1801243 (missense substitution: Ser406Ala), rs2147363 (intronic variant: c.1544-53A > C), rs1061472 (missense substitution: Lys832Arg) and rs732774 (missense substitution: Arg952Lys). We found high frequencies of the minor allele in two SNPs causing nonsynonymous substitutions: the rs1801243 (c.1216T > G) associated with amino acid change Serine to Alanine in position 406 and the rs1061472 (c.2495A > G) that causes the amino acid substitution of Lysine to Arginine in position 832. Subsequently, we studied another nonsynonymous change Arginine in Lysine in position 952 (rs732774). In a larger study population, we demonstrated a significant association of rs1061472 genotypes and AD risk and revealed an association for the rs772774.[59]

These studies demonstrated a linkage disequilibrium association of AD with the four informative SNPs and revealed that unknown spots within the gene region coding the transmembrane domains of the ATP7B ionic pump (Block 1 rs732774-rs1061472[47,48]) can have an association with the disease. These still elusive and probably rare loci in the *ATP7B* gene, along with those in modifier genes, such as *ATOX1* and *COMMD1*, can considerably impact the probability of developing a copper-related AD.

The AD Copper Subtype

As a multifactorial and complex disease, AD includes a broad spectrum of phenotypes. Unfavorable evolution of the cognitive function in AD has been associated with copper metabolism abnormalities.[36,42] However, the evidence of this association is stronger if the AD cohorts are stratified on the basis of a non-Cp-Cu content cut-off at base line. In fact, this stratification shows that subjects with a high non-Cp-Cu fraction have a higher risk of a more severe decline and of a greater rate of disease progression.[36,42] Summarizing the results of various previous studies of ours, this copper imbalance appears in 60%–65% of AD patients.[46,47,60]

Based on this evidence, we hypothesized the existence of an "AD copper subtype" and defined biological and statistical approaches suitable to detect it.[35,46,47]

Generally speaking, the comparison of demographic, clinical, genetic, and biological variables of patients stratified on a specific biomarker is a valid strategy for identifying subtypes of a disease,[46,47] {see [35] for an extensive discussion on this subject}. We have applied this strategy in recent studies[46,47,61] and demonstrated that single-locus and haplotype frequency of specific *ATP7B* gene variants are different in AD patients with high non-Cp-Cu than in patients with normal levels.[17,47,48] Also peculiar brain activity alterations, visible in the patient's electroencephalogram (EEG), can distinguish AD patients with abnormal non-Cp-Cu levels from patients with normal levels.[61] Furthermore, when comparing AD patients stratified for non-Cp-Cu content, cortical atrophy and cerebrovascular lesions appear different between the two groups, while MRI indexes of MTA were similar (work in progress). All this evidence demonstrates that AD heterogeneity can be detected by a copper marker that typifies a subgroup of individuals.

Our findings are supported by a 2013 case-report on an AD patient with Kayser-Fleischer rings showing MRI lesions predominantly located in the medial temporal lobe but not in the cortical region.[48] The patient had a marked brain atrophy of the temporal and parietal lobes, while cerebrovascular lesions and global cortical atrophy were under-represented. That case-report strongly suggests the existence of an AD copper subtype, as the patient exhibited an 11C-labeled Pittsburgh Compound-B ([11C]PIB) PET positive (strong binding to cortical fibrillar Aβ depositions in an AD-typical distribution) and a [18F] fluorodeoxyglucose (18F-FDG) PET altered with a typical AD topography (marked bilateral temporoparietal hypometabolism).[62]

CONCLUSIONS

Meta-analyses and systemic reviews point at a copper decrease in the brain, copper increase in the blood, and non-Cp-Cu increase in the serum as unequivocal signs of a breakdown of copper homeostasis in AD and MCI. The protein ATP7B, which loads copper into ceruloplasmin during its synthesis and escorts superfluous copper into the bile, appears to be a key actor in this copper failure. A faulty function of this ATPase is well known to be associated with WD, which is a well-established inborn error of copper metabolism. Several mutations of the *ATP7B* gene have been observed, involving different regions of the protein and thus resulting in a plethora of phenotypes in WD patients. The notion that a copper dysmetabolism occurs also in AD is now a consolidate one among researchers. Besides the assessment of molecular mechanisms relating copper to the protein hallmarks of this disease and more generally to neurodegeneration, new evidence of a role of the non-Cp-Cu fraction in accelerating the Aβ cascade has been recently added to the AD pathological picture.

References

1. Folstein MF, Folstein SEMP. "Mini-mental state". A practical method for grsading the cognitive state of patients for the clinician. *J Psychiatr Res*. 1975;12:189–198.
2. McKhann G, Drachman D, Folstein M, Katzman R, Price D, Stadlan EM. Clinical diagnosis of Alzheimer's disease: Report of the NINCDS-ADRDA Work Group* under the auspices of Department of Health and Human Services Task Force on Alzheimer's Disease. *Neurology*. 1984;34(7):939–1939.
3. Dubois B, Feldman HH, Jacova C, Dekosky ST, Barberger-Gateau P, Cummings J, Delacourte A, Galasko D, Gauthier S, Jicha G, Meguro K, O'brien J, Pasquier F, Robert P, Rossor M, Salloway S, Stern Y, Visser PJ, Scheltens P. Research criteria for the diagnosis of Alzheimer's disease: Revising the NINCDS-ADRDA criteria. *Lancet Neurol*. 2007;6:734–746.
4. Schrag M, Mueller C, Oyoyo U, Smith MA, Kirsch WM. Iron, zinc and copper in the Alzheimer's disease brain: a quantitative meta-analysis. Some insight on the influence of citation bias on scientific opinion. *Prog Neurobiol*. 2011;94(3):296–306.
5. Wang Z-X, Tan L, Wang H-F, et al. Serum iron, zinc, and copper levels in patients with Alzheimer's disease: a replication study and meta-analyses. *J Alzheimer's Dis*. 2015;47:565–581.
6. Squitti R, Simonelli I, Ventriglia M, et al. Meta-analysis of serum non-ceruloplasmin copper in Alzheimer's disease. *J Alzheimers Dis*. 2014;38(4):809–822.
7. Brewer GJ. Toxicity of copper in drinking water. *J Toxicol Env Heal B Crit Rev*. 2010;13:449–452:author reply: 453–449.
8. Squitti R, Siotto M, Polimanti R. Low-copper diet as a preventive strategy for Alzheimer's disease. *Neurobiol Aging*. 2014;35(Suppl. 2):1–11.
9. Turnlund JR. Human whole-body copper metabolism. *Am J Clin Nutr*. 1998;67:960S–964S.
10. Turnlund JR, Keyes WR, Anderson HL, Acord LL. Copper absorption and retention in young men at three levels of dietary copper by use of the stable isotope 65Cu. *Am J Clin Nutr*. 1989;49(5):870–878.
11. Salustri C, Barbati G, Ghidoni R, et al. Is cognitive function linked to serum free copper levels? A cohort study in a normal population. *Clin Neurophysiol*. 2010;121(4):502–507.
12. Scheinberg IH, Sternlieb I. Wilson disease and idiopathic copper toxicosis. *Am J Clin Nutr*. 1996;63(5).
13. Wenisch E1, De Tassigny A, Trocello JM, Beretti J, Girardot-Tinant NWF. Cognitive profile in Wilson's disease: a case series of 31 patients. *Rev Neurol (Paris)*. 2013;169:944–949.
14. Morris MC, Evans DA, Tangney CC, et al. Dietary copper and high saturated and trans fat intakes associated with cognitive decline. *Arch Neurol*. 2006;63(8):1085–1088.
15. Loef M, Walach H. Copper and iron in Alzheimer's disease: a systematic review and its dietary implications. *Br J Nutr*. 2012;107(1):7–19.
16. Zatta P1, Drago D, Zambenedetti P, Bolognin S, Nogara E, Peruffo ACB. Accumulation of copper and other metal ions, and metallothionein I/II expression in the bovine brain as a function of aging. *J Chem Neuroanat*. 2008;36:1–5.

17. Barnard ND, Bush AI, Ceccarelli A, et al. Dietary and lifestyle guidelines for the prevention of Alzheimer's disease. *Neurobiol Aging*. 2014;35(Suppl. 2):1–5.
18. Linder MC, Hazegh-Azam M. Copper biochemistry and molecular biology. *Am J Clin Nutr*. 1996;63(5):797S–811S.
19. Jacobs DS, Oxley DK DW. In: Hudson, ed. *Laboratory Test Handbook Concise with Disease Index, Hudson*. 5th ed. Cleveland, OH: Lexi-Comp; 2002.
20. Wyman S, Simpson RJ, McKie AT, Sharp PA. Dcytb (Cybrd1) functions as both a ferric and a cupric reductase in vitro. *FEBS Lett*. 2008;582(13):1901–1906.
21. Collins JF, Franck CA, Kowdley KV, Ghishan FK. Identification of differentially expressed genes in response to dietary iron deprivation in rat duodenum. *Am J Physiol Gastrointest Liver Physiol*. 2005;288(5):G964–G971.
22. Kim B-E, Nevitt T, Thiele DJ. Mechanisms for copper acquisition, distribution and regulation. *Nat Chem Biol*. 2008;4(3):176–185.
23. Bucossi S, Ventriglia M, Panetta V, et al. Copper in alzheimer's disease: a meta-analysis of serum, plasma, and cerebrospinal fluid studies. *J Alzheimer's Dis*. 2011;24(1):175–185.
24. Schlief M, Gitlin J. Copper homeostasis in the CNS. *Mol Neurobiol*. 2006;33(2):81–90.
25. Gaggelli E, Kozlowski H, Valensin D, Valensin G. Copper homeostasis and neurodegenerative disorders (Alzheimer's, prion, and Parkinson's diseases and amyotrophic lateral sclerosis). *Chem Rev*. 2006;106(6):1995–2044.
26. Bielli P, Calabrese L. Structure to function relationships in ceruloplasmin: a "moonlighting" protein. *Cell Mol Life Sci*. 2002;59:1413–1427.
27. Madsen E, Gitlin JD. Copper and iron disorders of the brain. *Annu Rev Neurosci*. 2007;30:317–337.
28. Vassiliev V, Harris ZL, Zatta P. Ceruloplasmin in neurodegenerative diseases. *Brain Res Rev*. 2005;49(3):633–640.
29. Hoogenraad TU. *Wilson's Disease*. Amsterdam/Rotterdam: Intermed Medical Publishers; 2001.
30. Miller LM1, Wang Q, Telivala TP, Smith RJ, Lanzirotti AMJ. Synchrotron-based infrared and X-ray imaging shows focalized accumulation of Cu and Zn co-localized with beta-amyloid deposits in Alzheimer's disease. *J Struct Biol*. 2006;155:30–37.
31. Bartzokis G, Tishler TA. MRI evaluation of basal ganglia ferritin iron and neurotoxicity in Alzheimer's and Huntingon's disease. *Cell Mol Biol*. 2000;46(4):821–833.
32. Bush AI, Tanzi RE. Therapeutics for Alzheimer's disease based on the metal hypothesis. *Neurotherapeutics*. 2008;5(3):421–432.
33. Atwood CS, Perry G, Zeng H, et al. Copper mediates dityrosine cross-linking of Alzheimer's amyloid-beta. *Biochemistry*. 2004;43(2):560–568.
34. Roberts BR, Ryan TM, Bush AI, Masters CL, Duce JA. The role of metallobiology and amyloid-beta peptides in Alzheimer's disease. *J Neurochem*. 2012;120(Suppl. 1):149–166.
35. Pal A, Siotto M, Prasad R, Squitti R. Towards a unified vision of copper involvement in Alzheimer's disease: a review connecting basic, experimental, and clinical research. *J Alzheimers Dis*. 2015;44(2):343–354.
36. Squitti R, Ghidoni R, Siotto M, et al. Value of serum nonceruloplasmin copper for prediction of mild cognitive impairment conversion to Alzheimer disease. *Ann Neurol*. 2014;75(4):574–580.
37. Fujiwara N, Iso H, Kitanaka N, et al. Effects of copper metabolism on neurological functions in Wistar and Wilson's disease model rats. *Biochem Biophys Res Commun*. 2006;349(3):1079–1086.
38. James SA, Volitakis I, Adlard PA, et al. Elevated labile Cu is associated with oxidative pathology in Alzheimer disease. *Free Radic Biol Med*. 2012;52(2):298–302.
39. George J. Brewer, Steve H. Kanzer, Earl A. Zimmerman, Dzintra F. Celmins SMH and RD. Copper and Ceruloplasmin Abnormalities in Alzheimer's Disease. *Am J Alzheimers Dis Other Demen*. 2010;25(6):490–497.
40. Squitti R, Quattrocchi CC, Salustri C, Rossini PM. Ceruloplasmin fragmentation is implicated in "free" copper deregulation of Alzheimer's disease. *Prion*. 2008;2(1):23–27:http://www.ncbi.nlm.nih.gov/pubmed/19164917.
41. Squitti R, Ventriglia M, Barbati G, et al. "Free" copper in serum of Alzheimer's disease patients correlates with markers of liver function. *J Neural Transm*. 2007;114(12):1589–1594.
42. Squitti R, Bressi F, Pasqualetti P, et al. Longitudinal prognostic value of serum "free" copper in patients with Alzheimer disease. *Neurology*. 2009;72(1):50–55.
43. Zappasodi F, Salustri C, Babiloni C, et al. An observational study on the influence of the APOE-??4 allele on the correlation between "free" copper toxicosis and EEG activity in Alzheimer disease. *Brain Res*. 2008;1215:183–189.
44. Squitti R, Barbati G, Rossi L, et al. Excess of nonceruloplasmin serum copper in AD correlates with MMSE, CSF [beta]-amyloid, and h-tau. *Neurology*. 2006;67(1):76–82.
45. Squitti R, Ventriglia M, Tecchio F. The role of copper in human diet and risk of dementia. *Curr Nutr Rep*. 2015;4:114–125.

46. Squitti R, Ventriglia M, Gennarelli M, et al. Non-ceruloplasmin copper distincts subtypes in Alzheimer's disease: a genetic study of ATP7B frequency. *Mol Neurobiol*. 2017;54(1):671–681.
47. Squitti R, Ventriglia M, Gennarelli M, et al. Erratum to: non-ceruloplasmin copper distincts subtypes in Alzheimer's disease: a genetic study of ATP7B frequency. *Mol Neurobiol*. 2017;54(1):671–681.
48. Liu H, Lin W, Wang W, et al. Genetic variability in copper-transporting P-type Triphosphatase (ATP7B) is associated with Alzheimer's Disease in a Chinese population. *J Biol Regul Homeost Agents*. 2013;27:319–327.
49. Lannfelt L, Blennow K, Zetterberg H, et al. Safety, efficacy, and biomarker findings of PBT2 in targeting A? as a modifying therapy for Alzheimer's disease: a phase IIa, double-blind, randomised, placebo-controlled trial. *Lancet Neurol*. 2008;7(9):779–786.
50. Brewer GJ, Kaur S. Zinc deficiency and zinc therapy efficacy with reduction of serum free copper in Alzheimer's disease. *Int J Alzheimers Dis*. 2013;2013:586365.
51. Evans DM, Zhu G, Dy V, et al. Genome-wide association study identifies loci affecting blood copper, selenium and zinc. *Hum Mol Genet*. 2013;22(19):3998–4006.
52. Ng E, Lind PM, Lindgren C, et al. Genome-wide association study of toxic metals and trace elements reveals novel associations. *Hum Mol Genet*. 2015;24(16):4739–4745.
53. Lord J, Lu AJ, Cruchaga C. Identification of rare variants in Alzheimer's disease. *Front Genet*. 2014;5:369.
54. Materia S, Cater MA, Klomp LWJ, Mercer JFB, La Fontaine S. Clusterin and COMMD1 independently regulate degradation of the mammalian copper ATPases ATP7A and ATP7B. *J Biol Chem*. 2012;287(4):2485–2499.
55. Squitti R. Copper dysfunction in Alzheimer's disease: from meta-analysis of biochemical studies to new insight into genetics. *J Trace Elem Med Biol*. 2012;26(2–3):93–96.
56. Squitti R, Polimanti R. Copper hypothesis in the missing hereditability of sporadic alzheimer's disease: ATP7B gene as potential harbor of rare variants. *J Alzheimer's Dis*. 2012;29(3):493–501.
57. Schushan M, Bhattacharjee A, Ben-Tal N, Lutsenko S. A structural model of the copper ATPase ATP7B to facilitate analysis of Wilson disease-causing mutations and studies of the transport mechanism. *Metallomics*. 2012;4(7):669.
58. Gupta A, Maulik M, Nasipuri P, et al. Molecular diagnosis of Wilson disease using prevalent mutations and informative single-nucleotide polymorphism markers. *Clin Chem*. 2007;53(9):1601–1608.
59. Bucossi S, Polimanti R, Ventriglia M, et al. Intronic rs2147363 variant in ATP7B transcription factor-binding site associated with Alzheimer's disease. *J Alzheimer's Dis*. 2013;37(2):453–459.
60. Squitti R, Pasqualetti P, Polimanti R, et al. Metal-score as a potential non-invasive diagnostic test for Alzheimer's disease. *Curr Alzheimer Res*. 2013;10(2):191–198:http://www.ncbi.nlm.nih.gov/pubmed/23036026.
61. Tecchio F, Vecchio F, Ventriglia M, et al. Non-ceruloplasmin copper appears a disctinct subtype of Alzheimer's disease: a study of EEG-derived brain activity. *Curr Alzheimer Res*. June 2016;13(12):1374–1384:http://www.ncbi.nlm.nih.gov/pubmed/27335037.
62. Torres J, Andreozzi E, Dunn J, et al. PET imaging of copper trafficking in a mouse model of Alzheimer disease. *J Nucl Med*. 2016;57:109–114.

CHAPTER

3

The Role of Selenium in Neurodegenerative Diseases

Bárbara R. Cardoso[*,†], Dominic J. Hare[*,**], Ashley I. Bush[*]*

[*]The Florey Institute of Neuroscience and Mental Health, The University of Melbourne, Parkville, VIC, Australia

[**]University of Technology Sydney, Broadway, NSW, Australia

[†]University of São Paulo, São Paulo, Brazil

OUTLINE

INTRODUCTION

Selenium was first identified as an essential element in mammals in 1957,[1] yet the first biological mechanism of selenium in normal physiology was reported in 1973 by Flohé et al.,[2] who identified that this micronutrient was the cofactor of the glutathione peroxidase (GPx) enzyme.

In the years following, studies of selenium biology have identified an elegant mechanism dictating the synthesis of selenoproteins, which incorporates the 21st amino acid selenocysteine (Sec) replacing cysteine (Cys). Sec features a selenol (SeH) moiety, which exhibits electrophilic properties, leading to greater reactivity via a decreased pK_a in comparison with Cys analogs.[3–5]

Selenium levels in the central nervous system are low in comparison with other organs, although they remain essential for brain function, as this organ, along with the reproductive and endocrine systems is atop a selenium hierarchy.[6,7] This priority for selenium retention explains why selenium concentrations in the brain are not significantly influenced by dietary

Biometals in Neurodegenerative Diseases. http://dx.doi.org/10.1016/B978-0-12-804562-6.00003-8

deficiency. For instance, selenium deficient rats presented approximately 29% lower selenium levels in the brain compared to animals with a sufficient supply, while liver and kidneys showed a 99% and 92% reduction in selenium levels, respectively.[8]

Selenium is differentially distributed across brain regions,[9] and in humans the highest concentration is found in gray matter, particularly the parietal inferior lobule, putamen and occipital cortex, while the lowest levels are observed in the cerebellum and medulla.[10] As the brain is the most metabolically active of all organs in the body and thus more vulnerable to oxidative stress as by-products of mitochondrial respiration,[11,12] it is believed that selenoproteins play essential roles in protecting vulnerable neurons from oxidative damage, and that this protective role is disrupted in neurodegenerative diseases.[13]

SELENOPROTEINS AND THE SELENOPROTEOME

Selenoprotein synthesis has a special machinery that codifies 25 different selenoproteins (Table 3.1).[14] As a first step, dietary selenium is converted to selenide (Se^{2-}), which is used to synthesize selenophosphate ($SePO_3^{3-}$) for incorporation into proteins via a unique tRNA pathway; a mechanism unique from typical protein synthesis. Sec is synthetized by a specific tRNA (RNAt[Ser]Sec) that presents a seryl (Ser) residue replaced by Sec and codifies a UGA codon to integrate selenium into the selenoprotein amino acid sequence. The decoding of UGA as Sec instead of a stop codon is possible due to the presence of a Sec insertion sequence

TABLE 3.1 Major Selenoproteins and Their Primary Neurological Functions

Selenoprotein (abbreviation)	Biological role(s)
Selenoprotein P (SelP)	• Se retention in brain. • Antioxidant role.
Glutathione peroxidase family (GPx)	• Protection against oxidative stress. • Modulation of other selenoprotein activities.
Selenoprotein H (SelH)	• Modulation of mitochondrial biogenesis. • Maintenance of genomic stability. • Induction of GSH de novo synthesis.
Selenoprotein M (SelM)	• Modulation of antioxidant activity. • Maintaining redox balance. • Activation of ERK MAPK signaling pathway. • Modulation of microglia activation. • Modulation of other gene expression.
Selenoprotein S (SelS)	• Modulation of astrocyte function.
Selenoprotein W (SelW)	• Antioxidant. • Mediation of synaptic adaptation.
Thioredoxin reductase family (TrxR)	• DNA protection. • Antioxidant. • Antiinflammatory. • Modulation of mitochondrial activity. • Regulation of growth and apoptosis.

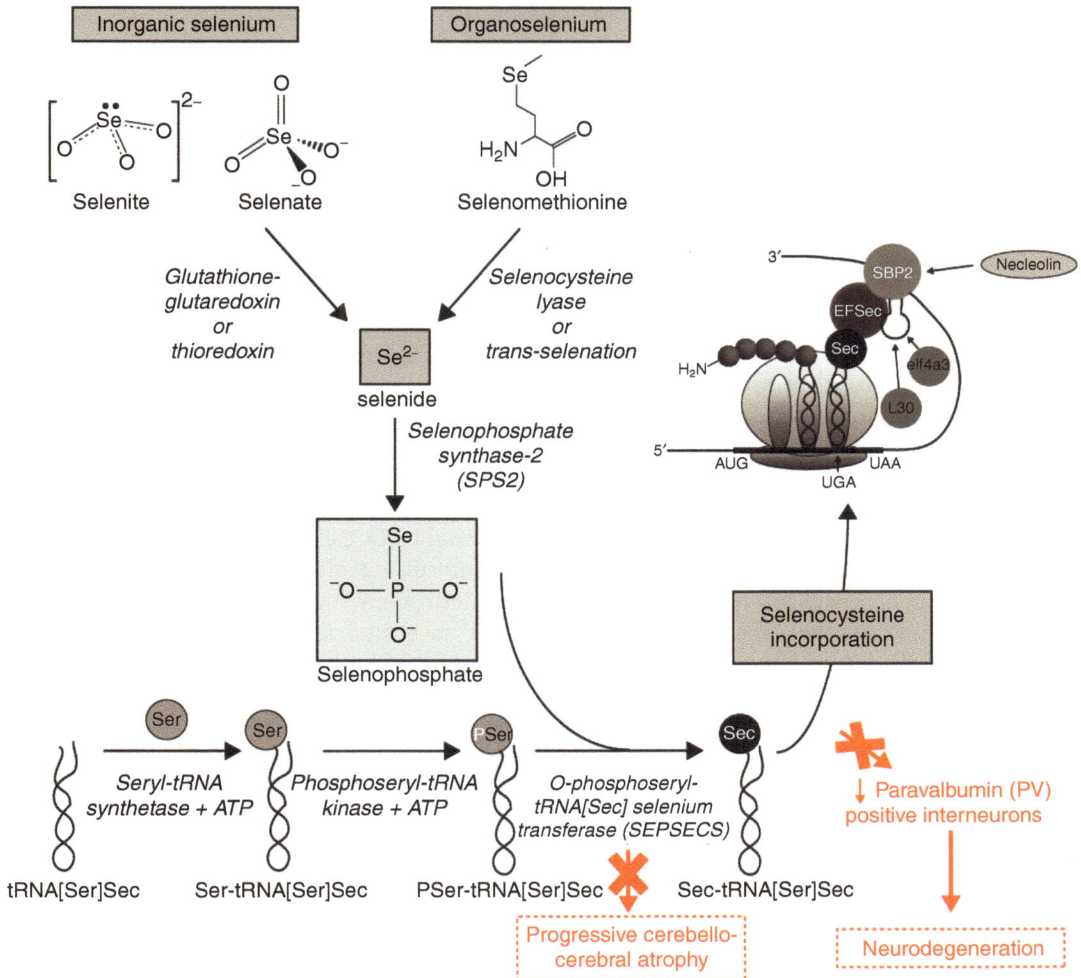

FIGURE 3.1 **Selenoprotein synthesis pathway.** Dietary Se intake, as either inorganic or organic species is metabolized to Se^{2-}, and the $SePO_3^{3-}$, which is incorporated into proteins via a unique tRNA pathway, where a seryl (Ser) residue is replaced with selenocysteine (Sec) prior to integration into mammalian proteins. Deficiencies in key metabolic factors involved in selenoprotein synthesis have been associated with specific neurological disorders, marked here in *red*. Abbreviations: *EFSec*, Sec elongation factor; *eIF4a3*, eukaryotic initiation factor; *L30*, ribosomal protein L30; *SBP2*, Sec insertion sequence (SCIS) binding protein-2. *Source: Reproduced from Cardoso BR, Roberts BR, Bush AI, Hare DJ. Selenium, selenoproteins and neurodegenerative diseases.* Metallomics. *2015;7(8):1213–1228. Published by The Royal Society of Chemistry.*

(SECIS) element in the 3′-untranslated region (UTR) of selenoprotein mRNA that is essential for RNA-binding proteins. To complete the selenoprotein synthesis machinery, the specific elongation factor (EFsec) interacts with SECIS binding protein 2 (SBP2) to employ tRNA[Ser] Sec and mediates insertion of Sec into nascent protein chains in response to the UGA codon (Fig. 3.1).[13,15]

Selenoprotein synthesis is essential for the central nervous system (CNS), as selective tRNA[Ser]Sec knockout in neurons of mice abolishes the developmental appearance of parvalbumin positive (PV) interneuron cells, characterizing progressive neurodegeneration.[16–18] In humans there are two mutations in the *O*-phosphoseryl-tRNA[Sec]:selenocysteinyl-tRNA[Sec] synthase (SepSecS) gene that result in deficient incorporation of selenium into selenoproteins, and development of progressive cerebellocerebral atrophy (PCCA), an autosomal-recessive phenotype of nondysmorphic profound mental retardation, severe spasticity, and microencephaly.[19]

Selenoprotein P (SelP) is the main mammalian selenium transporter. This selenoprotein presents ten SECIS forms, one of which is situated in the larger N-terminal region, which acts as an enzyme; and nine are located in a Sec-rich C-terminal domain, that provides a mechanism for transporting the highly reactive selenium atom.[20] The structure of plasma SelP remains unknown, and there is some dispute regarding how many circulating isoforms of the protein exist. Ballihaut et al.[21] recently reported three isoforms in a human plasma standard reference material, two of which incorporated selenium, and that the third is a truncated variant.

In the brain, selenium is delivered from SelP that is endocytosed following binding to the apolipoprotein E receptor-2 (apoER2) at the blood–brain barrier (BBB) in brain capillary endothelial cells (BCECs) and choroid plexus epithelial cells. Selenium is then taken up by brain cells via SelP synthesized by astrocytes on the abluminal side of BCECs.[22] ApoER2 mediates selenium levels in brain, including uptake by neurons, which has obvious implications for Alzheimer's disease (Fig. 3.2). Selenoprotein P is primarily expressed in astrocytes, although it is also found in neurons[23,24] in all the areas of the brain, mainly in the putamen and substantia nigra.[25] Selenoprotein P deprivation in brain, caused by either severe and chronic dietary selenium deficiency or gene deletion, causes progressive neurodegeneration and severe neurological dysfunction,[26–28] decreased density of PV interneurons in different brain areas, higher oxidative damage, and a behavioral phenotype characterized by impairments in contextual fear extinction, latent inhibition and sensorimotor gating, common of impaired GABAergic function of the inferior colliculus.[29]

The family of glutathione peroxidases (GPx) is comprised of eight sequentially numbered isoenzymes that catalyze the reduction of H_2O_2 of organic hydroperoxides by glutathione (GSH) or other biological reductants.[30] In the brain, GPx enzymes are expressed in neurons and glial cells,[31,32] and GPx4 is the most abundant; found in neurons of cerebellum, hippocampus and hypothalamus.[33] GPx4 is identified in reactive astrocytes after brain injury, which enhances its protective role against stress-induced oxidative damage and apoptosis.[34] This selenoenzyme seems to be a key regulator of other selenoproteins, as Wirth et al.[16] suggested that depletion of GPx4 may result in dysfunction in thioredoxin reductase (TrxR), selenoprotein M (SelM), and selenoprotein W (SelW) expression. Recently, GPx4 was recognized as a protective factor against ferroptosis, a newly discovered nonapoptotic programmed cell death pathway characterized by iron-dependent metabolic dysfunction that causes a rapid elevation in the levels of reactive oxygen species.[35] Ferroptosis has been described in cancerous,[35,36] hippocampal,[35] and renal cells.[37] This recently identified mechanism might also be involved in neurodegeneration, as it is believed that selenium supply to brain can minimize iron-mediated damage via increased GPx4 activity.[37a]

The TrxR family encompasses three different isoforms expressed in the cytosol or nucleus (TrxR1), mitochondria (TrxR2), and testes (TrxR3). These selenoenzymes maintain cells' redox

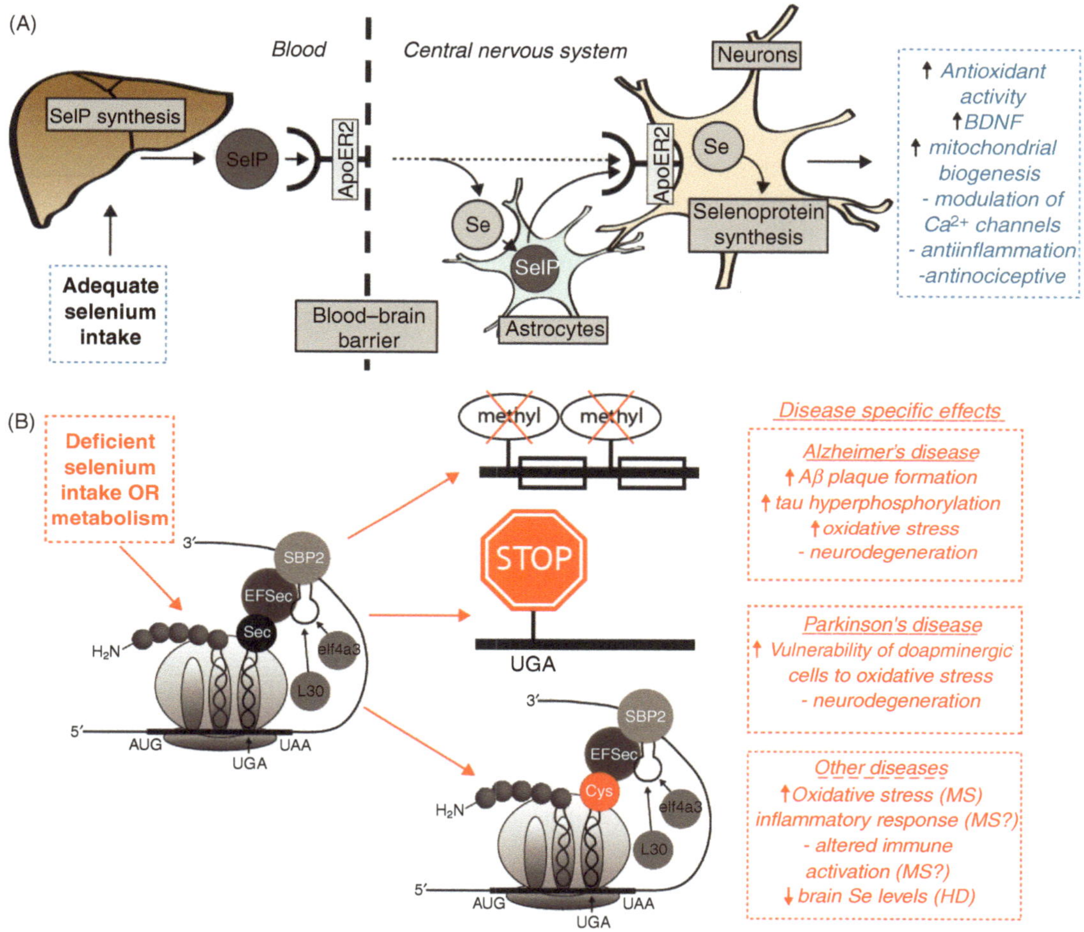

FIGURE 3.2 **Normal Se bioactivity and possible neurodegenerative effects of altered Se metabolism.** (A) Selenoprotein P (SelP), the master protein driving Se bioavailability is synthesized in the liver from both inorganic and organoselenium compounds accessible through dietary sources. At the blood–brain barrier, SelP releases Se into the CNS via the ApoER2 receptor, which is in turn incorporated into newly—formed SelP in astrocytes, or is transported directly to neurons *(dashed arrow)*. SelP is made available to neurons via the same membrane-bound ApoER2, where additional selenoproteins essential to neurological function *(blue box)* are biosynthesisised. (B) In cases of deficient Se intake Um34 methylation is downregulated, causing premature termination of protein synthesis via failure of tRNA[Ser]Sec to decode the UGA codon as Sec instead of a stop codon, and misincorpoartion of selenocysteine (Sec) as cysteine *(Cys; in red)*. These three pathological features may have downstream effects on a range of neurological disorders *(red boxes)*. *Source: Part A: Figure adapted from Burk RF, Hill KE, Motley AK, et al. Selenoprotein P and apolipoprotein E receptor-2 interact at the blood–brain barrier and also within the brain to maintain an essential selenium pool that protects against neurodegeneration.* FASEB Journal. *2014;28(8):3579–3588. Part B: Reproduced from Cardoso BR, Roberts BR, Bush AI, Hare DJ. Selenium, selenoproteins and neurodegenerative diseases.* Metallomics. *2015;7(8):1213–1228. Published by The Royal Society of Chemistry.*

balance, especially during ageing,[38] as they catalyze the reduction of thioredoxin or other proteins by NADPH.[39] Furthermore, TrxR enzymes regulate growth, apoptosis, and general cellular defense mechanisms, and the overexpression of this family may negatively contribute to astrocytomas and to resistance to therapy.[40] In the CNS, TrxR selenoenzymes are abundantly expressed. Animal models have shown that TrxR1 is mainly expressed in glial cells of the cerebellar white matter and the second isoform is primarily located in the cell bodies of neurons localized in the Purkinje and molecular cell layers in the cerebellum.[41] These enzymes were associated with protection of neuronal C6 cells against DNA damage under H_2O_2 challenge,[42] and demonstrated an anti-inflammatory and antiapoptotic role,[43] corroborating another study reporting that Trx2 is responsible for over 60% of the intramitochondrial H_2O_2 turnover, whereas the glutathione system contributes only about 20% to H_2O_2 detoxification reactions in the rat hippocampus.[44]

The iodothyronine deiodinase (DIO) family has three isoforms: isoforms I and II activate the prohormone 3,5,3′,5′-tetraiodo-L-thyronine (T_4) to 3,5,3′-triiodo-L-thyronine (T_3) by removing the 5′-iodine atom, whereas DIOs I and III inactivate T_3 hormone by deiodination on position 5. Deiodinase I is mainly found in the liver, kidneys and thyroid, and DIO II and DIO III are highly expressed in the CNS. It is believed that astrocytes generate active T_3, as they primarily express DIO II, whereas neurons degrade both T_4 and T_3 to inactive forms, as these cells express DIO III.[45] However, scant evidence suggested that deiodinase II has a role in developing brain, as deiodinase II-deficient and a deiodinase II/deiodinase I dual-knockout mice do not present evident defects in brain development or function,[46,47] suggesting that in absence of available T_3, T_4 can act as an active hormone in the brain by recruiting coactivators of TRα1.[48] Importantly, such DIO enzymes act in balance to protect the brain from damage caused either by hyper- or hypothyroidism.[49,50]

Selenoproteins typically have the conserved Cys-X-X-Sec redox motif, including selenoproteins H, W, T, O, and M. It is believed that these selenoproteins act as thiol-disulfide oxidoreductases that participate in the formation of disulfide bonds. Among them, SelM, an endoplasmic reticulum (ER)/Golgi-directing signaling peptide,[51] has been the most studied in brain. Although its precise mechanisms of action is not well understood, it has been associated with an antioxidant role by increasing the activity of other enzymes as superoxide dismutase-1 and GPx,[52–55] and in Ca^{2+} homeostasis in cortical neurons.[52] Neuroprotective roles for SelM seems also to be associated with interaction with galectin-1,[56] a β-galactoside-binding lectin associated with modulation of microglia activation in neuroinflammation, neuronal myelination and neuronal stem cell proliferation.[57,58] It has been hypothesized that SelM can modulate expression of other proteins, influencing cell viability indirectly.[55] Deletion of SelM does not cause morphological nor motor or cognitive deficits,[59] however it adversely affects hypothalamic thyrodoxin balance and causes metabolic dysfunction that leads to obesity, suggesting the participation of this selenoprotein in redox balance maintenance in brain areas associated with high metabolic output.[59]

As mentioned earlier, selenoproteins are at relatively low levels in brain cells, but are also of great interest for neuronal protection and normal brain function. For example, SelW is found in low levels in CNS, mainly in synapses, and in murine brain tissue is found in axons and dendrites of neurons from cortex, hippocampus, and cerebellum.[26,60,61] Deletion of SelP resulted in decreased expression of SelW, indicating that as the main Se transporter, SelP regulates the expression of SelW, just as other selenoproteins.[61] Although the role of SelW in the brain remains unclear, it is believed that it plays an essential mechanistic role in redox homeostasis, mediates synaptic plasticity[61] and protect neurons against oxidative stress.[62] Selenoprotein S is expressed mainly in neurons of hippocampus and cortex,[63–65] and it is also found in reactive astrocytes, where increased expression results in reduction of ER-stress and IL-6 release,[64,65] and thus mitigates inflammation.[66,67] Selenoprotein H has been associated with regulation of mitochondrial function, as studies showed that overexpression of this selenoprotein in HT-22 neurons increased the respiratory function of mitochondria, preserved UVB stress-induced mitochondrial membrane potential depolarization, improved mitochondrial biogenesis signaling via PGC-1α, NRF1 and mitochondrial transcription factor A (Tfam), probably mediated by modulation of CREB dependent PGC-1α activation.[68,69] In other cells, SelH has been associated with genomic stability under chronic oxidative stress either by a direct antioxidant role and for inducing de novo synthesis of GSH and phase II detoxification enzymes.[70]

Selenoprotein expression is modulated by selenium availability according to a hierarchical system, suggesting that they are classified according to their importance to the body. Selenium deficiency results in competition between transcripts of different selenoproteins,[71] and thus some proteins are maintained at a higher level than that of others. Iodothyronine deiodinase 1 is atop this hierarchy; glutathione peroxidases GPx2 and GPx4 are less vulnerable to selenium deficiency than GPx1 and GPx3; and SelP is in an intermediary position on this selenoprotein transcription ladder.[72] Selenoprotein hierarchy works through different mechanisms: (1) selenium deficiency causes downregulation of nonessential selenoproteins via nonsense-mediated mRNA decay, which decodes the UGA-Sec codon prematurely as a termination codon causing RNA degradation,[73,74] (2) selenium levels directly correlate with the degree of Um34 methylation, one step of maturation of tRNA[Ser]Sec which can be altered as a result of some mutations,[73] (3) selenium deficiency may result in replacement of Sec by Cys in the Sec biosynthetic organization, generating Cys-tRNA[Ser]Sec and the subsequent insertion of Cys in some selenoproteins.[75] This alteration may reduce the activity of different selenoproteins, although the impact seems specific and remains unclear.

Studies have pointed out diverse positive effects of selenium treatment on normal brain function through modulation of selenoprotein synthesis. Selenium treatment as organic selenomethionine and inorganic SeO_3^{2-} resulted in increased activity of antioxidant enzymes, scavenging of reactive oxygen species (ROS), and reduced protein carbonyl content of patulin-induced brain damaged rats,[76] and reduced the prooxidant effects of glyceryl trinitrate in a rat model of migraine headaches.[77] Other studies in animal models also demonstrated the antioxidant capacity of SeO_3^{2-} treatment that resulted in reduced degenerative changes in the granular cell layer of the dental gyrus,[78] increased levels of brain-derived neurothophic factor (BDNF) in the hippocampus and cerebellum[79] and corrected the neurobehavioral deficits caused by a protein-deficient diet.[80] Besides an antioxidant role, selenium treatment also seems to modulate different apoptotic pathways and mitochondrial biogenesis through regulation of Ca^{2+} channels,[81] reduction of caspases 3 and 9 activity,[82] activation of complexes I, II + III and IV, and positive regulation of peroxisome proliferator-activated receptor γ-coactivator-1α (PGC-1α) and nuclear respiratory factor 1 (NRF1), two important nuclear transcriptional factors associated with mitochondrial biogenesis.[68,69,83]

Synthetic organoselenium compounds have also been studied as potential antioxidant therapies due to their lower toxicity compared to inorganic forms of selenium. Diphenyl diselenide [$(PhSe)_2$] mimics GPx activity,[84] modified proteins involved in glutamate signaling damage to astrocytes,[85] and protected neurons in autoimmune encephalomyelitis and hypothyroidism animal models.[86,87] Other components, as m-trifluoromethyl (m-CF_3-PhSe)$_2$ and the selenium-containing salicylic acid derivative 5-5′-diselanediylbis-(2-hydroxybenzoic acid) demonstrated antinociceptive action by interaction with serotoninergic system, as well as an antiinflammatory role in mice[88,89]; and 3-methyl-1-pheny-2-(phenylseleno)oct-2-en-1-one appears to have immunomodulatory properties.[76]

SELENIUM AND ALZHEIMER'S DISEASE

Selenoprotein P seems to have direct relation with pathogenesis of Alzheimer's disease, as it was found to colocalize with senile plaques and neurofibrillary tangles,[90] and is elevated in the choroid plexus and cerebrospinal fluid of AD patients.[91] Selenoprotein P encodes two His-rich regions that act as high-affinity binding sites for transition metals, restricting metal-mediated $A\beta_{1-42}$ aggregation and subsequent ROS generation[92,93] and inhibiting aggregation of tau protein induced by Cu^+/Cu^{2+}.[94] These observations suggest that SelP might protect neurons against the classic pathogenic lesions either by its antioxidant role or transporting selenium to the synthesis of other selenoproteins. Selenoprotein M seems to also mitigate Alzheimer's disease, as when overexpressed it contributed to activation of ERK signaling, which induces a decrease in tau phosphorylation, α-secretase and γ-secretase activity and an increase in β-secretase.[53] Additionally, the overexpression of SelM reduced oxidative stress, mitochondrial damage, and Aβ aggregation,[54] besides increased γ-secretase activity.[55]

Different animal models and in vitro studies have shown different mechanisms through which selenium mitigates Alzheimer's disease. A selenium deficient diet was associated with increased Aβ plaque formation in the brains of *Tg2576* transgenic mice.[95] On the other side, treatment with sodium selenite resulted in antagonist effects on the protein phosphatase 2A inhibitor OA,[96] activated the protein phosphatase 2A and dephosphorylated tau in cells.[97] Sodium selenite improved tolerance to oxidative stress and prevented cognitive decline in a streptozotocin toxin model of mental impairment,[98] and decreased activity of α- and β-secretases and correspondingly reduced production of $A\beta_{1-40}$ and $A\beta_{1-42}$ in hippocampal cells.[99] Selenomethionine treatment of triple-transgenic AD mice expressing mutant forms of human APP_{swe}, $PS1_{M146V}$, and tau_{P301L} reduced total and phosphorylated tau, lowered inflammatory biomarkers, and improved cognition.[100] Organoselenium compounds also display interesting effects in improving AD pathology in murine models: *p,p′*-methoxyl-diphenyl diselenide treatment to streptozotocin-exposed mice slowed memory decline, reduced oxidative stress, and normalized acetyl-cholinesterase activity.[101] Selenium-containing 8-hydroxyquinoline derivatives bound to Cu^{2+}, Fe^{2+}, and Zn^{2+} inhibited aggregation and disassembled Cu^{2+}-induced aggregates of Aβ.[102]

In humans, selenium nutritional status has been positively associated with cognitive performance in older adults.[103,104] However, such correlation is observed more clearly in erythrocytes than in plasma,[105,106] suggesting that chronic deficiency correlates with cognition decline, as plasma is considered a biomarker of short exposure. These data are in agreement with previous studies that suggest that a lack of Se might increase the risk of dementia.[105,107] Corroborating the importance of selenium on cognitive performance, supplementation with selenium compounds has been associated with cognitive improvement, although this effect cannot be directly attributed to selenium alone.[108,109] Recently, mildly cognitively declined patients who were selenium deficient presented improved cognitive performance on two different tests (constructional praxis and animal naming) after consuming one Brazil nut, the most concentrated selenium food source which provided about 288 μg of this micronutrient daily over 6 months.[110] This study shows the importance of recovering nutritional status of selenium for cognition performance maintenance, which can be used as a strategy for prevention of Alzheimer's disease.

PARKINSON'S DISEASE

The use of selenium in the treatment of early Parkinson's disease was first reported in the 1980s,[111] however its mechanisms of action are not clear, and thus its utilization as a therapy has been poorly explored. Selenium treatment mitigated 1-methyl-4-phenyl-1,2,3,6-tetrahydropyridine (MPTP)-induced depletion of striatal dopamine in a dose dependent manner, though only a high dose of 3 mg/kg of selenium (as SeO_3^{2-}) produced a statistically significant effect.[112] Positive effects were also observed in a paraquat animal model of Parkinsonism treated with sodium selenite, as the animals presented normalization of motor activity when coadministered with the toxin.[113] It should be noted, however, that this effect may simply be due to mitigation of paraquat toxicity by sodium selenite, as opposed to a specific neuroprotective mechanism. The deficiency of selenium, on the other hand, seems to contribute to dopaminergic cell vulnerability,[114,115] particularly prior to exposure to Parkinsonian neurotoxins.[116]

Selenoprotein P and GPx4 are less expressed in Parkinson's disease patients compared with controls, although increased relative to cell density in surviving neurons.[25,117] It is believed that GPx4 metabolism is disrupted as part of the disease's pathogenesis, as this selenoenzyme is covalently modified by dopamine quinone, an oxidized and reactive metabolite of dopamine, and this deleterious product of neurotransmitter breakdown may result in degradation and reduced activity of this antioxidant selenoprotein.[118]

Observations in humans are not clear to associate selenium nutritional status with Parkinson's disease. Although one large study has reported an association between selenium levels and performance-based assessments of coordination,[119] another study from China showed that selenium levels were significantly increased in patients with idiopathic Parkinson's disease.[120]

OTHER NEURODEGENERATIVE DISEASES

As one third of selenoproteins have antioxidant roles, selenoproteins may participate in other neuroprotective mechanisms, and several neurodegenerative disorders have been studied with regard to a possible association with selenium metabolism. Studies have shown the patients with multiple sclerosis, the aetiology of which remains elusive, present lower levels of circulating selenium[121,122] and GPx activity.[123,124]

Amyotrophic lateral sclerosis has also been associated with selenium, however in this situation the excess exposure to inorganic selenium may interact with genetic susceptibility for the disease.[125] In a northern Italian village, where some inhabitants consumed drinking water with unusually high inorganic selenium content, a higher risk of amyotrophic lateral sclerosis was observed, with dose-response relationship.[126,127] In vitro studies confirm the negative effects of selenium toxicity to motor neuronal cells,[128] and to cholinergic and GABAergic neurons.[129–131]

There are only a few studies investigating selenium in Huntington's disease, however they suggest a potential protective role of this micronutrient against the pathogenesis. Total selenium levels in plasma was not different in Huntington's disease patients when compared with healthy individuals, but the distribution in different brain areas was not the same, as patients presented lower levels in the putamen, dorso-lateral prefrontal cortex, primary visual cortex, cingulate gyrus, and cerebellum.[132] Treatment with selenite of an animal model resulted in decreased brain weight and reduced Huntington protein aggregation and oxidized glutathione,[132] and treatment with *bis*-selenide improved locomotor activity and motor coordination, restored succinate dehydrogenase enzyme activity, and showed protection against oxidative stress.[133]

CONCLUSIONS

Selenium has an essential role in the brain; not only due to its direct antioxidant role, but also via its participation in maintaining redox balance, mitochondrial dynamics, regulation of Ca^{2+} channels, and modulation of neurogenesis. The relevance of selenium in the pathogenesis of different neurodegenerative disorders has been shown by several studies. However, future research is required to elucidate the role of different selenoproteins in brain, and the potential role of selenium on strategies for either prevention and treatment of these diseases.

References

1. Schwarz K, Foltz CM. Selenium as an integral part of factor 3 against dietary necrotic liver degeneration. *J Am Chem Soc*. 1957;79(12):3292–13292.
2. Flohe L, Günzler W, Schock H. Glutathione peroxidase: a selenoenzyme. *FEBS Lett*. 1973;32(1):132–134.
3. Huber RE, Criddle RS. Comparison of the chemical properties of selenocysteine and selenocystine with their sulfur analogs. *Arch Biochem Biophys*. 1967;122(1):164–173.
4. Nygard B. *Polarographic Investigations of Organic Selenium Compounds. Polarography of Selenocysteine-Selenocysteine. Polarographic Investigations of Organic Selenium Compounds. Polarography of Selenocysteine-Selenocysteine*. Stockholm: Almqvist and Wiksell; 1967.
5. Tan K-S, Arnold AP, Rabenstein DL. Selenium-77 nuclear magnetic resonance studies of selenols, diselenides, and selenenyl sulfides. *Can J Chem*. 1988;66(1):54–60.
6. Kühbacher M, Bartel J, Hoppe B, et al. The brain selenoproteome: priorities in the hierarchy and different levels of selenium homeostasis in the brain of selenium-deficient rats. *J Neurochem*. 2009;110(1):133–142.
7. Pitts MW, Kremer PM, Hashimoto AC, et al. Competition between the brain and testes under selenium-compromised conditions: insight into sex differences in selenium metabolism and risk of neurodevelopmental disease. *J Neurosci*. 2015;35(46):15326–15338.
8. Haratake M, Koga K, Inoue M, Fuchigami T, Nakayama M. Absorption and retention characteristics of selenium in dorsal root ganglion neurons. *Metallomics*. 2011;3(10):1019–1026.
9. Bishop DP, Clases D, Fryer F, et al. Elemental bio-imaging using laser ablation-triple quadrupole-ICP-MS. *J Anal At Spectrom*. 2016;31(1):197–202.
10. Ramos P, Santos A, Pinto NR, Mendes R, Magalhães T, Almeida A. Anatomical regional differences in selenium levels in the human brain. *Biol Trace Elem Res*. 2014;163(1–2):89–96.

11. Wang X, Michaelis EK. Selective neuronal vulnerability to oxidative stress in the brain. *Front Aging Neurosci.* 2010;2:12.
12. Bélanger M, Allaman I, Magistretti PJ. Brain energy metabolism: focus on astrocyte-neuron metabolic cooperation. *Cell Metab.* 2011;14(6):724–738.
13. Cardoso BR, Roberts BR, Bush AI, Hare DJ. Selenium, selenoproteins and neurodegenerative diseases. *Metallomics.* 2015;7(8):1213–1228.
14. Kryukov GV, Castellano S, Novoselov SV, et al. Characterization of mammalian selenoproteomes. *Science.* 2003;300(5624):1439–1443.
15. Gonzalez-Flores JN, Gupta N, DeMong LW, Copeland PR. The selenocysteine-specific elongation factor contains a novel and multi-functional domain. *J Biol Chem.* 2012;287(46):38936–38945.
16. Wirth EK, Conrad M, Winterer J, et al. Neuronal selenoprotein expression is required for interneuron development and prevents seizures and neurodegeneration. *FASEB J.* 2010;24(3):844–852.
17. Wirth EK, Bharathi BS, Hatfield D, Conrad M, Brielmeier M, Schweizer U. Cerebellar hypoplasia in mice lacking selenoprotein biosynthesis in neurons. *Biol Trace Elem Res.* 2014;158(2):203–210.
18. Seeher S, Carlson BA, Miniard AC, et al. Impaired selenoprotein expression in brain triggers striatal neuronal loss leading to co-ordination defects in mice. *Biochem J.* 2014;462(1):67–75.
19. Agamy O, Ben Zeev B, Lev D, et al. Mutations disrupting selenocysteine formation cause progressive cerebello-cerebral atrophy. *Am J Hum Genet.* 2010;87(4):538–544.
20. Ferguson LR, Karunasinghe N, Zhu S, Wang AH. Selenium and it's role in the maintenance of genomic stability. *Mutat Res.* 2012;733(1–2):100–110.
21. Ballihaut G, Kilpatrick LE, Kilpatrick EL, Davis WC. Multiple forms of selenoprotein P in a candidate human plasma standard reference material. *Metallomics.* 2012;4(6):533–538.
22. Burk RF, Hill KE, Motley AK, et al. Selenoprotein P and apolipoprotein E receptor-2 interact at the blood-brain barrier and also within the brain to maintain an essential selenium pool that protects against neurodegeneration. *FASEB J.*. 2014;28(8):3579–3588.
23. Steinbrenner H, Alili L, Bilgic E, Sies H, Brenneisen P. Involvement of selenoprotein P in protection of human astrocytes from oxidative damage. *Free Radic Biol Med.* 2006;40(9):1513–1523.
24. Scharpf M, Schweizer U, Arzberger T, Roggendorf W, Schomburg L, Köhrle J. Neuronal and ependymal expression of selenoprotein P in the human brain. *J Neural Trans.* 2007;114(7):877–884.
25. Bellinger FP, Raman AV, Rueli RH, et al. Changes in selenoprotein P in substantia nigra and putamen in Parkinson's disease. *J Parkinson's Dis.* 2012;2(2):115–126.
26. Raman AV, Pitts MW, Seyedali A, et al. Absence of selenoprotein P but not selenocysteine lyase results in severe neurological dysfunction. *Genes Brain Behav.* 2012;11(5):601–613.
27. Burk RF, Olson GE, Hill KE, Winfrey VP, Motley AK, Kurokawa S. Maternal-fetal transfer of selenium in the mouse. *FASEB J.* 2013;27(8):3249–3256.
28. Caito SW, Milatovic D, Hill KE, Aschner M, Burk RF, Valentine WM. Progression of neurodegeneration and morphologic changes in the brains of juvenile mice with selenoprotein P deleted. *Brain Res.* 2011;1398:1–12.
29. Pitts MW, Raman AV, Hashimoto AC, Todorovic C, Nichols RA, Berry MJ. Deletion of selenoprotein P results in impaired function of parvalbumin interneurons and alterations in fear learning and sensorimotor gating. *Neuroscience.* 2012;208:58–68.
30. Brigelius-Flohe R, Maiorino M. Glutathione peroxidases. *Biochimica et biophysica acta.* 2013;1830(5):3289–3303.
31. Garcia T, Esparza JL, Nogués MR, Romeu M, Domingo JL, Gómez M. Oxidative stress status and RNA expression in hippocampus of an animal model of Alzheimer's disease after chronic exposure to aluminum. *Hippocampus.* 2010;20(1):218–225.
32. Zhang S, Rocourt C, Cheng W-H. Selenoproteins and the aging brain. *Mech Ageing Dev.* 2010;131(4):253–260.
33. Pitts MW, Byrns CN, Ogawa-Wong AN, Kremer P, Berry MJ. Selenoproteins in nervous system development and function. *Biol Trace Elem Res.* 2014;161(3):231–245.
34. Savaskan NE, Borchert A, Bräuer AU, Kuhn H. Role for glutathione peroxidase-4 in brain development and neuronal apoptosis: Specific induction of enzyme expression in reactive astrocytes following brain injury. *Free Radic Biol Med.* 2007;43(2):191–201.
35. Dixon SJ, Lemberg KM, Lamprecht MR, et al. Ferroptosis: an iron-dependent form of nonapoptotic cell death. *Cell.* 2012;149(5):1060–1072.
36. Yang WS, SriRamaratnam R, Welsch ME, et al. Regulation of ferroptotic cancer cell death by GPX4. *Cell.* 2014;156(1–2):317–331.

37. Friedmann Angeli JP, Schneider M, Proneth B, et al. Inactivation of the ferroptosis regulator Gpx4 triggers acute renal failure in mice. *Nature Cell Biol*. 2014;16(12):1180–1191.
37a. Cardoso BR, Hare DJ, Bush AI, Roberts BR. Glutathione peroxidase 4: a new player in neurodegeneration?. *Mol Psychiatry*. 2016;:doi: 10.1038/mp.2016.196. [Epub ahead of print].
38. Ahn JH, Choi JH, Song JM, et al. Increase in Trx2/Prx3 redox system immunoreactivity in the spinal cord and hippocampus of aged dogs. *Exp Gerontol*. 2011;46(11):946–952.
39. Silva-Adaya D, Gonsebatt Mx, E a, Guevara J. Thioredoxin system regulation in the central nervous system: experimental models and clinical evidence. *Oxid Med Cell Longevity*. 2014;2014(1):1–13.
40. Esen H, Erdi F, Kaya B, Feyzioglu B, Keskin F, Demir LS. Tissue thioredoxin reductase-1 expression in astrocytomas of different grades. *J Neurooncol*. 2014;121(3):451–458.
41. Godoy JR, Funke M, Ackermann W, et al. Redox atlas of the mouse. Immunohistochemical detection of glutaredoxin-, peroxiredoxin-, and thioredoxin-family proteins in various tissues of the laboratory mouse. *Biochimica et biophysica acta.*. 2011;1810(1):2–92.
42. Mitozo PA, de Souza LF, Loch-Neckel G, et al. A study of the relative importance of the peroxiredoxin-, catalase-, and glutathione-dependent systems in neural peroxide metabolism. *Free Radic Biol Med*. 2011;51(1):69–77.
43. Cohen-Kutner M, Khomsky L, Trus M, et al. Thioredoxin-mimetic peptide CB3 lowers MAPKinase activity in the Zucker rat brain. *Redox Biol*. 2014;2:447–456.
44. Kudin AP, Augustynek B, Lehmann AK, Kovács R, Kunz WS. The contribution of thioredoxin-2 reductase and glutathione peroxidase to H2O2 detoxification of rat brain mitochondria. *Biochimica et Biophysica Acta (BBA)—Bioenergetics*. 2012;1817(10):1901–1906.
45. Tu HM, Kim SW, Salvatore D, et al. Regional distribution of type 2 thyroxine deiodinase messenger ribonucleic acid in rat hypothalamus and pituitary and its regulation by thyroid hormone. *Endocrinology*. 1997;138(8):3359–3368.
46. Galton VA, Schneider MJ, Clark AS, St Germain DL. Life without thyroxine to 3,5,3′-triiodothyronine conversion: studies in mice devoid of the 5′-deiodinases. *Endocrinology*. 2009;150(6):2957–2963.
47. Schneider MJ, Fiering SN, Pallud SE, Parlow AF, St Germain DL, Galton VA. Targeted disruption of the type 2 selenodeiodinase gene (DIO2) results in a phenotype of pituitary resistance to T4. *Mol Endocrinol*. 2001;15(12):2137–2148.
48. Schroeder AC, Privalsky ML. Thyroid Hormones, T3 and T4, in the Brain. *Front Endocrinol*. 2014;5:40.
49. Guadano-Ferraz A, Escamez MJ, Rausell E, Bernal J. Expression of type 2 iodothyronine deiodinase in hypothyroid rat brain indicates an important role of thyroid hormone in the development of specific primary sensory systems. *J Neurosci*. 1999;19(9):3430–3439.
50. Heuer H. The importance of thyroid hormone transporters for brain development and function. *Best Pract Res*. 2007;21(2):265–276.
51. Guariniello S, Colonna G, Raucci R, et al. Structure–function relationship and evolutionary history of the human selenoprotein M (SelM) found over-expressed in hepatocellular carcinoma. *Biochimica et Biophysica Acta (BBA)—Proteins and Proteomics*. 2014;1844(2):447–456.
52. Reeves MA, Bellinger FP, Berry MJ. The neuroprotective functions of selenoprotein m and its role in cytosolic calcium regulation. *Antioxid Redox Signal*. 2010;12(7):809–818.
53. Yim SY, Chae KR, Shim SB, et al. ERK activation induced by selenium treatment significantly downregulates β/γ-secretase activity and Tau phosphorylation in the transgenic rat overexpressing human selenoprotein M. *Int J Mol Med*. 2009;24(1):91–96.
54. Chen P, Wang R-R, Ma X-J, Liu Q, Ni J-Z. Different forms of selenoprotein M differentially affect Aβ aggregation and ROS generation. *Int J Mol Sci*. 2013;14(3):4385–4399.
55. Kim Y, Goo JS, Kim IY, et al. Identification of the responsible proteins for increased selenium bioavailability in the brain of transgenic rats overexpressing selenoprotein M. *Int J Mol Med*. 2014;34(6):1688–1698.
56. Qiao X, Tian J, Chen P, Wang C, Ni J, Liu Q. Galectin-1 is an interactive protein of selenoprotein M in the brain. *Int J Mol Sci*. 2013;14(11):22233–22245.
57. Starossom SC, Mascanfroni ID, Imitola J, et al. Galectin-1 deactivates classically activated microglia and protects from inflammation-induced neurodegeneration. *Immunity*. 2012;37(2):249–263.
58. Kajitani K, Kobayakawa Y, Nomaru H, Kadoya T, Horie H, Nakabeppu Y. Characterization of galectin-1-positive cells in the mouse hippocampus. *Neuro Rep*. 2014;25(3):171–176.
59. Pitts MW, Reeves MA, Hashimoto AC, et al. Deletion of selenoprotein M leads to obesity without cognitive deficits. *J Biol Chem*. 2013;288(36):26121–26134.
60. Cajigas IJ, Tushev G, Will TJ, Dieck St, Fuerst N, Schuman EM. The local transcriptome in the synaptic neuropil revealed by deep sequencing and high-resolution imaging. *Neuron*. 2012;74(3):453–466.

61. Raman AV, Pitts MW, Seyedali A, Hashimoto AC, Bellinger FP, Berry MJ. Selenoprotein W expression and regulation in mouse brain and neurons. *Brain Behav*. 2013;3(5):562–574.
62. Xiao-Long W, Chuan-Ping Y, Kai X, Ou-Jv Q. Selenoprotein W depletion in vitro might indicate that its main function is not as an antioxidative enzyme. *Biochemistry (Moscow)*. 2010;75(2):201–207.
63. Zhang Y, Zhou Y, Schweizer U, et al. Comparative analysis of selenocysteine machinery and selenoproteome gene expression in mouse brain identifies neurons as key functional sites of selenium in mammals. *J Biol Chem*. 2008;283(4):2427–2438.
64. Fradejas N, Serrano Perez MDel C, Tranque P, Calvo S. Selenoprotein S expression in reactive astrocytes following brain injury. *Glia*. 2011;59(6):959–972.
65. Liu LX, Zhou XY, Li CS, Liu LQ, Huang SY, Zhou SN. Selenoprotein S expression in the rat brain following focal cerebral ischemia. *Neurol Sci*. 2013;34(9):1671–1678.
66. Turanov AA, Shchedrina VA, Everley RA, et al. Selenoprotein S is involved in maintenance and transport of multiprotein complexes. *Biochem J*. 2014;462(3):555–565.
67. Du XA, Wang HM, Dai XX, et al. Role of selenoprotein S (SEPS1) -105G>A polymorphisms and PI3K/Akt signaling pathway in Kashin-Beck disease. *Osteoarthr Cartil*. 2015;23(2):210–216.
68. Mendelev N, Mehta SL, Witherspoon S, He Q, Sexton JZ, Li PA. Upregulation of human selenoprotein H in murine hippocampal neuronal cells promotes mitochondrial biogenesis and functional performance. *Mitochondrion*. 2011;11(1):76–82.
69. Mehta SL, Mendelev N, Kumari S, Andy Li P. Overexpression of human selenoprotein H in neuronal cells enhances mitochondrial biogenesis and function through activation of protein kinase A, protein kinase B, and cyclic adenosine monophosphate response element-binding protein pathway. *Int J Biochem Cell Biol*. 2013;45(3):604–611.
70. Wu RTY, Cao L, Chen BPC, Cheng W-H. Selenoprotein H suppresses cellular senescence through genome maintenance and redox regulation. *J Biol Chem*. 2014;289(49):34378–34388.
71. Schomburg L, Schweizer U. Hierarchical regulation of selenoprotein expression and sex-specific effects of selenium. *Biochimica et Biophysica Acta (BBA)—General Subjects*. 2009;1790(11):1453–1462.
72. Sunde R. Selenoproteins: hierarchy, requirements, and biomarkers. In: Hatfield DL, Berry M, Gladyshev VN, eds. *Selenium—Its Molecular Biology and Role in Human Health*. Springer; 2012:137–152.
73. Howard MT, Carlson BA, Anderson CB, Hatfield DL. Translational redefinition of UGA codons is regulated by selenium availability. *J Biol Chem*. 2013;288(27):19401–19413.
74. Seyedali A, Berry MJ. Nonsense-mediated decay factors are involved in the regulation of selenoprotein mRNA levels during selenium deficiency. *RNA*. 2014;20(8):1248–1256.
75. Xu X-M, Turanov AA, Carlson BA, et al. Targeted insertion of cysteine by decoding UGA codons with mammalian selenocysteine machinery. *Proc Natl Acad Sci USA*. 2010;107(50):21430–21434.
76. Bitencourt P, Belle L, Bonfanti G, et al. Differential effects of organic and inorganic selenium compounds on adenosine deaminase activity and scavenger capacity in cerebral cortex slices of young rats. *Hum Exp Toxicol*. 2013;32(9):942–949.
77. Nazıroğlu M, Çelik Ö, Uğuz AC, Bütün A. Protective effects of riboflavin and selenium on brain microsomal Ca^{2+}-ATPase and oxidative damage caused by glyceryl trinitrate in a rat headache model. *Biol Trace Elem Res*. 2015;164(1):72–79.
78. Ben Amara I, Fetoui H, Guermazi F, Zeghal N. Dietary selenium addition improves cerebrum and cerebellum impairments induced by methimazole in suckling rats. *Int J Dev Neurosci*. 2009;27(7):719–726.
79. Abedelhaffez AS, Hassan A. Brain derived neurotrophic factor and oxidative stress index in pups with developmental hypothyroidism: neuroprotective effects of selenium. *Acta Physiologica Hungarica*. 2013;100(2):197–210.
80. Adebayo OL, Adenuga GA, Sandhir R. Postnatal protein malnutrition induces neurochemical alterations leading to behavioral deficits in rats: prevention by selenium or zinc supplementation. *Nutr Neurosci*. 2014;17(6):268–278.
81. Uğuz AC, Nazıroğlu M. Effects of selenium on calcium signaling and apoptosis in rat dorsal root ganglion neurons induced by oxidative stress. *Neurochem Res*. 2012;37(8):1631–1638.
82. Nazıroğlu M, Şenol N, Ghazizadeh V, Yürüker V. Neuroprotection induced by *N*-acetylcysteine and selenium against traumatic brain injury-induced apoptosis and calcium entry in hippocampus of rat. *Cell Mol Neurobiol*. 2014;34(6):895–903.
83. Kumari S, Mehta SL, Li PA. Glutamate induces mitochondrial dynamic imbalance and autophagy activation: preventive effects of selenium. *PloS One*. 2012;7(6):e39382.
84. de Freitas AS, Rocha JBT. Diphenyl diselenide and analogs are substrates of cerebral rat thioredoxin reductase: A pathway for their neuroprotective effects. *Neurosci Lett*. 2011;503(1):1–5.

85. Ardais AP, Viola GG, Costa MS, et al. Acute treatment with diphenyl diselenide inhibits glutamate uptake into rat hippocampal slices and modifies glutamate transporters, SNAP-25, and GFAP immunocontent. *Toxicol Sci.* 2010;113(2):434–443.
86. Chanaday NL, de Bem AF, Roth GA. Effect of diphenyl diselenide on the development of experimental autoimmune encephalomyelitis. *Neurochem Int.* 2011;59(8):1155–1162.
87. Roseni Mundstock Dias G, Medeiros Golombieski R, de Lima Portella R, et al. Diphenyl diselenide modulates gene expression of antioxidant enzymes in the cerebral cortex, hippocampus and striatum of female hypothyroid rats. *Neuroendocrinology.* 2014;100(1):45–59.
88. Brüning CA, Gai BM, Soares SM, Martini F, Nogueira CW. Serotonergic systems are implicated in antinociceptive effect of m-trifluoromethyl diphenyl diselenide in the mouse glutamate test. *Pharmacol Biochem Behav.* 2014;125:15–20.
89. Chagas PM, Rosa SG, Sari MHM, et al. Evaluation of the pharmacological properties of salicylic acid-derivative organoselenium: 2-hydroxy-5-selenocyanatobenzoic acid as an anti-inflammatory and antinociceptive compound. *Pharmacol Biochemi Behav.* 2014;118:87–95.
90. Bellinger FP, He QP, Bellinger MT, Lin Y. Association of selenoprotein P with Alzheimer's pathology in human cortex. *J Alzheimer's Dis.* 2008;15:465–472.
91. Rueli RHLH, Parubrub AC, Dewing AST, et al. Increased selenoprotein p in choroid plexus and cerebrospinal fluid in Alzheimer's disease brain. *J Alzheimer's Dis.* 2015;44(2):379–383.
92. Du X, Li H, Wang Z, Qiu S, Liu Q, Ni J. Selenoprotein P and selenoprotein M block Zn^{2+}-mediated Aβ42 aggregation and toxicity. *Metallomics.* 2013;5(7):861–870.
93. Du X, Wang Z, Zheng Y, Li H, Ni J, Liu Q. Inhibitory effect of selenoprotein P on Cu^{+}/Cu^{2+}-induced Aβ42 aggregation and toxicity. *Inorg Chem.* 2014;53(3):1672–1678.
94. Du X, Zheng Y, Wang Z, et al. Inhibitory act of selenoprotein P on $Cu^{(+)}/Cu^{(2+)}$-induced tau aggregation and neurotoxicity. *Inorg Chem.* 2014;53(20):11221–11230.
95. Haratake M, Yoshida S, Mandai M, Fuchigami T, Nakayama M. Elevated amyloid-β plaque deposition in dietary selenium-deficient Tg2576 transgenic mice. *Metallomics.* 2013;5(5):479–483.
96. van Eersel J, Ke YD, Liu X, et al. Sodium selenate mitigates tau pathology, neurodegeneration, and functional deficits in Alzheimer's disease models. *Proc Natl Acad Sci USA.* 2010;107(31):13888–13893.
97. Corcoran NM, Martin D, Hutter-Paier B, et al. Sodium selenate specifically activates PP2A phosphatase, dephosphorylates tau and reverses memory deficits in an Alzheimer's disease model. *J Clin Neurosci.* 2010;17(8):1025–1033.
98. Ishrat T, Parveen K, Khan MM, et al. Selenium prevents cognitive decline and oxidative damage in rat model of streptozotocin-induced experimental dementia of Alzheimer's type. *Brain Res.* 2009;1281:117–127.
99. Gwon A-R, Park J-S, Park J-H, et al. Selenium attenuates Aβ production and Aβ-induced neuronal death. *Neurosci Lett.* 2010;469(3):391–395.
100. Song G, Zhang Z, Wen L, et al. Selenomethionine ameliorates cognitive decline, reduces tau hyperphosphorylation, and reverses synaptic deficit in the triple transgenic mouse model of Alzheimer's disease. *J Alzheimer's Dis.* 2014;41(1):85–99.
101. Pinton S, Brüning CA, Sartori Oliveira CE, Prigol M, Nogueira CW. Therapeutic effect of organoselenium dietary supplementation in a sporadic dementia of Alzheimer's type model in rats. *J Nutr Biochem.* 2013;24(1):311–317.
102. Wang Z, Wang Y, Li W, et al. Design, synthesis, and evaluation of multitarget-directed selenium-containing clioquinol derivatives for the treatment of Alzheimer's disease. *ACS Chem Neurosci.* 2014;5(10):952–962.
103. Cardoso BR, Silva Bandeira V, Jacob-Filho W, Franciscato Cozzolino SM. Selenium status in elderly: relation to cognitive decline. *J Trace Elem Med Biol.* 2014;28(4):422–426.
104. Gonzalez-Dominguez R, García-Barrera T, Gomez-Ariza JL. Homeostasis of metals in the progression of Alzheimer's disease. *BioMetals.* 2014;27(3):539–549.
105. Cardoso BR, Ong TP, Jacob-Filho W, Jaluul O, Freitas MIdaÁ, Cozzolino SMF. Nutritional status of selenium in Alzheimer's disease patients. *Br J Nutr.* 2010;103(06):803–806.
106. Paglia G, Miedico O, Cristofano A, et al. Distinctive pattern of serum elements during the progression of Alzheimer's disease. *Sci Rep.* 2016;6:22769.
107. Vural H, Demirin H, Kara Y, Eren I, Delibas N. Alterations of plasma magnesium, copper, zinc, iron and selenium concentrations and some related erythrocyte antioxidant enzyme activities in patients with Alzheimer's disease. *J Trace Elem Med Biol.* 2010;24(3):169–173.
108. Scheltens P, Kamphuis PJGH, Verhey FRJ, et al. Efficacy of a medical food in mild Alzheimer's disease: a randomized, controlled trial. *Alzheimer's Dementia.* 2010;6(1):1–10.

109. Kesse-Guyot E, Fezeu L, Jeandel C, et al. French adults' cognitive performance after daily supplementation with antioxidant vitamins and minerals at nutritional doses: a post hoc analysis of the supplementation in vitamins and mineral antioxidants (SU.VI.MAX) trial. *Am J Clin Nutr*. 2011;94(3):892–899.
110. Cardoso BR, Apolinário D, da Silva Bandeira V, et al. Effects of Brazil nut consumption on selenium status and cognitive performance in older adults with mild cognitive impairment: a randomized controlled pilot trial. *Eur J Nutr*. 2015;:1–10.
111. Cadet JL. The potential use of vitamin E and selenium in parkinsonism. *Medical Hypoth*. 1986;20(1):87–94.
112. Khan HA. Selenium partially reverses the depletion of striatal dopamine and its metabolites in MPTP-treated C57BL mice. *Neurochem Int*. 2010;57(5):489–491.
113. Ellwanger JH, Molz P, Dallemole DR, et al. Selenium reduces bradykinesia and DNA damage in a rat model of Parkinson's disease. *Nutrition (Burbank, Los Angeles County, Calif.)*. 2015;31(2):359–365.
114. Vizuete ML, Steffen V, Machado A, Cano J. 1-Methyl-4-phenylpyridinium has greater neurotoxic effect after selenium deficiency than after vitamin E deficiency in rat striatum. *Eur J Pharmacol*. 1994;270(2–3):183–187.
115. Kim H-C, Jhoo W-K, Shin E-J, Bing G. Selenium deficiency potentiates methamphetamine-induced nigral neuronal loss; comparison with MPTP model. *Brain Res*. 2000;862(1–2):247–252.
116. Hare DJ, Adlard PA, Doble PA, Finkelstein DI. Metallobiology of 1-methyl-4-phenyl-1,2,3,6-tetrahydropyridine neurotoxicity. *Metallomics*. 2013;5(2):91–109.
117. Bellinger FP, Bellinger MT, Seale LA, et al. Glutathione peroxidase 4 is associated with neuromelanin in substantia nigra and dystrophic axons in putamen of Parkinson's brain. *Mol Neurodegener*. 2011;6(1):8.
118. Hauser DN, Dukes AA, Mortimer AD, Hastings TG. Dopamine quinone modifies and decreases the abundance of the mitochondrial selenoprotein glutathione peroxidase 4. *Free Radic Biol Med*. 2013;65:419–427.
119. Shahar A, Patel KV, Semba RD, et al. Plasma selenium is positively related to performance in neurological tasks assessing coordination and motor speed. *Mov Disord*. 2010;25(12):1909–1915.
120. Zhao H-W, Lin J, Wang X-B, et al. Assessing plasma levels of selenium, copper, iron and zinc in patients of Parkinson's disease. *PloS One*. 2013;8(12):e83060.
121. Mehrpour M, Kyani A, Tafazzoli M, Fathi F, Joghataie MT. A metabonomics investigation of multiple sclerosis by nuclear magnetic resonance. *Magn Reson Chem*. 2013;51(2):102–109.
122. Socha K, Kochanowicz J, Karpińska E, et al. Dietary habits and selenium, glutathione peroxidase and total antioxidant status in the serum of patients with relapsing-remitting multiple sclerosis. *Nutr J*. 2014;13(1):62.
123. Ljubisavljevic S, Stojanovic I, Cvetkovic T, et al. Glutathione homeostasis disruption of erythrocytes, but not glutathione peroxidase activity change, is closely accompanied with neurological and radiological scoring of acute CNS inflammation. *Neuroimmunomodulation*. 2014;21(1):13–20.
124. Tasset I, Agüera E, Sánchez-López F, et al. Peripheral oxidative stress in relapsing–remitting multiple sclerosis. *Clin Biochem*. 2012;45(6):440–444.
125. Kilness AW, Hichberg FH. Amyotrophic lateral sclerosis in a high selenium environment. *J Am Med Assoc*. 1977;237(26):2843–2844.
126. Vinceti M, Bonvicini F, Rothman KJ, Vescovi L, Wang F. The relation between amyotrophic lateral sclerosis and inorganic selenium in drinking water: a population-based case-control study. *Environ Health*. 2010;9(1):77.
127. Vinceti M, Guidetti D, Pinotti M, et al. Amyotrophic lateral sclerosis after long-term exposure to drinking water with high selenium content. *Epidemiology*. 1996;7(5):529–532.
128. Maraldi T, Riccio M, Zambonin L, Vinceti M, De Pol A, Hakim G. Low levels of selenium compounds are selectively toxic for a human neuron cell line through ROS/RNS increase and apoptotic process activation. *Neuro Toxicol*. 2011;32(2):180–187.
129. Morgan KL, Estevez AO, Mueller CL, et al. The glutaredoxin GLRX-21 functions to prevent selenium-induced oxidative stress in caenorhabditis elegans. *Toxicol Sci*. 2010;118(2):530–543.
130. Estevez AO, Morgan KL, Szewczyk NJ, Gems D, Estevez M. The neurodegenerative effects of selenium are inhibited by FOXO and PINK1/PTEN regulation of insulin/insulin-like growth factor signaling in *Caenorhabditis elegans*. *Neuro Toxicol*. 2014;41(100):28–43.
131. Estevez AO, Mueller CL, Morgan KL, et al. Selenium induces cholinergic motor neuron degeneration in *Caenorhabditis elegans*. *Neuro Toxicol*. 2012;33(5):1021–1032.
132. Lu Z, Marks E, Chen J, et al. Altered selenium status in Huntington's disease: neuroprotection by selenite in the N171-82Q mouse model. *Neurobiol Dis*. 2014;71C:34–42.
133. Bortolatto CF, Jesse CR, Wilhelm EA, Chagas PM, Nogueira CW. Organoselenium bis selenide attenuates 3-nitropropionic acid-induced neurotoxicity in rats. *Neurotox Res*. 2012;23(3):214–224.

CHAPTER

4

Does HFE Genotype Impact Macrophage Phenotype in Disease Process and Therapeutic Response?

Anne M. Nixon, James R. Connor

The Pennsylvania State University College of Medicine, Hershey, PA, United States

OUTLINE

IRON

Iron is essential in the regulation of many biochemical and cellular processes within the body, including DNA synthesis, oxygen transport in blood, and energy metabolism in the mitochondria.[1,2] Too much or too little iron can have detrimental effects, therefore iron is tightly regulated. Once in the bloodstream, approximately two-thirds of transferrin-bound iron is absorbed by erythroid precursors where it becomes incorporated into hemoglobin, while the rest is circulated and utilized by muscle and other tissues including the brain.[2] Iron is stored primarily within the liver parenchymal cells and reticular endothelial cells, such as macrophages.[3]

Biometals in Neurodegenerative Diseases. http://dx.doi.org/10.1016/B978-0-12-804562-6.00004-X

HEMOCHROMATOSIS

Discovery

Hemochromatosis is an iron overload disorder that results in increased total body iron, primarily within the parenchymal cells. If not treated, the iron overload can lead to organ dysfunction and death.[4] The first studies describing hemochromatosis were in 1865 by Armand Trousseau, where he observed his diabetic patients had bronze pigmented skin, cirrhosis of the liver, and pancreatic fibrosis.[5] However, there was no pathological connection at this time to iron. It wasn't until 1889 that Friedrich Daniel von Recklinghausen associated these signs with iron. Upon sectioning and staining livers from deceased patients, he found increased iron pigmentation within liver cells. Believing that the iron was derived from blood, he in turn named the disorder hemochromatosis.[6] The cause of hemochromatosis was still unknown until Joseph Sheldon saw an increase in iron in all body regions including blood, brain, and colon. This, along with the increased frequency of hemochromatosis in males and familial incidence resulted in his belief that hemochromatosis was hereditary in nature.[7,8] Despite these early findings, the actual gene that causes hemochromatosis was not discovered until 1975. Simon discovered an association between hereditary hemochromatosis and HLA-A3 allele found on chromosome 6p.[9,10] It was not until 20 years later that the actual gene, HLA-H, was discovered by Feder and coworkers.[11] It was found within the major histocompatibility complex (MHC), located specifically on chromosome 6p21.3. From these studies two missense mutations were identified within this gene: C282Y and H63D.[11] Later HLA-H was renamed to HFE to avoid confusion with a previously found gene.[12] Although the HFE gene has been found to be directly associated with hemochromatosis, the precise mechanisms and functions of HFE are yet to be elucidated. The current state of knowledge for HFE function will be discussed later in the chapter.

Types

There are four types of hemochromatosis, each resulting in increased iron overload, by a mechanism unique to each. Hereditary hemochromatosis is type I hemochromatosis that results from a mutation within the HFE gene.[11] Type II hemochromatosis or juvenile hemochromatosis is a result of a mutation within the HAMP or HJV gene leading to misregulation of hepcidin.[13,14] Type III occurs due to a mutation within the transferrin receptor 2 gene, which is thought to contribute to the regulation of hepcidin.[15] Finally, type IV is an uncommon disorder with a mutation within the gene that encodes ferroportin synthesis.[16] Interestingly, the cause of hemochromatosis, despite which type, seems to be associated with low or inadequate levels of hepcidin.

HFE

Structure

The HFE gene encodes the HFE protein, a type I transmembrane glycoprotein resembling class I MHC molecules that associates with β_2-microglobulin(β_2M) molecule.[11] It contains an α chain broken down into three domains, two of which bend to form a peptide binding groove.

Despite MHC molecules classically being able to bind to peptides, HFE lacks this feature because the α_1 and α_2 domains are too close to one another, preventing peptide binding.[17] Instead, HFE binds to transferrin receptor-1 (TfR1) at a neutral pH through the α_1 and α_2 domains.[17–19] HFE and TfR1 form a complex within the endoplasmic reticulum and are transported together through the Golgi complex to the cell surface. Without TfR1, HFE is unable to be expressed on the cellular surface.[20] HFE forms a complex with TfR1 by binding to one or both of the binding sites, resulting in reduced affinity of TfR1 for diferric transferrin.[21] In addition, the α_2 and α_3 domains contain disulfide bridges that help stabilize HFE's tertiary structure and specifically the disulfide bridge of α_3 helps interact with β_2M as seen in other class I MHC molecules.[11,22]

Function

Due to HFE's ability to bind to TfR1, HFE indirectly regulates iron homeostasis.[17,19] The molecular mechanism by which HFE affects iron homeostasis is still not well understood. One proposal states binding of wildtype HFE to TfR1 limits the amount of iron imported into a cell because only one molecule of iron bound transferrin can bind to TfR1. Additionally, studies have shown that in the presence of HFE, cells express reduced levels of Fe_2-Tf uptake, decreased ferritin levels, and an increase in TfR1.[20,23–26] Therefore, a mutation within the gene results in parenchymal cells accumulating excess iron. Recent studies propose that HFE also interacts with another transferrin receptor found primarily in the liver, TfR2, after its dissociation from TfR1.[27] However, the interaction between HFE and TFR2 is at the α_3 domain and does not compete with transferrin.[28] This interaction is understood to regulate hepcidin expression through the bone morphogenetic protein (BMP) pathway; however, the underlying mechanism remains unidentified. Briefly, HFE may bind to the BMP type I receptor ALK3 or may bind to the BMP coreceptor, hemojuvelin (HJV), along with TfR2 resulting in phosphorylation of the Smad 1/5/8 proteins.[29–31] In turn, these proteins are transported to the cell's nucleus along with the protein Smad 4, resulting in hepcidin transcription.[32] Ultimately, hepcidin production is increased and will limit the amount of iron released by its previously described interaction with ferroportin.[33]

Polymorphisms

There are two main polymorphisms of HFE, C282Y, H63D, and one less commonly studied polymorphism, S65C. C282Y and H63D polymorphisms were elucidated through the discovery of the HFE gene and account for over 90% of the hemochromatosis alleles.[11,34] Not all cases of hemochromatosis are caused by these two missenses, which led to the discovery of the alternative S65C mutation.[34]

C282Y results from a substitution of a tyrosine with a cysteine at position 282. It is found to be homozygous in 80%–90% of patients with hemochromatosis, the most common mutation within the hemochromatosis population.[11,18,35,36] Unlike wildtype HFE, the C282Y mutation does not interact with the β_2M molecule as it is localized intracellularly and unable to migrate to the cellular membrane. Thus, it fails to interact with TfR1, resulting in increased iron import as more transferrin binding sites are available.[37–39] Additionally, the C282Y mutation is able to interact with ALK3, a receptor for BMP type 1(BMP1), similar to wildtype HFE. This interaction results in the inhibition of hepcidin expression even though ALK3 ubiquitination was not prevented. Despite not inhibiting ALK3 ubiquination, cell surface expression of ALK3 was not increased.[30]

The H63D mutation is caused by a replacement of histidine for aspartic acid at position 63.[11] It is the second most common mutation found in hemochromatosis patients with an allele frequency between 15%–20%.[40,41] Of note, H63D is the most common mutation within the Caucasian population even though it is not the most prevalent mutation in hemochromatosis patients.[11,40,42] A number of studies have examined the H63D mutation in neurodegenerative diseases which will be discussed later. Unlike the C282Y mutation, H63D is able to migrate to the cellular membrane through its association with β_2M and binds to TfR1 with the same affinity as wildtype HFE.[38,43] This may affect the interaction of HFE with associating proteins or ligands, nevertheless the mechanism is poorly understood.[18] However, it is known that H63D is able to interact with ALK3, and like the C282Y mutation it does not induce hepcidin expression.[30] Conversely, H63D causes ubiquination of ALK3 and thus results in decreased ALK3 protein levels.

The S65C mutation occurs with a lower frequency in hereditary hemochromatosis than C282Y and H63D mutations, affecting around 2% of the hemochromatosis population.[34,44] S65C is the resultant of a serine substitution for a cysteine on exon two, linked to HLA-32.[44] These patients rarely are homozygous and instead have one chromosome without a mutation, or in combination with the C282Y or H63D mutation. This may account for a milder iron overload in which patients present with normal transferrin saturation and the C282Y and H63D mutation may be needed to produce symptoms of hemochromatosis.[34,45] However, elevated transferrin saturation levels have been reported in S65C mutations, but it did not cause hepatic fibrosis or cirrhosis, the result of chronic iron overload.[34,46]

MACROPHAGES

Macrophages are components of the mononuclear phagocytic system, and critical regulators of the immune system. They are versatile cells that provide host defense, destroying invading pathogens, and initiating an immune response. Understanding the function of macrophages is critical because despite the macrophage's ability to protect the host, they can also contribute to inflammatory and degenerative diseases.

Macrophage and Iron Metabolism

Macrophages are a key component in the regulation of iron homeostasis as they recycle damaged erythrocytes and other senescent cells that can be used in the production of new erythrocytes and iron management proteins (IMPs).[47] Similar to other cell types, iron is able to enter macrophages through transferrin receptor-1 when bound to transferrin.[48,49] Macrophages also acquire iron through phagocytosis and endocytosis, consistent with their primary function of eliminating cellular debris and foreign particles. Within the macrophage, heme oxygenase-1(HO-1) releases iron through degradation of phagocytosed stressed and damaged erythrocytes, and endocytosed heme and hemoglobin.[50] Iron is then exported into the cytoplasm via DMT-1 and NRAMP-1 in phagolysomes[51]; the latter protein specific to macrophages. Once in the cytoplasm, iron can be stored within ferritin.[52] Ferritin can also be released from macrophages and microglia.[53] In the latter cell type, ferritin can be a trophic influence on oligodendrocytes.[54] The release of ferritin may occur through a lysosomal secretory pathway.[55] As macrophages and microglia are activated during inflammation, they release ferritin resulting in the increased serum ferritin levels found during inflammatory states.[56]

Macrophage Polarization

Macrophages also have a role in cell-mediated immunity and wound repair, and both are regulated through iron homeostasis.[57–59] Macrophages possess the unique ability to become polarized in response to different environmental stimuli.[60] Generally, polarized macrophages can be classified into two groups; classically activated (M1) or alternatively activated (M2) macrophages. M1 macrophages are activated for cell mediated immune response to provide host defense. During stress or infections, natural killer cells produce interferon gamma (IFNγ) that prime macrophages into classically activated macrophages, resulting in their secretion of proinflammatory cytokines, such as IL-6, IL-1, and TNF-α, and other innate immune mediators that help defend and kill off pathogens and infections.[61,62] M1 macrophages contain higher levels of ferritin and lower transferrin and ferroportin levels.[63] These findings may be attributed to their function, in which low levels of iron are exported to limit the growth of an infection and protect against oxidative damage. In addition, macrophages may be holding onto iron by increased hepcidin levels that occurs when IL-6 binds to it's receptor resulting in activation of Janus kinases, that in turn, phosphorylate STAT3. Subsequently, STAT3 is transported to the nucleus where it induces the transcription of many genes, including hepcidin.[64] This increase in hepcidin production attributes to the decreased levels of ferroportin, transferrin receptor, and iron export, and increased ferritin levels.[63] This elegant system for limiting the bioavailability of iron during infections was introduced in 1984 as the iron withholding defense.[65]

Alternatively activated M2 macrophages share some similarities to M1 macrophages. However, they are considered "healers" compared to the M1 "killer" macrophages. They are recruited in wound healing and debris scavenging, but have also play a role in promoting tumorigenesis.[66–71] The production of IL-4 from injured tissues activates M2 macrophages and causes them to secrete precursors and components of extracellular matrix.[66,67] M2 macrophages play a protumor role by promotion of angiogenesis. In fact, tumor associated macrophages are a subpopulation of M2.[71] In comparison to M1 macrophages, M2 macrophages have lower levels of ferritin, but higher levels of transferrin receptor and ferroportin. As previously stated, M1 macrophages secrete proinflammatory cytokines that attribute to their IMP characterization, whereas M2 macrophages secrete low levels of proinflammatory cytokines but high levels of antiinflammatory cytokines (IL-13). These low levels of proinflammatory cytokines subsequently result in a decrease in the production of hepcidin, thus leading to decreased levels of ferroportin.[63]

Macrophages and HFE

Reticuloendothelial cells, primarily macrophages, are reportedly iron poor in iron overload disorders, such as hereditary hemochromatosis, despite the high levels of iron within liver, spleen, and bone marrow.[72,73] Under normal conditions, the amount of iron within parenchymal cells is similar to that of reticuloendothelial cells. The mechanism behind macrophages' abnormal iron levels is poorly understood, but Montosi and coworkers[74] shows that HFE functions differently in macrophages when compared to parenchymal cells. Wild-type HFE macrophages have increased iron and ferritin expression following exposure to radiolabeled Fe-Tf. In addition, there were also decreased TfR-1 levels correlating with the increased levels of iron and ferritin.[74]

Drakesmith and coworkers[75] also found that wild-type HFE can increase iron levels within macrophages, through inhibition of iron export, and not enhanced iron uptake. Comparing the wild-type HFE macrophages to those transfected with the H63D mutation, the wild-type HFE was associated with an increased inhibition of iron release. Furthermore, it is proposed there is a homeostatic mechanism linking HFE binding to transferrin receptor-1 and ferroportin. When transferrin saturation levels are low, HFE remains bound to TfR-1, not ferroportin. Therefore, iron export is increased from macrophages and decreases intracellular iron concentration. The opposite occurs when transferrin saturation is high; HFE is blocked from binding to TfR-1 and instead binds to ferroportin, sequestering iron within the cell.[76] The loss of homeostasis between these two mechanisms decreases the capacity of iron storage within macrophages. In contrast to these results, Waheed and coworkers[38] showed an increase in iron uptake in Chinese hamster ovary cells transfected with wild-type HFE. Therefore, mutations with in the HFE gene would prevent enhanced iron uptake. Overall, the mechanism regarding macrophages as a function of HFE genotype is still unclear as there are many limitations to the studies presented. The previous studies described looked only at the role of HFE in wildtype macrophages, however, this still does not answer the question of why the mutated macrophages are iron deficient. Furthermore, the macrophages obtained by Drakesmith consisted of a monocytic cell line transfected with HFE, which may not accurately reflect the in situ process, leaving the role of HFE in macrophage iron management still undiscovered.

HFE and Neurodegenerative Diseases

The relationship between HFE status and the brain has been fraught with misinformation and misquoting of early literature. The prevailing paradigm was that the blood brain barrier kept the amount of iron static and protected the brain from increased iron accumulation. The initial autopsy reports on brains of patients with hemochromatosis reported brain iron accumulation not only in those areas unprotected by the blood–brain barrier (BBB), but also in regions protected by the BBB.[8,77] Supporting this, MRIs have shown increased iron accumulation within various brain regions,[78,79] and animal models of the HFE H63D mutation, unlike HFE knockout models (REF), also report increased iron in the brain.[80,81]

Mutations in HFE are associated with increased susceptibility to neurodegenerative diseases,[82] and also appear to disrupt other processes, such as myelination and cholesterol metabolism.[81] Loss of iron homeostasis leads to increased oxidative stress and neuronal death which are hallmarks of neurodegenerative disease.[80,83,84] The incidence of the HFE gene variants have been linked to Alzheimer's disease (AD), Amyotrophic Lateral Sclerosis (ALS), and Parkinson's disease (PD),[85–90] indicating a general critical contribution of the HFE protein in maintaining the brain in a healthy state. However, studies have also reported that the HFE gene variants maybe protective against neurodegenerative diseases and others have found no association between the gene and diseases.[88,91–94] The lack of agreement is likely associated with gene-environment interaction because, as pointed out earlier, iron is only obtained by the body via the diet, therefore variations in dietary access to iron are likely to impact the extent of HFE genotype effects on disease. Given the prevalence of the HFE mutations, especially the H63D variant in the general population it is likely that the presence of this mutation impacts disease processes and therapeutic response. For a more detailed review of HFE mutations and neurodegenerative disease, refer to Nandar and Connor (2011).[84] In this review, we will focus on microglial responses in various diseases and how their response may be impacted by the HFE genotype. Microglia are the resident macrophages in the brain and thus the impact of the HFE genotype on microglial function should be similar to that of macrophages in other organs. Microglial activation is reported as part of all neurodegenerative diseases.[95]

Alzheimer's Disease

In general, accumulation of iron within neurofibrillary tangles, senile plaques, and oxidative stress are pathological hallmarks of AD.[96–98] The oxidative stress in AD can cause degeneration of microglia, resulting in a limitation of neuroprotection.[99] In the presence of the HFE mutation, microglia could increase iron export which can lead to an increase in oxidative damage. Just like macrophages, microglia are phagocytic and should be able to clear amyloid-β (Aβ) plaques making them in sense neuroprotective. However, with age the function of microglia diminishes,[100] which would contribute to the accumulation of Aβ plaques. Furthermore, cell culture studies have shown that even though microglia may initially phagocytose Aβ plaques this phenomenon does not continue and the amount of degradation is limited.[101–103] In cell culture models, expression of H63D mutation within neuroblastoma cells caused an increase in tau phosphorylation and decreased levels of Prolylpeptidyl isomerase-1, which is involved in the production of neurofibrillary tangles and phosphorylation of APP and tau, respectively.[104] The presence of the H63D variant increases cellular sensitivity to Aβ toxicity. Furthermore, HFE is increased within the area of Aβ plaques of AD brains.[105]

Amyotrophic Lateral Sclerosis

In ALS, the HFE mutation is associated with a fourfold increase in risk for ALS[85,86] and present in up to 30% of cases.[85,86,106,107] Neuronal cell culture models and a mouse model that carries the H63D gene variant have shown increased levels of oxidative stress, glutamate, and endoplasmic reticulum stress which are consistent findings in models of ALS.[80,108–110] Additionally, when combined with the SOD1 mutation, the H63D gene variant accelerates disease progression and shorten life expectancy in the mouse model. Furthermore, microglia within this model contain increased levels of L-ferritin and overall had more activated microglia than the wildtype counterpart.[111] The increase in L-ferritin could indicate increased levels of iron and proinflammatory cytokines and ultimately lead to increase in oxidative stress, microglia toxicity, and accelerated disease progression.[112] Just as with Alzheimer's Disease, microglia may have a protective effect of motor neurons during early stages of ALS due to low levels of microglia present in spinal cord.[113] However, in later stages there are significantly increased levels of activated microglia which may lead to accelerated disease progression through their secretion of proinflammatory cytokines and reactive oxygen species.[114,115]

Parkinson's Disease

There have been many clinical studies looking at the incidence between HFE and PD, however, the results are conflicting. Multiple studies have shown an increase in frequency between the HFE mutation, C282Y, and PD,[89,90] however, others have shown no association of HFE genotypes and PD.[116–118] In PD, the HFE gene variant is associated with an increase in α-synuclein, which enhances the generation of Lewy bodies, a pathological hallmark of PD.[119,120] Just as in AD and ALS, PD has an increase in activated microglia. This activation in PD, however, can come from α-synuclein through subsequent activation of the toll-like receptor.[121] Furthermore, characterization of PD is the loss of dopaminergic neurons which may be mediated through the production of inflammation and ROS from activated microglia.[122]

HFE and Cancer

HFE gene variants have been linked to an increased risk for certain cancers.[123] Despite the fact that studies looking at the relationship between HFE and cancer have tended to focus on iron overload in the liver and hepatic cancer, associations with many other cancers have been found. Several studies have found HFE mutations can be cytoprotective, suggesting a tumor suppressive role.[98,110,124–127] Opposing this, the H63D mutation has also been shown to be significantly increased in breast cancer, hepatocellular carcinoma, and gliomas,[128–131] suggesting the loss of function of HFE increases tumor progression. It was also found that patients expressing this mutation had an increased risk of pediatric acute lymphocytic leukemia (ALL), colorectal cancer, gastric cancer, and hepatocellular carcinoma.[132–136] Similarly, increased C282Y mutations have been found in breast cancer, colorectal cancer, hepatocellular carcinoma, and pediatric ALL.[130,132,137–140] Furthermore, those with a C282Y have increased risk for developing pediatric ALL, breast cancer, colorectal cancer, hepatocellular carcinoma, and ovarian cancer.[132,134,141–145] However, there are also studies that have reported neither an association of the HFE variants to patients with cancer, nor their risk for developing cancer.[136,146–149] The differences in these studies may be attributed to their differences in methodologies, such as a lack of controls and limited patient population but also the question of gene and environment interaction mentioned earlier.

A key question lacking from these studies is how macrophages are influencing particularly solid tumors. As discussed previously, macrophages can be activated and polarized into two different populations, of which M2 (alternatively-activated macrophages) are most commonly associated with tumor promotion. M2 macrophages play a key role in tumor growth and progression through an increase in iron release that in turn promotes cellular growth and DNA replication. Tumor associated macrophages (TAMs) secrete components that aide in the angiogenesis, recruitment of additional macrophages, and lymphangiogensis.[150,151] These all allow the tumors to become highly vascularized and increase their growth and migration. In those reports where the HFE mutation has been shown be protective, one wonders if the tumoricidal activity of macrophages was activated differently. Weston and coworkers showed that upon incubating conditioned media from H67D (H63D mouse homolog) macrophages on B16F10 cells, there was significantly smaller tumor growths compared to B16F10 cells incubated with wildtype macrophages.[152] Corresponding to these results, other studies have shown TAMs to secrete proinflammatory cytokines which can destroy tumor cells, and initiate a T-cell antitumor response.[153]

The ability of macrophages to take up iron is being explored, for imaging of brain tumors. Superparamagnetic iron oxide nanoparticles are under consideration as image enhancing agents for CNS brain tumors by taking advantage of macrophages and their aggressive iron uptake in the tumor microenvironment.[92] Given the utilization of iron by the macrophages for proinflammatory activity, some caution should be given until we learn how iron loading macrophages in tumors may impact the tumor or how the HFE genotype affects the phenotype of tumor associated macrophages.

HFE ANIMAL MODELS

A number of mouse models and cell lines have been created in an attempt to model the impact of HFE gene variants and identify the mechanisms involved. The HFE gene found in mice is structurally similar to the human HFE gene and contains a 66% conserved sequence between the two species.[154] Different mouse models disrupting the HFE gene include, HFE knockout, C294Y knockin (mouse homolog for C282Y), and H67D knockin (mouse homolog for H63D).[47,80,155–157] All of the models containing a knockout of HFE result in significant iron overload compared to the control mice, in addition to increased transferrin saturation and plasma levels. Predominately, iron accumulation was found in liver localized in the hepatocytes. There was not a significant change in iron levels found in other organs, such as the spleen, kidneys, and heart.[47,155,156] In comparison to HFE null mice, HFE knockin mice also have increased iron loading however it is not as significant as the null mice.[156,157] Furthermore, the H67D mutation did not induce as severe iron loading as C294Y, however the amount of iron was significantly greater than wildtype mice.[157] This observation could be relevant to the clinical data where C282Y is much more common in hemochromatosis than the H63D mutation.[11,158] Few studies have examined changes in the brain with the HFE gene variants. Nandar and coworkers[111] found their H67D knockin model to have increased levels of ferritin, HFE, and oxidative stress along with decreased transferrin. Furthermore, Ali-Rahmani[81] found increased caspase-3 levels, decreased synaptic proteins and lower spatial memory and recognition in the same H67D knockin model. These mice showed structural changes in the brain similar to that seen in aging humans with an H63D mutation.[159] These results clearly establish that the HFE genotype is relevant to human neurological disease and provide models for studying the role of macrophages and microglia in iron management in disease.

CONCLUSIONS

A key cellular component of neurodegenerative disease and cancer is the role of iron as a determining factor in the function of macrophage/microglia; not only in the phenotype of these cells but in the manner in which they influence disease process. The HFE genotype alters the incidence and the disease course in a number of diseases. In this review, we proposed that altered macrophage function as a result of HFE genotype could underlie the impact of HFE genotype on disease pathogenesis.

References

1. Wang J, Pantopoulos K. Regulation of cellular iron metabolism. *Biochem J*. 2011;434(3):365–381.
2. Andrews NC. Disorders of iron metabolism. *N Engl J Med*. 1999;341(26):1986–1995.
3. Bothwell TH, Charlton RW, Cook JD, Finch CA. *Iron metabolism in man*. Oxford, England: Blackwell Scientific Publications; 1979.
4. Piperno A. Classification and diagnosis of iron overload. *Haematologica*. 1998;83(5):447–455.
5. Trousseau A. Glycosurie; diabete sucre. *Clinique Med de l'Hotel de Paris*. 1865;2:663–698.
6. von Recklinghausen F. Uber Hamochromatose. *Tagebl Versamml Natur Artze Heidelberg*. 1889;62:324–325.
7. Ramage H, Sheldon J. Haemochromatosis. *Quart J Med*. 1934;4:121–129.
8. Sheldon J. *Haemochromatosis*. London: Oxford University Press; 1935.
9. Simon M, Pawlotsky Y, Bourel M, Fauchet R, Genetet B. Hemochromatose idiopathique: maladie associee a l'anligine tissulaire HLA 3? *La Nouvelle presse medicale*. 1975;4(19):1432.
10. Simon M, Bourel M, Fauchet R, Genetet B. Association of HLA-A3 and HLA-B14 antigens with idiopathic haemochromatosis. *Gut*. 1976;17(5):332–334.
11. Feder JN, Gnirke A, Thomas W, Tsuchihashi Z, Ruddy DA, Basava A, Dormishian F, Domingo R, Ellis MC, Fullan A, Hinton LM, Jones NL, Kimmel BE, Kronmal GS, Lauer P, Lee VK, Loeb DB, Mapa FA, McClelland E, Meyer NC, Mintier GA, Moeller N, Moore T, Morikang E, Prass CE, Quintana L, Starnes SM, Schatzman RC, Brunke KJ, Drayna DT, Risch NJ, Bacon BR, Wolff RK. A novel MHC class I-like gene is mutated in patients with hereditary haemochromatosis. *Nat Genet*. 1996;13(4):399–408.
12. Bodmer JG, Marsh SGE, Albert ED, Bodmer WF, Bontrop RE, Charron D, Dupont B, Erlich HA, Fauchet R, Mach B, Mayr WR, Parham P, Sasazuki T, Schreuder GMT, Strominger JL, Svejgaard A, Terasaki PI. Nomenclature for factors of the HLA system, 1996. *Hum Immunol*. 1997;53(1):98–128.
13. Roetto A, Papanikolaou G, Politou M, Alberti F, Girelli D, Christakis J, Loukopoulos D, Camaschella C. Mutant antimicrobial peptide hepcidin is associated with severe juvenile hemochromatosis. *Nat Genet*. 2003;33(1):21–22.
14. Papanikolaou G, Samuels ME, Ludwig EH, MacDonald MLE, Franchini PL, Dube M-P, Andres L, MacFarlane J, Sakellaropoulos N, Politou M, Nemeth E, Thompson J, Risler JK, Zaborowska C, Babakaiff R, Radomski CC, Pape TD, Davidas O, Christakis J, Brissot P, Lockitch G, Ganz T, Hayden MR, Goldberg YP. Mutations in HFE2 cause iron overload in chromosome 1q-linked juvenile hemochromatosis. *Nat Genet*. 2004;36(1):77–82.
15. Nemeth E, Roetto A, Garozzo G, Ganz T, Camaschella C. Hepcidin is decreased in TFR2 hemochromatosis. *Blood*. 2004;105(4):1803–1806.
16. De Domenico I, Ward DM, Nemeth E, Vaughn MB, Musci G, Ganz T, Kaplan J. The molecular basis of ferroportin-linked hemochromatosis. *Proc Natl Acad Sci USA*. 2005;102(25):8955–8960.
17. Lebrón JA, Bennett MJ, Vaughn DE, Chirino AJ, Snow PM, Mintier GA, Feder JN, Bjorkman PJ. Crystal structure of the hemochromatosis protein HFE and characterization of its interaction with transferrin receptor. *Cell*. 1998;93(1):111–123.
18. Feder JN, Penny DM, Irrinki A, Lee VK, Lebrón JA, Watson N, Tsuchihashi Z, Sigal E, Bjorkman PJ, Schatzman RC. The hemochromatosis gene product complexes with the transferrin receptor and lowers its affinity for ligand binding. *Proc Natl Acad Sci USA*. 1998;95(4):1472–1477.
19. Bennett MJ, Lebron JA, Bjorkman PJ. Crystal structure of the hereditary haemochromatosis protein HFE complexed with transferrin receptor. *Nature*. 2000;403(6765):46–53.
20. Salter-Cid L, Brunmark A, Li Y, Leturcq D, Peterson PA, Jackson MR, Yang Y. Transferrin receptor is negatively modulated by the hemochromatosis protein HFE: implications for cellular iron homeostasis. *Proc Natl Acad Sci USA*. 1999;96(10):5434–5439.
21. Giannetti AM, Björkman PJ. HFE and transferrin directly compete for transferrin receptor in solution and at the cell surface. *J Biol Chem*. 2004;279(24):25866–25875.
22. Bjorkman PJ, Parham P. Structure, function, and diversity of class I major histocompatibility complex molecules. *Ann Rev Biochem*. 1990;59(1):253–288.
23. Roy CN, Penny DM, Feder JN, Enns CA. The hereditary hemochromatosis protein, HFE, specifically regulates transferrin-mediated iron uptake in HeLa cells. *J Biol Chem*. 1999;274(13):9022–9028.
24. Corsi B, Levi S, Cozzi A, Corti A, Altimare D, Albertini A, Arosio P. Overexpression of the hereditary hemochromatosis protein, HFE, in HeLa cells induces an iron-deficient phenotype. *FEBS Lett*. 1999;460(1):149–152.
25. Roy CN, Carlson EJ, Anderson EL, Basava A, Starnes SM, Feder JN, Enns CA. Interactions of the ectodomain of HFE with the transferrin receptor are critical for iron homeostasis in cells. *FEBS Lett*. 2000;484(3):271–274.

26. Gross CN, Irrinki A, Feder JN, Enns CA. Co-trafficking of HFE, a nonclassical major histocompatibility complex class I protein, with the transferrin receptor implies a role in intracellular iron regulation. *J Biol Chem.* 1998;273(34):22068–22074.
27. Gao J, Chen J, Kramer M, Tsukamoto H, Zhang A-S, Enns CA. Interaction of the hereditary hemochromatosis protein, HFE, with transferrin receptor 2 is required for transferrin-induced hepcidin expression. *Cell Metabol.* 2009;9(3):217–227.
28. Chen J, Chloupková M, Gao J, Chapman-Arvedson TL, Enns CA. HFE modulates transferrin receptor 2 levels in hepatoma cells via interactions that differ from transferrin receptor 1-HFE interactions. *J Biol Chem.* 2007;282(51):36862–36870.
29. D'Alessio F, Hentze MW, Muckenthaler MU. The hemochromatosis proteins HFE, TfR2, and HJV form a membrane-associated protein complex for hepcidin regulation. *J Hepatol.* 2012;57(5):1052–1060.
30. Wu X-g, Wang Y, Wu Q, Cheng W-H, Liu W, Zhao Y, Mayeur C, Schmidt PJ, Yu PB, Wang F, Xia Y. HFE interacts with the BMP type I receptor ALK3 to regulate hepcidin expression. *Blood.* 2014;124(8):1335–1343.
31. Ryan JD, Ryan E, Fabre A, Lawless MW, Crowe J. Defective bone morphogenic protein signaling underlies hepcidin deficiency in HFE hereditary hemochromatosis. *Hepatology.* 2010;52(4):1266–1273.
32. Heldin C-H, Miyazono K, ten Dijke P. TGF-[beta] signalling from cell membrane to nucleus through SMAD proteins. *Nature.* 1997;390(6659):465–471.
33. Nemeth E, Tuttle MS, Powelson J, Vaughn MB, Donovan A, Ward DM, Ganz T, Kaplan J. Hepcidin regulates cellular iron efflux by binding to ferroportin and inducing its internalization. *Science.* 2004;306(5704):2090–2093.
34. Mura C, Raguenes O, Férec C. HFE mutations analysis in 711 hemochromatosis probands: evidence for S65C implication in mild form of hemochromatosis. *Blood.* 1999;93(8):2502–2505.
35. Jouanolle AM, Gandon G, Jezequel P, Blayau M, Campion ML, Yaouanq J, Mosser J, Fergelot P, Chauvel B, Bouric P, Carn G, Andrieux N, Gicquel I, Le Gall J-Y, David V. Haemochromatosis and HLA-H. *Nat Genet.* 1996;14(3):251–252.
36. Beutler E, Gelbart T, West C, Lee P, Adams M, Blackstone R, Pockros P, Kosty M, Venditti CP, Phatak PD, Seese NK, Chorney KA, Ten Elshof AE, Gerhard GS, Chorney M. Mutation analysis in hereditary hemochromatosis. *Blood Cells Mol Dis.* 1996;22(2):187–194.
37. Feder JN, Tsuchihashi Z, Irrinki A, Lee VK, Mapa FA, Morikang E, Prass CE, Starnes SM, Wolff RK, Parkkila S, Sly WS, Schatzman RC. The hemochromatosis founder mutation in HLA-H disrupts β2-microglobulin interaction and cell surface expression. *J Biol Chem.* 1997;272(22):14025–14028.
38. Waheed A, Parkkila S, Zhou XY, Tomatsu S, Tsuchihashi Z, Feder JN, Schatzman RC, Britton RS, Bacon BR, Sly WS. Hereditary hemochromatosis: effects of C282Y and H63D mutations on association with β(2)-microglobulin, intracellular processing, and cell surface expression of the HFE protein in COS-7 cells. *Proc Natl Acad Sci USA.* 1997;94(23):12384–12389.
39. Feeney GP, Worwood M. The effects of wild-type and mutant HFE expression upon cellular iron uptake in transfected human embryonic kidney cells. *Biochim Biophys Acta.* 2001;1538(2–3):242–251.
40. Burt MJ, George PM, Upton JD, Collett JA, Frampton CMA, Chapman TM, Walmsley TA, Chapman BA. The significance of haemochromatosis gene mutations in the general population: implications for screening. *Gut.* 1998;43(6):830–836.
41. Steinberg KK, Cogswell ME, Chang JC, Caudill SP, McQuillian GM, Bowman BA, Grummer-Strawn LM, Sampson EJ, Khoury MJ, Gallagher ML. Prevalence of C282Y and H63D mutations in the hemochromatosis (HFE) gene in the United States. *JAMA.* 2001;285(17):2216–2222.
42. Marshall DS, Linfert DR, Tsongalis GJ. Prevalence of the C282Y and H63D polymorphisms in a multi-ethnic control population. *Int J Mol Med.* 1999;4(4):389–393.
43. Lebron JA, Bjorkman PJ. The transferrin receptor binding site on HFE, the class I MHC-related protein mutated in hereditary hemochromatosis. *J Mol Biol.* 1999;289(4):1109–1118.
44. Barton JC, Sawada-Hirai R, Rothenberg BE, Acton RT. Two novel missense mutations of the HFE gene (I105T and G93R) and identification of the S65C mutation in Alabama hemochromatosis probands. *Blood Cells Mol Dis.* 1999;25(3):147–155.
45. Arya N, Chakrabrati S, Hegele RA, Adams PC. HFE S65C variant is not associated with increased transferrin saturation in voluntary blood donors. *Blood Cells Mol Dis.* 1999;25(6):354–357.
46. Holmström P, Marmur J, Eggertsen G, Gåfvels M, Stål P. Mild iron overload in patients carrying the HFE S65C gene mutation: a retrospective study in patients with suspected iron overload and healthy controls. *Gut.* 2002;51(5):723–730.

47. Zhou XY, Tomatsu S, Fleming RE, Parkkila S, Waheed A, Jiang J, Fei Y, Brunt EM, Ruddy DA, Prass CE, Schatzman RC, O'Neill R, Britton RS, Bacon BR, Sly WS. HFE gene knockout produces mouse model of hereditary hemochromatosis. *Proc Natl Acad Sci*. 1998;95(5):2492–2497.
48. Warner RC, Weber I. The cupric and ferric citrate complexes1. *J Am Chem Soc*. 1953;75(20):5086–5094.
49. Dautry-Varsat A, Ciechanover A, Lodish HF. pH and the recycling of transferrin during receptor-mediated endocytosis. *Proc Natl Acad Sci*. 1983;80(8):2258–2262.
50. Brittenham G. The red cell cycle. In: Brock J, ed. *Iron Metabolism in Health and Disease*. London: W.B. Saunders Company Ltd; 1994:31–62.
51. Soe-Lin S, Apte SS, Mikhael MR, Kayembe LK, Nie G, Ponka P. Both Nramp1 and DMT1 are necessary for efficient macrophage iron recycling. *Exp Hematol*. 2010;38(8):609–617.
52. Harrison PM, Arosio P. The ferritins: molecular properties, iron storage function and cellular regulation. *Biochim Biophys Acta*. 1996;1275(3):161–203.
53. Connor JR, Zhang X, Nixon AM, Webb B, Perno JR. Comparative evaluation of nephrotoxicity and management by macrophages of intravenous pharmaceutical iron formulations. *PLoS One*. 2015;10(5):e0125272.
54. Zhang X, Surguladze N, Slagle-Webb B, Cozzi A, Connor JR. Cellular iron status influences the functional relationship between microglia and oligodendrocytes. *Glia*. 2006;54(8):795–804.
55. Cohen LA, Gutierrez L, Weiss A, Leichtmann-Bardoogo Y, Zhang D-l, Crooks DR, Sougrat R, Morgenstern A, Galy B, Hentze MW, Lazaro FJ, Rouault TA, Meyron-Holtz EG. Serum ferritin is derived primarily from macrophages through a nonclassical secretory pathway. *Blood*. 2010;116(9):1574–1584.
56. Zhang X, Haaf M, Todorich B, Grosstephan E, Schieremberg H, Surguladze N, Connor JR. Cytokine toxicity to oligodendrocyte precursors is mediated by iron. *Glia*. 2005;52(3):199–208.
57. Goodman GT, Koprowski H. Macrophages as a cellular expression of inherited natural resistance. *Proc Natl Acad Sci USA*. 1962;48(2):160–165.
58. Mackaness GB. Cellular resistance to infection. *J Exp Med*. 1962;116:381–406.
59. Gratchev A, Guillot P, Hakiy N, Politz O, Orfanos CE, Schledzewski K, Goerdt S. Alternatively activated macrophages differentially express fibronectin and its splice variants and the extracellular matrix protein betaIG-H3. *Scand J Immunol*. 2001;53(4):386–392.
60. Mackaness GB. Cellular immunity and the parasite. *Adv Exp Med Biol*. 1977;93:65–73.
61. Nathan CF, Murray HW, Wiebe ME, Rubin BY. Identification of interferon-gamma as the lymphokine that activates human macrophage oxidative metabolism and antimicrobial activity. *J Exp Med*. 1983;158(3):670–689.
62. Arango Duque G, Descoteaux A. Macrophage cytokines: involvement in immunity and infectious diseases. *Front Immunol*. 2014;5:491.
63. Corna G, Campana L, Pignatti E, Castiglioni A, Tagliafico E, Bosurgi L, Campanella A, Brunelli S, Manfredi AA, Apostoli P, Silvestri L, Camaschella C, Rovere-Querini P. Polarization dictates iron handling by inflammatory and alternatively activated macrophages. *Haematologica*. 2010;95(11):1814–1822.
64. Wrighting DM, Andrews NC. Interleukin-6 induces hepcidin expression through STAT3. *Blood*. 2006;108(9):3204–3209.
65. Weinberg ED. Iron withholding: a defense against infection and neoplasia. *Physiol Rev*. 1984;64(1):65–102.
66. Edwards JP, Zhang X, Frauwirth KA, Mosser DM. Biochemical and functional characterization of three activated macrophage populations. *J Leukoc Biol*. 2006;80(6):1298–1307.
67. Albina JE, Mills CD, Henry Jr WL, Caldwell MD. Temporal expression of different pathways of 1-arginine metabolism in healing wounds. *J Immunol*. 1990;144(10):3877–3880.
68. Nagaoka T, Kaburagi Y, Hamaguchi Y, Hasegawa M, Takehara K, Steeber DA, Tedder TF, Sato S. Delayed wound healing in the absence of intercellular adhesion molecule-1 or L-selectin expression. *Am J Pathol*. 2000;157(1):237–247.
69. Subramaniam M, Saffaripour S, Van De Water L, Frenette PS, Mayadas TN, Hynes RO, Wagner DD. Role of endothelial selectins in wound repair. *Am J Pathol*. 1997;150(5):1701–1709.
70. Martin P, D'Souza D, Martin J, Grose R, Cooper L, Maki R, McKercher SR. Wound healing in the PU.1 null mouse—tissue repair is not dependent on inflammatory cells. *Curr Biol*. 2003;13(13):1122–1128.
71. Sica A, Schioppa T, Mantovani A, Allavena P. Tumour-associated macrophages are a distinct M2 polarised population promoting tumour progression: potential targets of anti-cancer therapy. *Eur J Cancer*. 2006;42(6):717–727.
72. Valberg LS, Simon JB, Manley PN, Corbett WE, Ludwig J. Distribution of storage iron as body iron stores expand in patients with hemochromatosis. *J Lab Clin Med*. 1975;86(3):479–489.

73. Brink B, Disler P, Lynch S, Jacobs P, Charlton R, Bothwell T. Patterns of iron storage in dietary iron overload and idiopathic hemochromatosis. *J Lab Clin Med*. 1976;88(5):725–731.
74. Montosi G, Paglia P, Garuti C, Guzman CA, Bastin JM, Colombo MP, Pietrangelo A. Wild-type HFE protein normalizes transferrin iron accumulation in macrophages from subjects with hereditary hemochromatosis. *Blood*. 2000;96(3):1125–1129.
75. Drakesmith H, Sweetland E, Schimanski L, Edwards J, Cowley D, Ashraf M, Bastin J, Townsend ARM. The hemochromatosis protein HFE inhibits iron export from macrophages. *Proc Natl Acad Sci USA*. 2002;99(24):15602–15607.
76. Townsend A, Drakesmith H. Role of HFE in iron metabolism, hereditary haemochromatosis, anaemia of chronic disease, and secondary iron overload. *Lancet*. 2002;359(9308):786–790.
77. Cammermyer J. Deposition of iron in paraventricular areas of the human brain in hemochromatosis. *J Neuropathol Exp Neurol*. 1947;6(2):111–127.
78. Nielsen JE, Jensen LN, Krabbe K. Hereditary haemochromatosis: a case of iron accumulation in the basal ganglia associated with a parkinsonian syndrome. *J Neurol Neurosurg Psychiatry*. 1995;59(3):318–321.
79. Berg D, Hoggenmuller U, Hofmann E, Fischer R, Kraus M, Scheurlen M, Becker G. The basal ganglia in haemochromatosis. *Neuroradiology*. 2000;42(1):9–13.
80. Nandar W, Neely EB, Unger E, Connor JR. A mutation in the HFE gene is associated with altered brain iron profiles and increased oxidative stress in mice. *Biochim Biophys Acta*. 2013;1832(6):729–741.
81. Ali-Rahmani F, Grigson PS, Lee S, Neely E, Connor JR, Schengrund CL. H63D mutation in hemochromatosis alters cholesterol metabolism and induces memory impairment. *Neurobiol Aging*. 2014;35(6):1511.e1–1511.e12.
82. Salvador GA. Iron in neuronal function and dysfunction. *Biofactors*. 2010;36(2):103–110.
83. Rouault TA, Cooperman S. Brain iron metabolism. *Semin Pediatr Neurol*. 2006;13(3):142–148.
84. Nandar W, Connor JR. HFE gene variants affect iron in the brain. *J Nutr*. 2011;141(4):729S–739S.
85. Wang X-S, Lee S, Simmons Z, Boyer P, Scott K, Liu W, Connor J. Increased incidence of the Hfe mutation in amyotrophic lateral sclerosis and related cellular consequences. *J Neurol Sci*. 2004;227(1):27–33.
86. Goodall EF, Greenway MJ, van Marion I, Carroll CB, Hardiman O, Morrison KE. Association of the H63D polymorphism in the hemochromatosis gene with sporadic ALS. *Neurology*. 2005;65(6):934–937.
87. Moalem S, Percy ME, Andrews DF, Kruck TP, Wong S, Dalton AJ, Mehta P, Fedor B, Warren AC. Are hereditary hemochromatosis mutations involved in Alzheimer disease? *Am J Med Genet*. 2000;93(1):58–66.
88. Blázquez L, De Juan D, Ruiz-Martínez J, Emparanza JI, Sáenz A, Otaegui D, Sistiaga A, Martínez-Lage P, Lamet I, Samaranch L, Buiza C, Etxeberria I, Arriola E, Cuadrado E, Urdaneta E, Yanguas J, López de Munain A. Genes related to iron metabolism and susceptibility to Alzheimer's disease in Basque population. *Neurobiol Aging*. 2007;28(12):1941–1943.
89. Dekker MC, Giesbergen PC, Njajou OT, van Swieten JC, Hofman A, Breteler MM, van Duijn CM. Mutations in the hemochromatosis gene (HFE), Parkinson's disease and parkinsonism. *Neurosci Lett*. 2003;348(2):117–119.
90. Guerreiro R, Bras J, Santana I, Januario C, Santiago B, Morgadinho A, Ribeiro M, Hardy J, Singleton A, Oliveira C. Association of HFE common mutations with Parkinson's disease. Alzheimer's disease and mild cognitive impairment in a Portuguese cohort. *BMC Neurol*. 2006;6(1):24.
91. Buchanan DD, Silburn PA, Chalk JB, Le Couteur DG, Mellick GD. The Cys282Tyr polymorphism in the HFE gene in Australian Parkinson's disease patients. *Neurosci Lett*. 2002;327(2):91–94.
92. Correia AP, Pinto JP, Dias V, Mascarenhas C, Almeida S, Porto G. CAT53 and HFE alleles in Alzheimer's disease: a putative protective role of the C282Y HFE mutation. *Neurosci Lett*. 2009;457(3):129–132.
93. Li M, Wang L, Wang W, Qi XL, Tang ZY. Mutations in the HFE gene and sporadic amyotrophic lateral sclerosis risk: a meta-analysis of observational studies. *Braz J Med Biol Res*. 2014;47(3):215–222.
94. Ali-Rahmani F, Hengst JA, Connor JR, Schengrund CL. Effect of HFE variants on sphingolipid expression by SH-SY5Y human neuroblastoma cells. *Neurochem Res*. 2011;36(9):1687–1696.
95. Lull ME, Block ML. Microglial activation & chronic neurodegeneration. *Neurotherapeutics*. 2010;7(4):354–365.
96. Lovell MA, Robertson JD, Teesdale WJ, Campbell JL, Markesbery WR. Copper, iron and zinc in Alzheimer's disease senile plaques. *J Neurol Sci*. 1998;158(1):47–52.
97. Good PF, Perl DP, Bierer LM, Schmeidler J. Selective accumulation of aluminum and iron in the neurofibrillary tangles of Alzheimer's disease: a laser microprobe (LAMMA) study. *Ann Neurol*. 1992;31(3):286–292.
98. Smith MA, Harris PLR, Sayre LM, Perry G. Iron accumulation in Alzheimer disease is a source of redox-generated free radicals. *Proc Natl Acad Sci USA*. 1997;94(18):9866–9868.

99. Lopes KO, Sparks DL, Streit WJ. Microglial dystrophy in the aged and Alzheimer's disease brain is associated with ferritin immunoreactivity. *Glia*. 2008;56(10):1048–1060.
100. Streit WJ, Sammons NW, Kuhns AJ, Sparks DL. Dystrophic microglia in the aging human brain. *Glia*. 2004;45(2):208–212.
101. Paresce DM, Chung H, Maxfield FR. Slow degradation of aggregates of the Alzheimer's disease amyloid beta-protein by microglial cells. *J Biol Chem*. 1997;272(46):29390–29397.
102. Chung H, Brazil MI, Soe TT, Maxfield FR. Uptake, degradation, and release of fibrillar and soluble forms of Alzheimer's amyloid beta-peptide by microglial cells. *J Biol Chem*. 1999;274(45):32301–32308.
103. Majumdar A, Chung H, Dolios G, Wang R, Asamoah N, Lobel P, Maxfield FR. Degradation of fibrillar forms of Alzheimer's amyloid beta-peptide by macrophages. *Neurobiol Aging*. 2008;29(5):707–715.
104. Hall 2nd EC, Lee SY, Simmons Z, Neely EB, Nandar W, Connor JR. Prolyl-peptidyl isomerase, Pin1, phosphorylation is compromised in association with the expression of the HFE polymorphic allele, H63D. *Biochim Biophys Acta*. 2010;1802(4):389–395.
105. Connor JR, Snyder BS, Beard JL, Fine RE, Mufson EJ. Regional distribution of iron and iron-regulatory proteins in the brain in aging and Alzheimer's disease. *J Neurosci Res*. 1992;31(2):327–335.
106. Restagno G, Lombardo F, Ghiglione P, Calvo A, Cocco E, Sbaiz L, Mutani R, Chiò A. HFE H63D polymorphism is increased in patients with amyotrophic lateral sclerosis of Italian origin. *J Neurol Neurosurg Psychiatry*. 2007;78(3):327.
107. Praline J, Blasco H, Vourc'h P, Rat V, Gendrot C, Camu W, Andres CR. Group FASStudy of the HFE gene common polymorphisms in French patients with sporadic amyotrophic lateral sclerosis. *J Neurol Sci*. 2012;317(1-2):58–61.
108. Lee SY, Patton SM, Henderson RJ, Connor JR. Consequences of expressing mutants of the hemochromatosis gene (HFE) into a human neuronal cell line lacking endogenous HFE. *FASEB J*. 2007;21(2):564–576.
109. Mitchell RM, Lee SY, Simmons Z, Connor JR. HFE polymorphisms affect cellular glutamate regulation. *Neurobiol Aging*. 2011;32(6):1114–1123.
110. Liu Y, Lee SY, Neely E, Nandar W, Moyo M, Simmons Z, Connor JR. Mutant HFE H63D protein is associated with prolonged endoplasmic reticulum stress and increased neuronal vulnerability. *J Biol Chem*. 2011;286(15):13161–13170.
111. Nandar W, Neely EB, Simmons Z, Connor JR. H63D HFE genotype accelerates disease progression in animal models of amyotrophic lateral sclerosis. *Biochim Biophys Acta*. 2014;1842(12 Part A):2413–2426.
112. Rathore KI, Redensek A, David S. Iron homeostasis in astrocytes and microglia is differentially regulated by TNF-α and TGF-β1. *Glia*. 2012;60(5):738–750.
113. Gerber YN, Sabourin JC, Rabano M, Vivanco M, Perrin FE. Early functional deficit and microglial disturbances in a mouse model of amyotrophic lateral sclerosis. *PLoS One*. 2012;7(4):e36000.
114. Wang WY, Tan MS, Yu JT, Tan L. Role of pro-inflammatory cytokines released from microglia in Alzheimer's disease. *Ann Transl Med*. 2015;3(10):136.
115. Keller JN, Hanni KB, Gabbita SP, Friebe V, Mattson MP, Kindy MS. Oxidized lipoproteins increase reactive oxygen species formation in microglia and astrocyte cell lines. *Brain Res*. 1999;830(1):10–15.
116. Akbas N, Hochstrasser H, Deplazes J, Tomiuk J, Bauer P, Walter U, Behnke S, Riess O, Berg D. Screening for mutations of the HFE gene in Parkinson's disease patients with hyperechogenicity of the substantia nigra. *Neurosci Lett*. 2006;407(1):16–19.
117. Aamodt AH, Stovner LJ, Thorstensen K, Lydersen S, White LR, Aasly JO. Prevalence of haemochromatosis gene mutations in Parkinson's disease. *J Neurol Neurosurg Psychiatry*. 2007;78(3):315–317.
118. Halling J, Petersen MS, Grandjean P, Weihe P, Brosen K. Genetic predisposition to Parkinson's disease: CYP2D6 and HFE in the Faroe Islands. *Pharmacogenet Genomics*. 2008;18(3):209–212.
119. Golts N, Snyder H, Frasier M, Theisler C, Choi P, Wolozin B. Magnesium inhibits spontaneous and iron-induced aggregation of α-synuclein. *J Biol Chem*. 2002;277(18):16116–16123.
120. Castellani RJ, Siedlak SL, Perry G, Smith MA. Sequestration of iron by Lewy bodies in Parkinson's disease. *Acta Neuropathol*. 2000;100(2):111–114.
121. Roodveldt C, Labrador-Garrido A, Gonzalez-Rey E, Lachaud CC, Guilliams T, Fernandez-Montesinos R, Benitez-Rondan A, Robledo G, Hmadcha A, Delgado M, Dobson CM, Pozo D. Preconditioning of microglia by α-synuclein strongly affects the response induced by toll-like receptor (TLR) stimulation. *PLoS ONE*. 2013;8(11):e79160.

122. Gao HM, Kotzbauer PT, Uryu K, Leight S, Trojanowski JQ, Lee VM. Neuroinflammation and oxidation/nitration of alpha-synuclein linked to dopaminergic neurodegeneration. *J Neurosci*. 2008;28(30):7687–7698.
123. Connor JR, Lee SY. Iron and cancer. In: Milner J, Donato F, eds. *Bioactive Compounds and Cancer*. New York: Humana Press; 2010:469–496.
124. Hann HW, Stahlhut MW, Menduke H. Iron enhances tumor growth. Observation on spontaneous mammary tumors in mice. *Cancer*. 1991;68(11):2407–2410.
125. Luanpitpong S, Talbott SJ, Rojanasakul Y, Nimmannit U, Pongrakhananon V, Wang L, Chanvorachote P. Regulation of lung cancer cell migration and invasion by reactive oxygen species and caveolin-1. *J Biol Chem*. 2010;285(50):38832–38840.
126. Stevens RG, Morris JE, Cordis GA, Anderson LE, Rosenberg DW, Sasser LB. Oxidative damage in colon and mammary tissue of the HFE-knockout mouse. *Free Radic Biol Med*. 2003;34(9):1212–1216.
127. de Almeida SF, Picarote G, Fleming JV, Carmo-Fonseca M, Azevedo JE, de Sousa M. Chemical chaperones reduce endoplasmic reticulum stress and prevent mutant HFE aggregate formation. *J Biol Chem*. 2007;282(38):27905–27912.
128. Gunel-Ozcan A, Alyılmaz-Bekmez S, Guler EN, Guc D. HFE H63D mutation frequency shows an increase in Turkish women with breast cancer. *BMC Cancer*. 2006;6:37–137.
129. Gharib AF, Karam RA, Pasha HF, Radwan MI, Elsawy WH. Polymorphisms of hemochromatosis, and alpha-1 antitrypsin genes in Egyptian HCV patients with and without hepatocellular carcinoma. *Gene*. 2011;489(2):98–102.
130. Elmberg M, Hultcrantz R, Ekbom A, Brandt L, Olsson S, Olsson R, Lindgren S, Lööf L, Stål P, Wallerstedt S, Almer S, Sandberg-Gertzén H, Askling J. Cancer risk in patients with hereditary hemochromatosis and in their first-degree relatives. *Gastroenterology*. 2003;125(6):1733–1741.
131. Martinez di Montemuros F, Tavazzi D, Salsano E, Piepoli T, Pollo B, Fiorelli G, Finocchiaro G. High frequency of the H63D mutation of the hemochromatosis gene (HFE) in malignant gliomas. *Neurology*. 2001;57(7):1342–11342.
132. Dorak MT, Mackay RK, Relton CL, Worwood M, Parker L, Hall AG. Hereditary hemochromatosis gene (HFE) variants are associated with birth weight and childhood leukemia risk. *Pediatr Blood Cancer*. 2009;53(7):1242–1248.
133. Shi Z, Johnstone D, Talseth-Palmer BA, Evans T-J, Spigelman AD, Groombridge C, Milward EA, Olynyk JK, Suchy J, Kurzawski G, Lubinski J, Scott RJ. Haemochromatosis HFE gene polymorphisms as potential modifiers of hereditary nonpolyposis colorectal cancer risk and onset age. *Int J Cancer*. 2009;125(1):78–83.
134. Shaheen NJ, Silverman LM, Keku T, Lawrence LB, Rohlfs EM, Martin CF, Galanko J, Sandler RS. Association between hemochromatosis (HFE) gene mutation carrier status and the risk of colon cancer. *J Natl Cancer Inst*. 2003;95(2):154–159.
135. Agudo A, Bonet C, Sala N, Muñoz X, Aranda N, Fonseca-Nunes A, Clavel-Chapelon F, Boutron-Ruault MC, Vineis P, Panico S, Palli D, Tumino R, Grioni S, Quirós J, Molina E, Navarro C, Barricarte A, Chamosa S, Allen NE, Khaw K-T, Bueno-de-Mesquita H, Siersema PD, Numans ME, Trichopoulou A, Lagiou P, Trichopoulos D, Kaaks R, Canzian F, Boeing H, Meidtner K, Johansson M, Sund M, Manjer J, Overvad K, Tjonneland A, Lund E, Weiderpass E, Jenab M, Fedirko V, Offerhaus GA, Riboli E, González CA, Jakszyn P. Hemochromatosis (HFE) gene mutations and risk of gastric cancer in the European Prospective Investigation into Cancer and Nutrition (EPIC) study. *Carcinogenesis*. 2013;34(6):1244–1250.
136. Ropero P, Briceno O, Lopez-Alonso G, Agundez JA, Gonzalez Fernandez FA, Garcia-Hoz F, Villegas Martinez A, Diaz-Rubio M, Ladero JM. The H63D mutation in the HFE gene is related to the risk of hepatocellular carcinoma. *Rev Esp Enferm Dig*. 2007;99(7):376–381.
137. Kallianpur AR, Hall LD, Yadav M, Christman BW, Dittus RS, Haines JL, Parl FF, Summar ML. Increased prevalence of the HFE C282Y hemochromatosis allele in women with breast cancer. *Cancer Epidemiol Biomarkers Prev*. 2004;13(2):205–212.
138. Chen W, Zhao H, Li T, Yao H. HFE gene C282Y variant is associated with colorectal cancer in Caucasians: a meta-analysis. *Tumour Biol*. 2013;34(4):2255–2259.
139. Lauret E, Rodriguez M, Gonzalez S, Linares A, Lopez-Vazquez A, Martinez-Borra J, Rodrigo L, Lopez-Larrea C. HFE gene mutations in alcoholic and virus-related cirrhotic patients with hepatocellular carcinoma. *Am J Gastroenterol*. 2002;97(4):1016–1021.

140. Fargion S, Stazi MA, Fracanzani AL, Mattioli M, Sampietro M, Tavazzi D, Bertelli C, Patriarca V, Mariani C, Fiorelli G. Mutations in the HFE gene and their interaction with exogenous risk factors in hepatocellular carcinoma. *Blood Cells Mol Dis*. 2001;27(2):505–511.
141. Asberg A, Thorstensen K, Irgens WO, Romundstad PR, Hveem K. Cancer risk in HFE C282Y homozygotes: results from the HUNT 2 study. *Scand J Gastroenterol*. 2013;48(2):189–195.
142. Osborne NJ, Gurrin LC, Allen KJ, Constantine CC, Delatycki MB, McLaren CE, Gertig DM, Anderson GJ, Southey MC, Olynyk JK, Powell LW, Hopper JL, Giles GG, English DR. HFE C282Y homozygotes are at increased risk of breast and colorectal cancer. *Hepatology*. 2010;51(4):1311–1318.
143. Nahon P, Sutton A, Rufat P, Ziol M, Thabut G, Schischmanoff PO, Vidaud D, Charnaux N, Couvert P, Ganne-Carrie N, Trinchet JC, Gattegno L, Beaugrand M. Liver iron, HFE gene mutations, and hepatocellular carcinoma occurrence in patients with cirrhosis. *Gastroenterology*. 2008;134(1):102–110.
144. Willis G, Wimperis JZ, Lonsdale R, Fellows IW, Watson MA, Skipper LM, Jennings BA. Incidence of liver disease in people with HFE mutations. *Gut*. 2000;46(3):401–404.
145. Gannon PO, Medelci S, Le Page C, Beaulieu M, Provencher DM, Mes-Masson A-M, Santos MM. Impact of hemochromatosis gene (HFE) mutations on epithelial ovarian cancer risk and prognosis. *Int J Cancer*. 2011;128(10):2326–2334.
146. Rodriguez-Lopez R, Donoso M, Fernandez-Cavada M, Gonzalez LM, Margallo A, Corral C, Gallego M, Garcia de Caceres MT, Herrera T, Gonzalez C, Vagace JM, Gervasini G. Diagnostic utility of HFE variants in Spanish patients: association with HLA alleles and role in susceptibility to acute lymphoblastic leukemia. *Gene*. 2013;514(1):31–35.
147. Abraham BK, Justenhoven C, Pesch B, Harth V, Weirich G, Baisch C, Rabstein S, Ko YD, Bruning T, Fischer HP, Haas S, Brod S, Oberkanins C, Hamann U, Brauch H. Investigation of genetic variants of genes of the hemochromatosis pathway and their role in breast cancer. *Cancer Epidemiol Biomarkers Prev*. 2005;14(5):1102–1107.
148. Altes A, Gimferrer E, Capella G, Barcelo MJ, Baiget M. Colorectal cancer and HFE gene mutations. *Haematologica*. 1999;84(5):479–480.
149. Boige V, Castéra L, de Roux N, Ganne-Carrié N, Ducot B, Pelletier G, Beaugrand M, Buffet C. Lack of association between HFE gene mutations and hepatocellular carcinoma in patients with cirrhosis. *Gut*. 2003;52(8): 1178–1181.
150. Guruvayoorappan C. Tumor versus tumor-associated macrophages: how hot is the link? *Integr Cancer Ther*. 2008;7(2):90–95.
151. Kzhyshkowska J, Riabov V, Gudima A, Wang N, Orekhov A, Mickley A. Role of tumor associated macrophages in tumor angiogenesis and lymphangiogenesis. *Front Physiol*. 2014;5(75).
152. Weston C, Hund W, Nixon A, Neely E, Webb B, Alkhateeb A, Connor J. Host H67D genotype affects tumor growth in mouse melanoma. *J Cancer Sci Ther*. 2015;7:216–223.
153. Ong SM, Tan YC, Beretta O, Jiang D, Yeap WH, Tai JJ, Wong WC, Yang H, Schwarz H, Lim KH, Koh PK, Ling KL, Wong SC. Macrophages in human colorectal cancer are pro-inflammatory and prime T cells towards an anti-tumour type-1 inflammatory response. *Eur J Immunol*. 2012;42(1):89–100.
154. Hashimoto K, Hirai M, Kurosawa Y. Identification of a mouse homolog for the human hereditary haemochromatosis candidate gene. *Biochem Biophys Res Commun*. 1997;230(1):35–39.
155. Bahram S, Gilfillan S, Kühn LC, Moret R, Schulze JB, Lebeau A, Schümann K. Experimental hemochromatosis due to MHC class I HFE deficiency: immune status and iron metabolism. *Proc Natl Acad Sci USA*. 1999;96(23):13312–13317.
156. Levy JE, Montross LK, Cohen DE, Fleming MD, Andrews NC. The C282Y mutation causing hereditary hemochromatosis does not produce a null allele. *Blood*. 1999;94(1):9–11.
157. Tomatsu S, Orii KO, Fleming RE, Holden CC, Waheed A, Britton RS, Gutierrez MA, Velez-Castrillon S, Bacon BR, Sly WS. Contribution of the H63D mutation in HFE to murine hereditary hemochromatosis. *Proc Natl Acad Sci USA*. 2003;100(26):15788–15793.
158. Merryweather-Clarke AT, Pointon JJ, Shearman JD, Robson KJ. Global prevalence of putative haemochromatosis mutations. *J Med Genet*. 1997;34(4):275–278.
159. Pulliam JF, Jennings CD, Kryscio RJ, Davis DG, Wilson D, Montine TJ, Schmitt FA, Markesbery WR. Association of HFE mutations with neurodegeneration and oxidative stress in Alzheimer's disease and correlation with APOE. *Am J Med Genet B Neuropsychiatr Genet*. 2003;119B(1):48–53.

CHAPTER

5

Chemical Elements and Oxidative Status in Neuroinflammation

Michela Ferraldeschi, Silvia Romano*, Maria C. Buscarinu*, Arianna Fornasiero*, Rosella Mechelli*, Benedetta Cerasoli*, Anna Pino**, Sonia Brescianini†, Carlo Mattei*, Maria A. Stazi**, Alessandro Alimonti**, Marco Salvetti*, Giovanni Ristori**

*Center for Experimental Neurological Therapies, S. Andrea Hospital, "Sapienza" University of Rome, Rome, Italy

**National Institute of Health, Rome, Italy

†Center for Epidemiology, Surveillance and Health Promotion, National Institute of Health, Rome, Italy

OUTLINE

INTRODUCTION

Metals are widely found in our environment and humans are exposed to these metals from numerous sources, including contaminated air, water, soil, and food. The metals are divided into two groups: essential metals, such as chromium (Cr), cobalt (Co), copper (Cu), iron (Fe),

Biometals in Neurodegenerative Diseases. http://dx.doi.org/10.1016/B978-0-12-804562-6.00005-1

magnesium (Mg), manganese (Mn), molybdenum (Mo), nickel (Ni), and zinc (Zn); nonessential metals like cadmium (Cd), mercury (Hg), lead (Pb). Essential metals play important roles in the human body being involved in principal cellular functions. They are indeed required for optimal central nervous system (CNS) function, and the maintenance of their fine balance is vital, because both deficiency and excess can result in aberrant function of CNS and other main organs.

Excessive metal accumulation in the CNS may be toxic inducing oxidative stress, mitochondrial dysfunction, DNA fragmentation, protein misfolding, endoplasmic reticulum (ER) stress, autophagy dysregulation, and activation of apoptosis.[1] Many studies have shown that metals increase the production of reactive oxygen species (ROS) as superoxide ion, hydrogen peroxide, and hydroxyl radical resulting in a condition known as "oxidative stress" (OS). As a consequence, cells under OS display various dysfunctions due to lesions caused by ROS to lipids, proteins, and DNA. Consequently, it is suggested that the toxicities associated with metals might be partially due to oxidative tissue damage.[2,3] Neurotoxicity induced by metals is suspected of being involved in the pathogenesis of various neurological disorders including, among others, multiple sclerosis (MS), Alzheimer's disease (AD), amyotrophic lateral sclerosis (ALS), Guillain–Barré disease (GBD), Huntington's disease (HD), and Parkinson's disease (PD).[1]

MS is a chronic inflammatory disease of the CNS leading to demyelination and neurodegeneration of as yet unknown aetiology. The disease is plurifactorial, being assumed that it is caused by an interplay between environmental factors and susceptibility genes. An international consensus has defined four different categories of MS: relapsing-remitting MS (RRMS), secondary progressive MS (SPMS), primary progressive MS (PPMS), and progressive-relapsing (PRMS).[4] Most patients (80%–85%) have an initial course with episodes of neurological dysfunction followed by partial or complete recovery (the relapsing-remitting -RR- form of MS); over time in a majority of patients the course of the disease becomes secondary progressive (SPMS) with a progressive accumulation of disability. In the primary progressive (PPMS; 10%–15% of all cases), the disease progression is observed from onset, while in the PRMS subtype, the disease is progressive from onset but patients also refer with clear acute relapses. In these patients, periods between relapses are characterized by continuing progression.[5,6]

Accumulating data, based on the biochemical analysis of cerebrospinal fluid, blood samples, tissue homogenates, and animal models of MS, indicate that OS plays a central role in the pathogenesis of MS being implicated as mediator of demyelination and axonal damage.[7–13] Overproduction of ROS and reactive nitrogen species by macrophages/microglia can cause cellular damage and subsequent cell death by necrosis or apoptosis by oxidizing cardinal cellular components, such as lipids, proteins, and nucleic acids.[14] Oxidized DNA molecules, lipid, and protein adducts are found in active MS lesions and are associated spatially and quantitatively with apoptotic oligodendrocytes and neurodegeneration in the brain of MS patients.[15,16]

Reported evidences suggests that exposure to some heavy metals may alter immune responses and may contribute to induce autoimmune disorders.[17–22] Considering the complexity of their interaction with the immune system, several mechanisms have been proposed to explain the roles of metals in the possible induction of autoimmunity: direct binding to major histocompatibility complex (MHC) molecules or even to the clonotypic receptors, that is, T-cell receptor may cause aberrant MHC expression on target cells, inhibition of T regulatory cells, changes of cytokine production; and other mechanisms of metal-induced tolerance breakdown.

Several studies assessed metal imbalance and OS in MS and other neurological diseases. Here we will discuss the results of our previous studies evaluating the levels of many chemical elements and oxidative status in the serum of patients with MS and clinically isolated syndrome (CIS). We also review the other reported data on the role of metals with supposed etiologic relevance on MS pathogenesis.

METAL-INDUCED NEUROTOXICITY AND MULTIPLE SCLEROSIS

Zn is an essential trace element, it is required for essential catalytic functions in > 300 enzymes and is involved in a variety of general cellular functions, including signal transduction, transcription, and replication.[23,24] It is abundantly present in the brain, mainly in presynaptic vesicles in neurons, where it plays an important role in maintaining normal brain functions. It is believed that the abnormality of Zn plays a role in neuronal damage observed in cerebral ischemia, brain trauma, epilepsy, vascular type dementia, and neurodegenerative disease, such as AD.[25,26] Neurotoxicity caused by an excess of Zn appears to be related to the mitochondrial production of ROS, alteration of the normal activity of metabolic enzymes, activation of apoptotic processes, and increased formation of fibrillar beta amyloid aggregation.[27–29]

The link between Zn and MS may also be connected to the consequences that the zinc alterations have on the immune system. Zn deficiency impairs both the innate and the adaptive immune system while high dosages induce altered immune cell functions. T-cell count and function are delicately regulated by the concentration (high or low) of zinc in the cell or plasma. Natural killer (NK) cell activity, phagocytosis of macrophage, and neutrophils are also impaired by decreased zinc concentrations.[30] Higashi and coworkers[31] investigated how Zn causes the sequential activation of microglia, that is known to be an essential step of MS immunopathogenesis. Indeed after the exposure of microglia to zinc, the authors demonstrated that a plasma membrane-type Zn transporter increased the extracellular ATP concentration, triggering microglial activation via the NADPH oxidase, and poly(ADP-ribose) polymerase (PARP)-1. Zn is the cofactor of all matrix metalloproteinases (MMPs) that are a group of proteases with a wide spectrum of activities, such as remodeling of the extracellular matrix and modifying cell-matrix interactions.[32] Being myelin basic protein (MBP), components of blood-brain barrier (BBB), and neural/glial antigen 2 (NG2) substrates of these proteases,[33–35] changes of the local Zn levels could induce typical alterations of the MS pathogenic loop (T cell migration across the BBB and breakdown of MBP).[36]

There are several published studies evaluating plasma or serum Zn levels in MS compared to healthy subjects since 1980, with the evidence of heterogeneity in their results: some showed significant reduction[37–42] or increase of Zn concentration,[43,44] and in other cases significant differences have not been shown.[45–50] A systematic review and a meta-analysis of the published results of Zn measuring studies was performed by Bredholt and coworkers and reported a significant reduction in overall serum or plasma Zn levels in MS patient versus healthy controls (95% CI of $-3.66, -0.93$ $p = 0.001$).[51] The heterogeneity in the results on serum or plasma levels in MS patients of the studies seen earlier may be due to the influence of many confounders or the uncritical mixing of patients with different age, sex, disease subtype, duration, and disability that might interfere with the correct interpretation of the results. It is unclear if there is a possible beneficial effect of Zn supplementation on inhibition of the MS exacerbation. Some evidences have reported beneficial effects of Zn aspartate on experimental autoimmune encephalomyelitis (EAE), an animal model for MS.[52,53] In a randomized, double-blind, placebo-controlled clinical trial by Salari and coworkers patients who received the zinc sulfate for 12 week compared to placebo group had no improvement of neurological signs.[54]

Cu is an essential transition metal present in all tissues that acts as a cofactor for numerous enzymes in CNS (tyrosinase, peptidylglycine α-amidating mono-oxygenase, copper/zinc superoxide dismutase, ceruloplasmin, hephaestin, dopamine-β-hydoxylase, and cytochrome *c* oxidase) and plays an important role in CNS development;[55] indeed excessive Cu has been associated with multiple neurological diseases, such as prion disease, ALS, PD, AD, HD, and Wilson's disease (WD).[55–57] Elevated Cu levels may be involved in ROS production, that results in mitochondrial damage, DNA breakage, neuronal injury,[55,58] and Cu interaction with β-amyloid peptide and α-synuclein could result in AD and PD respectively.[59–61] The physiological basis of a link between Cu and pathogenesis of MS has not been completely clarified. The results derived from studies comparing the serum Cu levels in MS patients and controls are conflicting: in some studies, a significant difference was not demonstrated,[47] while in others significantly higher[39,42,44] or lower levels[38,48] of Cu in plasma or serum were found in MS patients. In a study in which Cu values in whole blood of MS patients were compared with healthy persons, only a minor difference was observed.[62] In a study by Melø and coworkers, Cu concentrations were significantly elevated in cerebrospinal fluid (CSF) of MS patients compared to the levels in the control group.[63] A study by Choi and coworkers was aimed at evaluating the therapeutic potential of clioquinol (CQ), an antifungal and antiprotozoal drug with chelating properties for Cu and Zn ions. After induction in female mice of EAE by immunization with myelin oligodendrocyte glycoprotein (MOG35-55), CQ was given by gavage once per day for the whole duration of the experiment. The authors observed a reduction of the daily clinical score and incidence rate of EAE mice, suppression of demyelination, reduction of inflammatory cell infiltration, inhibition of BBB disruption, and decreased MMP-9 activation.[64] This study suggests that the transition metals may play a role at different levels in the pathogenesis of neuroinflammation.

Fe is an essential metal involved in many crucial processes including oxygen transport, a variety of redox reactions, myelin production, glucose metabolism, neurotransmitter production, and DNA replication.[65] Brain iron uptake is regulated by the expression of transferrin receptor 1 in endothelial cells of the BBB. Transferrin-bound iron in the systemic circulation is endocytosed after binding with this receptor, and, after crossing BBB, it is released from transferrin into the interstitium.[65,66] Abnormal Fe homeostasis with increased iron deposition in the brain has been implicated in the pathophysiology of many neurological disorders including MS.[65] An increased level of brain iron may promote neurotoxicity due to free radical formation, dopamine autoxidation, and mitochondrial fragmentation.[65,67–70]

As previously said, the OS induced by ROS, plays a major role in the pathogenesis of demyelination and axonal damage in both MS and EAE.[14] In 1982, Craelius and coworkers conducted a histological study on postmortem cerebral samples of MS patients: they observed iron depositions in sections surrounding demyelinated plaque; myelinated white matter near the lesion contained numerous iron-laden ovoid bodies and axons that stained positively for iron: positive reactions were also found within blood vessels of gray matter near the lesion.[71] Hametner and coworkers recently examined the nonheme iron distribution and the expression of the iron-related proteins ferritin, hephaestin, and ceruloplasmin in relation to the oxidative damage in the brain tissue of 33 MS and 30 control cases. They found significant decrease of iron in the normal-appearing white matter (NAWM) correlating with disease duration. In MS lesions, iron was apparently released from dying oligodendrocytes, resulting in extracellular accumulation of iron and uptake into macrophages and microglia that showed signs of cell degeneration. Accumulation of iron was observed at edges and within centers of lesions, in astrocytes and axons.[72]

Conventional and advanced magnetic resonance imaging (MRI) techniques has aided characterization of Fe deposits in both gray matter (GM) and white matter of patients with MS. Brain Fe accumulation may result in signal loss or hypointensity on T2-weighted images and hyperintensity on T1-weighted images. Cortical and subcortical GM hypointensities on T2 images, suggestive of excessive iron deposition, are relatively common in MS patients and have been associated to disease duration, brain atrophy, disability progression, and cognitive impairment.[73–83] The relevance of abnormal Fe deposition in cortical and deep GM was also confirmed by use of recent advanced MRI techniques.[84–92] Similar findings have been shown also in CIS patients.[93,94] In a study by Hagemeier and coworkers performed using susceptibility-weighted filtered phase imaging, patients with CIS showed significantly increased content and volume of Fe in various subcortical deep GM structures and these findings precede structure-specific atrophy.[95]

Significantly lower serum Fe concentration in the blood of MS patients compared with healthy people emerged in some clinical studies.[39–41,49–50] The altered systemic Fe metabolism (namely changes in serum levels of ferritin, transferrin, and transferrin receptors) showed by Sfagos and coworkers[96] are in agreement with these findings and may suggest an increased Fe turnover or presence of mechanisms that facilitate the dislocation of Fe from the peripheral fluids into the brain of patients with neurological diseases. Further investigations using antioxidants or iron chelation are needed to assess the beneficial effect in treating MS patients.[65]

Aluminum (Al) is a nonessential metal, highly abundant and ubiquitously distributed as environmental and industrial toxicant that is also contained in many food products. Toxic levels of Al have been involved in many neurological diseases, such as AD, ALS, GBD, and MS.[97] The Al neurotoxicity may be due to induction of oxidative stress and mitochondrial dysfunction.[98–103] Al is also able to mimic biological functions of metals, such as Mg, calcium (Ca), and Fe triggering many biochemical alterations. Evidence suggested that Al toxicity is mediated through ROS production and Fe accumulation.[104]

Exley and coworkers demonstrated that urinary concentrations of Al were significantly increased in RRMS and SPMS with levels of Al excretion similar to those seen in Al intoxication.[105] These findings are consistent with the results from another group reporting that, after the use of a chelating agent, MS patients showed significantly higher levels of urinary Al compared to healthy subjects.[106] Few and conflicting forms of evidence emerged from studies examining the Al blood concentration in MS patients.[39–40,49–50] Further studies have to be conducted to assess if Al is involved in development of MS.

Mg may affect the maintenance and function of nerve cells as well as the proliferation and synthesis of lymphocytes. Moreover, Mg interacts with other minerals, such as Al, Ca, and Zn in biological systems, supporting the assumption that modification of this element may be a cofactor in the development of the disease.[107] Mg concentration has been shown to decrease in the CNS of MS patients.[108] Additional studies have shown variations in Mg concentrations in serum and cerebrospinal fluid from patients with MS.[39–40,48,49]

A long studied metal, as a possible contributor in MS development, has been Hg. Methylmercury (MeHg) is a toxic organic metal considered an environmental contaminant for which the primary exposure source for humans is fish consumption.[109] Hg can have toxic effects on many organs[110] and the neurological disorders related to its exposure in acute cases are due to its ability to cross the BBB and accumulate in the CNS.[111] MeHg can induce an extensive array of pathogenic mechanisms affecting CNS functions: ROS generation,[112] tau phosphorylation, mitochondrial dysfunction,[110] alteration of the flow of calcium,[113] inhibition of neuronal differentiation of rodent embryonic neural stem cells,[114] caspase-dependent apoptosis and autophagy in the NSCs,[115] impairment of dopamine metabolism.[116] Its involvement as a possible risk factor in MS was related to the supposed long term release of Hg vapor from Hg containing dental amalgam tooth fillings; however, there are controversial results from case series and the role of mercury has not been confirmed.[117–119] In a metaanalysis the pooled odds ratio(OR) for the risk of MS among amalgam users was consistent, with a slight, but not significant increase of MS risk.[120] The studies that evaluated the serum Hg concentration in MS patients in comparison with healthy subjects gave different results: in some, serum mercury levels were significantly higher than controls,[121] in others, this elevation was not significant,[49–50] and finally few studies showed lower levels in MS patients.[39–40,45]

Pb is a nonessential heavy metal whose neurotoxicity is well known. After ingestion or inhalation this metal can accumulate in different regions of the CNS and impaired various neurological functions with mechanisms comparable to those of Hg.[122–124] The link between exposure to Pb and Hg and neurotoxicity in MS is mediated also by immunological mechanisms and this is suggested by the presence of autoantibodies, primarily IgG, against neuronal cytoskeletal proteins, neurofilaments (NFs), and MBP in humans and animals exposed to either metal. Titers of IgG against NFs and MBP significantly correlated with blood Pb or urinary Hg, the typical indices of exposure. In rats exposed to metals, histopathology findings indicated that both central and peripheral nervous system are damaged. In addition there was evidence of astrogliosis, which is indicative of neuronal damage in the CNS, and the presence of IgG along the BBB, with disruption of BBB.[125–127] As for Hg, conflicting evidence emerges from studies examining the Pb blood level in MS patients.[39–41,44,45,49,50]

METALS AND OXIDATIVE STATUS IN MULTIPLE SCLEROSIS

After the suggestion by various authors on the role of some chemical elements in neurodegeneration and the presence of few and controversial studies on serum, in 2006 we conducted a study to obtain a profile of chemical elements and oxidative status in three complex neurological diseases: AD and PD, with a prevalent neurodegenerative component, and MS, with prevalent inflammatory immunopathogenesis.[40]

We enrolled 308 patients: 53 patients with AD, 71 with PD, 60 affected by MS, and 124 healthy individuals living in the same urban area. The strict exclusion criteria were as follows: severe cardiological, respiratory, kidney, or liver disease; absorption abnormalities; infections; thyroid hormone therapy; lithium therapy; vitamin or mineral supplement intake; vegetarian diet; artificial metallic bodies.

The MS group included 60 patients (38 females and 22 males; mean age 38.5 ± 10.4 years, range 24–66 years) with definite MS diagnosed according to the revised McDonald criteria.[128] Forty-nine patients had RRMS, while the remaining eleven had a secondary progressive form. Mean expanded disability status scale (EDSS) was 1.9 ± 1.7 (range 1–8) and mean disease duration was 105.3 ± 102.9 months (range 12–636 months). All the patients were clinically stable at the time of sample collection and had not taken steroid therapy for at least 3 months. Forty-two patients were taking disease-modifying therapies (25 interferon beta, 10 mitoxantrone, 6 glatiramer acetate and 1 azathioprine).

We have measured the serum concentration of 26 elements: Al, barium (Ba), beryllium (Be), bismuth (Bi), Cd, Ca, Cu, Co, Cr, Fe, Hg, lithium (Li), Mg, molybdenum (Mo), nickel (Ni), Pb, antimony (Sb), silicon (Si), tin (Sn), strontium (Sr), Tl, vanadium (V), tungsten (W), Zn, and zirconium (Zr). Both serum oxidative status (SOS) and serum antioxidant capacity (SAC) were spectrophotometrically determined as the serum concentration of hydroperoxides and serum ability to oppose the oxidative action of a hypochlorous acid solution. Patient groups were compared with controls using the Mann-Whitney U-test with a p value corrected by means of Bonferroni's method, as multiple independent statistical analyses were carried out simultaneously.[129] The statistical analysis applied was a forward discriminant analysis (FDA), which is a well-known multivariate statistical classification technique used to determine which variables discriminate between two or more groups.

We found numerous significant differences in the concentration of chemical element and oxidative parameter values in the MS group compared to healthy subjects (Table 5.1).

TABLE 5.1 Significant Differences Between MS Patients and Controls in Element Concentration and Oxidative Status

Parameter[a]	Controls	MS	Profile[b]
Be	0.21 (0.13–0.32)	034 (0.21–0.45)	+
Ca	64,236 (59,380–68,34)	73,039 (68,786–76,417)	+
Cd	0.09 (0.06–0.12)	0.16 (0.08–0.20)	+
Fe	1610 (1228–1995)	920 (752–1294)	−
Ni	0.39 (0.19–0.76)	0.81 (0.41–1.37)	+
Sb	0.09 (0.06–0.14)	0.17 (0.11–0.33)	+
Si	137 (96–224)	314 (226–385)	+
Sn	0.53 (0.35–0.88)	1.39 (0.96–2.32)	+
W	0.03 (0.02–0.05)	0.06 (0.03–0.08)	+
Zn	795 (703–897)	650 (591–710)	−
Zr	0.10 (0.08–0.14)	0.36 (0.08–0.66)	+
SOS	272 (242–300)	331 (306–349)	+
SAC	363 (340–387)	326 (305–340)	−

[a] *Medians (25%–75%) of elements (in μg/L), SOS (in U.CARR, where 1 U.CARR corresponds to 0.08 mg of peroxyl radicals for 100 mL of hydrogen peroxide) and SAC (in μmol of HClO/mL of sample).*
[b] *Higher or lower concentrations than controls (P ≤ 0.0003 according to Bonferroni's correction).*

A significant increase in Be, Ca, Cd, Ni, Sb, Sn, Si, W, Zr, and SOS and a decrease in Fe, Zn, and SAC were detected in MS patients. We also found numerous significant differences between the other two neurological diseases considered and healthy status, highlighting in particular a significant decrease in Fe, Zn, and SAC and an increase in SOS that were shared by all the diseases. The imbalance in serum chemical elements and oxidative status observed in our study is greater than previously believed and this was especially evident in MS, where as many as 13 out of 28 parameters were different. This finding suggests that there are complex profiles of altered elements for each disease, rather than single chemical element imbalances, which is in keeping with the multifactorial etiology of the three neurological diseases studied.

Furthermore, the evidence of a shared imbalance (reduction in Fe, Zn, and SAC and increase in SOS) detected in all diseases can suggest a common mechanism that, in the context of complex disease-specific profiles of element changes, contributes to disease status. Oxidative damage is one of the most plausible mechanisms underlying this shared imbalance because SAC and SOS changes are a direct expression of oxidative stress and the findings on reduction of Zn and Fe are consistent with data emerging from the other studies as seen earlier.

FDA identified unprecedented disease-specific profiles of element imbalances. Each profile included the aforementioned shared imbalance (reduction in Fe, Zn, and SAC and increase in SOS) plus element changes (positively or negatively correlated with the discriminant functions) that characterized each disease: in the case of MS we found high values of Ca and Zr. The fact that Ca levels in patients were significantly higher than those in controls might be link to the pathogenic impact of Ca on T-cell function[130] and axonal damage.[131–132] The potential pathogenetic and predictive value of changes in Zr concentration, emerging in this study and confirmed in other, our studies[39,49,50] are yet to be evaluated.

METALS AND OXIDATIVE STATUS IN CLINICALLY ISOLATED SYNDROMES

The vast majority of MS cases start with a CIS that is generally reversible. Approximately half of these cases convert to clinically definite MS (CDMS) within two years of the diagnosis, while about 10% of CIS people remain free of further neurological events, even in the presence of a brain and spinal cord MRI compatible with MS.

After the evidence in our previous study[40] that it's possible to detect a complex imbalance in serum chemical elements and oxidative status in patients with MS, we conducted a study with the same approach to understand whether this imbalance affects people with CIS and, if so, whether it predicts conversion to clinically definite MS (CDMS).[50]

We compared serum concentration of 22 chemical elements Al, Ca, Cd, Co, Cr, Cu, Fe, Hg, Li, Mg, Mn, Mo, Ni, Pb, Sb, Sn, Sr, Tl, V, W, Zn, and Zr, (SOS and SAC) in 49 CIS people who were matched for age-class, sex, and geographic origin with two control groups, consisting of 49 patients with CDMS and 49 healthy donors (HD).

Inclusion criteria included: (1) a single clinical episode suggestive of MS with monofocal or multifocal onset; (2) a baseline brain MRI scan supporting a diagnosis of MS (i.e., with at least three lesions on the T2W images so as to include only patients in whom evolution to CDMS was more likely); (3) age between 18 and 50 years; (4) no steroid treatment in the 2 months prior to inclusion in the study and no disease modifying therapies (DMT). Eligible patients underwent triple-dose Gd-enhanced MRI and venous puncture for the study of serum chemical elements and oxidative status at the same time point.

A one-way ANOVA, using Bonferroni's adjustment, was performed to compare the trace elements and the oxidative status of the three groups (CIS people, CDMS patients, and HD). In order to investigate which of the variables accounted for the main differences in the average score profiles of each of the groups, a discriminant analysis (DA) was applied.

To identify predictors of a second demyelinating episode, a logistic regression analysis was performed using three models. Besides age and gender, these models were based on brain MRI data, that is, number of T2W and T1W Gd-enhancing lesions (1st model), serum element profile, and oxidative status, that is, the score obtained from elements that best discriminate CIS people with and those without a relapse at the DA (2nd model), and MRI data combined with the score (3rd model). The third model yielded an equation that can be used to estimate the probability of having a relapse, given the age, gender, and baseline characteristics of a CIS person, on the basis of the MRI findings, serum element profile, and oxidative status. Receiver operating characteristic (ROC) curves of the first and third models were compared to test whether the score improved the predictive potential of the MRI data. The area under the curve was estimated for each model.

Differences emerged in several of the elements and in the oxidative status in our three groups ($P < 0.0007$): the CIS people and CDMS patients, when compared with HD, shared an increase in Ca, Cd, Mo, Sn, Zr, and SOS, as well as a decrease in Fe and SAC; moreover, Al, Ca, Cr, Cu, Mg, and Zn values were significantly higher in CIS people than in CDMS patients; last, we observed a relationship between changes in Fe and SAC levels (CDMS < CIS <HD) as well as in Sn and SOS levels (CDMS > CIS > HD) and the status of the demyelinating process. Since this univariate analysis strongly suggested distinct serum chemical element and oxidative status profiles in each group, we applied the DA as a multivariate approach that revealed a major contribution of Ca, Fe, Sn, Zn, SOC, and SAC.

By the end of the follow-up (36 months), 24 people with CIS remained relapse-free, while 25 had reported a second episode, thus converting to CDMS. To identify the baseline predictors of relapse, we used a logistic regression approach identifying three models.

In the first model we introduced, along with age and gender, the MRI data: T2W lesions were < 9 in 8 (16.3%) subjects, 9–20 in 21 (42.8%) subjects, > 20 in the remaining 20 (40.8%) subjects; active scans were present in 21 (43%) subjects. T2W lesion > 20 or ≤ 20 and presence or absence of T1W Gd-enhancing lesions proved to be the best predictive findings, although they did not reach significance; the area under the ROC curve was 61.3%.

The second model was based on the baseline profile of the serum chemical elements and oxidative status of CIS people. For this purpose, DA was performed on four groups: HD, CDMS, and CIS people with and those without a relapse over the follow-up period. As the third function discriminates between people with and those without a relapse, a score (a summary measure based on the best discriminating elements) was calculated using the canonical discriminant function coefficients obtained from the third function (F3 score: see Appendix e-1 on the neurology website at www.neurology.org). In this logistic model, the OR was 0.42 (95%CI 0.2–0.8; $P = 0.01$): for each score unit increase, the odds of having a second episode decreased by 58% (i.e., high Ca, Fe, Sn, and SAC values as well as low Cr, Zn, and Zr values reduced the probability of having a relapse); the area under the ROC curve was 74.2%.

The third regression model integrated the MRI data and F3 score, along with age and sex: defining the contribution of the serum chemical elements and oxidative status to the MRI findings. The third model improved the predictive potential of the first model, particularly as regards to the high sensitivity and specificity. The area under the ROC curve in the third model was 78.9%. Subjects with T2W lesion > 20 had a higher, albeit nonsignificant, risk of a second demyelinating episode (OR = 3.78, $P = 0.109$), although the odds of a relapse decreased by 63% for each unit increase in the score, after adjusting for the number of lesions, age and gender (OR 0.37; 95% CI 0.18– 0.76; $P = 0.007$). Using these results, we calculated by an equation (see Appendix e-2 on the neurology website at www.neurology.org), the probability of a second demyelinating episode that, if applied to our sample of CIS people, would correctly predict conversion to CDMS in as many as 70% of the cases.

CONCLUSIONS

Our study in MS and other neurodegenerative diseases (AD and PD) allowed us to draw several interesting points: descriptive statistics revealed numerous differences between each disease and healthy status; a concordant imbalance (reduction in Fe, Zn, and SAC, and increase in SOS) was shared by AD, PD, and MS; multivariate statistical approach (FDA) yielded three significant discriminant functions based on age, SOS, Ca, Fe, Si, Sn, V, Zn, and Zr, and identified disease-specific profiles of element imbalances.

The peculiar imbalance in serum elements and oxidative status that characterizes CIS people may predict conversion to CDMS, suggesting the contribution of chemical elements and oxidative stress to disease causation and providing complex biomarkers, that, associated to neuroimaging, may help predict disease evolution or treatment response.

References

1. Chen P, Miah MR, Aschner M. Metals and Neurodegeneration. *F1000Res*. 2016;17(5).
2. Stohs SJ, Bagchi D. Oxidative mechanisms in the toxicity of metal ions. *Free Radic Biol Med*. 1995;18(2):321–336.
3. Ercal N, Gurer-Orhan H, Aykin-Burns N. Toxic metals and oxidative stress part I: mechanisms involved in metal-induced oxidative damage. *Curr Top Med Chem*. 2001;1(6):529–539.
4. Lublin FD, Reingold SC. Defining the clinical course of multiple sclerosis: results of an international survey. *Neurology*. 1996;46(4):907–911.
5. Compston A, Coles A. Multiple sclerosis. *Lancet*. 2008;372(9648):1502–1517.
6. Confavreux C, Vukusic S. The clinical course of multiple sclerosis. *Handb Clin Neurol*. 2014;122:343–369.
7. Koch M, Ramsaransing GS, Arutjunyan AV, Stepanov M, Teelken A, Heersema DJ, De Keyser J. Oxidative stress in serum and peripheral blood leukocytes in patients with different disease courses of multiple sclerosis. *J Neurol*. 2006;253(4):483–487.
8. Vladimirova O, O'Connor J, Cahill A, Alder H, Butunoi C, Kalman B. Oxidative damage to DNA in plaques of MS brains. *Mult Scler*. 1998;4(5):413–418.
9. Hammann KP, Hopf HC. Monocytes constitute the only peripheral blood cell population showing an increased burst activity in multiple sclerosis patients. *Int Arch Allergy Appl Immunol*. 1986;81(3):230–234.
10. Greco A, Minghetti L, Sette G, Fieschi C, Levi G. Cerebrospinal fluid isoprostane shows oxidative stress in patients with multiple sclerosis. *Neurology*. 1999;53(8):1876–1879.
11. Nikic´ I, Merkler D, Sorbara C, et al. A reversible form of axon damage in experimental autoimmune encephalomyelitis and multiple sclerosis. *Nat Med*. 2011;17(4):495–499.

12. van Horssen J, Witte ME, Schreibelt G, de Vries HE. Radical changes in multiple sclerosis pathogenesis. *Biochim Biophys Acta*. 2011;1812(2):141–150.
13. Haider L. Inflammation, iron, energy failure, and oxidative stress in the pathogenesis of multiple sclerosis. *Oxid Med Cell Longev*. 2015;2015:725370.
14. Gilgun-Sherki Y, Melamed E, Offen D. Oxidative stress induced-neurodegenerative diseases: the need for antioxidants that penetrate the blood brain barrier. *Neuropharmacology*. 2001;40(8):959–975.
15. van Horssen J, Schreibelt G, Drexhage J, et al. Severe oxidative damage in multiple sclerosis lesions coincides with enhanced antioxidant enzyme expression. *Free Radic Biol Med*. 2008;45(12):1729–1737.
16. Haider L, Fischer MT, Frischer JM, et al. Oxidative damage in multiple sclerosis lesions. *Brain*. 2011;134(Pt. 7):1914–1924.
17. Pearson HA, Robinson JE. The role of iron in host resistance. *Adv Pediatr*. 1976;23:1–33.
18. Mishra KP. Lead exposure and its impact on immune system: a review. *Toxicol In Vitro*. 2009;23(6):969–972.
19. Suzuki Y, Inoue T, Ra C. Autoimmunity-inducing metals (Hg, Au and Ag) modulate mast cell signaling, function and survival. *Curr Pharm Des*. 2011;17(34):3805–3814.
20. Silbergeld EK, Silva IA, Nyland JF. Mercury and autoimmunity: implications for occupational and environmental health. *Toxicol Appl Pharmacol*. 2005;207(2 Suppl.):282–292.
21. Rowley B, Monestier M. Mechanisms of heavy metal-induced autoimmunity. *Mol Immunol*. 2005;42(7):833–838.
22. Goldman M, Druet P, Gleichmann E. Th2 cells in systemic autoimmunity: insights from allogeneic diseases and chemically-induced autoimmunity. *Immunol Today*. 1991;12(7):223–227.
23. Coleman JE. Zinc proteins: enzymes, storage proteins, transcription factors and replication proteins. *Annu Rev Biochem*. 1992;16:897–946.
24. Vallee BL, Falchuk KH. The biochemical basis of zinc physiology. *Physiol Rev*. 1993;73:79–118.
25. Mizuno D, Kawahara M. The molecular mechanisms of zinc neurotoxicity and the pathogenesis of vascular type senile dementia. *Int J Mol Sci*. 2013;14(11):22067–22081.
26. Jomova K, Vondrakova D, Lawson M, et al. Metals, oxidative stress and neurodegenerative disorders. *Mol Cell Biochem*. 2010;345(1-2):91–104.
27. Wright RO, Baccarelli A. Metals and neurotoxicology. *J Nutr*. 2007;137(12):2809–2813.
28. Frederickson CJ, Maret W, Cuajungco MP. Zinc and excitotoxic brain injury: a new model. *Neuroscientist*. 2004;10(1):18–25.
29. Cuajungco MP, Fagét KY. Zinc takes the center stage: its paradoxical role in Alzheimer's disease. *Brain Res Rev*. 2003;41(1):44–56.
30. Rink L, Kirchner H. Zinc-altered immune function and cytokine production. *J Nutr*. 2000;130(5S Suppl.): 1407S–1411S.
31. Higashi Y, Segawa S, Matsuo T, et al. Microglial zinc uptake via zinc transporters induces ATP release and the activation of microglia. *Glia*. 2011;59(12):1933–1945.
32. Murphy G, Nagase H. Progress in matrix metalloproteinase research. *Mol Aspects Med*. 2008;29(5):290–308.
33. Chandler S, Coates R, Gearing A, Lury J, Wells G, Bone E. Matrix metalloproteinases degrade myelin basic protein. *Neurosci Lett*. 1995;201(3):223–226.
34. Larsen PH, Wells JE, Stallcup WB, Opdenakker G, Yong VW. Matrix metalloproteinase-9 facilitates remyelination in part by processing the inhibitory NG2 proteoglycan. *J Neurosci*. 2003;23(35):11127–11135.
35. Ram M, Sherer Y, Shoenfeld Y. Matrix metalloproteinase-9 and autoimmune diseases. *J Clin Immunol*. 2006;26(4):299–307.
36. Leppert D, Waubant E, Galardy R, Bunnett NW, Hauser SL. T cell gelatinases mediate basement membrane transmigration in vitro. *J Immunol*. 1995;154(9):4379–4389.
37. Wong Jr EK, Enomoto H, Leopold IH, et al. Plasma zinc levels in multiple sclerosis. *Metab Pediatr Ophthalmol*. 1980;4(1):3–8.
38. Palm R, Hallmans G. Zinc and copper in multiple sclerosis. *J Neurol Neurosurg Psychiatry*. 1982;45(8):691–698.
39. Forte G, Visconti A, Santucci S, et al. Quantification of chemical elements in blood of patients affected by multiple sclerosis. *Ann Ist Super Sanita*. 2005;41(2):213–216.
40. Alimonti A, Ristori G, Giubilei F, et al. Serum chemical elements and oxidative status in Alzheimer's disease. Parkinson disease and multiple sclerosis. *Neurotoxicology*. 2007;28(3):450–456.
41. Moradi A, Honarjoo N, Etemadifar M, Fallahzade J. Bio-accumulation of some heavy metals in blood serum of residents in Isfahan and Shiraz, Iran. *Environ Monit Assess*. 2016;188(5):269.

42. Ghazavi A, Kianbakht S, Ghasami K, Mosayebi G. High copper and low zinc serum levels in Iranian patients with multiple sclerosis: a case control study. *Clin Lab*. 2012;58(1-2):161–164.
43. Dore-Duffy P, Catalanotto F, Donaldson JO, Ostrom KM, Testa MA. Zinc in multiple sclerosis. *Ann Neurol*. 1983;14(4):450–454.
44. Ghoreishi A, Mohseni M, Amraei R, Alizadeh AM, Mazloomzadeh S. Investigation the amount of copper, lead, zinc and cadmium levels in serum of Iranian multiple sclerosis patients. *J Chem Pharm Sci*. 2015;8:40–45.
45. Giacoppo S, Galuppo M, Calabrò RS, et al. Heavy metals and neurodegenerative diseases: an observational study. *Biol Trace Elem Res*. 2014;161(2):151–160.
46. Smith DK, Feldman EB, Feldman DS. Trace element status in multiple sclerosis. *Am J Clin Nutr*. 1989;50(1): 136–140.
47. Sedighi B, Ebrahimi HA, Haghdoost AA, Abotorabi M. Comparison of serum levels of copper and zinc among multiple sclerosis patients and control group. *Iran J Neurol*. 2013;12(4):125–128.
48. Kapaki E, Segditsa J, Papageorgiou C. Zinc, copper and magnesium concentration in serum and CSF of patients with neurological disorders. *Acta Neurol Scand*. 1989;79(5):373–378.
49. Visconti A, Cotichini R, Cannoni S, et al. Concentration of elements in serum of patients affected by multiple sclerosis with first demyelinating episode: a six-month longitudinal follow-up study. *Ann Ist Super Sanita*. 2005;41(2):217–222.
50. Ristori G, Brescianini S, Pino A, et al. Serum elements and oxidative status in clinically isolated syndromes: imbalance and predictivity. *Neurology*. 2011;76(6):549–555.
51. Bredholt M, Frederiksen JL. Zinc in multiple sclerosis: a systematic review and meta-analysis. *ASN Neuro*. 2016;8(3):pii.
52. Stoye D, Schubert C, Goihl A, et al. Zinc aspartate suppresses T cell activation in vitro and relapsing experimental autoimmune encephalomyelitis in SJL/J mice. *Biometals*. 2012;25(3):529–539.
53. Schubert C, Guttek K, Grüngreiff K, et al. Oral zinc aspartate treats experimental autoimmune encephalomyelitis. *Biometals*. 2014;27(6):1249–1262.
54. Salari S, Khomand P, Arasteh M, Yousefzamani B, Hassanzadeh K. Zinc sulphate: a reasonable choice for depression management in patients with multiple sclerosis: a randomized, double-blind, placebo-controlled clinical trial. *Pharmacol Rep*. 2015;67(3):606–609.
55. Desai V, Kaler SG. Role of copper in human neurological disorders. *Am J Clin Nutr*. 2008;88(3):855S–858S.
56. Gaggelli E, Kozlowski H, Valensin D, Valensin G. Copper homeostasis and neurodegenerative disorders (Alzheimer's, prion, and Parkinson's diseases and amyotrophic lateral sclerosis). *Chem Rev*. 2006;106(6):1995–2044.
57. Waggoner DJ, Bartnikas TB, Gitlin JD. The role of copper in neurodegenerative disease. *Neurobiol Dis*. 1999;6(4):221–230.
58. Rotilio G, Carrì MT, Rossi L, Ciriolo MR. Copper-dependent oxidative stress and neurodegeneration. *IUBMB Life*. 2000;50(4-5):309–314.
59. Rasia RM, Bertoncini CW, Marsh D, et al. Structural characterization of copper(II) binding to alpha-synuclein: insights into the bioinorganic chemistry of Parkinson's disease. *Proc Natl Acad Sci USA*. 2005;102(12):4294–4299.
60. Binolfi A, Lamberto GR, Duran R, et al. Site-specific interactions of Cu(II) with alpha and beta-synuclein: bridging the molecular gap between metal binding and aggregation. *J Am Chem Soc*. 2008;130(35):11801–11812.
61. Paik SR, Shin HJ, Lee JH, Chang CS, Kim J. Copper(II)-induced self-oligomerization of alpha-synuclein. *Biochem J*. 1999;340(Pt 3):821–828.
62. Rieder HP, Schoettli G, Seiler H. Trace elements in whole blood of multiple sclerosis. *Eur Neurol*. 1983;22(2): 85–92.
63. Melø TM, Larsen C, White LR, Aasly J, Sjøbakk TE, Flaten TP, Sonnewald U, Syversen T. Manganese, copper, and zinc in cerebrospinal fluid from patients with multiple sclerosis. *Biol Trace Elem Res*. 2003;93(1-3):1–8.
64. Choi BY, Jang BG, Kim JH, et al. Copper/zinc chelation by clioquinol reduces spinal cord white matter damage and behavioral deficits in a murine MOG-induced multiple sclerosis model. *Neurobiol Dis*. 2013;54:382–391.
65. Stankiewicz JM, Neema M, Ceccarelli A. Iron and multiple sclerosis. *Neurobiol Aging*. 2014;35(Suppl 2):S51–S58.
66. Rouault TA, Cooperman S. Brain iron metabolism. *Semin Pediatr Neurol*. 2006;13(3):142–148.
67. Nohl H, Kozlov AV, Gille L, Staniek K. Cell respiration and formation of reactive oxygen species: facts and artefacts. *Biochem Soc Trans*. 2003;31(Pt 6):1308–1311.
68. Salvador GA, Uranga RM, Giusto NM. Iron and mechanisms of neurotoxicity. *Int J Alzheimers Dis*. 2010;2011:720658.

69. Shen XM, Dryhurst G. Iron- and manganese-catalyzed autoxidation of dopamine in the presence of L-cysteine: possible insights into iron- and manganese-mediated dopaminergic neurotoxicity. *Chem Res Toxicol.* 1998;11(7):824–837.
70. Park J, Lee DG, Kim B, et al. Iron overload triggers mitochondrial fragmentation via calcineurin-sensitive signals in HT-22 hippocampal neuron cells. *Toxicology*. 2015;337:39–46.
71. Craelius W, Migdal MW, Luessenhop CP, Sugar A, Mihalakis I. Iron deposits surrounding multiple sclerosis plaques. *Arch Pathol Lab Med*. 1982;106(8):397–399.
72. Hametner S, Wimmer I, Haider L, Pfeifenbring S, Brück W, Lassmann H. Iron and neurodegeneration in the multiple sclerosis brain. *Ann Neurol*. 2013;74(6):848–861.
73. Bakshi R, Benedict RH, Bermel RA, et al. T2 hypointensity in the deep gray matter of patients with multiple sclerosis: a quantitative magnetic resonance imaging study. *Arch. Neurol*. 2002;59(1):62–68.
74. Bakshi R, Dmochowski J, Shaikh ZA, Jacobs L. Gray matter T2 hypointensity is related to plaques and atrophy in the brains of multiple sclerosis patients. *J Neurol Sci*. 2001;185(1):19–26.
75. Bakshi R, Shaikh ZA, Janardhan V. MRI T2 shortening ('black T2') in multiple sclerosis: frequency, location, and clinical correlation. *Neuroreport*. 2000;11(1):15–21.
76. Bermel RA, Puli SR, Rudick RA, et al. Prediction of longitudinal brain atrophy in multiple sclerosis by gray matter magnetic resonance imaging T2 hypointensity. *Arch Neurol*. 2005;62(9):1371–1376.
77. Brass SD, Benedict RH, Weinstock-Guttman B, Munschauer F, Bakshi R. Cognitive impairment is associated with subcortical magnetic resonance imaging grey matter T2 hypointensity in multiple sclerosis. *Mult Scler*. 2006;12(4):437–444.
78. Drayer BP, Burger P, Hurwitz B, et al. Magnetic resonance imaging in multiple sclerosis: decreased signal in thalamus and putamen. *Ann Neurol*. 1987;22(4):546–550.
79. Drayer B, Burger P, Hurwitz B, Dawson D, Cain J. Reduced signal intensity on MR images of thalamus and putamen in multiple sclerosis: increased iron content? *AJR Am J Roentgenol*. 1987;149(2):357–363.
80. Neema M, Arora A, Healy BC, et al. Deep gray matter involvement on brain MRI scans is associated with clinical progression in multiple sclerosis. *J Neuroimaging*. 2009;19(1):3–8.
81. Tjoa CW, Benedict RH, Weinstock-Guttman B, Fabiano AJ, Bakshi R. MRI T2 hypointensity of the dentate nucleus is related to ambulatory impairment in multiple sclerosis. *J Neurol Sci*. 2005;234(1-2):17–24.
82. Zhang Y, Metz LM, Yong VW, Mitchell JR. 3T deep gray matter T2 hypointensity correlates with disability over time in stable relapsing-remitting multiple sclerosis: a 3-year pilot study. *J Neurol Sci*. 2010;297(1-2):76–81.
83. Khalil M, Enzinger C, Langkammer C, et al. Quantitative assessment of brain iron by R(2)* relaxometry in patients with clinically isolated syndrome and relapsing-remitting multiple sclerosis. *Mult Scler*. 2009;15(9):1048–1054.
84. Bagnato F, Hametner S, Welch EB. Visualizing iron in multiple sclerosis. *Magn Reson Imaging*. 2013;31(3):376–384.
85. Ge Y, Jensen JH, Lu H, et al. Quantitative assessment of iron accumulation in the deep gray matter of multiple sclerosis by magnetic field correlation imaging. *Am J Neuroradiol*. 2007;28(9):1639–1644.
86. Habib CA, Liu M, Bawany N, et al. Assessing abnormal iron content in the deep gray matter of patients with multiple sclerosis versus healthy controls. *Am J Neuroradiol*. 2012;33(2):252–258.
87. Hagemeier J, Yeh EA, Brown MH, et al. Iron content of the pulvinar nucleus of the thalamus is increased in adolescent multiple sclerosis. *Mult Scler*. 2013;19(5):567–576.
88. Hagemeier J, Heininen-Brown M, Poloni GU, et al. ron deposition in multiple sclerosis lesions measured by susceptibility-weighted imaging filtered phase: a case control study. *J Magn Reson Imaging*. 2012;36(1):73–83.
89. Zivadinov R, Heininen-Brown M, Schirda CV, et al. Abnormal subcortical deep-gray matter susceptibility-weighted imaging filtered phase measurements in patients with multiple sclerosis: a case-control study. *Neuroimage*. 2012;59(1):331–339.
90. Hammond KE, Metcalf M, Carvajal L, Okuda DT, Srinivasan R, Vigneron D, Nelson SJ, Pelletier D. Quantitative in vivo magnetic resonance imaging of multiple sclerosis at 7 Tesla with sensitivity to iron. *Ann Neurol*. 2008;64(6):707–713.
91. Lebel RM, Eissa A, Seres P, Blevins G, Wilman AH. Quantitative high-field imaging of sub-cortical gray matter in multiple sclerosis. *Mult Scler*. 2012;18(4):433–441.
92. Walsh AJ, Blevins G, Lebel RM, Seres P, Emery DJ, Wilman AH. Longitudinal MR imaging of iron in multiple sclerosis: an imaging marker of disease. *Radiology*. 2014;270(1):186–196.

93. Al-Radaideh AM, Wharton SJ, Lim SY, et al. Increased iron accumulation occurs in the earliest stages of demyelinating disease: an ultra-high field susceptibility mapping study in clinically isolated syndrome. *Mult Scler*. 2013;19(7):896–903.
94. Ceccarelli A, Rocca MA, Neema, et al. Deep gray matter T2 hypointensity is present in patients with clinically isolated syndromes suggestive of multiple sclerosis. *Mult Scler*. 2010;16(1):39–44.
95. Hagemeier J, Weinstock-Guttman B, Bergsland N, et al. Iron deposition on SWI-filtered phase in the subcortical deep gray matter of patients with clinically isolated syndrome may precede structure-specific atrophy. *Am J Neuroradiol*. 2012;33(8):1596–1601.
96. Sfagos C, Makis AC, Chaidos A, et al. Serum ferritin, transferrin and soluble transferrin receptor levels in multiple sclerosis patients. *Mult Scler*. 2005;11(3):272–275.
97. Shaw CA, Tomljenovic L. Aluminum in the central nervous system (CNS): toxicity in humans and animals, vaccine adjuvants, and autoimmunity. *Immunol Res*. 2013;56(2–3):304–316.
98. Campbell A, Bondy SC. Aluminum induced oxidative events and its relation to inflammation: a role for the metal in Alzheimer's disease. *Cell Mol Biol*. 2000;46(4):721–730.
99. Bondy SC, Guo-Ross SX, Pien J. Mechanisms underlying the aluminum-induced potentiation of the pro-oxidant properties of transition metals. *Neurotoxicology*. 1998;19(1):65–71.
100. Strong MJ, Garruto RM, Joshi JG, Mundy WR, Shafer TJ. Can the mechanisms of aluminum neurotoxicity be integrated into a unified scheme? *J Toxicol Environ Health*. 1996;48(6):599–613.
101. Lukiw WJ, Pogue AI. Induction of specific micro RNA (miRNA) species by ROS-generating metal sulfates in primary human brain cells. *J Inorg Biochem*. 2007;101(9):1265–1269.
102. De Marchi U, Mancon M, Battaglia V, Ceccon S, Cardellini P, Toninello A. Influence of reactive oxygen species production by monoamine oxidase activity on aluminum-induced mitochondrial permeability transition. *Cell Mol Life Sci*. 2004;61(19-20):2664–2671.
103. Niu PY, Niu Q, Zhang QL, et al. Aluminum impairs rat neural cell mitochondria in vitro. *Int J Immunopathol Pharmacol*. 2005;18(4):683–689.
104. Wu Z, Du Y, Xue H, Wu Y, Zhou B. Aluminum induces neurodegeneration and its toxicity arises from increased iron accumulation and reactive oxygen species (ROS) production. *Neurobiol Aging*. 2012;33(1):199.e1–199.e12.
105. Exley C, Mamutse G, Korchazhkina O, et al. Elevated urinary excretion of aluminium and iron in multiple sclerosis. *Mult Scler*. 2006;12(5):533–540.
106. Fulgenzi A, Vietti D, Ferrero ME. Aluminium involvement in neurotoxicity. *Biomed Res Int*. 2014;2014:758323.
107. Yasui M, Ota K. Experimental and clinical studies on dysregulation of magnesium metabolism and the aetiopathogenesis of multiple sclerosis. *Magnes Res*. 1992;5(4):295–302.
108. Yasui M, Yase Y, Ando K, Adachi K, Mukoyama M, Ohsugi K. Magnesium concentration in brains from multiple sclerosis patients. *Acta Neurol Scand*. 1990;81(3):197–200.
109. Sheehan MC, Burke TA, Navas-Acien A, Breysse PN, McGready J, Fox MA. Global methylmercury exposure from seafood consumption and risk of developmental neurotoxicity: a systematic review. *Bull World Health Organ*. 2014;92(4):254F–269F.
110. Rice KM, Walker Jr EM, Wu M, Gillette C, Blough ER. Environmental mercury and its toxic effects. *J Prev Med Public Health*. 2014;47(2):74–83.
111. Aschner M, Aschner JL. Mercury neurotoxicity: mechanisms of blood-brain barrier transport. *Neurosci Biobehav Rev*. 1990;14(2):169–176.
112. Petroni D, Tsai J, Agrawal K, Mondal D, George W. Low-dose methylmercury-induced oxidative stress, cytotoxicity, and tau-hyperphosphorylation in human neuroblastoma (SH-SY5Y) cells. *Environ Toxicol*. 2012;27(9):549–555.
113. Sadiq S, Ghazala Z, Chowdhury A, Büsselberg D. Metal toxicity at the synapse: presynaptic, postsynaptic, and long-term effects. *J Toxicol*. 2012;2012:132671.
114. Tamm C, Duckworth JK, Hermanson O, Ceccatelli S. Methylmercury inhibits differentiation of rat neural stem cells via Notch signalling. *Neuroreport*. 2008;19(3):339–343.
115. Chang SH, Lee HJ, Kang B, Yu KN, Minai-Tehrani A, Lee S, Kim SU, Cho MH. Methylmercury induces caspase-dependent apoptosis and autophagy in human neural stem cells. *J Toxicol Sci*. 2013;38(6):823–831.
116. Tiernan CT, Edwin EA, Hawong HY, et al. Methylmercury impairs canonical dopamine metabolism in rat undifferentiated pheochromocytoma (PC12) cells by indirect inhibition of aldehyde dehydrogenase. *Toxicol Sci*. 2015;144(2):347–356.

117. Casetta I, Invernizzi M, Granieri E. Multiple sclerosis and dental amalgam: case-control study in Ferrara. *Italy Neuroepidemiol*. 2001;20(2):134–137.
118. Siblerud RL, Kienholz E. Evidence that mercury from silver dental fillings may be an etiological factor in multiple sclerosis. *Sci Total Environ*. 1994;142(3):191–205.
119. Bangsi D, Ghadirian P, Ducic S, et al. Dental amalgam and multiple sclerosis: a case-control study in Montreal, Canada. *Int J Epidemiol*. 1998;27(4):667–671.
120. Aminzadeh KK, Etminan M. Dental amalgam and multiple sclerosis: a systematic review and meta-analysis. *J Public Health Dent*. 2007;67(1):64–66.
121. Attar AM, Kharkhaneh A, Etemadifar M, Keyhanian K, Davoudi V, Saadatnia M. Serum mercury level and multiple sclerosis. *Biol Trace Elem Res*. 2012;146(2):150–153.
122. Zheng W, Aschner M, Ghersi-Egea JF. Brain barrier systems: a new frontier in metal neurotoxicological research. *Toxicol Appl Pharmacol*. 2003;192(1):1–11.
123. Nava-Ruiz C, Méndez-Armenta M, Ríos C. Lead neurotoxicity: effects on brain nitric oxide synthase. *J Mol Histol*. 2012;43(5):553–563.
124. Audesirk G. Electrophysiology of lead intoxication: effects on voltage-sensitive ion channels. *Neurotoxicology*. 1993;14(2-3):137–147.
125. Struzyñska L, Bubko I, Walski M, Rafałowska U. Astroglial reaction during the early phase of acute lead toxicity in the adult rat brain. *Toxicology*. 2001;165(2-3):121–131.
126. El-Fawal HA, Waterman SJ, De Feo A, Shamy MY, Neuroimmunotoxicology: humoral assessment of neurotoxicity and autoimmune mechanisms. *Environ Health Perspect*. 1999;107(Suppl 5):767–775.
127. Stejskal J, Stejskal VD. The role of metals in autoimmunity and the link to neuroendocrinology. *Neuro Endocrinol Lett*. 1999;20(6):351–364.
128. Polman CH, Reingold SC, et al. Diagnostic criteria for multiple sclerosis: 2005 revisions to the "McDonald Criteria". *Ann Neurol*. 2005;58(6):840–846.
129. Bonferroni CE. Teoria statistica delle classi e calcolo delle probabilità. *Ist Super Scienze Econom Comm Firenze*. 1936;8:3–62.
130. Martino G, Clementi E, Brambilla E, Moiola L, Comi G, Meldolesi J, Grimaldi LM. Gamma interferon activates a previously undescribed Ca2+ influx in T lymphocytes from patients with multiple sclerosis. *Proc Natl Acad Sci USA*. 1994;91(11):4825–4829.
131. Kornek B, Storch MK, Bauer J, et al. Distribution of a calcium channel subunit in dystrophic axons in multiple sclerosis and experimental autoimmune encephalomyelitis. *Brain*. 2001;124:1114–1124.
132. Stirling DP, Stys PK. Mechanisms of axonal injury: internodal nanocomplexes and calcium deregulation. *Trends Mol Med*. 2010;16:160–170.

CHAPTER

6

Metals and Neuroinflammation

Stephen C. Bondy

Center for Occupational and Environmental Health, University of California, Irvine, CA, United States

OUTLINE

INTRODUCTION

Inflammation represents the reaction of the body to factors that may be harmful and is a protective attempt to minimize damage by materials with potentially injurious qualities. The goal is to remove the harmful processes including aberrant cells, bacterial pathogens, and irritating materials. Inflammation is a constituent of both the innate and the adaptive immune systems and can be an important component of healing processes. Ideally, inflammation is an acute event lasting for only a few days, triggered by infection or physical injury. A less desirable event is chronic inflammation, which can be triggered in autoimmune disorders, nondegradable pathogens, or by long-lasting pathological conditions. Such detrimental extended responses can lead to tissue destruction and infiltration of affected areas by fibrous cells.

Biometals in Neurodegenerative Diseases. http://dx.doi.org/10.1016/B978-0-12-804562-6.00006-3

In the brain, in addition to disease-related extended inflammation, there is evidence that aging is associated with an enduring elevation of inflammatory changes, even in the absence of known provocative factors.[1] These heightened immune events appear even further exacerbated in several neurodegenerative disorders found with senescence. These include Alzheimer's and Parkinson's disease and also stroke.[2,3] The cause of most age-related neurological disease is unclear. Overall, such disorders cannot be accounted for in genetic terms and they are thus likely to involve environmental influences. A range of laboratory-based studies, together with epidemiological findings, suggest that such deleterious environmental materials provoking excess immune activity within the brain, are likely to include several metals.

MECHANISMS BY WHICH METAL ELEMENTS CAN INCITE IMMUNE ACTIVITY

There are several means by which metal species may provoke disproportionate immune reactions. Although there is a distinctive sequence of events characterizing each mode of action, discussed later, several metals belong to more than one of these groupings.

Metals as Haptens

Some xenobiotic metals can act as haptens by complexing with normal proteins. Such complexes can then stimulate the production of antibodies that may not only interact with the complex but also the original tissue protein can now act as an antigen. This can develop into a widespread autoimmune activation. While metals can act as haptens and provoke inflammatory activity, they largely involve tissues coming into direct contact with exogenous metals, such as skin and lung.[4] There are few reports on this type of toxicity affecting the nervous system. However, developmental exposure to methyl mercury or mercuric chloride can lead to autoimmune responses to brain antigens.[5]

Metal Elements with Valence Instability

Some metals can change valence under physiological conditions and these fluxes can catalyze the production of reactive oxygen species. Most of these metals, including iron, copper, and manganese also have essential biological roles, which can also depend on this property. Under normal physiological conditions, this attribute allows safe flow of electrons through the electron transport chain and a means of performing protected oxidation and reduction reactions. However, in the unregulated presence of these free ions, the production of oxidant radicals (ROS, reactive oxygen species) can take place, by promoting redox activity. This can then activate immune activity and empower unchecked inflammatory processes.

Major metals in this grouping are Fe, Cu, Mn, and Cr, all of which are also essential for normal cell metabolism. The intracellular distribution and binding of these metals is tightly controlled under normal circumstances and so only under pathological conditions are these constraints disrupted. Abnormal homeostasis of Fe and Cu appears associated with both Alzheimer's and Parkinson's diseases.[6] Both Cu and Fe levels are elevated in the Alzheimer's brain.[7]

Copper (Cu)

The harmful effects of excessive levels of copper are very apparent in Wilson's disease. This is a genetic disorder in which excessive copper, normally excreted or tightly bound to ceruloplasmin, accumulates in tissues.[8] In addition to a range of systemic effects, this disorder involves extensive brain damage.[9] The levels of markers of oxidative stress correspond with the clinical severity of the disease.[10] Environmental levels of copper may also be neurologically harmful. Low levels of copper in the drinking water of experimental animals can cause an inflammatory response in the brain[11] and also enhances levels of amyloidogenesis in a mouse model of Alzheimer's disease.[12] The processes underlying this include activation of microglial NF-κB and consequent release of TNF-α and nitric oxide and superoxide.[13]

Iron (Fe)

Similarly, in situations where intracellular iron concentrations are abnormally elevated, elevated levels of generation of damaging ROS are found.[14,15] The heightened neuroinflammation found in multiple sclerosis may be associated with excess iron deposition.[16]

The potency of iron in catalyzing redox-related ROS production is greatly enhanced by its partial sequestration on the surfaces of colloidal and particulate material, discussed in a later section.

Manganese

This metal differs from Fe and Cu in that both oxidant and reductive properties have been observed. Unlike the reduced forms of Cu and Fe, Mn^{2+} is resistant to oxidation and does not have strong reducing activity. The symmetry of its half-filled 3d shell may account for the reluctance of Mn^{2+} to lose one of its 5 d-electrons, and for its poor reducing ability.[17] However, in the presence of Mn^{3+} at 1/500 of the concentration of Mn^{2+}, Fenton redox cycling with strong ROS producing capacity can take place.[18,19] The ability of Mn^{3+} to dismutate into the divalent and tetravalent forms can lead to formation of Mn oxo-bridged complexes[20]. These may form a colloidal suspension providing a large surface area thus further promoting oxidant reactions, described in a following section.

Metals Attaching to Sulfhydryl Residues

Metals, such as mercury and cadmium, which have a high affinity for sulfhydryl groups, can bind to important antioxidant molecules, such as lipoate and glutathione, effectively blocking their free radical quenching ability. This can result in a reduced detoxification of, and thus excessive presence of short-lived ROS. In addition to damaging macromolecules, such oxidant species can summon and activate immune-competent cell types, represented in the nervous system by microglia, astroglia, and mast cells. Mast cells are found in sites of demyelination within the plaques of patients with multiple sclerosis and thus can also promote inflammation within the brain.[21] In addition, mast cells are found in the CNS. Like microglia, mast cells are derived from hematopoietic cells that migrate to the brain before closure of the blood brain barrier.[22] By this means, oxidant events can enhance the development of inflammation. Important metals with strong affinity for –SH groups include Hg, Cd, and Pb. The neurological consequences of exposure to these metals include initiation of glial immune reactions.[23]

Lead (Pb)

Exposure of neonatal primates to lead can result in amyloid and tau deposition several decades later, in aged animals long after the cessation of any contact with Pb.[24,25] These changes are associated with upregulation of genes associated with the proinflammatory proteins related to the immune response.[26] Permanent functional sequelae following neonatal exposure to lead or methyl mercury have also been reported.[27] Since Nrf-2, which facilitates expression of several antioxidant enzymes, appears to be protective,[28] it is likely that any inflammatory effects, such as induction of GFAP and release of inflammatory cytokines, are preceded by oxidative events leading to activation of phospholipase A2.[29,30] While these are generally considered harmful events, glial release of graded amounts of these cytokines in response to heavy metals may activate neurons in a protective manner.[31,32] Both the extent and duration of the inflammatory response can determine whether it results in a beneficial or deleterious outcome. Neonatal exposure to lead has been reported to disrupt microglial development without leading to neuroinflammation,[33] but a very similar study has found Pb to upregulate inflammatory genes.[34] There appears to be a fine balance between the disruption of ontogenesis by Pb and its ability to enhance inflammatory processes in surviving cells.

Lead is undoubtedly a significant competitor with calcium and zinc and has an affinity for –SH groups. These may lie beneath its capacity for disruption of mitochondrial function, and inhibition of many key enzymes including synthesis of biopterin (essential for synthesis of catecholamine neurotransmitters). The complexity of lead toxicity and large range of targets impacted makes difficult the assigning of the relative importance of neuroinflammation in contributing to its overall harmfulness. However, lead has a much greater affinity for Zn than for Ca binding sites and this makes zinc finger proteins and δ-aminolevulinic acid dehydratase vulnerable to femtomolar concentrations of lead.[35] These levels are several orders of magnitude below those required to disturb calcium metabolism. The GATA zinc finger protein that restrains autoimmune events and confines inflammatory events, binds Pb tightly, leading to a decreased ability to bind to DNA and activate transcription.[36]

Both lead and mercury induce glial cell reactivity; a hallmark of brain inflammation and this may form the basis for promotion of Alzheimer's disease.[37] While there is a barrier preventing many materials crossing from the circulation to the CNS, there is nonetheless a continual interplay between glial elements and the peripheral immune system.[3]

Mercury (Hg)

Mercury has a high affinity for thiol (–SH) and seleno groups (–SeH) that are present in cysteine (a precursor for the biosynthesis of glutathione, the most prevalent intracellular antioxidant), lipoic acid, proteins, and enzymes. Selenium is critical for brain function and is present in 25 proteins that have selenocysteine at their active center. This element has both antioxidant and antiinflammatory properties.[38] Selenium administration may have clinical utility in the treatment of mercurial poisoning.[39]

All forms of mercury, elemental, inorganic, and organic are able to induce formation of ROS and inflammatory responses within the brain. Thus inhaled HgO depressed levels of antioxidant enzymes, superoxide dismutase, and peroxidase and increased levels of oxidized glutathione in the mouse brain and this was accompanied by release of inflammatory IL-6.[40] The antiinflammatory, salicylic acid was protective and blocked these changes. Administration of either mercuric chloride or methylmercury to neonates can also evoke inflammatory changes in the brain but the underlying mechanisms may differ since only $HgCl_2$ induced the production of autoantibodies, which appear in the brain.[5] Pretreatment with dexamethasone can totally block some enzyme changes resulting from exposure to MeHg.[41] Methyl mercury has been shown to both induce expression of genes for proteins related to inflammation (such as GFAP) and to inhibit expression of antioxidant genes (such as glutathione peroxidase).[42] This simultaneous change in gene expression and the ability of both antioxidant and antiinflammatory agents to be protective against mercurials, illustrates the close linkage between immune and oxidant events and the difficulty of establishing a sequential relation between them.

$HgCl_2$ is able to stimulate liberation of inflammatory cytokines from human mast cells, and this together with the use of methylmercury as a preservative in some vaccines, has been suggested as a means by which low levels of Hg might contribute to the pathogenesis of autism spectrum disorder perhaps by way of activation of inflammatory mast cells.[43] However, the evidence for this is very limited.

Dimethyl mercury (Me_2Hg) is several orders of magnitude more lethal to humans and experimental animals than is monomethyl mercury (MeHgCl).[44] However, in isolated cell systems, the opposite is true, MeHgCl being much more toxic.[45,46] This apparent contradiction illustrates the importance of two independent features of chemical neurotoxicity:

1. The partition coefficients of toxicants will determine the rapidity of their accessing the brain. Generally, it is amphiphilic compounds, such as ethanol and nicotine that exhibit maximal penetrance.
2. The rate of biotransformation of absorbed materials is another key determinant of their toxicity. Such metabolism may enhance or diminish toxicity, or may initially increase harmfulness and then act in a detoxifying manner.

Lipophilic Me_2Hg is absorbed across the skin or gut very rapidly and stored in fatty tissues, where gradually converted to the more toxic MeHgCl which ultimately accesses the brain. The penetrance of MeHgCl across tissue membranes is much lower but over time, it can gradually accumulate in tissues. This would account for the very long latencies encountered both after a single brief exposure to Me_2Hg or after extended low level exposure to MeHgCl.[47]

Metals Associated with Particulate and Colloidal Materials

A final class of metals appear rather inert, possessing no powerful affinity for sulfhydryl resides and no ability to change valence and little obvious reactivity. The key feature of this class is their presence in colloidal materials or nanoparticles, materials both endowed with a very large surface area. This can provide a site for the binding of traces of more redox-active metals whose incomplete sequestration greatly magnifies their redox-cycling abilities leading to major production of ROS.[48]

Aluminum (Al)

A common metal of this class is aluminum, which exists within the cell either in colloidal form or as nanoparticles. Aluminum can promote amyloidogenesis by activation of NF-kB and a specific miRNA.[49] Very low levels of Al in drinking water, paralleling those found in reservoir supplies in some areas, have been found to promote neuroinflammation in experimental animals.[11,50]

An important factor in enhancing the ROS producing potential of colloidal aluminum, is the presence of trace amounts of iron adhering to these particles. This is deduced from the finding that aluminum sulfate which has no ability in itself to promote ROS, can strongly stimulate the ROS-producing potential of very low concentrations of iron.[51] A similar interactive situation between a colloidal and a transition metal may pertain in the case of aluminum and copper.[52]

Titanium, Silver and Gold (Ti, Ag, Au)

Titanium dioxide nanoparticles can lead to oxidative stress in isolated microglial cell lines[53] and this can activate NF-κB and lead to inflammation.[54] Parallel findings have been reported using treated experimental animals.[55]

A wide range of metallic oxide nanoparticles, including oxides of Ti, Fe, Zn, Cu, and elemental Ag and Au, are able to cross the blood brain barrier and are suspected to be potentially neurotoxic. Both the surface chemistry and the shape of particles are relevant in establishing their degree of toxicity.[56] The major mechanism of toxicity of these particles involves generation of oxidant free radicals which then activate transcription factors, such as NF-κB that precede inflammation.[54] In the case of elemental Ag and Au, it is not established whether inflammatory changes caused by these elements are preceded by ROS production or not[57] especially as Au particles can also inhibit neuroinflammation in animal models of brain injury under some circumstances.[58] The ability of Ag salts to bring about necrotic cell death may also be causal to the onset of inflammation.[59]

The means by which these metals can promote ROS production and thence inflammation, is not readily apparent, but probably involves their colloidal nature under physiological conditions. The presence of such finely distributed colloids can have two major consequences. First, as they may be mistaken by the immune system for bacteria or material of bacterial origin, such dispersions are likely to promote phagocytic and oxidant activity. Since the particles cannot be cleared, such events can lead to a chronic inflammatory focus. A good parallel for this is found in the case of silicosis of the lung where an irresolvable mineral particle forms the basis for a source of persistent inflammation.[60] Second, the large surface area of such colloidal particles, lends itself to the absorption of many materials on their outer surfaces. These materials may include redox active metals, such as iron and copper. The prooxidant nature of such transition metals is greatly enhanced by their incomplete sequestration on surfaces of particulate materials. Again, silica can provide a useful example of the power of such interactions. Silica nanoparticles also only produce ROS in the presence of trace amounts of iron.[61] The toxicity of silica particles is strongly reduced by their prior washing in deferoxamine, a potent iron chelator. Thus traces of iron are likely to contribute powerfully to the ability of silica to promote inflammation. This attribute may be shared by other particles with a large surface area.

Metals Which Lead to Oxidative Stress and Inflammation by Means that are not yet Understood

Some metals, such as rare earths cerium (Ce) and lanthanum (Ln) can lead to the appearance of elevated levels of lipid peroxidation, inflammation, and apoptosis in many tissues including the brain. While this involves major changes in gene expression including upregulation of a range of immune-related genes, the sequence of events by which this takes place remains unknown.[62] However, it is possible that transcriptional pathways other than NFκB mediate between oxidative and inflammatory events.[63]

THE RELATION BETWEEN REACTIVE OXYGEN AND NITROGEN SPECIES AND INFLAMMATION

There is a bidirectional connection between oxidant and inflammatory events. On the one hand inflammation often involves activation of microglial and astroglial elements within the brain, and this is associated with elevated levels of NADPH oxidase, which is a major source of superoxide anion production.[64] Such superoxide, while relatively stable, if not rapidly detoxified by superoxide dismutase, can be converted to the very reactive hydroxyl radical.

On the other hand, there are several means by which a prooxidant milieu can be translated into activation of immune events. The transcription factor NFκB is at the crossroads between oxidative stress and derepression of proinflammatory genes. Several stimuli including reactive oxidizing species, effect the activation and translocation to the nucleus of NFκB, leading to enhanced glial expression of a broad range of genes relating to regulation of immune function. This includes genes for immunoreceptors, cytokines, chemokines, proteins involved in antigen presentation, acute phase genes, and stress response genes (such as iNOS). Increasing production of reactive oxidant species can upregulate expression of diverse inflammatory mediators and the combination of these events can lead to brain injury.[65] The glial inflammatory response that Cu^{2+} causes, includes release of nitric oxide, TNFα, activation of NF-κB and its migration to the nucleus. All these changes can be blocked by the antioxidant n-acetylcysteine,[14] indicating that at least in this case, oxidative stress precedes inflammatory changes. This report also implicates mitochondrial production of superoxide and thence hydrogen peroxide as the target of Cu. However, it must be borne in mind that the composition of NF-κB dimers is critical in determining whether this transcription factor exerts predominantly beneficial and antiapoptotic or inflammatory and proapoptotic effects. The NF-κB/c-Rel dimer is predominantly protective while the NF-κB/RelA dimer triggers expression of genes relating to apoptosis and neuroinflammation.[66]

While oxidative stress and inflammation can interact in a synergistic manner, harmful events are generally limited by opposing homeostatic regulatory processes. One of these counterbalancing elements is the transcription factor Nrf2 which is redox-sensitive, activated under oxidant conditions and which reacts to these events by derepression of genes for antioxidant and detoxifying enzymes contained within the antioxidant response element (ARE).[67] Nrf2 is the predominant mediator of cellular responses to redox stress and is activated by cysteine thiols present as thiolate anions (S^-), which are more reactive toward oxidant species than are sulfhydryl groups (–SH).[40] When homeostatic processes are overwhelmed, the prolonged appearance of highly ROS caused by mechanisms based on the chemistry of various metals, described earlier, can all lead to neuroinflammation.

CONCLUSIONS

The tight relation between oxidant and inflammatory events, also discussed in the section on mercury, makes difficult their clear separation. Metal-induced neuroinflammation and oxidative stress are inextricably intertwined, often rendering discussion of causal relationships speculative rather than definitive. It is however, certain that metals can provoke undesirable inflammatory events that have a negative health outcome. The immune system is very sophisticated and its subtlety makes it prone to misinterpret events or to over-react to them. The evolution of the immune system has been largely determined by the development of a means to detoxify and remove adverse biological materials. These may be of exogenous origin (viruses and bacteria) or may have an endogenous source (abnormal cells). Many metal-based materials are not readily detoxified by immune mechanisms and their persistence can give rise to a detrimental chronic inflammatory state. The isolated nature of cerebral immune processes can make the brain especially vulnerable to such prolonged periods of immune hyperactivity.

References

1. Deleidi M, Jäggle M, Rubino G. Immune aging, dysmetabolism, and inflammation in neurological diseases. *Front Neurosci*. 2015;9:172.
2. Heneka MT, Carson MJ, El Khoury J, Landreth GE, Brosseron F, Feinstein DL, Jacobs AH, Wyss-Coray T, Vitorica J, Ransohoff RM, Herrup K, Frautschy SA, Finsen B, Brown GC, Verkhratsky A, Yamanaka K, Koistinaho J, Latz E, Halle A, Petzold GC, Town T, Morgan D, Shinohara ML, Perry VH, Holmes C, Bazan NG, Brooks DJ, Hunot S, Joseph B, Deigendesch N, Garaschuk O, Boddeke E, Dinarello CA, Breitner JC, Cole GM, Golenbock DT, Kummer MP. Neuroinflammation in Alzheimer's disease. *Lancet Neurol*. 2015;14:388–405.
3. Su X, Federoff HJ. Immune responses in Parkinson's disease: interplay between central and peripheral immune systems. *Biomed Res Int*. 2014;2014:275178.
4. Raghavan B, Martin SF, Esser PR, Goebeler M, Schmidt M. Metal allergens nickel and cobalt facilitate TLR4 homodimerization independently of MD2. *EMBO Rep*. 2012;13:1109–1115.
5. Zhang Y, Gao D, Bolivar VJ, Lawrence DA. Induction of autoimmunity to brain antigens by developmental mercury exposure. *Toxicological Sci*. 2011;119:270–280.
6. Myhre O, Utkilen H, Duale N, Brunborg G, Hofer T. Metal dyshomeostasis and inflammation in Alzheimer's and Parkinson's diseases: possible impact of environmental exposures. *Oxid Med Cell Longev*. 2013;2013:726954.
7. Jomova K, Vondrakova D, Lawson M, Valko M. Metals, oxidative stress and neurodegenerative disorders. *Mol Cell Biochem*. 2010;345:91–104.
8. Dusek P, Roos PM, Litwin T, Schneider SA, Flaten TP, Aaseth J. The neurotoxicity of iron, copper and manganese in Parkinson's and Wilson's diseases. *J Trace Elem Med Biol*. 2015;31:193–203.
9. Brewer GJ. The risks of free copper in the body and the development of useful anticopper drugs. *Curr Opin Clin Nutr Metab Care*. 2008;1:727–732.
10. Kalita J, Kumar V, Misra UK, Ranjan A, Khan H, Konwar R. A study of oxidative stress, cytokines and glutamate in Wilson disease and their asymptomatic siblings. *J Neuroimmunol*. 2014;274:141–148.
11. Campbell A, Becaria A, Lahiri DK, Sharman K, Bondy SC. Chronic exposure to aluminum in drinking water increases inflammatory parameters selectively in the brain. *J Neurosci Res*. 2004;75:565–672.
12. Kitazawa M, Cheng D, LaFerla FM. Chronic copper exposure exacerbates both amyloid and tau pathology and selectively dysregulates cdk5 in a mouse model of AD. *J. Neurochem*. 2009;108:1550–1560.
13. Hu Z, Yu F, Gong P, Qiu Y, Zhou W, Cui Y, Li J, Chen H. Subneurotoxic copper(II)-induced NF-κB-dependent microglial activation is associated with mitochondrial ROS. *Toxicol Appl Pharmacol*. 2014;276:95–103.
14. Barbeito AG, Garringer HJ, Baraibar MA, Gao X, Arredondo M, Nunez MT, Smith MA, Ghetti B, Vidal R. Abnormal iron metabolism and oxidative stress in mice expressing a mutant form of the ferritin light polypeptide gene. *J Neurochem*. 2009;109:1067–1078.

15. Deng X, Vidal R, Englander EW. Accumulation of oxidative DNA damage in brain mitochondria in mouse model of hereditary ferritinopathy. *Neurosci Lett*. 2010;479:44–48.
16. Williams R, Buchheit CL, Berman NE, LeVine SM. Pathogenic implications of iron accumulation in multiple sclerosis. *J Neurochem*. 2012;120:7–25.
17. HaMai D, Bondy SC, Becaria A, Campbell A. The chemistry of transition metals in relation to their role in neurodegenerative disease. *Curr Top Med Chem*. 2001;1(6):541–551.
18. HaMai D, Campbell A, Bondy SC. Modulation of oxidative events by multivalent manganese complexes in brain tissue. *Free Rad Biol Med*. 2001;31:763–768.
19. HaMai D, Bondy SC. Oxidative basis of manganese neurotoxicity. *Ann N Y Acad Sci*. 2004;1012:129–141.
20. Wekesa M, Uddin J, Sobhi HF. An insight into Mn (II) chemistry: a study of reaction kinetics under alkaline conditions. *Int J Chem Res*. 2011;2:34–37.
21. Rottem M, Mekori YA. Mast cells and autoimmunity. *Autoimmun Rev*. 2005;4:21–27.
22. Aguirre A, Maturana CJ, Harcha PA, Sáez JC. Possible involvement of TLRs and hemichannels in stress-induced CNS dysfunction via mastocytes, and glia activation. *Mediators Inflamm*. 2013;2013:893521.
23. Struzynska L, Dabrowska-Bouta B, Koza K, Sulkowski G. Inflammation-like glial response in lead-exposed immature rat brain. *Toxicol Sci*. 2007;95:156–162.
24. Wu J, Basha MR, Brock B, Cox DP, Cardozo-Pelaez F, McPherson CA, et al. Alzheimer's disease (AD)-like pathology in aged monkeys after infantile exposure to environmental metal lead (Pb): evidence for a developmental origin and environmental link for AD. *J Neurosci*. 2008;28:3–9.
25. Bihaqi SW, Bahmani A, Adem A, Zawia NH. Infantile postnatal exposure to lead (Pb) enhances tau expression in the cerebral cortex of aged mice: relevance to AD. *Neurotoxicology*. 2014;44:114–120.
26. Dosunmu R, Alashwal H, Zawia NH. Genome-wide expression and methylation profiling in the aged rodent brain due to early-life Pb exposure and its relevance to aging. *Mech Ageing Dev*. 2012;133:435–443.
27. Fox DA, Grandjean P, de Groot D, Paule M. Developmental origins of adult diseases and neurotoxicity: epidemiological and experimental studies. *Neurotoxicology*. 2012;33:810–816.
28. Rand MD, Dao JC, Clason TA. Methylmercury disruption of embryonic neural development in Drosophila. *Neurotoxicology*. 2009;30:794–802.
29. Sun GY, Xu J, Jensen MD, Yu S, Wood WG, González FA, Simonyi A, Sun AY, Weisman GA. Phospholipase A2 in astrocytes: Responses to oxidative stress, inflammation, and G protein-coupled receptor agonists. *Mol Neurobiol*. 2005;31:27–41.
30. Chang JY. Methylmercury-induced IL-6 release requires phospholipase C activities. *Neurosci Lett*. 2011;496: 152–156.
31. Eskes C, Honegger P, Juillerat-Jeanneret L, Monnet-Tschudi F. Microglial reaction induced by noncytotoxic methylmercury treatment leads to neuroprotection via interactions with astrocytes and IL-6 release. *Glia*. 2002;37: 43–52.
32. Malfa GA, Tomasello B, Sinatra F, Villaggio G, Amenta F, Avola R, Renis M. "Reactive" response evaluation of primary human astrocytes after methylmercury exposure. *J Neurosci Res*. 2014;92:95–103.
33. Sobin C, Montoya MG, Parisi N, Schaub T, Cervantes M, Armijos RX. Microglial disruption in young mice with early chronic lead exposure. *Toxicol Lett*. 2013;220:44–52.
34. Kasten-Jolly J, Pabello N, Bolivar VJ, Lawrence DA. Developmental lead effects on behavior and brain gene expression in male and female BALB/cAnNTac mice. *Neurotoxicology*. 2012;33:1005–1020.
35. Magyar JS, Weng TC, Stern CM, Dye DF, Rous BW, Payne JC, Bridgewater BM, Mijovilovich A, Parkin G, Zaleski JM, Penner-Hahn JE, Godwin HA. Reexamination of lead(II) coordination preferences in sulfur-rich sites: implications for a critical mechanism of lead poisoning. *J Am Chem Soc*. 2005;127:9495–9505.
36. Ghering AB, Jenkins LM, Schenck BL, Deo S, Mayer RA, Pikaart MJ, Omichinski JG, Godwin HA. Spectroscopic and functional determination of the interaction of Pb2+ with GATA proteins. *J Am Chem Soc*. 2005;127: 3751–3759.
37. Monnet-Tschudi F, Zurich MG, Boschat C, Corbaz A, Honegger P. Involvement of environmental mercury and lead in the etiology of neurodegenerative diseases. *Rev Environ Health*. 2006;21:105–117.
38. Solovyev ND. Importance of selenium and selenoprotein for brain function: from antioxidant protection to neuronal signalling. *J Inorg Biochem*. 2015;153:1–12.
39. Heath JC, Banna KM, Reed MN, Pesek EF, Cole N, Li J, Newland MC. Dietary selenium protects against selected signs of aging and methylmercury exposure. *Neurotoxicology*. 2010;31:169–179.
40. Ma Q. Role of nrf2 in oxidative stress and toxicity. *Annu Rev Pharmacol Toxicol*. 2013;53:401–426.

41. Cambier S, Gonzalez P, Mesmer-Dudons N, Brèthes D, Fujimura M, Bourdineaud JP. Effects of dietary methylmercury on the zebrafish brain: histological, mitochondrial, and gene transcription analyses. *Biometals.* 2012;25:165–180.
42. Kumagai Y, Mizukado S, Nagafune J, Shinyashiki M, Homma-Takeda S, Shimojo N. Post-transcriptional elevation of mouse brain Mn-SOD protein by mercuric chloride. *Brain Res.* 1997;769:178–182.
43. Kempuraj D, Asadi S, Zhang B, Manola A, Hogan J, Peterson E, Theoharides TC. Mercury induces inflammatory mediator release from human mast cells. *J Neuroinflammation.* 2010;7:20.
44. Nierenberg DW, Nordgren RE, Chang MB, Siegler RW, Blayney MB, Hochberg F, Toribara TY, Cernichiari E, Clarkson T. Delayed cerebellar disease and death after accidental exposure to dimethylmercury. *N Engl J Med.* 1998;338:1672–1676.
45. Chao ES, Gierthy JF, Frenkel GD. A comparative study of the effects of mercury compounds on cell viability and nucleic acid synthesis in HeLa cells. *Biochem Pharmacol.* 1984;33:1941–1945.
46. Oyama Y, Nakata M, Sakamoto M, Chikahisa L, Miyoshi N, Satoh M. Methylmercury toxicity in dissociated rat brain neurons: modification by l-cysteine and trimethylbenzylmercaptan and comparison with dimethylmercury and N-ethylmaleimide. *Environ Toxicol Pharmacol.* 1998;6:221–227.
47. Weiss B, Clarkson TW, Simon W. Silent latency periods in methylmercury poisoning and in neurodegenerative disease. *Environ Health Perspect.* 2002;110(Suppl 5):851–854.
48. Bondy SC. Nanoparticles and colloids as contributing factors in neurodegenerative disease. *Int J Environ Res Public Health.* 2011;8:2200–2211.
49. Alexandrov PN, Zhao Y, Jones BM, Bhattacharjee S, Lukiw WJ. Expression of the phagocytosis-essential protein TREM2 is down-regulated by an aluminum-induced miRNA-34a in a murine microglial cell line. *J Inorg Biochem.* 2013;128:267–269.
50. Becaria A, Lahiri DK, Bondy SC, Chen D, Hamadeh A, Li H, Taylor R, Campbell A. Aluminum and copper in drinking water enhance inflammatory or oxidative events specifically in the brain. *J Neuroimmunol.* 2006;176: 16–23.
51. Bondy SC, Kirstein S. The promotion of iron-induced generation of reactive oxygen species in nerve tissue by aluminum. *Mol Chem Neuropath.* 1996;27:185–194.
52. Becaria A, Bondy SC, Campbell A. Aluminum and copper interact in the promotion of oxidative but not inflammatory events: implications for Alzheimer's disease. *J Alz Dis.* 2003;5:31–38.
53. Long TC, Saleh N, Tilton RD, Lowry GV, Veronesi B. Titanium dioxide (P25) produces reactive oxygen species in immortalized brain microglia (BV2): implications for nanoparticle neurotoxicity. *Environ Sci Technol.* 2006;40:4346–4352.
54. Xue Y, Wu J, Sun J. Four types of inorganic nanoparticles stimulate the inflammatory reaction in brain microglia and damage neurons in vitro. *Toxicol Lett.* 2012;214:91–98.
55. Ze Y, Sheng L, Zhao X, Hong J, Ze X, Yu X, Pan X, Lin A, Zhao Y, Zhang C, Zhou Q, Wang L, Hong F. TiO_2 nanoparticles induced hippocampal neuroinflammation in mice. *PLoS One.* 2014;9:e92230.
56. Migliore L, Uboldi C, Di Bucchianico S, Coppedè F. Nanomaterials and neurodegeneration. *Environ Mol Mutagen.* 2015;56:149–170.
57. Trickler WJ, Lantz-McPeak SM, Robinson BL, Paule MG, Slikker Jr W, Biris AS, Schlager JJ, Hussain SM, Kanungo J, Gonzalez C, Ali SF. Porcine brain microvessel endothelial cells show pro-inflammatory response to the size and composition of metallic nanoparticles. *Drug Metab Rev.* 2014;46:224–231.
58. Pedersen MO, Larsen A, Pedersen DS, Stoltenberg M, Penkowa M. Metallic gold reduces TNFalpha expression, oxidative DNA damage and pro-apoptotic signals after experimental brain injury. *Brain Res.* 2009;1271:103–113.
59. Inoue T, Suzuki Y, Yoshimaru T, Ra C. Ca2+-dependent mast cell death induced by Ag (I) via cardiolipin oxidation and ATP depletion. *J Leukoc Biol.* 2009;86:167–179.
60. Peeters PM, Eurlings IM, Perkins TN, Wouters EF, Schins RP, Borm PJ, Drommer W, Reynaert NL, Albrecht C. Silica-induced NLRP3 inflammasome activation in vitro and in rat lungs. *Part Fibre Toxicol.* 2014;11:58.
61. Napierska D, Rabolli V, Thomassen LC, Dinsdale D, Princen C, Gonzalez L, Poels KL, Kirsch-Volders M, Lison D, Martens JA, Hoet PH. Oxidative stress induced by pure and iron-doped amorphous silica nanoparticles in subtoxic conditions. *Chem Res Toxicol.* 2012;25:828–837.
62. Cheng Z, Zhao H, Ze Y, Su J, Li B, Sheng L, Zhu L, Guan N, Gui S, Sang X, Zhao X, Sun Q, Wang L, Cheng J, Hu R, Hong F. Gene-expression changes in cerium chloride-induced injury of mouse hippocampus. *PLoS One.* 2013;8:e60092.

63. Wilson D, Zaqout M, Heo JH, Park EK, Oak CH, Ueno S. Nuclear factor-kappa B is not involved in titanium dioxide-induced inflammation. *J UOEH*. 2012;34:183–191.
64. Qin L, Crews FT. NADPH oxidase and reactive oxygen species contribute to alcohol-induced microglial activation and neurodegeneration. *J Neuroinflammation*. 2012;9:5.
65. Hsieh HL, Yang CM. Role of redox signaling in neuroinflammation and neurodegenerative diseases. *Biomed Res Int*. 2013;2013:484613.
66. Lanzillotta A, Porrini V, Bellucci A, Benarese M, Branca C, Parrella E, Spano PF, Pizzi M. NF-κB in innate neuroprotection and age-related neurodegenerative diseases. *Front Neurol*. 2015;6:98.
67. Singh S, Vrishni S, Singh BK, Rahman I, Kakkar P. Nrf2-ARE stress response mechanism: a control point in oxidative stress-mediated dysfunctions and chronic inflammatory diseases. *Free Radic Res*. 2010;44:1267–1288.

CHAPTER

7

Metals and Prions: Twenty Years of Mining the Awe

David R. Brown

University of Bath, Bath, United Kingdom

OUTLINE

PRION DISEASES

It could be forgiven in the current age to be highly confused about what constitutes a prion disease. The reason for this is because of the unique concept that a disease can be transmitted on the basis of a misfolded protein being transferred between individuals.[1] However, the terminology has also been used for the transmission of a misfolded protein between cells, which results in those cells generating further misfolded protein from their own protein synthesis machinery.[2,3] This confusing picture has meant that the original concept has been broadened too widely to include diseases that previously never fell under the umbrella of prion diseases. It also means that some kinds of proteins are described as prions, not because they can cause disease, but because they transfer a protein conformation between cells via a non-Mendelian mechanism.[4] This includes proteins widely accepted in their description, such as "yeast prions."[5] For the purpose of this review, the term prion disease will be limited to those that

Biometals in Neurodegenerative Diseases. http://dx.doi.org/10.1016/B978-0-12-804562-6.00007-5

involve the prion protein. These diseases are also widely known as the transmissible spongiform encephalopathies.

Transmissible spongiform encephalopathies are a group of neurodegenerative diseases afflicting both humans and animals that share a number of features, including experimental transmissibility, a long delay following transmission to symptom onset, distinctive neuropathological changes, and a rapid decline following early symptoms up until morbidity.[6–9] Development of prion diseases follows significant cell loss in specific CNS areas. However, other changes are quite common, such as the appearance of vacuoles in CNS tissue sections otherwise known as spongiform changes. There is often gliosis, including the proliferation of astrocytes and microglia. The distinctive change specific to prion diseases is the deposition of an abnormal, protease resistant isoform of the prion protein.[1] This protease resistance distinguishes it from the normal cellular isoform (PrP^c) and it is commonly termed PrP^{Sc}.

There are three general classes of prion disease related to the mechanism that results in a change in protein structure.[10] In sporadic cases, the cause remains unknown but may be a result of spontaneous protein conversion. There are also inherited forms of human prion disease in which mutations (either insertions or point mutations) result in protein that has an increased probability of either undergoing spontaneous conversion or is inappropriately associated with the cell membrane. Lastly, prion diseases can be transmitted. In this case, prion protein from an exogenous source is able to pass into the host either through the digestive tract or another point (such as transplanted material). The introduced material is then able to catalyze host prion protein to become the disease associated isoform.[11] All three process are believed to be associated with a change in structure of the prion protein.

The prion diseases of animals include scrapie a disease of sheep with low incidence but tightly associated with specific locations and even specific farms.[12,13] While largely considered sporadic, the disease may be caused by low level environmental factors in these specific locations. Sheep scrapie has been widely studied in rodent models as it is easily transmitted to mice.[14] Sheep scrapie has numerous strains characterized by unique reproducible differences in incubation time, location, and extent of pathology and minor conformational/glycosylation differences in PrP^{Sc}.[15] Another sporadic animal prion disease is chronic wasting disease (CWD) which is a disease of elk and deer, environmentally restrict to areas of the United States and Canada.[16] The disease has a very low incidence in native animals but occurs at high incidence in farmed animals, which suggests that factors associated with close confinement enhance incidence of the disease. Bovine spongiform encephalopathy (BSE), the so called "mad cow" disease is possibly the best-known animal disease, although its incidence has fallen to very low level due to various restrictions.[17] BSE was largely believe to be caused by the feeding of rendered animals remains back to cattle. Interestingly, BSE still has not disappeared despite the cessation of these practice more than 15 years ago (https://www.gov.uk/government/statistics/cattle-tse-surveillance-statistics). It is quite possible that BSE was originally a low incidence sporadic diseases similar to scrapie.

Of greater interest are the human prion diseases. Chief among these is sporadic Creutzfeldt-Jakob disease (sCJD) which has the highest incidence, accounts for 80% of all human cases, occurs at the same incidence worldwide and has no known cause.[18] This disease mostly affects individuals of at around 60 years of age. The most advertised form of human prion diseases is variant Creutzfeldt-Jakob disease (vCJD).[19] This disease affects people significantly younger than sCJD patients and is believed to be caused by the transmission of BSE through the consumption of contaminated food sources. The incidence has dramatically declined with the reduction in BSE incidence and currently there are no living vCJD cases. The last patient died in 2013. Other forms of transmitted prion disease include iatrogenic CJD which resulted from the use of contaminated growth hormone or from transplanted tissue, such as dura mater. There are numerous inherited forms of prion disease which include Fatal Familial Insomnia (FFI), Gerstmann-Sträussler-Scheinker syndrome (GSS), and familiar CJD (fCJD).[7] The differences between these diseases lie in the point mutations in the prion protein gene and the exact resulting symptoms. Some diseases have similar point mutations but, in addition, differences in polymorphism at codon 129 which can be either valine or methionine. With all these diseases, presentational differences appear to depend on slight differences in the prion protein. These differences often appear to be a result of changes in single amino acid residues. Such an astonishing effect indicates how vital it is to understand the molecular behavior of the prion protein, its normal function and metabolism and how small changes in its sequences can impact on its cellular role.

PRION PROTEIN

The prion protein was first identified as a mammalian protein but homologs have been found in all vertebrates including fish.[20–22] Other proteins also have homology to the prion protein and these are Doppel and Shadoo.[23,24] These proteins are all cell surface associated glycoproteins.[25] The cellular isoform of the prion protein (PrP^c) is largely globular with a long unstructured N-terminal tail.[26,27] A glycosyl-phosphotidyl-inositol (GPI) anchor attaches the protein to the outer surface of the cell membrane.[28] The protein has a short half-life at the surface of the cell of approximately 1 h.[29] The globular domain is formed principally of three alpha helices, two of which are linked by a disulfide bridge formed between two cysteines. The cellular protein is also glycosylated at two asparagine residues and can exist as di-, mono-, and nonglycosylated forms. The primary sequence is highly conserved in all mammals. This is important as only mammals develop prion diseases.[21] The unglycosylated form of the protein is 25 kD and has two highly conserved domains. The octameric repeat region, within the N-terminal domain has 4–6 repeats (depending on species) of 8 amino acid residues and includes one histidine in each repeat. The second conserved region is a hydrophobic region toward the end of the N-terminal domain which contains a palendromic sequence (Ala-Gly-Ala-Ala-Ala-Ala-Gly-Ala). It is within this region that the protein is cleaved during metabolic break down.[30,31] This site is lost during conversion to abnormal isoform (PrP^{Sc}) and endows protease resistance. A second cleavage site occurs at the end of the octameric repeat region.[32]

Initial identification of the prion protein was as an aggregated protein in brains of rodents infected with scrapie.[33] Analyses of the protein primary structure eventually lead to the identification of the Prnp gene.[34] It was subsequent to this that PrP^c was identified, as it had the same protein sequence. PrP^{Sc} is the aggregated form, although variations exist in its naming, such as PrP* and PrP^d.[35] The abnormal isoform has higher beta-sheet content and is protease resistant.[36] PrP^{Sc} is also often cleaved at the N-terminus around residue 90. In sCJD, the sequence of the protein is no different suggesting that the disease is principally a protein conformation disorder. The abnormal isoform of PrP is considered the agent of disease as transference of the protein between individuals appears to be sufficient for disease transmission.[37] Additionally, mice knocked out for the prion protein are resistant to prion disease, suggesting that host expression of PrP^c is essential for disease.[38] This highlights the critical nature of conversion of host, PrP^c to the abnormal isoform to the cause of prion disease. Therefore, understanding this process, and factors that influence this process, are at the heart of research strategies to understand the cause and possible treatment of prion diseases.

PRION PROTEIN FUNCTION

Despite the understanding of the critical requirement of PrP^c to prion diseases, the function of the protein in cells still remains controversial. While some reviews continue to describe this function as "unknown," this is a ludicrous statement given the huge volume of data that has been published on this subject.[39–52] Initial attempts to identify the function by the standard "knockout mouse" approach failed, because of the apparent lack of obvious phenotype displayed by the mice.[53] Further knockout mice generated by other researchers muddied the water as it was found different knockout methods could result in the upregulation of another protein (Doppel) that caused a severe phenotype that manifested with increased age.[23] Increased study of the supposed "no phenotype" PrP knockout mice resulted in the identification of a host of minor changes which have not gained much critical acceptance.[54] Similarly, studies have also been carried out on cell lines derived from PrP-knockout mice which have showed considerable differences to wild-type cells but despite these studies[55] there is still no agreement on PrP function.

There has been a huge range of suggestions concerning the nature of the function. Many of these functions are inferred by studies of complex systems. A recent entry into such a list is the suggestion that PrP^c is involved in long term memory in the hippocampus.[56] However, this study was not a molecular study and as such the implication is that the molecular PrP^c somehow causes a change in an emergent phenomenon (i.e., plasticity) which has far more complexity than can be applied to a single molecule. Similarly, the study of stem cells from PrP-knockout mice led some researchers to suggest that it is required for the ability of stem cells to replicate.[57] While this might be what is observed in stem cell populations in vitro this is again an emergent phenomenon and not a molecular function. There have been a variety of similar studies over the years and include measured changes in a range of systems. These changes can range from altered electrophysiological parameters,[58] altered sleep patterns,[59] modified cell adhesion characteristics,[60,61] and disturbed cell signaling pathways.[62] While all these studies provide some insight into what PrP^c does, none of them exactly indicates what PrP^c does in the cell to cause the changes measured.

The largest amount of literature on PrP^c function suggests that it plays a role in cellular viability and resistance to oxidative stress.[39,63–76] Indeed, any of the other proposed functions for PrP^c could be explained through an indirect relationship between cell viability/oxidative resistance and the system being measured (e.g., plasticity). While many of the roles of PrP^c in emergent phenomena have a small number of papers supporting them, the role of PrP^c in cellular protection continues to pour forth. Recent work has shown that PrP^c protects against hypoxia and ischemia and other forms of stress.[77,78] With continued publication of evidence that PrP^c alters cell viability and protects against oxidative damage, it is difficult to understand why there is continued resistance to accepting this as the cellular function of PrP^c.

Delving deeper into how PrP^c protects cells from oxidative damage throws up even further controversy. As will be discussed in later sections, one of the most accepted aspects of PrP^c biology is its role in copper binding.[79] Therefore, it is logical to conclude that a cellular function for PrP^c may require copper binding to the protein. Following enzymatic analysis of copper-bound PrP^c, it was suggested that the protein can cause superoxide dismutation when provided with a low concentration source of superoxide radicals.[63] The original studies were based on purified recombinant protein using a variety of different assays including different sources of superoxide radicals and different reporting techniques and were not based on kits originally (and specifically) designed to detect Cu/Zn superoxide dismutase activity. The finding was also confirmed in vivo[65] and verified by other laboratories.[80,81] Despite this, some research groups have published data reportedly showing that PrP^c does not have superoxide dismutase-like activity. The reports either include high concentrations of chelators that strip copper from PrP^c,[82,83] use inappropriate kits with similar high affinity chelators,[84] or generate recombinant PrP where no attempt to chelate copper to the protein has been undertaken.[85] In comparison, research that has shown categorically that PrP with copper bound can channel electrons and generate hydrogen peroxide[86,87] renders studies disregarding metallochemistry and copper affinity as futile. The ability to electrochemically transfer electrons in this manner means that when a protein with this capacity encounters a high electron donor, such as superoxide, electron transfer will occur and the highly spontaneous dismutation reaction will be catalyzed. Therefore, the potential of PrP^c to be a superoxide dismutase-like protein remains firmly plausible with little credible evidence to the contrary.

COPPER AND PrP

The original suggestion that the prion protein binds copper was similarly contentious. Twenty years have passed since the original suggestions that peptides based on the octameric and hexameric repeats of mammalian and avian prion proteins can chelate copper.[88,89] The original work based on peptides was considered to be unconvincing because of the low dissociation constants (low μM) and the fact that a short peptide with four histidines has a high probability of binding copper without this being of any consequence for the full-length protein. The high profile study that followed was based on a large fragment and initial work suggested that the dissociation would occur in the low nM range but the final published work again reported μM dissociation.[79] Subsequent studies generated a large range of affinities ranging all the way down to femtoM.[90–93] While the octameric repeat region was considered the "copper binding site", even this did not remain fixed as new data demonstrated that two histidines outside the octameric repeat region could contribute to copper binding.[94] This was not inconsistent with early data which suggested that PrP could bind up to five copper atoms.[79] This gave rise to the so called "5th site." Further analysis indicated that the mode of copper binding of PrP changes with the degree of copper binding.[93] In other words one copper atom was coordinated differently than when the protein bound four. Furthermore, PrP demonstrates both sequential copper binding[86] and positive cooperativity when binding copper.[79] It was also demonstrated that native (glycosylated) PrP^c bound copper similarly to recombinant protein with no significant change in affinity.[86] Eventually, mapping of the affinity of all possible binding sites led to a clear definition of the affinity of each site and the extent

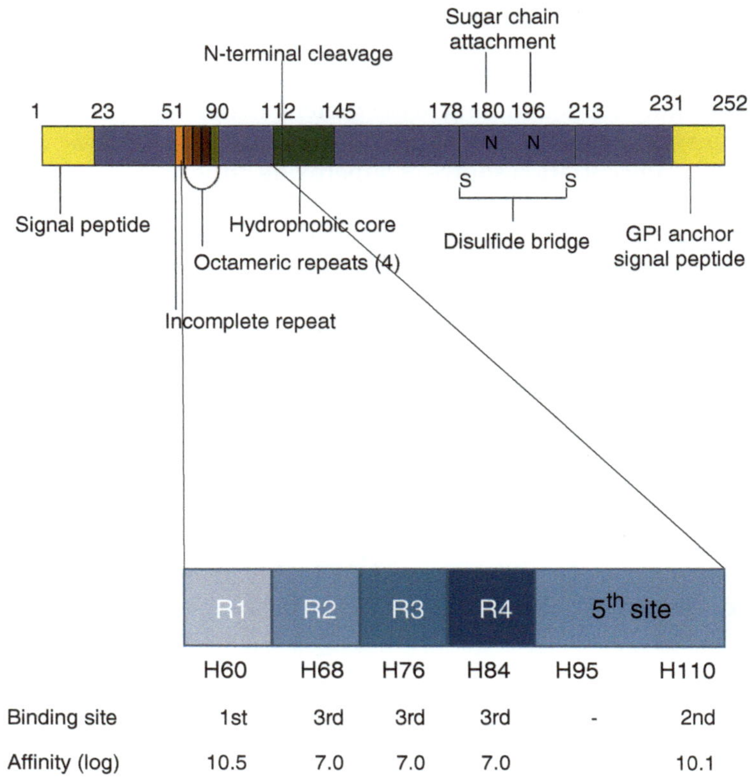

FIGURE 7.1 **Copper binding to PrP.** The mammalian prion protein has numerous features common across all species. For this illustration the mouse prion protein has been chosen. The protein has two signal peptides. The first is for export from the cell and the second is associate with the addition of a GPI anchor to the C-terminus. The protein also has sites for attachment of carbohydrate chains and two cysteine residues that form a disulfide bridge in the mature protein. A highly conserved hydrophobic core protects the site for cleavage of the N-terminus during metabolic breakdown. Another conserved domain is the octameric repeat region which has four complete and one incomplete repeats. The expansion of the figure shows the octameric repeat region and a distal region of the protein to this. This region contains six histidine residues. One each for each repeat and two within the distal area. These two distal histidines constitute the so called 5th site for copper binding. The relative affinity of each of these sites has been assessed using isothermal titration calorimetry.[95] The first binding site is within the octameric repeat region and the second site is to the 5th site. In vivo it has been shown that PrP binds 3 copper atoms per molecule and this third atom can bind to either of the remaining histdines within the octameric repeat region. The relative affinities of the sites are shown (log of M). A fourth atom of copper binds to PrP at one of the remaining octameric repeats with a slightly lower affinity of 6.0 (log M).

to which there was cooperativity with other sites.[95] It was then clear that the first site where copper bound was within the octameric repeat region and that the second site of binding was at the 5th site but with cooperativity of the octameric repeat region (Fig. 7.1). It now appears to be agreed that the high affinity site of PrP^c for copper is in the low nM range.[96]

While the mechanism by which PrP^c binds copper has received considerable attention, there is also considerable research looking at the effect of copper on PrP metabolism. It has been shown that copper binding to PrP^c at the cell surface increases its rate of internalization.[29]

The N-terminus was indicated to be necessary for this, but it was specifically shown that altering the copper binding domain could prevent internalization induced by concentrations as low as 100 nM.[97] Work on the internalization process has focused on sites required for the internalization[98] and the destination of the protein following internalization, which appears to be early endosomes.[99] Disease associated mutations have also been shown to alter internalization.[100] Despite this research, it has not been determined why this process occurs or what its consequence is. It has been shown that the N-terminus with metals bound is cleaved in the presence of oxidative stress.[31] Therefore, it has also been suggested that both events may be associated with signaling into the cell that oxidative processes are ongoing.[101]

One of the consequences of internalization of copper-bound PrP^c is the uptake of copper. Studies with radioactive copper demonstrated that the expression of PrP^c at the cell surface is associated with the copper uptake by both neurons and astrocytes.[102,103] The copper taken up by neurons could be released by veratridine, a depolarizing agent, suggesting that the copper associated with PrP^c is released synaptically.[102] Furthermore, it was shown that copper taken up by astrocytes was associated with PrP^c.[103] Astrocytes have a role in clearance of extracellular copper.[104] This suggests that secreted PrP^c or its N-terminus could play a role in sequestering and removing excess copper.

One of the consequences of increased copper delivery related to PrP^c appears to be altered expression of a host of proteins associated with copper metabolism.[105] These proteins include copper transporting proteins, such as CTR2 and chaperones, such as Atox1. Also other proteins were altered when PrP was knocked out. These include several proteins involved in other neurodegenerative diseases, such as APP, alpha-synucein, Cu/Zn SOD, and the Menkes' disease ATPase. Altered expression of PrP^c also alters copper concentrations found at synapses and copper levels in brains in general with increased age.[106] Some aspects of this have been disputed by others,[107] such as synaptic copper content or copper uptake.[108] However, differences in these data probably relate to incomparable techniques.

As discussed earlier, the main role copper has in regards to PrP^c is as a cofactor for a potential enzymatic activity as an antioxidant. In this regard, the binding of copper is essential for its ability to protect cells. Alteration in copper binding decreases or abolishes the SOD-like activity of PrP^c.[109] It has been demonstrated that copper binding alters the structure of PrP^c.[110–112] Therefore it is highly likely that these structural changes are necessary for the enzymatic activity. Copper binding is strongly influenced by pH[86] and this is again likely to impact biological activity associated with the copper binding. The ability of PrP^c to function as electron transferring protein, is dependent on its copper binding. As mentioned earlier, the copper-PrP complex is redox active and copper is able to cycle between oxidized and reduced forms while bound to the protein.[95] In some complexes, a protein is able to redox silence copper, but this is not the case for PrP where the copper centers remain redox active.[113,114]

ZINC AND PrP

While the vast majority of research relating metals and PrP has focused on copper, there has been substantial investigation of potential interactions of PrP and other metals. The metals of significance in this regard are zinc, iron, and manganese. Some studies have looked at the potential of recombinant PrP to bind other metals.[115] The most effective metals in replacing copper appeared to be nickel and manganese where four atoms were bound per molecule.

However, there was also evidence that around two atoms of zinc could bind to a molecule of PrP. While only trace amounts of magnesium and iron were found to bind. Calorimetric studies were also carried out which demonstrated reasonable binding of manganese, nickel, iron, and zinc at pH 7.[86,116] However, binding of most of these metals was quite pH sensitive with only manganese and iron binding at more acidic pHs. There is also some evidence to suggest that zinc binding to PrP can alter copper binding.[117]

Evidence for a relation between zinc and PrP has emerged from only a small number of publications. First, it was reported, that like copper, zinc can alter PrP^c turnover at the cell surface.[100] More recently it has been suggested that altered expression of PrP results in a change in zinc flux into cells.[118] Also, it was suggested in the same work that the octameric repeat region of the N-terminus of PrP was required for this effect. While increased PrP expression had no effect on zinc retention, effects of PrP expression on basal zinc concentrations were not determined in this study. In contrast, studies of zinc concentration in cells with different expression levels of PrP^c showed no effect on zinc.[119] PrP^c expression had no effect on zinc transporters. Overall no relation between PrP^c and zinc was identified.[119] This suggests that any effect of PrP^c expression on zinc transport is likely to be transient with no lasting effect on cellular zinc levels.

IRON AND PrP

While there is only scant evidence for any real relation between PrP^c and zinc, there is even less for iron. However, there has been recent interest in a possible enzymatic relation between PrP^c and iron. As noted earlier, PrP-complexes are redox active and able to transfer electrons from possible electron donor sources. The process of reduction involves such transfer. The research group of Nina Singh has extensively studied the links between iron and the prion protein. Initial findings suggested that PrP could influence iron uptake.[120] PrP overexpressing cells showed increased levels of intracellular iron. Further studies suggested that CJD patients have increased levels of iron while PrP knockout mice have decrease iron levels.[121,122] A number of studies have shown that the divalent metal transporter-1 (DMT-1), which is known to transport iron, is altered in both PrP-knockout and prion disease.[105] Changes in this protein could explain changes in intracellular iron. Change in iron storage could result from changes in proteins also involved in copper metabolism as DMT-1 can also influence copper. It has also been suggested that PrP^c itself is a ferrireductase.[123] This fits with the suggestion that PrP^c could play a role in electron transfer. The implication is that PrP^c causes conversion of Fe^{3+} to Fe^{2+} which is then more likely to be transported into the cell thus resulting in increased cellular iron. However, unlike studies on alpha-synuclein where kinetic studies on purified protein suggested that an enzymatic catalysis is involved in iron reduction,[124] studies on the ferrireductase activity of PrP^c have only been performed on cell extracts.[123] Our own investigations with recombinant mouse PrP show no activity in a standard ferrireductase assay that measures ferrireductase activity from a known ferriereductase, diaporase (D. R. Brown personal communication, Fig. 7.2). As PrP^c has already been suggested to be associated with redox balance in cells,[39] this observation may only be reporting a secondary effect rather than a direct function of PrP^c in iron reduction.

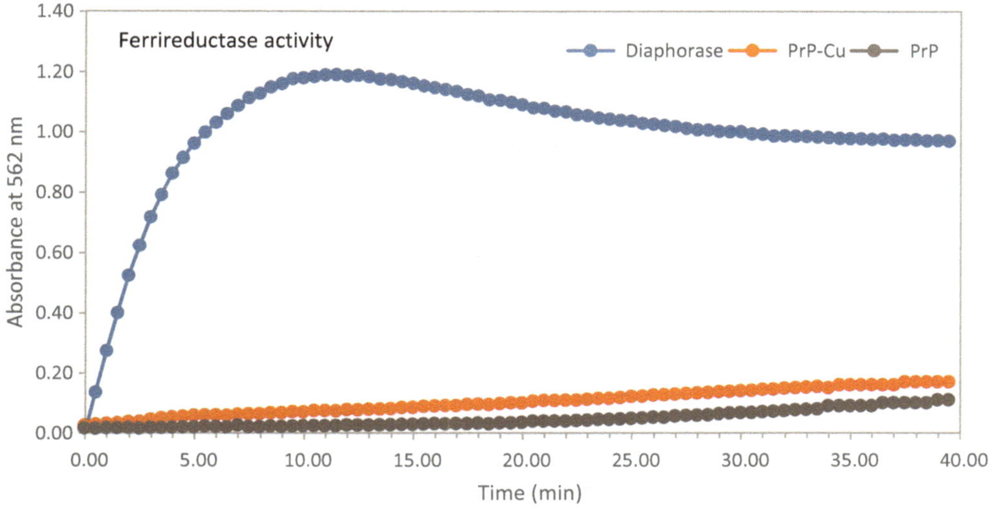

FIGURE 7.2 **Is PrP a ferrireductase?** We used a standard ferrireductase assay based on the ability of ferrozine to detect Fe(II).[124] Recombinant mouse PrP was generated and purified from bacteria.[86] The protein was refolded to form metal free PrP or refolded in the presence of Cu (II) to form copper bound PrP (PrP-Cu). As a positive control we used commercial human diaphorase (Sigma), which is a known ferrireductase. Diaphorase at 0.1 mg/mL or PrP and PrP-Cu at 0.5 mg/mL were reacted with a pure source of Fe(III) in the presence of NADH. Absorbance was measured at 562 nm over 40 minutes. While diaphorase showed strong ferrireductase activity, neither form of PrP showed any significant activity. This suggests that PrP is not a ferrireductase.

MANGANESE AND PrP

As indicated earlier, manganese was identified as a metal that could bind to PrP instead of copper.[115] More detailed analysis of manganese binding to PrP lead to the identification of a binding site associated with a histidine outside of the octameric repeat region (H95).[116] The affinity at this site was equivalent to the affinity of Mn for other known manganese binding proteins. More interestingly, when PrP was saturated with copper, manganese was still able to bind to the site at H95.[116] This indicates that copper binding does not prevent the interaction of the protein with manganese even when the octameric repeat region is occupied by copper. Further analysis showed that when manganese binds to PrP, the protein undergoes a conformational change that is quite different to that when it binds copper. There is considerable compacting of the structure. When PrP^c is isolated from the brain, it contains around three copper atoms per molecule.[65] However, when PrP is isolated from the brains of an animal with prion disease there is an observed change in occupancy to manganese.[125] This would suggest that during the disease process there is a loss of copper binding and an increase in manganese binding to PrP.

There have been only a few other studies that have looked at the affinity of manganese for PrP. One of these studies confirmed manganese binding but indicated a slightly lower affinity.[90] Another study was based on a peptide of the octameric repeat region but showed no binding, but this is no surprise given the main binding site is outside the octameric repeat region.[126] A third study suggested that binding occurs within the 106–126 region of PrP, centered on histidine 111.[127] A study using surface plasmon resonance indicated that while peptides from the octameric repeat did not bind manganese, that the full length protein may possess a conformational binding site with a nanomolar dissociation constant.[128] These differences are likely due to the different techniques used or the use of nonphysiological peptides. There is currently little known about the exact coordination of manganese by full length PrP but this is likely to be quite different to that of copper.

When PrP is occupied by manganese the protein undergoes a conformational change.[111,129] This process occurs slowly over time and results in a unique aggregated form of the protein. Studies with PrP generated this way have shown that the protein is toxic and mimics PrP^{Sc} in the mechanism by which it kills cells.[130] It also mimics PrP^{Sc} in the mechanism by which it is able to seed aggregation of more PrP.[131] The core domain of PrP necessary to generate a seed of PrP using interaction with manganese was found to be residues 90–171, which is similar to that of the "mini-prion."[132] Additionally, it was found that certain kinds of prion proteins that defy conversion in animals models could generate prion seeds when interacted with manganese.[131] These included chicken prion protein and sheep prion protein with the ARR polymorphism. In the latter case prion seeds generated with ARR protein generated seeds with the highest catalytic potential.[131] Analysis of the "seed" generated from PrP and manganese indicated that the size of the oligomer was around 200 kD and consisted of about eight monomers of PrP.[131]

Analysis using recombinant protein has shown that this manganese-bound PrP will become protease resistant.[31,115] As well as change in the conformation of PrP, the expression of PrP also has an influence on the expression of manganese transporting proteins, such as DMT-1 also known as NRAMP-2.[105] Such changes could alter the manganese retained in cells and increase the rate at which manganese and PrP interact. Furthermore, cells grown in the presence of manganese occasionally showed expression of protease resistant PrP.[115] This result has also been observed in a yeast based system.[133] Conformational changes do not necessarily result in aggregation. However, binding manganese with/instead of copper causes different conformational changes as indicated earlier.[111,129] With different exposure of key residues to the environment, the protein is more able to be influenced by oxidative radicals, which potentially play a role in structural changes. Analysis with cyclic voltammetry clearly illustrates the difference in this regard because of the high propensity of the metal to be oxidized to Mn(III) irreversibly.[116] The response of PrP to manganese in terms of change in protease resistance and aggregation is altered by the number of octameric repeats present. This might alter the number of manganese atoms bound by the protein and increase the rate of its oxidation.[134]

Aggregated PrP while potentially toxic and able to catalyze in vitro aggregation assays is more interesting because of its association with prion infection. The spontaneous appearance of aggregated PrP in cultured cells as mentioned earlier is not proof of infection. However, the ability of cell lines that maintain production of protease resistant PrP have been termed persistently infected cell lines, such as the SMB cell line.[135] Treatment of SMB cells with manganese increases both the level of PrP^{Sc} the cells generate and decreases the amount of infectious agent required to establish continuous PrP^{Sc} from the cells.[136] This clearly creates a link between manganese and the rate of conversion of PrP^{c} to PrP^{Sc}. This is supported by experiments with a manganese chelator that reduced the PrP^{Sc} load in experimental mice infected with prion disease.[137] Given the possible relation between manganese and the maintenance of "prion infection" in cells, a strategy that could remove manganese from cells could be beneficial in reducing or "curing" this infection. We identified that an interesting mutant of a manganese transporting protein termed SPCA (secretory pathway calcium ATPase-1) is able to increase manganese efflux from cells. We transfected SMB cells to overexpress the mutant SPCA protein and showed that this abolished detectible PrP^{Sc} in the cells.[119] SMB cells, as well having high levels of PrP^{Sc} also show elevated levels of manganese. Mutant SPCA caused a reduction in manganese, but only in the SMB cells. Furthermore control cells expressing mutant SPCA could not be infected with prions.[119] The implication is that without the increased levels of manganese the infected cells could not continue to produce PrP^{Sc} and that uninfected cells required manganese for the infection to be established (Fig. 7.3). Astonishingly, this amazing result has largely been ignored by the scientific community. However,

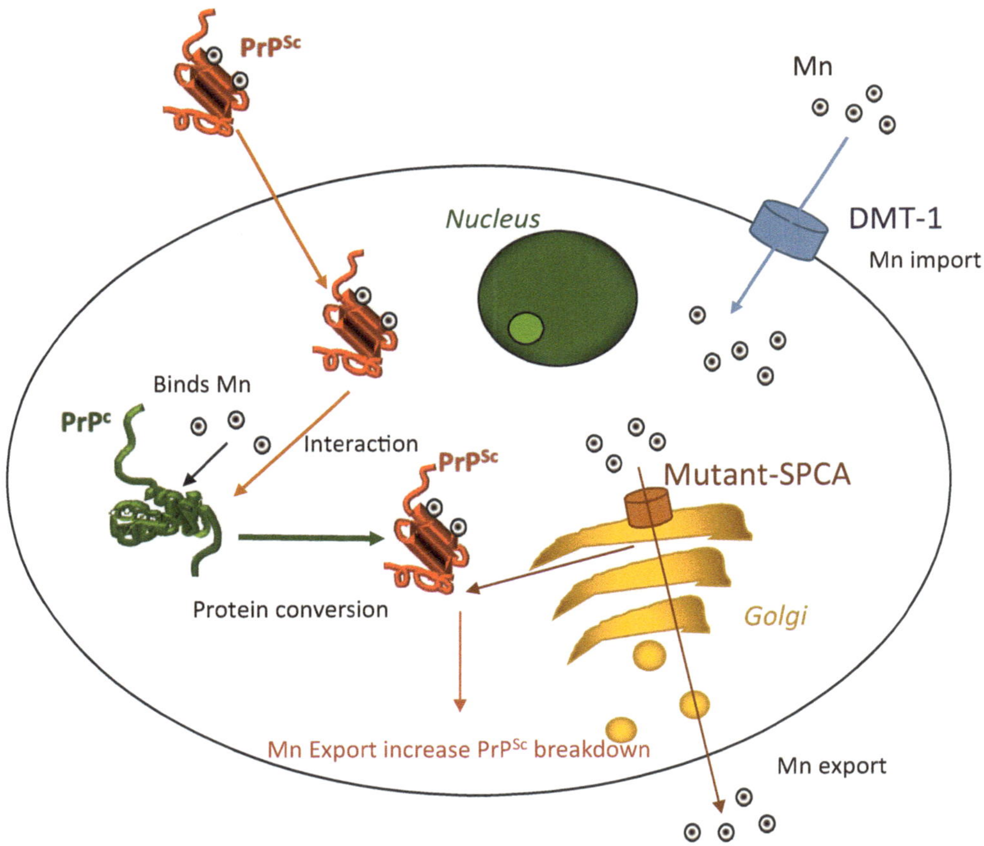

FIGURE 7.3 **Altering copper in prion disease.** Cellular response to prion infection leads to an increase in manganese present in cells. This is likely due to increased uptake through the main manganese import route, via DMT-1. Increased manganese in cells increases the rate of conversion of PrP^{c} to PrP^{Sc}. PrP^{Sc} also binds manganese and this appears to be necessary for prion infection. When cells overexpress a mutant form of the manganese exporting protein, SPCA, this leads to a decrease in manganese in prion infected cells and a reduction in detectible PrP^{Sc}.

the implication is that there is an approachable path to the treatment of prion diseases involving chelation therapy. This is especially astonishing as there have already been in vivo experiments showing the benefit of chelation therapy.[137] While the majority of the evidence discussed is from in vitro studies there is also good evidence for a link between prion diseases and alter metal homeostasis.

METALS IN PRION DISEASE

Studies of the mechanism that leads to prion disease have focused on a small number of models. They are either cell culture based with permanently infected cell lines, employ recombinant protein to study aggregation, or use rodent/animal/insect models to study the infection process and progress of the pathology. In all such models, metal concentrations have been shown to have an influence on the outcome or the concentrations metals themselves have been altered due to the disease process. What remains inconclusive is what actual role metals have in the disease process. Does dyshomeostasis of metallobiology cause the disease or occur as part of the pathology?

Studies looking at the levels of trace elements in the brains of animals with BSE, sheep scrapie, patients with CJD or vCJD, and rodents experimentally infected with scrapie all show a similar trend.[125,138,139] The studies show reduced levels of copper and increased levels of manganese in select CNS regions. There have been similar reports for altered manganese concentrations associated with chronic wasting disease in elk[140] and deer[141] but one study on deer showed no correlation.[142] A recent study has shown increased manganese in prion plaques in experimental hamsters.[143] As indicated earlier there is a change in the metal occupancy of PrP in prion disease which favors manganese. However, it is not clear from any of these studies as to whether the change in PrP metal binding causes the change in trace element concentrations. Changes in blood manganese have also been observed in cattle, sheep, experimental mice, and CJD patients.[125,138,139] This was of considerable interest because of the possibility for diagnosis. However, this possibility has never been pursued.

Given the binding of manganese to PrP in vitro, elevated manganese levels observed in the CNS and blood of patients suffering from prion disease is interesting. Therefore, Mn dyshomeostasis has attracted interest as a possible early diagnostic tool.[139] Similar to the findings with experimental rodents discussed earlier,[125] metal occupancy of PrP in sporadic CJD patients differed from PrP purified from normal brains and an elevation of associated manganese was detected.[144] The reason for the change in metal balance in prion-infected brains remains unclear, although with regard to the BSE epidemic in the United Kingdom, it was hypothesized that cattle exposed to high absorbable forms of manganese from excess in the environment may create a situation where manganese could bind more easily to PrP.[145] Research into the possible association of high environmental manganese with sites of higher prion diseases incidence in general support a correlation[146] although another study did not find a relation.[147] There has been some attempt to treat cattle with special diets to try to induce a prion disease but these were unsuccessful.[148,149] However, given the incidence of these diseases in areas with appropriate metal concentration is very low, then the number of animals needed for such a study would be in the hundreds and beyond any research budget. Such studies are unlikely to be conclusive as attempting to find a correlation between a particular disease aetiology and such a ubiquitous element as manganese is unlikely to lead to meaningful data. More meaningful data has come from studies taking a different approach. In this case the hypothesis was that increased soil manganese would increase prion survival in soils. This study showed that manganese increases the survival of the infectious prion protein in soil by almost 100-fold when compared to normal soil.[136] This implies that prions trapped in manganese rich soils are more likely to survive the harsh conditions in the environment than elsewhere, potentially explaining the association between prion disease and manganese-rich soil areas.

CHELATION THERAPY AND PRION DISEASE

While there is no conclusive explanation for why metal concentrations change in patients and animals with prion disease, there is at least a skeletal view of how altering the metal association of PrP could create cells that generate PrP^{Sc}. From this point of view, an attempt to alleviate prion disease by rebalancing brain trace element status might be beneficial or at least enlightening in terms of mechanistic relations.

One of the consequences of altered metal concentrations in the brain is the possibility of oxidative damage as a result of increased Fenton-like reactions catalyzed by divalent metals. There have been quite a few observations of damage from oxidative stress in prion disease.[150–156] As indicated earlier, there are changes in metals in the brain in prion diseases and such changes have been demonstrated to be accentuated in preparations of neuronal synaptosomes from the brains of mice infected with scrapie prions, with significant changes in metal content occurring as early as 100 days postinoculation.[157]

Investigations into the efficacy of antioxidant and metal chelation-based therapeutics have unfortunately offered only limited benefit in combating prion disease. One study employed an antioxidant therapeutic, EUK-189, a Mn-SOD (SOD2) mimetic with additional catalase activity.[158] Mice inoculated intracerebrally with a low dose of prions treated with EUK-189 were shown to survive approximately 10% longer than cognate, untreated controls and these treated mice displayed a significantly reduced brain vacuolar lesion profile in particular regions.

There have also been attempts at copper and manganese chelation therapies producing slight increases in survival times. A study applying D-penicillamine to a mouse model of prion disease achieved an approximately 10% extension to the survival times of low dose inoculated-mice but not with mice given a high dose inoculum.[159] Another study using clioquinol (another copper chelator) reported a similar effect.[160] A transgenic approach to reduce brain copper by mutating a copper transporting ATPase also increased survival of scrapie infection by around 10%.[161] However, it is important to note that none of these methods, involving copper reduction/chelation prevented formation of PrP^{Sc} or saved the life of a single infected animal. A study of manganese chelation therapy utilizing the disodium calcium salt of CDTA in a mouse model of prion infection has also shown an extension of survival by approximately 10% but only in mice inoculated with a low-dose of infectious prions.[137] While these studies showed only small changes and small reductions in associated metals, there was clear evidence of an effect on disease progression. To this point, several other treatments have been tested with possibly greater effect, but none have actually resulted in a cure. Only switching off prion protein expression results in cessation of prion disease progression.[162] Altering metal content of diets also can change the levels of trace elements in the brain and studies of such diets have shown a reduction in the level of expression of PrP^{C}.[105]

Altering metal content of diet to treat prion disease has generated interesting results (Fig. 7.4). In some experiments a low-copper diet fed before inoculation with prions and

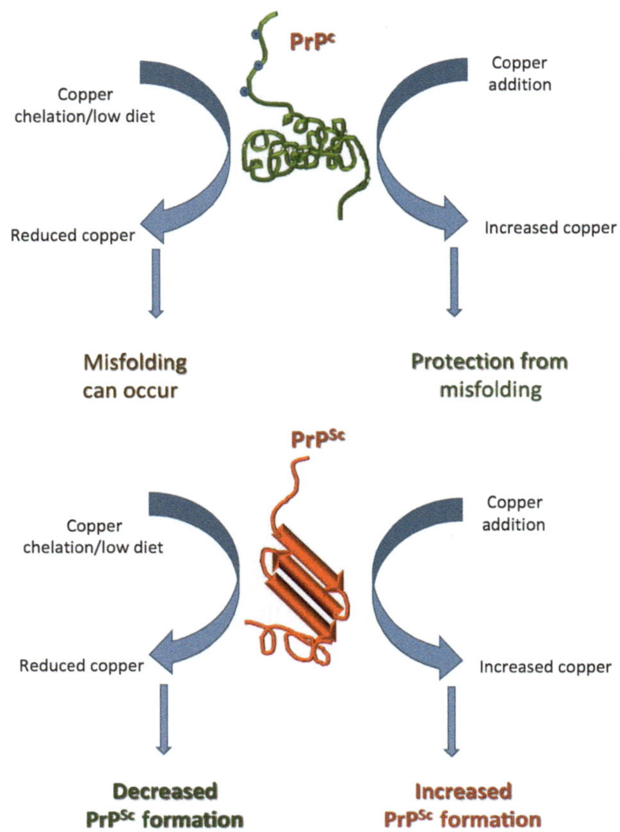

FIGURE 7.4 **Manganese removal reduces PrP^{Sc} formation.** The impact of altering the levels of brain copper on prion disease depend on when the alteration occurs. Neither increase nor decreasing copper levels prevent prion disease entirely. However, different researchers have found that both increasing and decreasing copper levels can have similar effects. This figure offers a possible rationalization for this. Before infection of experimental animals, addition of extra copper in the diet increase the amount available to bind to PrP^{c}. This plays a protective role maintaining the normal conformation of the protein. If chelation or low copper diets are applied, the opposite effect occurs increasing the rate at which PrP^{c} can misfold. Once prion infection occurs and PrP^{Sc} has formed, a low copper diet or chelation has the opposite effect, because interaction of PrP^{Sc} with copper increases its aggregation rate. Therefore, although the diet might initially increase the rate at which PrP^{c} misfold, it decreases the aggregation rate of PrP^{Sc} once it has formed, leading to a longer incubation period for the disease. In contrast, an increase copper diet increases the rate of PrP^{Sc} formation. So, while a high copper diet might initially be protective, once a source of prions is introduced and host conversion can occur, the additional copper is no longer protective. In this case a longer incubation period might still be observed even with the opposite diet.

during the incubation period resulted in worsened symptoms and a shorter incubation period.[157,163] In another set of experiments, a diet high in copper has been shown to delay the onset of the symptoms and extended the incubation period of scrapie prion-infected mice.[164] In this context copper appears to be protective. What is important to note is that the interaction of copper with PrP^{Sc} is different to that of PrP^{c}. While copper binding to PrP^{c} is needed for its function and may prevent protein conversion, interaction with PrP^{Sc} increases aggregation and infectivity.[165] This is not surprising as the interaction of transition metals with beta-sheet is known to increase stacking associated with aggregation. Increasing manganese in diet increases neuronal loss and makes symptoms of prion disease worse.[157,163] Thus the overall picture arising from these animal studies reflects findings from molecular and in vitro studies. Manganese interactions in prion disease increase the likelihood of pathological change. Therefore reduction in manganese is beneficial. Overall ensuring normal copper levels is protective while reduction in copper is not beneficial and may increase susceptibility to prion disease. Increasing copper is less likely to be beneficial as this may cause additional changes to PrP^{Sc}. Copper chelation appears beneficial possibly because it prevents inappropriate interactions of copper and PrP^{Sc}. This is not contradictory, but reflects the complexity of the interaction of copper and PrP (Fig. 7.4).

CONCLUSIONS

The relation of neurodegenerative diseases to metal homeostasis has been firmly established. The copper-prion interaction is now considered to be solid and irrefutable. However, many aspects of prions and metals remain in the periphery of research in the area. This is somewhat bizarre given the mounting data from multiple sources. However, as funding for research in these areas has massively declined and is largely focused on the black hole of diagnostics and therapeutics, further significant advance on this subject may take considerable time. Only time will tell if a new vein can be opened and further awe can flow.

References

1. Prusiner SB. Prions. *Proc Natl Acad Sci USA*. 1998;95(23):13363–13383.
2. Uchihara T, Giasson BI, Paulus W. Propagation of Abeta, tau and alpha-synuclein pathology between experimental models and human reality: prions, propagons and propaganda. *Acta Neuropathol*. 2016;131(1):1–3.
3. Angot E, Steiner JA, Hansen C, Li JY, Brundin P. Are synucleinopathies prion-like disorders?. *Lancet Neurol*. 2010;9(11):1128–1138.
4. Woerman AL, Stohr J, Aoyagi A, et al. Propagation of prions causing synucleinopathies in cultured cells. *Proc Natl Acad Sci USA*. 2015;112(35):E4949–E4958.
5. Rowley A. Prion-mediated diversity in yeast. *Trends Genet*. 2000;16(12):543.
6. Ironside JW, Bell JE. Infective dementias. *Panminerva Med*. 2007;49(4):209–225.
7. Lloyd S, Mead S, Collinge J. Genetics of Prion Disease. *Top Curr Chem*. 2011;305:1–22.
8. Collinge J. Molecular neurology of prion disease. *J Neurol Neurosurg Psychiatry*. 2005;76(7):906–919.
9. Imran M, Mahmood S. An overview of human prion diseases. *Virol J*. 2011;8:559.
10. Prusiner SB. Biology and genetics of prions causing neurodegeneration. *Annu Rev Genet*. 2013;47:601–623.
11. Acevedo-Morantes CY, Wille H. The structure of human prions: from biology to structural models-considerations and pitfalls. *Viruses*. 2014;6(10):3875–3892.
12. Windl O, Dawson M. Animal prion diseases. *Subcell Biochem*. 2012;65:497–516.

13. Gough KC, Baker CA, Simmons HA, Hawkins SA, Maddison BC. Circulation of prions within dust on a scrapie affected farm. *Vet Res*. 2015;46:40.
14. Fernandez-Borges N, Erana H, Venegas V, Elezgarai SR, Harrathi C, Castilla J. Animal models for prion-like diseases. *Virus Res*. 2015;207:5–24.
15. Telling GC. Transgenic mouse models and prion strains. *Top Curr Chem*. 2011;305:79–99.
16. Haley NJ, Hoover EA. Chronic wasting disease of cervids: current knowledge and future perspectives. *Annu Rev Animal Biosci*. 2015;3:305–325.
17. Balkema-Buschmann A, Fast C, Kaatz M, et al. Pathogenesis of classical and atypical BSE in cattle. *Prev Vet Med*. 2011;102(2):112–117.
18. Knight R. Creutzfeldt-Jakob disease: a rare cause of dementia in elderly persons. *Clin Infect Dis*. 2006;43(3): 340–346.
19. Diack AB, Head MW, McCutcheon S, et al. Variant CJD: 18 years of research and surveillance. *Prion*. 2014;8(3):286–295.
20. Calzolai L, Lysek DA, Perez DR, Guntert P, Wuthrich K. Prion protein NMR structures of chickens, turtles, and frogs. *Proc Natl Acad Sci USA*. 2005;102(3):651–655.
21. Wopfner F, Weidenhofer G, Schneider R, et al. Analysis of 27 mammalian and 9 avian PrPs reveals high conservation of flexible regions of the prion protein. *J Mol Biol*. 1999;289(5):1163–1178.
22. Cotto E, Andre M, Forgue J, Fleury HJ, Babin PJ. Molecular characterization, phylogenetic relationships, and developmental expression patterns of prion genes in zebrafish (Danio rerio). *FEBS J*. 2005;272(2):500–513.
23. Moore RC, Lee IY, Silverman GL, et al. Ataxia in prion protein (PrP)-deficient mice is associated with upregulation of the novel PrP-like protein doppel. *J Mol Biol*. 1999;292(4):797–817.
24. Premzl M, Sangiorgio L, Strumbo B, Marshall Graves JA, Simonic T, Gready JE. Shadoo, a new protein highly conserved from fish to mammals and with similarity to prion protein. *Gene*. 2003;314:89–102.
25. Meyer RK, McKinley MP, Bowman KA, Braunfeld MB, Barry RA, Prusiner SB. Separation and properties of cellular and scrapie prion proteins. *Proc Natl Acad Sci USA*. 1986;83(8):2310–2314.
26. Riek R, Hornemann S, Wider G, Billeter M, Glockshuber R, Wuthrich K. NMR structure of the mouse prion protein domain PrP(121-321). *Nature*. 1996;382(6587):180–182.
27. Riek R, Hornemann S, Wider G, Glockshuber R, Wuthrich K. NMR characterization of the full-length recombinant murine prion protein, mPrP(23-231). *FEBS Lett*. 1997;413(2):282–288.
28. Stahl N, Baldwin MA, Hecker R, Pan KM, Burlingame AL, Prusiner SB. Glycosylinositol phospholipid anchors of the scrapie and cellular prion proteins contain sialic acid. *Biochemistry*. 1992;31(21):5043–5053.
29. Pauly PC, Harris DA. Copper stimulates endocytosis of the prion protein. *J Biol Chem*. 1998;273(50):33107–33110.
30. Vincent B, Paitel E, Saftig P, et al. The disintegrins ADAM10 and TACE contribute to the constitutive and phorbol ester-regulated normal cleavage of the cellular prion protein. *J Biol Chem*. 2001;276(41):37743–37746.
31. Abdelraheim SR, Kralovicova S, Brown DR. Hydrogen peroxide cleavage of the prion protein generates a fragment able to initiate polymerisation of full length prion protein. *Int J Biochem Cell Biol*. 2006;38(8): 1429–1440.
32. Mange A, Beranger F, Peoc'h K, Onodera T, Frobert Y, Lehmann S. Alpha- and beta- cleavages of the amino-terminus of the cellular prion protein. *Biol Cell*. 2004;96(2):125–132.
33. Bolton DC, McKinley MP, Prusiner SB. Identification of a protein that purifies with the scrapie prion. *Science*. 1982;218(4579):1309–1311.
34. Basler K, Oesch B, Scott M, et al. Scrapie and cellular PrP isoforms are encoded by the same chromosomal gene. *Cell*. 1986;46(3):417–428.
35. Jeffrey M, Gonzalez L. Classical sheep transmissible spongiform encephalopathies: pathogenesis, pathological phenotypes and clinical disease. *Neuropathol Appl Neurobiol*. 2007;33(4):373–394.
36. Pan KM, Baldwin M, Nguyen J, et al. Conversion of alpha-helices into beta-sheets features in the formation of the scrapie prion proteins. *Proc Natl Acad Sci USA*. 1993;90(23):10962–10966.
37. Prusiner SB. Novel proteinaceous infectious particles cause scrapie. *Science*. 1982;216(4542):136–144.
38. Bueler H, Aguzzi A, Sailer A, et al. Mice devoid of PrP are resistant to scrapie. *Cell*. 1993;73(7):1339–1347.
39. Brown DR. Prion and prejudice: normal protein and the synapse. *Trends Neurosci*. 2001;24(2):85–90.
40. Zeng L, Zou W, Wang G. Cellular prion protein (PrP(C)) and its role in stress responses. *Int J Clin Exp Med*. 2015;8(5):8042–8050.
41. Westergard L, Christensen HM, Harris DA. The cellular prion protein (PrP(C)): its physiological function and role in disease. *Biochim Biophys Acta*. 2007;1772(6):629–644.

42. Baumann F, Pahnke J, Radovanovic I, et al. Functionally relevant domains of the prion protein identified in vivo. *PLoS One*. 2009;4(9):e6707.
43. Del Rio JA, Gavin R. Functions of the cellular prion protein, the end of Moore's law, and Ockham's razor theory. *Prion*. 2016;10(1):25–40.
44. McCulloch L, Brown KL, Mabbott NA. Ablation of the cellular prion protein, PrPC, specifically on follicular dendritic cells has no effect on their maturation or function. *Immunology*. 2013;138(3):246–257.
45. Alfaidy N, Chauvet S, Donadio-Andrei S, et al. Prion protein expression and functional importance in developmental angiogenesis: role in oxidative stress and copper homeostasis. *Antioxid Redox Signal*. 2013;18(4): 400–411.
46. Guillot-Sestier MV, Checler F. Cellular prion and its catabolites in the brain: production and function. *Curr Mol Med*. 2012;12(3):304–315.
47. Wilson DA, Nixon RA. Sniffing out a function for prion proteins. *Nat Neurosci*. 2009;12(1):7–8.
48. Sakudo A, Ikuta K. Prion protein functions and dysfunction in prion diseases. *Curr Med Chem*. 2009;16(3): 380–389.
49. Millhauser GL. Copper and the prion protein: methods, structures, function, and disease. *Annu Rev Phys Chem*. 2007;58:299–320.
50. Varela-Nallar L, Toledo EM, Chacon MA, Inestrosa NC. The functional links between prion protein and copper. *Biol Res*. 2006;39(1):39–44.
51. Yu G, Chen J, Yu H, et al. Functional disruption of the prion protein gene in cloned goats. *J Gen Virol*. 2006;87(Pt 4):1019–1027.
52. Kretzschmar HA, Tings T, Madlung A, Giese A, Herms J. Function of PrP(C) as a copper-binding protein at the synapse. *Arch Virol Suppl*. 2000;(16):239–249.
53. Bueler H, Fischer M, Lang Y, et al. Normal development and behaviour of mice lacking the neuronal cell-surface PrP protein. *Nature*. 1992;356(6370):577–582.
54. Onodera T, Sakudo A, Tsubone H, Itohara S. Studies for normal function of prion protein using knockout mice under the immunological or pathophysiological stress. *Microbiol Immunol*. 2014;58:361–374.
55. Sakudo A, Onodera T. Prion protein (PrP) gene-knockout cell lines: insight into functions of the PrP. *Front Cell Dev Biol*. 2014;2:75.
56. Caiati MD, Safiulina VF, Fattorini G, Sivakumaran S, Legname G, Cherubini E. PrPC controls via protein kinase A the direction of synaptic plasticity in the immature hippocampus. *J Neurosci*. 2013;33(7):2973–2983.
57. Zhang CC, Steele AD, Lindquist S, Lodish HF. Prion protein is expressed on long-term repopulating hematopoietic stem cells and is important for their self-renewal. *Proc Natl Acad Sci USA*. 2006;103(7):2184–2189.
58. Collinge J, Whittington MA, Sidle KC, et al. Prion protein is necessary for normal synaptic function. *Nature*. 1994;370(6487):295–297.
59. Huber R, Deboer T, Tobler I. Sleep deprivation in prion protein deficient mice sleep deprivation in prion protein deficient mice and control mice: genotype dependent regional rebound. *Neuroreport*. 2002;13(1):1–4.
60. Graner E, Mercadante AF, Zanata SM, et al. Cellular prion protein binds laminin and mediates neuritogenesis. *Brain Res Mol Brain Res*. 2000;76(1):85–92.
61. Graner E, Mercadante AF, Zanata SM, Martins VR, Jay DG, Brentani RR. Laminin-induced PC-12 cell differentiation is inhibited following laser inactivation of cellular prion protein. *FEBS Lett*. 2000;482(3):257–260.
62. Chiarini LB, Freitas AR, Zanata SM, Brentani RR, Martins VR, Linden R. Cellular prion protein transduces neuroprotective signals. *EMBO J*. 2002;21(13):3317–3326.
63. Brown DR, Wong BS, Hafiz F, Clive C, Haswell SJ, Jones IM. Normal prion protein has an activity like that of superoxide dismutase. *Biochem J*. 1999;344(Pt 1):1–5.
64. Davies P, Brown DR. The chemistry of copper binding to PrP: is there sufficient evidence to elucidate a role for copper in protein function?. *Biochem J*. 2008;410(2):237–244.
65. Brown DR, Clive C, Haswell SJ. Antioxidant activity related to copper binding of native prion protein. *J Neurochem*. 2001;76(1):69–76.
66. Frederikse PH, Zigler Jr SJ, Farnsworth PN, Carper DA. Prion protein expression in mammalian lenses. *Curr Eye Res*. 2000;20(2):137–143.
67. Milhavet O, Lehmann S. Oxidative stress and the prion protein in transmissible spongiform encephalopathies. *Brain Res Brain Res Rev*. 2002;38(3):328–339.
68. Mitteregger G, Vosko M, Krebs B, et al. The role of the octarepeat region in neuroprotective function of the cellular prion protein. *Brain Pathol*. 2007;17(2):174–183.

69. Oh JM, Choi EK, Carp RI, Kim YS. Oxidative stress impairs autophagic flux in prion protein-deficient hippocampal cells. *Autophagy*. 2012;8(10):1448–1461.
70. Paterson AW, Curtis JC, Macleod NK, Complex I. specific increase in superoxide formation and respiration rate by PrP-null mouse brain mitochondria. *J Neurochem*. 2008;105(1):177–191.
71. Vassallo N, Herms J. Cellular prion protein function in copper homeostasis and redox signalling at the synapse. *J Neurochem*. 2003;86(3):538–544.
72. Walz R, Castro RM, Velasco TR, et al. Cellular prion protein: implications in seizures and epilepsy. *Cell Mol Neurobiol*. 2002;22(3):249–257.
73. Watt NT, Routledge MN, Wild CP, Hooper NM. Cellular prion protein protects against reactive-oxygen-species-induced DNA damage. *Free Radic Biol Med*. 2007;43(6):959–967.
74. White AR, Collins SJ, Maher F, et al. Prion protein-deficient neurons reveal lower glutathione reductase activity and increased susceptibility to hydrogen peroxide toxicity. *Am J Pathol*. 1999;155(5):1723–1730.
75. Wong BS, Liu T, Li R, et al. Increased levels of oxidative stress markers detected in the brains of mice devoid of prion protein. *J Neurochem*. 2001;76(2):565–572.
76. Zomosa-Signoret V, Arnaud JD, Fontes P, Alvarez-Martinez MT, Liautard JP. Physiological role of the cellular prion protein. *Vet Res*. 2008;39(4):9.
77. Guitart K, Loers G, Buck F, Bork U, Schachner M, Kleene R. Improvement of neuronal cell survival by astrocyte-derived exosomes under hypoxic and ischemic conditions depends on prion protein. *Glia*. 2016;64(6):896–910.
78. Guitart K, Loers G, Schachner M, Kleene R. Prion protein regulates glutathione metabolism and neural glutamate and cysteine uptake via excitatory amino acid transporter 3. *J Neurochem*. 2015;133(4):558–571.
79. Brown DR, Qin K, Herms JW, et al. The cellular prion protein binds copper in vivo. *Nature*. 1997;390(6661):684–687.
80. Treiber C, Pipkorn R, Weise C, Holland G, Multhaup G. Copper is required for prion protein-associated superoxide dismutase-I activity in Pichia pastoris. *FEBS J*. 2007;274(5):1304–1311.
81. Stanczak P, Kozlowski H. Can chicken and human PrPs possess SOD-like activity after beta-cleavage?. *Biochem Biophys Res Commun*. 2007;352(1):198–202.
82. Hutter G, Heppner FL, Aguzzi A. No superoxide dismutase activity of cellular prion protein in vivo. *Biol Chem*. 2003;384(9):1279–1285.
83. Wadsworth JD, Hill AF, Joiner S, Jackson GS, Clarke AR, Collinge J. Strain-specific prion-protein conformation determined by metal ions. *Nat Cell Biol*. 1999;1(1):55–59.
84. Jones S, Batchelor M, Bhelt D, Clarke AR, Collinge J, Jackson GS. Recombinant prion protein does not possess SOD-1 activity. *Biochem J*. 2005;392(Pt 2):309–312.
85. Sakudo A, Nakamura I, Tsuji S, Ikuta K. GPI-anchorless human prion protein is secreted and glycosylated but lacks superoxide dismutase activity. *Int J Mol Med*. 2008;21(2):217–222.
86. Davies P, Marken F, Salter S, Brown DR. Thermodynamic and voltammetric characterization of the metal binding to the prion protein: insights into pH dependence and redox chemistry. *Biochemistry*. 2009;48(12):2610–2619.
87. Liu L, Jiang D, McDonald A, Hao Y, Millhauser GL, Zhou F. Copper redox cycling in the prion protein depends critically on binding mode. *J Am Chem Soc*. 2011;133(31):12229–12237.
88. Hornshaw MP, McDermott JR, Candy JM. Copper binding to the N-terminal tandem repeat regions of mammalian and avian prion protein. *Biochem Biophys Res Commun*. 1995;207(2):621–629.
89. Hornshaw MP, McDermott JR, Candy JM, Lakey JH. Copper binding to the N-terminal tandem repeat region of mammalian and avian prion protein: structural studies using synthetic peptides. *Biochem Biophys Res Commun*. 1995;214(3):993–999.
90. Jackson GS, Murray I, Hosszu LL, et al. Location and properties of metal-binding sites on the human prion protein. *Proc Natl Acad Sci USA*. 2001;98(15):8531–8535.
91. Thompsett AR, Abdelraheim SR, Daniels M, Brown DR. High affinity binding between copper and full-length prion protein identified by two different techniques. *J Biol Chem*. 2005;280(52):42750–42758.
92. Stockel J, Safar J, Wallace AC, Cohen FE, Prusiner SB. Prion protein selectively binds copper(II) ions. *Biochemistry*. 1998;37(20):7185–7193.
93. Walter E.D, Chattopadhyay M, Millhauser GL. The affinity of copper binding to the prion protein octarepeat domain: evidence for negative cooperativity. *Biochemistry*. 2006;45(43):13083–13092.
94. Jones CE, Abdelraheim SR, Brown DR, Viles JH. Preferential Cu2+ coordination by His96 and His111 induces beta-sheet formation in the unstructured amyloidogenic region of the prion protein. *J Biol Chem*. 2004;279(31):32018–32027.

95. Davies P, McHugh PC, Hammond VJ, Marken F, Brown DR. Contribution of individual histidines to prion protein copper binding. *Biochemistry*. 2011;50(50):10781–10791.
96. Nadal RC, Davies P, Brown DR, Viles JH. Evaluation of copper2+ affinities for the prion protein. *Biochemistry*. 2009;48(38):8929–8931.
97. Haigh CL, Edwards K, Brown DR. Copper binding is the governing determinant of prion protein turnover. *Mol Cell Neurosci*. 2005;30(2):186–196.
98. Nunziante M, Gilch S, Schatzl HM. Essential role of the prion protein N terminus in subcellular trafficking and half-life of cellular prion protein. *J Biol Chem*. 2003;278(6):3726–3734.
99. Brown LR, Harris DA. Copper and zinc cause delivery of the prion protein from the plasma membrane to a subset of early endosomes and the Golgi. *J Neurochem*. 2003;87(2):353–363.
100. Perera WS, Hooper NM. Ablation of the metal ion-induced endocytosis of the prion protein by disease-associated mutation of the octarepeat region. *Curr Biol*. 2001;11(7):519–523.
101. Haigh CL, McGlade AR, Collins SJ. MEK1 transduces the prion protein N2 fragment antioxidant effects. *Cell Mol Life Sci*. 2015;72(8):1613–1629.
102. Brown DR. Prion protein expression aids cellular uptake and veratridine-induced release of copper. *J Neurosci Res*. 1999;58(5):717–725.
103. Brown DR. Role of the prion protein in copper turnover in astrocytes. *Neurobiol Dis*. 2004;15(3):534–543.
104. Dringen R, Scheiber IF, Mercer JF. Copper metabolism of astrocytes. *Front Aging Neurosci*. 2013;5:9.
105. Kralovicova S, Fontaine SN, Alderton A, et al. The effects of prion protein expression on metal metabolism. *Mol Cell Neurosci*. 2009;41(2):135–147.
106. Brown DR. Prion protein expression modulates neuronal copper content. *J Neurochem*. 2003;87(2):377–385.
107. Waggoner DJ, Drisaldi B, Bartnikas TB, et al. Brain copper content and cuproenzyme activity do not vary with prion protein expression level. *J Biol Chem*. 2000;275(11):7455–7458.
108. Rachidi W, Mange A, Senator A, et al. Prion infection impairs copper binding of cultured cells. *J Biol Chem*. 2003;278(17):14595–14598.
109. Cui T, Daniels M, Wong BS, et al. Mapping the functional domain of the prion protein. *Eur J Biochem*. 2003;270(16):3368–3376.
110. Thompsett AR, Brown DR. Dual polarisation interferometry analysis of copper binding to the prion protein: evidence for two folding states. *Biochim Biophys Acta*. 2007;1774(7):920–927.
111. Zhu F, Davies P, Thompsett AR, et al. Raman optical activity and circular dichroism reveal dramatic differences in the influence of divalent copper and manganese ions on prion protein folding. *Biochemistry*. 2008;47(8): 2510–2517.
112. Younan ND, Klewpatinond M, Davies P, Ruban AV, Brown DR, Viles JH. Copper(II)-induced secondary structure changes and reduced folding stability of the prion protein. *J Mol Biol*. 2011;410(3):369–382.
113. Nadal RC, Abdelraheim SR, Brazier MW, Rigby SE, Brown DR, Viles JH. Prion protein does not redox-silence Cu2+, but is a sacrificial quencher of hydroxyl radicals. *Free Radic Biol Med*. 2007;42(1):79–89.
114. Zhou F, Millhauser GL. The Rich Electrochemistry and Redox Reactions of the Copper Sites in the Cellular Prion Protein. *Coord Chem Rev*. 2012;256(19–20):2285–2296.
115. Brown DR, Hafiz F, Glasssmith LL, et al. Consequences of manganese replacement of copper for prion protein function and proteinase resistance. *EMBO J*. 2000;19(6):1180–1186.
116. Brazier MW, Davies P, Player E, Marken F, Viles JH, Brown DR. Manganese binding to the prion protein. *J Biol Chem*. 2008;283(19):12831–12839.
117. Stellato F, Minicozzi V, Millhauser GL, et al. Copper-zinc cross-modulation in prion protein binding. *Eur Biophys J*. 2014;43(12):631–642.
118. Watt NT, Taylor DR, Kerrigan TL, et al. Prion protein facilitates uptake of zinc into neuronal cells. *Nat Commun*. 2012;3:1134.
119. Pass R, Frudd K, Barnett JP, Blindauer CA, Brown DR. Prion infection in cells is abolished by a mutated manganese transporter but shows no relation to zinc. *Mol Cell Neurosci*. 2015;68:186–193.
120. Singh A, Mohan ML, Isaac AO, et al. Prion protein modulates cellular iron uptake: a novel function with implications for prion disease pathogenesis. *PLoS One*. 2009;4(2):e4468.
121. Singh A, Isaac AO, Luo X, et al. Abnormal brain iron homeostasis in human and animal prion disorders. *PLoS Pathog*. 2009;5(3):e1000336.
122. Singh A, Kong Q, Luo X, Petersen RB, Meyerson H, Singh N. Prion protein (PrP) knock-out mice show altered iron metabolism: a functional role for PrP in iron uptake and transport. *PLoS One*. 2009;4(7):e6115.

123. Singh A, Haldar S, Horback K, et al. Prion protein regulates iron transport by functioning as a ferrireductase. *J Alzheimers Dis*. 2013;35(3):541–552.
124. Davies P, Moualla D, Brown DR. Alpha-synuclein is a cellular ferrireductase. *PLoS One*. 2011;6(1):e15814.
125. Thackray AM, Knight R, Haswell SJ, Bujdoso R, Brown DR. Metal imbalance and compromised antioxidant function are early changes in prion disease. *Biochem J*. 2002;362(Pt 1):253–258.
126. Garnett AP, Viles JH. Copper binding to the octarepeats of the prion protein. Affinity, specificity, folding, and cooperativity: insights from circular dichroism. *J Biol Chem*. 2003;278(9):6795–6802.
127. Gaggelli E, Bernardi F, Molteni E, et al. Interaction of the human prion PrP(106-126) sequence with copper(II), manganese(II), and zinc(II): NMR and EPR studies. *J Am Chem Soc*. 2005;127(3):996–1006.
128. Treiber C, Thompsett AR, Pipkorn R, Brown DR, Multhaup G. Real-time kinetics of discontinuous and highly conformational metal-ion binding sites of prion protein. *J Biol Inorg Chem*. 2007;12(5):711–720.
129. Tsenkova RN, Iordanova IK, Toyoda K, Brown DR. Prion protein fate governed by metal binding. *Biochem Biophys Res Commun*. 2004;325(3):1005–1012.
130. Uppington KM, Brown DR. Resistance of cell lines to prion toxicity aided by phospho-ERK expression. *J Neurochem*. 2008;105(3):842–852.
131. Hesketh S, Thompsett AR, Brown DR. Prion protein polymerisation triggered by manganese-generated prion protein seeds. *J Neurochem*. 2012;120(1):177–189.
132. Supattapone S, Bouzamondo E, Ball HL, et al. A protease-resistant 61-residue prion peptide causes neurodegeneration in transgenic mice. *Mol Cell Biol*. 2001;21(7):2608–2616.
133. Treiber C, Simons A, Multhaup G. Effect of copper and manganese on the de novo generation of protease-resistant prion protein in yeast cells. *Biochemistry*. 2006;45(21):6674–6680.
134. Li XL, Dong CF, Wang GR, et al. Manganese-induced changes of the biochemical characteristics of the recombinant wild-type and mutant PrPs. *Med Microbiol Immunol*. 2009;198(4):239–245.
135. Birkett CR, Hennion RM, Bembridge DA, et al. Scrapie strains maintain biological phenotypes on propagation in a cell line in culture. *EMBO J*. 2001;20(13):3351–3358.
136. Davies P, Brown DR. Manganese enhances prion protein survival in model soils and increases prion infectivity to cells. *PLoS One*. 2009;4(10):e7518.
137. Brazier MW, Volitakis I, Kvasnicka M, et al. Manganese chelation therapy extends survival in a mouse model of M1000 prion disease. *J Neurochem*. 2010;114(2):440–451.
138. Hesketh S, Sassoon J, Knight R, Hopkins J, Brown DR. Elevated manganese levels in blood and central nervous system occur before onset of clinical signs in scrapie and bovine spongiform encephalopathy. *J Anim Sci*. 2007;85(6):1596–1609.
139. Hesketh S, Sassoon J, Knight R, Brown DR. Elevated manganese levels in blood and CNS in human prion disease. *Mol Cell Neurosci*. 2008;37(3):590–598.
140. White SN, O'Rourke KI, Gidlewski T, et al. Increased risk of chronic wasting disease in Rocky Mountain elk associated with decreased magnesium and increased manganese in brain tissue. *Can J Vet Res*. 2010;74(1):50–53.
141. Wolfe LL, Conner MM, Bedwell CL, Lukacs PM, Miller MW. Select tissue mineral concentrations and chronic wasting disease status in mule deer from North-central Colorado. *J Wildl Dis*. 2010;46(3):1029–1034.
142. Rivera NA, Novakofski J, Weng HY, et al. Metals in obex and retropharyngeal lymph nodes of Illinois white-tailed deer and their variations associated with CWD status. *Prion*. 2015;9(1):48–58.
143. Johnson CJ, Gilbert PU, Abrecht M, et al. Low copper and high manganese levels in prion protein plaques. *Viruses*. 2013;5(2):654–662.
144. Wong BS, Chen SG, Colucci M, et al. Aberrant metal binding by prion protein in human prion disease. *J Neurochem*. 2001;78(6):1400–1408.
145. Purdey M. Ecosystems supporting clusters of sporadic TSEs demonstrate excesses of the radical-generating divalent cation manganese and deficiencies of antioxidant co factors Cu, Se, Fe, Zn. Does a foreign cation substitution at prion protein's Cu domain initiate TSE?. *Med Hypotheses*. 2000;54(2):278–306.
146. Imrie CE, Korre A, Munoz-Melendez G. Spatial correlation between the prevalence of transmissible spongiform diseases and British soil geochemistry. *Environ Geochem Health*. 2009;31(1):133–145.
147. Chihota CM, Gravenor MB, Baylis M. Investigation of trace elements in soil as risk factors in the epidemiology of scrapie. *Vet Rec*. 2004;154(26):809–813.
148. Legleiter LR, Liu HC, Lloyd KE, Hansen SL, Fry RS, Spears JW. Exposure to low dietary copper or low copper coupled with high dietary manganese for one year does not alter brain prion protein characteristics in the mature cow. *J Anim Sci*. 2007;85(11):2895–2903.

149. Legleiter LR, Spears JW, Liu HC. Copper deficiency in the young bovine results in dramatic decreases in brain copper concentration but does not alter brain prion protein biology. *J Anim Sci*. 2008;86(11):3069–3078.
150. Guentchev M, Voigtlander T, Haberler C, Groschup MH, Budka H. Evidence for oxidative stress in experimental prion disease. *Neurobiol Dis*. 2000;7(4):270–273.
151. Guentchev M, Siedlak SL, Jarius C, et al. Oxidative damage to nucleic acids in human prion disease. *Neurobiol Dis*. 2002;9(3):275–281.
152. Choi SI, Ju WK, Choi EK, et al. Mitochondrial dysfunction induced by oxidative stress in the brains of hamsters infected with the 263 K scrapie agent. *Acta Neuropathol*. 1998;96(3):279–286.
153. Andreoletti O, Levavasseur E, Uro-Coste E, et al. Astrocytes accumulate 4-hydroxynonenal adducts in murine scrapie and human Creutzfeldt-Jakob disease. *Neurobiol Dis*. 2002;11(3):386–393.
154. Petersen RB, Siedlak SL, Lee HG, et al. Redox metals and oxidative abnormalities in human prion diseases. *Acta Neuropathol*. 2005;110(3):232–238.
155. Wong BS, Brown DR, Pan T, et al. Oxidative impairment in scrapie-infected mice is associated with brain metals perturbations and altered antioxidant activities. *J Neurochem*. 2001;79(3):689–698.
156. Milhavet O, McMahon HE, Rachidi W, et al. Prion infection impairs the cellular response to oxidative stress. *Proc Natl Acad Sci USA*. 2000;97(25):13937–13942.
157. Mitteregger G, Korte S, Shakarami M, Herms J, Kretzschmar HA. Role of copper and manganese in prion disease progression. *Brain Res*. 2009;1292:155–164.
158. Brazier MW, Doctrow SR, Masters CL, Collins SJ. A manganese-superoxide dismutase/catalase mimetic extends survival in a mouse model of human prion disease. *Free Radic Biol Med*. 2008;45(2):184–192.
159. Sigurdsson EM, Brown DR, Alim MA, et al. Copper chelation delays the onset of prion disease. *J Biol Chem*. 2003;278(47):46199–46202.
160. Pollera C, Lucchini B, Formentin E, Bareggi S, Poli G, Ponti W. Evaluation of anti-prionic activity of clioquinol in an in vivo model (Mesocricetus auratus). *Vet Res Commun*. 2005;29(Suppl 2):253–255.
161. Siggs OM, Cruite JT, Du X, et al. Disruption of copper homeostasis due to a mutation of Atp7a delays the onset of prion disease. *Proc Natl Acad Sci USA*. 2012;109(34):13733–13738.
162. Mallucci G, Dickinson A, Linehan J, Klohn PC, Brandner S, Collinge J. Depleting neuronal PrP in prion infection prevents disease and reverses spongiosis. *Science*. 2003;302(5646):871–874.
163. Hortells P, Monleon E, Acin C, et al. The effect of metal imbalances on scrapie neurodegeneration. *Zoonoses Public Health*. 2010;57(5):358–366.
164. Hijazi N, Shaked Y, Rosenmann H, Ben-Hur T, Gabizon R. Copper binding to PrPC may inhibit prion disease propagation. *Brain Res*. 2003;993(1-2):192–200.
165. McKenzie D, Bartz J, Mirwald J, Olander D, Marsh R, Aiken J. Reversibility of scrapie inactivation is enhanced by copper. *J Biol Chem*. 1998;273(40):25545–25547.

CHAPTER

8

Manganese and Neurodegeneration

Dinamene Marques dos Santos, Michael Aschner***, *Ana P. Marreilha dos Santos**

*University of Lisbon, Lisboa, Portugal

**Albert Einstein College of Medicine, Bronx, NY, United States

OUTLINE

Biometals in Neurodegenerative Diseases. http://dx.doi.org/10.1016/B978-0-12-804562-6.00008-7

BACKGROUND

Manganese (Mn; atomic no. 25, weight = 54.94 g/mol, density = 7.43 at 20°C) is a transitional metal (Group VIIa),[1] isolated in 1774, by the Swedish chemist Scheele.[2,3] Mn is the 12th most abundant element in the earth's crust, naturally present in rocks, soil, water, and food.[2,4] Mn is known to be an essential trace element for animals since 1931,[5] required for normal mammalian physiological processes, such as bone growth, development of cartilage and connective tissues,[6] reproductive,[7,8] neuronal,[9,10] immune, and antioxidant[7,11] functions. It can exist in 11 oxidation states from −3 to +7, being the normally encountered valences +2 (the most common form in nature), +4 (in dioxide Mn) and +7 (in permanganate ion).[12]

Parenteral nutrition (PN) is a method of supplying nutrients by parenteral route to patients that cannot meet their nutritional requirements from the gastrointestinal (GI) tract.[13] Mn supplementation in PN patients is essential[14] to prevent the depletion of endogenous stores and deficiency symptoms.[15] In humans, despite the classification of Mn as an essential trace element, there is little evidence of Mn deficiency being clinically relevant as no cases of deficiency have been described receiving unsupplemented PN.[16] Most of the evidence for human Mn deficiency is derived from experimental studies where subjects received Mn depleted diets.[14] The first case of suspected Mn deficiency was in a male subject who was fed with a chemically defined diet as part of an investigation for determining vitamin-K requirements. Mn was inadvertently omitted from the diet for 17 weeks; the subject developed mild dermatitis, reddening of his black hair and beard, slowed growth of hair, nails, and beard, occasional nausea and vomiting, and moderate weight loss. His total diet (food and water) provided only 0.35 mg Mn/d, resulting in 55% and 85% reduction in serum and stool Mn levels, respectively.[17,18] Friedman and coworkers investigated experimental Mn depletion in seven healthy male subjects, 19–22 years of age. The subjects were fed with a Mn-adequate diet (2.59 mg Mn/d) for 3 weeks to establish baseline data, followed by a purified diet containing 0.11 mg Mn/d for 39 days (depletion), followed by two 5 days periods of 1.53 and 2.55 mg Mn/d (repletion). The appearance of dermatitis, termed Miliaria crystallina (prickly heat), developed in five of the seven subjects at the end of depletion period, but disappeared as Mn repletion began. They also had increased serum calcium (Ca) and phosphorous concentrations and increased alkaline phosphate activity, suggestive of bone resorption.[19]

Although PN was introduced into medical practice in the 1960s,[20,21] the iatrogenic risk of Mn-induced neurotoxicity associated to PN was only recognized in 1990, when Mehta and Reilly reported a case of a 32 year old woman medicated with haloperidol, receiving daily Mn (0.3 mg). After 4 months of Mn supplementation, the patient developed extrapyramidal signs, which were irreversible after haloperidol discontinuation. Whole blood (WB) Mn level was significantly increased, and 3 days after Mn-free PN all symptoms resolved. WB Mn level fell to normal limits within 1 month after its discontinuation in the PN solution.[22]

The recent PN guidelines recommend the biomonitoring of Mn in patients receiving PN for >30 days.[13] Biomonitoring is based on a systematic collection of biological samples for analysis of concentrations of compounds, metabolites, or specific nonadverse biological effect parameters, with the objective of assessing exposure and health risk in exposed subjects, comparing the data observed with the reference level and—if necessary—leading to corrective actions.[23] The data in the literature are conflicting about the optimal method for assessing Mn stores in humans. A definitive biomarker of Mn exposure or Mn-induced neurotoxicity has yet to be identified.

The biomonitoring of Mn relies on the analysis of whole blood Mn (WB Mn) levels, which are highly variable among human population and are not correlated with Mn-induced neurotoxicity.[24–26] Increased brain Mn levels can be detected by T1-weighted magnetic resonance imaging (MRI). Accordingly, periodic brain MRI examination may be required to monitor excess Mn accumulation in the brain of patients receiving PN.[27] However, MRI is not used as a routine method of diagnosis due to high costs and the need to examine the relationships between hyperintensities in the basal ganglia and the onset of subclinical Mn neurotoxicity.[28] Alterations in dopaminergic (DAergic)[29–32] and catecholaminergic[33–35] metabolism have been studied as predictive biomarkers of Mn-induced neurotoxicity.

Since the first report of Mn-induced neurotoxicity, numerous other cases of Parkinsonian-like symptoms associated with Mn exposure from parenteral admixtures have been reported.[24–27,36–45] Mn toxicity upon ingestion is rare as homeostatic mechanisms tightly regulate its absorption and excretion,[4,46] ensuring adequate supplies. In contrast, Mn delivered intravenously (IV) bypasses homeostatic mechanisms regulating Mn absorption.[22,24,25,36–38,40,47,48] Tables 8.1 and 8.2 show several reports on hypermanganesemia and induced-neurotoxicity in patients fed by parenteral route.

Mn ESSENTIALITY AND METABOLIC FUNCTIONS

The criteria for essentiality for human health is that the absence or deficiency of the nutrient from the diet produces either functional or structural abnormalities, and that these abnormalities are related to, or a consequence of, specific biochemical changes that may be reversed by the presence of the essential nutrient.[4] Mn is an essential trace element required for a variety of important enzymatic reactions.[14] Mn is involved in oxidation-reduction processes,[49] phosphorylation,[50] and the synthesis of cholesterol, fatty acids, mucopolysaccharides,[51] and chondroitin sulfate.[52] Mn functions as a constituent of metalloenzymes and also as an enzyme activator.[53] Mn is a cofactor of important metalloenzymatic systems, such as arginase, pyruvate carboxylase, and Mn superoxide dismutase (Mn-SOD).[51,54] Arginase, the cytosolic enzyme responsible for urea production, contains 4 mol Mn (II) per mol enzyme.[53,55] The enzyme is found in high concentrations in the liver, the site of the urea cycle. Low-Mn diets in animals have been shown to decrease arginase activity.[56] Pyruvate carboxylase, a ligase that contains four Mn atoms converts pyruvate to the tricarboxylic acid (TCA) cycle intermediate oxaloacetate.[57,58] Because magnesium (Mg) can replace Mn in pyruvate carboxylase, minimal changes in pyruvate carboxylase activity occur with Mn deficiency.[59] Mn is also a cofactor of the antioxidant mitochondrial Mn-SOD that catalyzes the dismutation of two molecules of superoxide anion (O_2^-), into hydrogen peroxide (H_2O_2) and oxygen (O_2). H_2O_2 is further detoxified to water (H_2O) by catalase and glutathione peroxidase.[60,61] Decreased Mn-SOD levels may lead to increased reactive oxygen species (ROS) levels in mitochondria, thus increasing the susceptibility of cells to oxidative stress.[62] Mn-deficient animals have low Mn-SOD activity in several tissues including liver, brain, heart, and kidney.[63]

In contrast to the relatively few metalloenzymes, there are a large number of Mn-activated enzymes, including oxidoreductases, transferases, hydrolases, lyases, isomerases, and ligases.[64] Mn activation of these enzymes can occur as a direct consequence of Mn binding to the protein, causing a subsequent conformation change, or by binding to the substrate. However, largely because the activation of these enzymes is not Mn specific, Mn deficiency

TABLE 8.1 Selected Reports of Hypermanganesemia in Parenterally Fed Adult Patients

References	*n*	Age (years)	Disease/ condition	Type of PN	Mn daily dose and duration of intake	Laboratory findings	Radiological findings	Clinical symptoms
Ejima et al. (1992)[26]	1	62	SBS	PN	2.2 mg (2.3 mo)	WB Mn decr after 15 wk of Mn-free PN	Incr MRI signal (basal ganglia, especially globus pallidus, tectum, and tegmentum of midbrain and pons); MRI signal decr after 22 wk of Mn-free PN.	Parkinsonism with dysarthria, mild rigidity, hypokinesia, masked face, halting gate
Mirowitz et al. (1991)[24]	9	58.9 (5174)	Numerous	PN	0.30.4 mg 5.3 y (5 mo 11 y)	NR	Incr MRI signal (basal ganglia)	5 pts with neurologic symptoms: memory loss, confusion weakness, fatigue, and imbalance
Mirowitz and Westrich (1992)[37]	1	61	GI dyskinesia	PN	0.4 mg 3 y	NR	Incr MRI signal (globus pallidus); 12 mo after d/c Mn, complete regression MRI signals	No symptoms
Alves et al. (1997)[38]	1	63	SBS	PN	1–2 mg 19 mo	Incr serum and urine Mn	Incr MRI signal (basal ganglia and white matter); 6 mo after d/c Mn, decr MRI signals	Gait disturbance, dystonic movements

Nagatomo et al. (1999)[39]	1	68	Ulcerative colitis	PN	20 μmol 3 mo	Incr serum (4.2 mg/dL) and urine (9.0 mg/dL) Mn	Incr MRI signal (basal ganglia)	Psychiatric symptoms and gait disturbance
	1	70	Aspiration pneumonia	PN	20 μmol 4 mo	Incr serum (5.1 mg/dL) and urine (1.0 mg/dL) Mn	Incr MRI signal (basal ganglia)	Progressive gait disturbance and confusion
Fitzgerald et al. (1999)[36]	36 30 21	1487	Numerous	PN PN HPN	500 μg < 48 h 500 μg 228 d 500 μg 365075 d	RBC Mn: low to normal Incr RBC Mn in 2 pts Incr RBC Mn in 15/21 pts	3 selected cases of abnormal MRI	1 HPN pt was noted to exhibit petit mal seizures, vertigo, gait disturbances, and peripheral neuropathy
Bertinet et al. (2000)[25]	15	54 (3274)	Numerous	HPN	Mg 3.8 (1.710) y	WB, plasma, and RBC Mn within normal limits	10/15 incr MRI signal (basal ganglia)	No symptoms

d, days; Decr, decreased; GI, gastrointestinal; HPN, home parenteral nutrition; h, hours; Incr, increased; MRI, magnetic resonance imaging; mo, month; NR, not reported, PN, parenteral nutrition; pts, patients; RBC, red blood cells; SBS, short-bowel disease, wk, weeks; y, years.

TABLE 8.2 Selected Reports of Hypermanganesemia in Parenterally Fed Children and Adolescent Patients

References	n	Age (years)	Disease/condition	Type of PN	Mn daily dose and duration of intake	Laboratory findings	Radiological findings	Clinical symptoms
Fell et al. (1992)	57	9 mo (0.5–162)	Numerous 46/57 w/o cholestasis	HPN	<10 kg 0.17 mg/kg 10 kg 0.14 mg/kg (0.5–17) mo <10 kg 0.17 mg/kg 10 kg 0.14 mg/kg 7/57 PN for > 2 y	45/57 incr WB Mn Higher Mn associated with cholestasis; 8 mo after d/c Mn, decr WB Mn 6/7 incr WB Mn	Selected cases of abnormal MRI Incr MRI signal (globus pallidus, nuclei subthalamic) 4/7 selected cases of abnormal MRI	Pts with dystonic limb movements and abnormal posturing; 4 pts died No symptoms
Reynolds et al. (1994)[41]	1 53	7 mo	SBS, PN associated liver disease numerous	NR	44–55 µg/kg 17 mo 44–55 µg/kg > 6 wk	Incr WB Mn (1740 nmol/L) Incr WB Mn in those with evidence of cholestatic liver disease (n = 35); highest conc found in those < 2 y	MRI abnormalities compatible with deposition of a paramagnetic metal NR	Developmental delay, abnormal dystonic movements of both arms, microcephaly
Ono et al. (1995)[42]	1	5 y	Intractable diarrhea and recurrent pancreatitis	PN	2 mg > 2y	Incr WB (135 µg/dL) Mn, 5 mo after d/c Mn, decr WB Mn to 20 µg/dL	Incr MRI signal (basal ganglia)	Nonspecific headache and amnesia

Komaki et al. (1998)	1	2 y	Intractable vomiting and diarrhea	PN	mg (82 μg/kg) 14 mo	Incr WB (9.7 μg/dL) Mn, 3 mo after d/c Mn, decr WB Mn to normal levels	Incr MRI signal (globus pallidus, thalamus) 3 mo after d/c Mn MRI abnormalities regressed	Tremor and generalized tonic seizures, psychomotor retardation, hyperactivity; 3 mo after d/c Mn, seizures and tremor completely disappeared
Hsieh et al. (2007)[44]	1	10 y	SBS	PN	8 μg/kg mo	Incr WB (3.7 μg/dL) Mn	Incr MRI signal (basal ganglia)	Tonic-clonic seizures
Iinuma et al. (2003)[27]	7	10 (3–20)	Numerous	HPN	15.7–91.5 μg/kg 93 (18–179) mo	4/7 Incr WB (5.1 μg/dL) Mn	Incr MRI signal; 12 mo after d/c Mn, 5/7 pts decr MRI signals	No symptoms

conc, Concentration; decr, decreased; d/c, discontinuation; GI, gastrointestinal; HPN, home parenteral nutrition; incr, increased; MRI, magnetic resonance imaging; mo, month; NR, not reported; PN, parenteral nutrition; RBC, red blood cells; SBS, short-bowel disease; wk, weeks; w/o, without; y, years.

does not impair the activity of most of these enzymes. One exception to this apparent lack of specificity is the Mn specific activation of glycosyl transferases,[53] that is especially important for the synthesis of glycosaminoglycans, such as chondroitin sulfate. Mn deficiency is associated with impaired glycosyl transferase activity.[59] Mn is also a cofactor of glutamine synthetase (GS), an enzyme found exclusively in the astrocytes, which catalyzes the conversion of glutamate, an excitotoxic amino acid, into glutamine.[65] GS contains four Mn ions per octamer and accounts for approximately 80% of total Mn in brain.[66] Brain GS activity can be normal even in severely Mn deficient animals, suggesting that the enzyme either has a high priority for this element or Mg can act as a substitute when Mn is lacking.[53]

Mn BIOKINETICS AND HOMEOSTATIC CONTROL

Routes and Sources of Mn Exposure

Absorption of Airborne Mn

Occupational exposure to Mn is linked to the majority of the reported cases of Mn intoxication.[67] Neurotoxicity due to inhalation exposure to airborne Mn has been reported in Mn dioxide miners,[68] smelters,[69] and welders.[70] Health risks of exposure to Mn have also been associated with organic Mn-containing pesticides, such as Mn ethylenebis-dithiocarbamate (MANEB). Currently, there is a significant concern on Mn toxicity due to use of the organometallic compound methylcyclopentadienyl Mn tricarbonyl (MMT), an octane improver in unleaded gasoline.[71–73] Increased usage of Mn-containing products results in greater exposure of large populations to Mn.[67] Average levels of Mn in ambient air are approximately 5 and 33 ng Mn/m^3 in nonurban and urban air, respectively.[74] The daily intake of Mn from the ambient air is estimated to be < 2 μg Mn/d in the general population.[11] Cellular mechanisms involved with Mn absorption within the respiratory tract are unknown.[11]

Parenteral Exposure to Mn

Parenteral exposure may pose a much higher risk for Mn toxicity since the bioavailability of Mn in parenteral fluids is much higher than that observed following oral route (100% vs. 5%). Moreover, normal regulation mechanisms for Mn metabolism are largely bypassed, and there is a greater danger of toxicity.[11] Mn is added to PN in the water soluble forms, sulfate or chloride, usually in a fixed-concentration trace elements (TE) supplement containing several TE.[75] Another potential source of Mn exposure by the parenteral route is the inclusion of Mn in the radiological contrast agents, such as Mn dipyridoxil diphosphate (Mn-DPDP), useful in MRI diagnosis of pancreatic adenocarcinoma or pancreatitis.[50,76,77] There have been no reported cases of Mn intoxication following administration of one or more doses of Mn containing contrast agents. The low incidence of Mn toxicity following systemic administration of Mn containing contrast agents is probably owing to acute, less frequent exposure, fast elimination, and low body burden of Mn in clinical diagnosis.[67]

Oral Absorption of Mn From Food and Water

The main route responsible for Mn absorption is the GI tract[60]; in steady state conditions, the GI tract absorbs ~5% of the total oral intake of Mn.[50,78] Whole grain cereals, dried fruits, nuts, and leafy vegetables are among the common Mn rich foods.[79] Dietary supplements provide Mn in the gluconate, sulfate, ascorbate, and amino acid chelates forms.[59] The mean and upper range dietary Mn exposure for adults from United kingdom (UK) consumers estimated from the UK 1994 *Total Diet Study* were 4.5 and 8.2 mg/d, respectively.[80] In an earlier review, World Health Organization (WHO) reported the average daily consumption of Mn to range from 2.0 to 8.8 mg Mn/d.[81]

Mn absorption is equally efficient in the small intestine.[82] Mn absorption may occur also in the large intestine via a nonsaturable process consistent with passive diffusion,[60,83] that may come into play when intakes are high.[82] The mechanism by which Mn is absorbed from the GI tract is not completely understood. Some studies suggest that Mn is absorbed through an active transport mechanism,[84] that most likely involves the metal divalent transporter 1, referred as DMT1 (also known as DCT-1 or nramp-2).[85]

Mn Biodistribution and Elimination

Once in blood, Mn rapidly distributes into other tissues.[67] The normal whole-body content in humans is 12–20 mg (218–364 μmol) with a daily turnover of 5–8 mg.[86] Mn is found in all mammalian tissues, with concentrations ranging from 0.3 to 2.9 μg Mn/g tissue of wet-weight (ww) and little variation among species with regard to tissue Mn concentrations.[87] The highest Mn concentrations in humans were found in liver (1.2–2.1 mg/Kg = 21.8–38.2 μmol/L), kidneys (0.6–0.9 mg/Kg = 10.9–16.4 μmol/L), endocrine glands, and intestines.[1,50,88] Few studies have addressed the kinetics of Mn in the body upon PN administration.[89] Malecki and coworkers maintained male Sprague-Dawley rats on PN (0.5+/− 0.2 or 16+/−3 nmol Mn/g for 7 days) and compared tissue concentrations of Mn with rats maintained on a reference diet (1.3 mmol Mn/g/d). Concentrations of Mn in tibia, spleen, and pancreas were increased in the PN high Mn dose group compared to the PN low Mn dose or the normal diet groups.[90]

Within the plasma, approximately 80% of Mn is bound to β-globulin and albumin, and a small fraction of Mn is bound to transferrin (Tf).[11,91,92] When complexed with Tf, Mn is exclusively present in the trivalent oxidation-state.[91] At normal plasma iron (Fe) concentrations (0.9– 2.8 μg/ml), Fe binding capacity (2.5–4 μg/mL) and plasma Tf concentration (3 mg/mL), with two metal–ion-binding sites per molecule, of which only 30% are occupied by Fe (III)), Tf has 50 μmol/L of unoccupied Mn(III) binding sites.[93,94] The protein binding is a key determinant of both Mn retention in the body and brain Mn delivery.[95] The Tf null mice have more rapid loss of Mn from the body.[96]

Biliary secretion is the main pathway for Mn excretion.[48,97] Pancreatic excretion of Mn contributes only a small fraction of the absorbed Mn dose.[97] Urinary excretion of Mn is generally low.[51] In the liver, Mn is removed from the blood, conjugated with bile, and excreted into the intestine.[78] Mn concentration in bile can exceed plasma by 100-fold, suggesting active transport.[98] Recently, solute carrier 30A10 (SLC30A10) has been identified as a human Mn transporter, highly expressed in the liver. The autosomal recessively inherited disorder associated SLC30A10 deficiency leads to Mn accumulation in brain and liver.[99]

A small fraction of Mn in the intestine is reabsorbed, establishing de facto an enterohepatic circulation.[2] Biliary elimination is dose-dependent.[48] The rate of Mn radioactivity elimination following an IV injection of a tracer dose in bile duct ligated rats was enhanced by IV injection of large amounts of unlabeled Mn, indicating inducible intestinal excretion of Mn.[100]

Dose-dependent elimination of tracer doses of Mn has also been reported in Mn-exposed miners from Chile as compared to control populations. The terminal blood half-time for the active (i.e., Mn-exposed) miners was 15 ± 2 days, compared to 37.5 ± 7.5 days for control individuals and 28.3 ± 8 days for exminers with chronic Mn toxicity who had stopped working in mining 2–25 years previously.[101]

Biokinetics of Mn in Brain

Mn Transport Into Brain

Physiological concentrations of Mn range from 2 to 8 μM in brain tissue,[102] but can increase several-fold upon overexposure.[67,103] Entry of Mn to brain can occur via three known pathways: through the capillary endothelial cells of the blood–brain barrier (BBB), by the choroid plexus (CP) of the blood–cerebrospinal fluid (CSF) barrier, or via the olfactory nerve from the nasal cavity directly to brain.[67] The CP epithelium exists between blood and ventricular CSF, which is secreted by CP in the lateral, third and fourth ventricles.[104] The exact role of the CP in the regulation of cerebral Mn uptake is still uncertain.[105] The BBB is responsible for the regulation of exchange of Mn between the blood and brain parenchyma.[106] The endothelial cells of adult mammal brain are continuously linked by tight junctions (*zonula occludens*),[106] to form the BBB,[107] which contributes in the restriction of passage of water-soluble molecules from blood to brain; the endothelium of the CP is leaky (no tight junctions).[108]

There are multiple mechanisms for Mn transport across the BBB,[109] which involve different transport systems including facilitated diffusion and active transport[106,109]; the relative contribution of each of these transporters remains unknown, and it is likely that optimal tissue Mn concentrations are maintained by the concordant involvement of many of these transporters.[110] Chua and coworkers[111] reported that DMT1 mediates the transport of Mn across the BBB, as it was noted that the uptake of ^{54}Mn, as well as ^{59}Fe by the brain was decreased in homozygous Belgrade b/b rats comparatively to heterozygous +/b rats, suggesting that the defective DMT1 allele affects the distribution of both metals, and that Mn(II) and Fe(II) might share DMT1 transporters in the BBB.[111] DMT1 is a symporter energized by the proton-motive force generated by the vacuolar ATPase, which extrudes protons from the cell. Upon acidification, Mn(III) ions released by the Tf receptor system are converted to Mn(II) ions available for transport by DMT1.[110] Yokel and Crossgrove, using in situ rat brain perfusion, showed that Mn(II) uptake was not inhibited by the absence of DMT1 expression, suggesting an Fe-transporter-independent mechanism at the BBB.[112] In vitro studies, using bovine brain capillary endothelial cells (BCEC) showed that Mn uptake was reduced by vanadate, a Ca transport inhibitor, suggesting that Ca-dependent mechanisms mediate Mn(II) ion uptake across the BBB.[113] Some of these transporters include the DMT1,[114] ZIP-8,[115] transferrin receptor (TfR),[95,116] voltage regulated (VR),[117] and store-operated Ca channels[118] and N-methyl-D-aspartate (NMDA) channels.[119]

Mn may also be transported as a citrate complex, and candidates for this transporter include the organic anion transporter or a monocarboxylate transporter (MCT) and/or members of the organic anion transporter polypeptide (OATP) or ATP-binding cassette (ABC) super-families.[120]

Regional Delivery of Mn in the Brain

Mn accumulates primarily in those areas known to contain high concentrations of nonheme Fe, especially the globus pallidus (GP) and striatum.[106] The neuronal circuit of the basal ganglia consists of an interconnected set of neuronal clusters, in the subcortical region of the brain[121] that control motor function.[122] The circuitry of basal ganglia is comprised of the following discrete nuclei: globus pallidus, substantia nigra, subthalamic nucleus, and the striatum (caudate and putamen). This circuit sends and receives information from the cortex and thalamus.[123]

Recent in vivo studies suggest that dopamine active transporter (DAT) plays an important role in Mn accumulation in the striatum.[124] Inhibition of DAT function in weanling male Sprague–Dawley rats attenuates Mn accumulation in the globus pallidus during chronic exposure.[125]

Tracqui and coworkers examined brain Mn concentrations in three control subjects, and reported that globus pallidus, putamen, fifth gyrus temporalis and thalamus Mn concentrations were 0.39 ± 0.05, 0.43 ± 0.11, 0.27 ± 0.05, and 0.33 ± 0.07 μg/g, respectively.[126] These investigators also reported a 63 year-old woman maintained on PN for 19 months, with higher globus pallidus, putamen, and fifth gyrus temporalis Mn concentrations (0.95, 1.00, and 0.44 μg/g, respectively) compared with normal subjects.

The use of MRI has also revealed that Mn-poisoned humans and macaque monkeys develop elevated striatum, globus pallidus, and substantia nigra brain Mn concentrations.[11,39,127–129] The paramagnetic properties of Mn are due to its unpaired electrons that can interact with water protons.[50] The paramagnetic properties of Mn cause shortening of T1 relaxation times of hydrogen nuclei in water molecules,[130] which results in a detectable increase of signal intensities in T1-weighted sequences.[50]

Mn Elimination From Brain Compartment

Once Mn has crossed the BBB, the average half-life of Mn in the rat brain is 51–74 days.[131] In nonhuman primates, available data suggest that the rate of elimination in the brain has region specificity and estimates of half-life range from $\leq$ 33 days[132] to 53 days[133] after inhalational and subcutaneous Mn exposure, respectively. Cotzias and coworkers noted brain elimination half-life for Mn of 53 days in humans dosed intravenously with tracer ^{54}Mn.[101] In contrast to the evidence for brain Mn influx, less is known about Mn movement out from the brain into blood.[67] The brain efflux of Mn across the BBB does not appear to occur through a transporter and is likely to occur slowly by diffusion.[134] The brain uptake of Mn is unidirectional and in light of transporter-mediated brain influx but not efflux, it would be anticipated that repeated, excessive, Mn exposure might result in brain Mn accumulation over time.[135]

Subcellular Distribution of Mn in Brain

Mn can be taken up into astrocytes and neurons. Astrocytic uptake of Mn takes place at least in part via DMT1[54]; neuronal uptake of Mn involves Tf,[136] as well as utilization of specific transporter systems, such as DAT.[125] In cystosol, Mn can either be complexed by cytosolic proteins, phosphates, adenosine triphosphate (ATP), or it can enter cellular compartments, such as the mitochondria, the endoplasmic reticulum, or the Golgi complex.[137] Mn accumulation in the mitochondria, capillaries, synaptosomes, and cytosol has been demonstrated by instrumental neutron activation analysis.[138] Mn is trafficked to mitochondria by an ATP-dependent Ca uniporter; Mn loading into mitochondria is essential for being incorporated in Mn-SOD.[139,140] Electron paramagnetic resonance (EPR) shows that over 97% of the Mn(III) in the mitochondrial matrix is normally bound to the membrane or to matrix proteins.[140] Mn(II) is transported out of mitochondria via the very slow sodium [Na(I)]-independent Ca(II) efflux mechanism, which is an active (energy-requiring) mechanism; Mn(II) is not significantly transported over the Na(I)-dependent Ca (II) efflux mechanism, which is the dominant efflux mechanism in heart and brain mitochondria.[140]

Homeostatic Control of Mn

With Mn, as with other essential minerals, there is a dichotomy of response according to the body levels and adverse health effects that can occur when body stores of Mn are either too low (deficiency) or too high (toxicity).[11] Between illnesses caused by too much or too little Mn and optimum functioning, the relationship between Mn intake, well-being, and performance is probably similar to an inverted U-shaped curve.[141]

The "region of homeostasis" is defined as the dose range that results in neither deficiency or toxicity.[142] Mn is widespread in human diets, thus Mn deficiency is generally not recognized.[11] Below the threshold value, Mn deficiency has been shown to affect reproductive function, carbohydrate metabolism,[143] bone growth,[144] and brain function[145,146] in animals. Most of the evidence for human Mn deficiency is derived from experimental studies where subjects received Mn depleted diets.[14] The absorbed dose of Mn is kept within a certain range by homeostatic mechanisms that prevent large fluctuations of Mn concentrations in blood through changes in absorption and excretion rates.[87,147] The Mn absorption rate depends on the ingested amount.[79] When dietary Mn levels are high, adaptive changes include reduced GI absorption of Mn, enhanced Mn liver metabolism, and increased biliary and pancreatic excretion of Mn.[97,148] For example, the relative amount of Mn retained in the rats liver, kidney, spleen, and other systemic tissues decreased as the concentration of Mn in the diet increased from 4 to 2000 ppm.[149]

Above the threshold value, health progressively deteriorates with increasing Mn exposure leading to neurotoxicity.[141] The risks of Mn neurotoxicity by oral route are also minimal because of the homeostatic mechanisms regulate Mn concentrations and prevent retention.[79] When Mn is administered to patients by parenteral route there is a bypass of the homeostatic mechanisms[22,45] and once Mn has been deposited in the brain, it is cleared slowly, even after parental administration has ceased.[24,25,38]

Influence of Age and Gender on Mn Metabolism

Influence of Age on Mn Metabolism

In female rats, Mn concentration decreased with age in lung, heart, liver, kidney, and muscle but increased in brain.[150] Schroeder and coworkers reported no tendency for decrease or increase in Mn concentrations in human tissues with age.[1] Analyses of a variety of tissues taken from humans of various ages have indicated that there is no tendency for either a decrease or an increase in Mn accumulation throughout most of the life cycle.[1]

The pharmacokinetics of Mn in infants is known to be different from the adults. Balance studies show that there is high retention of Mn during the neonatal period.[151,152] There is some limited evidence that prenatal or neonatal exposure of animals to elevated levels of Mn can lead to neurological changes in the newborn.[151,153] To study the sensitivity of neonatal and adult rats to Mn-induced neurotoxicity, Dorman and coworkers,[155] administered Mn chloride ($MnCl_2$) doses (0, 25, or 50 mg/Kg /d) throughout lactation [postnatal day (PND) 1 through 21] and found increased striatal, hippocampal, hindbrain, and cortical Mn concentrations in all Mn-exposed neonates on PND 21. Increased striatal, cerebellar, and brain residue Mn concentrations were observed only in adult rats from the high-dose group.[154,155] The increased Mn absorption in the neonatal period may also be a compensatory mechanism due to the low concentration of Mn in mother's milk[151,153] and to the increased metabolic needs of infants as compared to adults, since Mn is required for adequate bone mineralization, as well as for connective tissue synthesis.[154] The developing brain takes up a significant proportion of Mn retained by the body during the early neonatal period. Keen and coworkers report that ~ 8% of total oral Mn dose is retained in rats' brain.[155–158] However, the relative higher net increase in brain Mn concentrations in the neonates (vs. adults) should not necessarily be construed as evidence for heightened neurotoxicity in developing animals, given the known requirement for Mn for optimal central nervous system (CNS) development in the neonate.

Influence of Gender on Mn Metabolism

Finley and coworkers reported that men absorbed significantly less Mn than women from the GI tract. The decreased Mn absorption in GI is related to Fe status and the lower ferritin concentrations found in men,[159] as DMT1 mediates uptake of both cations and is upregulated in dietary Fe deficiency (ID).[114]

Toxicological Evaluation Mn Levels in Nutrition

Safe and adequate levels of Mn in PN are unknown.[38] PN guidelines are based on Mn oral reference dose (RfD) considering Mn bioavailability by the oral route. The United States Environmental Protection Agency (US EPA) used estimates of Mn levels in typical western and vegetarian diets to calculate Mn RfD in food. The RfD represents an estimate of the daily exposure to which the human population (including sensitive subpopulations) may be continually exposed over a lifetime without an appreciable risk of deleterious effects.[146] The RfD for Mn was calculated by dividing the no-observed-adverse-effect level (NOAEL) by the product of the total amount of uncertainty and modifying factors.[160] The NOAEL is the highest experimental dose at which there is no statistically or biologically significant increase in frequency or severity of adverse health effects, as seen in the exposed population compared with an appropriate unexposed population.[161] In contrast to numerous reports describing Mn toxicity following inhalation exposure at high doses in humans, there are relatively few reports on manganism arising from water or dietary sources. Four studies have reported toxicity from ingestion of drinking water containing high levels of Mn. Kawamura and coworkers documented outbreaks of manganism in Japan and Greece, respectively, due to consumption of well-water contaminated with extremely high levels of Mn (1.8–14 mg/L).[162] Wasserman and coworkers[163,164] also reported adverse impact of Mn exposure associated with water consumption on child developmental outcomes in Bangladesh.[163,164] In another study, neurologic symptoms were reported in individuals who consumed drinking water with Mn levels of 1.8–2.3 mg/mL in Greece.[165] Mn toxicity has been also reported in an individual who consumed high amounts of Mn supplements for several years[166]. In animals, the toxicity of ingested Mn is low and signs of a toxic response generally appear only after concentrations higher than 1,000 μg/g diet are fed.[167]

Based on a composite of data from several epidemiological studies, the NOAEL for Mn was derived at 10 mg/day (0.14 mg/kg-day for 70 kg adult) for chronic human consumption of Mn in the diet using uncertainty and modifying factors of 1.[168] However, the US EPA stated that there are significant concerns about possible adverse neurological effects at doses not far from the range of essentiality. Because of this concern, the EPA recommended that a modifying factor of three be applied when assessing risk from Mn in drinking water or soil. A modified RfD of 0.05 mg/kg/d is recommended for Mn from drinking water or soil.[146]

Dietary reference Intakes (DRI) are established by the US Food and Nutrition Board of the National Research Council (US NRC) to provide quantitative estimates of nutrient intakes for use in a variety of settings.[169]

Progress in the field of Mn nutrition has been hampered because of the lack of a practical method for assessing Mn status as interindividual variations in Mn retention can be large.[170] Consistent changes in blood or plasma Mn levels have not been observed in depleted or repleted human subjects.[19,171]

Mn ADI was established for Mn intake based on median intake because data are insufficient to calculate the RDA.[59] The US National Research Council (NRC) has established an estimated safe and acceptable dietary intake (ESADDI) of 2–5 mg/day for adults.[172] Table 8.3 shows ADI and UL values for different age groups.[173]

The first guidelines for Mn supplementation in PN were developed by the American Medical Association Nutrition Advisory Group (AMA NAG).[174] In 1988, the pediatric parenteral trace element requirements were reevaluated by the Committee on Clinical Practice Issues of the American Society for Clinical Nutrition (ASCN) and the pediatric dosage of Mn was reduced to 1 μg/kg/d (from 2 to 10 μg/kg/d) about 10 years after the original AMA NAG recommendations were published.[175] The European Society of Pediatric Gastroenterology Hepatology and Nutrition (ESPGHAN) and the European Society for Clinical Nutrition and Metabolism (ESPEN) recommend 1 μg/kg/d with a maximum of 50 μg/d for children receiving long-term PN.[176] Table 8.4 summarizes the guidelines issued for administration of Mn by parenteral route.

In 2002, the published literature indicated a broad range in adults Mn supplementation in PN. Takagi and coworkers suggested a safe optimal Mn dose for adult patients undergoing PN at 1 μmol/d, based on MRI observations.[89] Later, in 2004 the AMA guidelines were revisited by the American Society of Parenteral and Enteral Nutrition (ASPEN) and the daily intake of Mn for adults was reduced to 60–100 μg/d.[13] Although based on toxicological data, the recent ASPEN guidelines do not pose a significant risk for Mn overexposure in patients without risk factors, other sources of exposure should be accounted in PN patients, such as the contamination of PN with Mn from raw components.[21,48,144,177]

TABLE 8.3 ADI and UL Levels for Mn

Life stage group		ADI of Mn (mg/d)	UL (mg/d)
Infants	0–6 mo	0.003	ND
	6–12 mo	0.6	ND
Children	1–3 y	1.2	2
	4–8 y	1.5	3
Females	9–13 y	1.6	6
	14–18 y	1.6	9
	19–30 y	1.8	11
	31–50 y	1.8.	11
	51–70 y	1.8	11
	> 70 y	1.8	11
Males	9–13 y	1.9	6
	14–18 y	2.2	9
	19–30 y	2.3	11
	31–50 y	2.3	11
	51–70 y	2.3	11
	> 70 y	2.3	11
Pregnancy	14–18 y	2.0	9
	19–50 y	2.0	11
Lactation	14–18 y	2.6	9
	19–50 y	2.6	11

ND, Not determinable due to lack of data of adverse effects in this age group and concern with regard to lack of ability to handle excess amounts. Source of intake should be from food only to prevent high levels of intake.

TABLE 8.4 Guidelines Issued for Administration of Mn by Parenteral Route

AMA (1979)[174]	Children	2–10 μg/kg/d
	Adults	0.15 and 0.8 mg/d
ASCN (1988)	Infants (preterm and term) and children	1 μg/Kg/d
ASPEN (2004)	Infants (preterm and term) and children	1 μg/Kg/d
	Adults	60–100 μg/d

AMA, American Medical Association; ASCN, American Society for Clinical Nutrition; ASPEN, American Society of Parenteral and Enteral Nutrition.

NEUROTOXICOLOGY OF Mn

Deficient Exposure

The most common presentations of Mn deficiency are abnormalities of bone growth in mice, rats, rabbits, pigs, cattle, and poultry, caused by defective synthesis of the mucopolysaccharide organic matrix of cartilage.[1] Mn deficiency is also associated with abnormal lipid metabolism characterized by high liver fat, hypocholesterolemia, and low high-density lipoprotein (HDL) concentrations.[178] In female rats, Mn deficiency is associated with deficiency in their young, stillbirths, early deaths, and sterility. Males of various species show sterility, absence of libido, and seminal tubular degeneration, indicating a requirement of Mn for spermatogenesis.[1] Deficient Mn concentrations are associated with convulsions.[179] Lower Mn concentrations were found in epileptic patients compared with controls.[180,181] A study in genetically epilepsy-prone rats (GEPR) chronically exposed to induced seizures showed that the rats susceptible to epilepsy had WB Mn levels and GS activity significantly lower than the control group.[182]

Mn Overexposure

Clinical Features

Changes in neuromotor domain, referred to as Mn-induced Parkinsonism, have been described in some patients fed with parenteral admixtures supplemented with Mn.[26,38,41,43,45] In humans, excess brain Mn produces neurotoxicity that may develop into a Parkinsonian syndrome (manganism).[11,71] Mn neurotoxicity is a progressive disorder,[183] that is generally considered to have two phases[141]: (1) the first stage is characterized by nonspecific symptoms, such as asthenia, anorexia, apathy, headaches, spasms, weariness of the legs, arthralgia, and irritability[184,185]; (2) the second stage is characterized by signs of basal ganglia dysfunction and may include expressionless face, speech disturbance, staggering gait (cock walk), muscular rigidity, and fine tremor.[141] Other, nonclassical symptoms of manganism, such as acute dystonias (spasms of the muscles of the tongue, face, neck, and back)[41,45] and epilepsy[43] were also reported in patients receiving Mn by parenteral route.

Modulating Factors of Mn Induced Neurotoxicity

MN DOSAGE

The dosage of parenteral Mn is recognized as an important risk factor for the development of hypermanganesemia and subsequent neurotoxicity. A broad range of daily adult Mn dosages, extending from a low dose of 0.18–0.91 μmol/d (0.01–0.05 mg/d) to a high dose of 40 μmol/d (2.2 mg/d)[186] has been previously recommended. Most of the case reports of Mn intoxication were in adults receiving > 500 μg/d of parenteral Mn[26,38,42,47,144,187] or pediatric patients receiving > 40 μg/kg/d.[41,45] The above adult dosage is significantly greater than the total estimated Mn absorbed dose of ~115 μg/d from food and drinking water, and 0.5 μg/d from inhaled Mn.[4,74]

DURATION OF MN SUPPLEMENTATION

Several reports describe an association between long-term PN and increased WB Mn levels[27,38,43] and brain Mn accumulation, particularly in the basal ganglia.

A recent analysis of *postmortem* data describes the cumulative effect of Mn supplementation in patients who received long-term PN for short bowel syndrome (SBS).[188] Hypermanganesemia may also be observed after a short course of PN, in patients receiving > 500 μg daily; for example, elevated Mn levels in red blood cells (RBC) of two patients were detected after 14 and 18 days of PN.[36] These findings suggest a potential toxicity from the administration of high Mn doses in PN and argue that the routine addition of doses higher than 500 μg daily may pose a risk of Mn-induced neurotoxicity even after short-term administration.

CO-MORBIDITIES ASSOCIATED WITH MN EXPOSURE

Hypermanganesemia can occur as a result of liver disease and decreased biliary excretion,[189] as bile is the major excretory route for Mn.[147] Elevated Mn levels have also been noted in patients suffering from chronic liver failure (with inability to excrete Mn via the biliary system) and as well as PN supplementation.[22,190] Patients on long-term PN may develop biliary stasis or obstructive jaundice,[191,192] which has been attributed to inhibitory effect of amino acid solutions on bile flow and bile composition.[193,194] Hepatic steatosis PN related is associated with the administration of lipid emulsions[191,192] and carbohydrate solutions.[195,196] Despite the clinical epidemiological evidence, the cause–effect relationships linking PN with the hepatobiliary system are largely unknown.[197]

ID can increase brain Mn levels,[198] as it is associated with increased expression of serum transferrin and cellular receptors (TfR),[60,199] a transporter present at the BBB that mediates brain influx of both Fe and Mn.[200,201]

Individuals with ID (low serum ferritin) are likely to absorb greater amounts of Mn.[202] Animal studies have demonstrated that ID enhances Mn absorption across the GI tract, independent of body Mn stores.[203,204] DMT1 is a transporter that mediates brain influx of both Fe and Mn[79] An inverse association has been also demonstrated between DMT1 levels and Mn absorption in humans.[148] Competition between Mn and Fe for intestinal absorption likely occurs by way of DMT1.[79] DMT1 expression is regulated by Fe status[205] as its levels strongly increase in the duodenum in response to ID.[206] DMT1 is also present in the astrocytes plasma membranes.[110] Erikson and Aschner showed that increased Mn uptake in primary astrocyte cultures, with altered Fe status is predominantly mediated by DMT1.[207]

Neuropathological Features

Neuropathological changes associated with Mn intoxication are predominantly localized in the basal ganglia[208,209]; the substantia nigra is occasionally affected, but generally to a lesser extent.[209,210] Human manganism is characterized by neuronal loss and reactive gliosis in the globus pallidus and substantia nigra pars reticulata without Lewy bodies (intraneuronal protein aggregates).[209] Neuronal loss in the substantia nigra pars compacta with the appearance of Lewy bodies is a neuropathological hallmark in idiopathic Parkinson Disease (PD).[102]

A key feature of the reactive gliosis observed in human and experimental manganism is the presence of Alzheimer type II astrocytosis.[129,211,212] A study conducted in adult rhesus monkeys showed gliosis with extensive glial fiber production in the globus pallidus and to a lesser extent in the substantia nigra par reticulata after 7 IV injections of $MnCl_2$. In the globus pallidus, astrocytes with an enlarged irregular nuclear outline with watery nucleochromatin consistent with the appearance of Alzheimer type II astrocytes have been described.[213]

Selected Mechanisms of Mn-Induced Neurotoxicity

ALTERATIONS OF GLUTAMATERGIC, GABAERGIC AND DOPAMINERGIC (DAERGIC) SYSTEMS

Classically, Mn neurotoxicity is characterized by deregulation of glutamatergic,[214,215] GABAergic,[123,199,214,216] and DAergic[123,216,217] systems. The mechanism by which Mn alters the levels of glutamate, γ-aminobutyric acid (GABA), and dopamine (DA) is not clear.[218] Motor impairment is associated with the degeneration of inhibitory GABAergic input from the globus pallidus to the subthalamic nucleus resulting in decreased inhibitory GABA input to the subthalamic nucleus.[218] This would potentially lead to disinhibition of the down-stream glutamate output to the substantia nigra leading to chronic over-stimulation.[123]

A study in nonhuman primates dosed IV with manganese sulfate ($MnSO_4$) (10–15 mg $MnSO_4$/kg or 3.26–4.89 mg Mn/kg) once per week, during 39.6 ± 1.0 weeks, showed a marked decrease of in vivo DA release in the absence of changes of DA receptors in the striatum.[219] A subacute study in mice injected subcutaneously with $MnCl_2$ (50 mg/Kg) for 1, 7, and 21 days, showed that Mn exposure does not deplete intracellular DA (as total tissue DA levels in the striatum were unchanged), despite reductions in extracellular DA levels.[220] Another study in Wistar rats after subchronic oral exposure to $MnCl_2$ (50–100–150 mg/kg) showed that DA levels were decreased in striatum.[221] Other studies showed that Mn accumulation is associated with striatal DA depletion.[222–225] Recent studies have indicated that GABAergic nuclei of the basal ganglia, such as the globus pallidus and the striatum may be early, more sensitive targets of Mn.[226–228] These findings are also consistent with a recent review on animal model studies suggesting that Mn produces an effect on striatal GABA levels over a wide range of cumulative doses, while decreased striatal DA is observed only at very high exposures.[229]

There is considerable evidence suggesting that Mn can alter DA D2 receptor binding and protein expression, but the lack of consistent findings across Mn treatments and animal models has made it difficult to ascertain the exact interaction between excess Mn and DA D2 receptors[220]. In vivo examination of DA metabolism in asymptomatic intoxicated patients using ^{18}Fluor-dopa positron emission tomography (^{18}F-dopa PET) did not show any reduction in DA uptake in manganism,[226] however abnormal in people with PD.[127,226,230–232]

The glutamatergic system of the basal ganglia is also disrupted in manganism, due to the involvement of either the thalamus or the subthalamic nucleus.[123] Glutamate deregulation can lead to excitotoxicity and significant oxidative stress.[233] ROS are also known to decrease activity of Na^+/K^+-ATPase[234] leading to alterations in transmembrane ion gradients that may contribute to reversal of glutamate transporter and possibly underlie the basis of net reduction in glutamate uptake in primary astrocyte cultures upon addition of Mn to the culture medium,[235] leading to increased extra cellular glutamate concentrations.[236]

IMPAIRED ENERGY METABOLISM

Another established mechanism responsible for Mn-induced neurotoxicity is impaired energy metabolism.[218] Mn decreases intracellular ATP in rat astrocytes.[237] As a consequence, ATP depletion or a perturbation in energy metabolism might diminish the ATP-requiring neuroprotective effect in astrocytes, decreasing glutamate uptake and free radical scavenging.[238] Experimental studies demonstrate that Mn inhibits in rat brain TCA enzymes, such as succinate dehydrogenase[239] and aconitase.[240] Mn also inhibits oxidative phosphorylation in isolated mitochondria preparations.[140] In the DAergic neuronal-derived cell line (PC12), Mn inhibits mitochondrial complexes of the respiratory chain, but the mitochondrial complex I in a more pronounced manner,[241] while in the glial-derived cell line (C6) this effect was not observed; Mn (III) has a stronger affinity for complex I than divalent Mn, however Mn (II) is the most predominant species in vivo.[242] Mn is putatively transported into cells in its divalent state and oxidized intracellularly, via reaction with the O_2^- to the trivalent state.[223] In primary striatal neuron cultures, Mn inhibits the mitochondrial complex II in a dose-dependent manner.[243] In vivo studies with rats have shown that Mn intoxication leads to the inhibition of all four respiratory chain complexes,[244] thereby leading to altered oxidative phosphorylation.[140,223,245,246]

OXIDATIVE STRESS

In the mitochondria, the nonenzymatic production of O_2^- occurs when a single electron is directly transferred to O_2 by reduced coenzymes or prosthetic groups (e.g., flavins or iron sulfur clusters).[247] When proteins or quinones that participate in transfer of electrons are damaged, the chain begins to donate electrons directly to O_2, thereby creating the highly reactive O_2^-.[248] Ali and coworkers demonstrated that in vitro exposure of rats' brain to $MnCl_2$ resulted in a dose-dependent increase in ROS in the striatum. Whereas, in vivo exposure to Mn acetate (MnOAc, Mn III) produced significant increases of ROS in caudate nucleus and hippocampus.[246] The relatively high rate of oxidative phosphorylation in the globus pallidus may account for the relative susceptibility of this region.[213] O_2^- inactivates enzymes (e.g., aconitase) that include iron–sulfur centers, releasing Fe (II) iron, which catalyzes production of $OH^{\bullet}$ from the H_2O_2 by the Fenton reaction.[249]

Free radicals can remove hydrogen atoms from polyunsaturated fatty acyl chains (linoleic, linolenic, arachidonic, docosahexaenoic, others) of membrane phospholipids, generating carbon-centered fatty acyl radicals that react with O_2 to form peroxyl radicals.[250] ROS can also lead to oxidation of amino acid residue side chains, formation of protein–protein cross-linkages, and oxidation of the protein backbone, resulting in protein fragmentation.[251]

BIOMONITORING OF Mn IN PATIENTS UNDERGOING PN

Biomarkers of Exposure, Effect, and Susceptibility

WHO defined biomarkers as a chemical, its metabolite, or the product of an interaction between a chemical and some target molecule or cell that is measurable in the human body.[252] Biomarker research assumes that toxicant-induced diseases are progressive and that injury proceeds from entry of the toxicant into target cells, which induces subcellular biochemical events, to cell- and organ-level events that eventually induce irreversible or persistent organism dysfunction[253]; such effect markers are generally preclinical indicators of abnormalities.[254]

Biomarkers may be classified into three types: biomarkers of exposure (internal dose), of effect and of susceptibility.[255,256] Exposure biomarkers reflect the internal dose of a xenobiotic and may be an exogenous compound (or a metabolite) within the body, an interactive product between the compound (or metabolite) and an endogenous component, or another event related to the exposure.[254] A biomarker of effect is a characteristic that is objectively measured and evaluated as an indicator of normal or pathogenic biologic processes.[257] Biomarkers of susceptibility serve as indicators of a particular sensitivity of individuals to the effect of a xenobiotic or to the effects of a group of such compounds.[257] Biochemical events can be modified by genetically determined individual differences, which may play a role as modifiers not only of long-term outcomes, but also of early biochemical changes. Examples of biomarkers of individual susceptibility to Mn include Fe status and markers of redox status,[259] the latter playing a key role in Mn neurotoxicity.

Classical Approach of Mn Biomonitoring in PN Patients: Biomarkers of Exposure

Mn Concentration in Body Fluids

WB Mn levels are linked to external administration of Mn by the PN route; for example, a study in adult patients receiving PN showed that WB Mn changed in a dose-dependent manner. Takagi and coworkers reported that WB Mn was significantly higher when PN patients were administered 2 or 20 μmol Mn/d compared to 0 or 1 μmol/d during PN exposure.[89]

A reasonable biomarker of Mn exposure should display an acceptable threshold or cut-off value above which a Mn exposed individual can be differentiated from unexposed individuals.[260] Although WB Mn analysis is the preferred screening method, the high variability in human normal Mn levels, makes it unsuitable for individual biological monitoring.[261]

Accordingly, reference intervals of what is considered a "normal" Mn level vary not much between different populational studies. A review by Iyengar and Woittiez[262] reported median Mn values of 13.6 (8.0–18.7) μg/L in WB, 0.63 (0.54–1.76) μg/L in serum, and 0.6 (0.5–9.8) μg/L in urine from a population covering 100,000 individuals from 55 countries.[262] A comprehensive review on Mn from the United States of America quotes 4–15 μg/L for WB, whereas a more recent North American publication quotes a slightly higher range of 7–16 μg/L as the normal levels in WB.[14] A study from Japan measured WB and plasma Mn levels in healthy volunteers and considered a range of 5.2–24.0 μg/L in WB and 1.9–5.8 μg/L in plasma as normal.[89] In contrast, a UK study quotes a reference range of 7–27 nmol/L (0.38–1.4 μg/L) as the normal plasma Mn level.[263] Australasian hospitals consider that the normal values range between 140–220 nmol/L (7.7–12.1 μg/L) in WB. Despite the high variability in WB Mn levels, an association between higher WB Mn (above 7.5 μg/L) levels and motor deficits.[264]

Lauwerys and Hoet[265] reported urinary levels of Mn in the general population <3 mg/L. Minoia and coworkers[266]suggested an average value of 1.02 mg/L. Other authors consider normal levels of Mn in urine <2.0 mg/dL.[39] Elevated urine Mn concentrations (> 25 μg/L) may confirm recent acute exposure.[267] However, given that urinary excretion of Mn is very low (<5%) the value of urinary Mn levels as a biomarker of exposure and toxicity is questionable.

The utility of serum Mn has been questioned as a marker for whole body Mn as it was reported that intracerebral Mn levels were increased in the presence of normal serum values.[38] Several authors do not consider serum and WB Mn levels to be suitable indicators and suggest that the Mn content of RBC may better reflect tissue accumulation as it is not directly influenced by current IV supplementation. WB-Mn is not a homogenous matrix and it is affected by IV delivery of Mn.[268] Accordingly, in patients receiving PN, WB Mn is influenced by the pattern of PN (i.e., intermittent PN vs. continuous whole-day PN), as it may lead to changes in the distribution of Mn between tissues and blood and result in individual variation in response to parenterally administered Mn.[27] RBC account for about 60%–80% of Mn in the WB,[24,269,270] and because their turnover is slower than that of other cellular components,[271] they are not directly dependent on current IV supplementation making it a better indicator of Mn exposure.[25]

Urinary Mn levels may also serve as a biomarker of exposure. However, biliary excretion is the main pathway by which Mn is excreted with most of the element ultimately being excreted in the feces.[11,97] Mn urinary excretion is low, representing only about 0.01 ±1% of the absorbed dose,[261] and about 6% of the total excreted amount.[259] Greger and coworkers and Davis and Greger failed to demonstrate a correlation between urinary Mn concentration and dietary intake in adult male and female volunteers.[272,273] Mn in urine shows a poor correlation with either recent or cumulative dose.[259,274]

Magnetic Resonance Imaging (MRI)

MRI intensity in the globus pallidus is a useful means for the detection of brain Mn accumulation.[28,89] The Mn (II) ion has five unpaired electrons in the 3d orbit, causing the shortening of T1-relaxation time and an increase in signal intensity on T1-weighted MRI.[275] In clinical settings, most patients undergoing PN are asymptomatic and diagnosed only on the basis of abnormal T1 signal intensity in the globus pallidus and occasionally in the tegmentum of the brainstem.[24,276] However, MRI is not used as a routine method for diagnosis due to high costs and the need to examine the relationships between hyperintensities in the basal ganglia and the onset of subclinical Mn neurotoxicity.[28] Some authors also suggest that Mn accumulation detected by MRI does not necessarily correlate with the degree of clinically apparent neurological abnormalities.[277] For example, Alves and coworkers[38] and Iinuma and coworkers[27] reported on patients parenterally fed Mn with MRI abnormalities, absent abnormal neurological signs.[27,38]

Alternative Approaches: Subclinical Biomarkers Predictive of Mn-Induced Neurotoxicity

Neurobehavioral Tests

During the early stages of pathogenesis, Mn-induced neuropsychological impairment is subtle,[141,185,278] characterized by alterations in motor function and response speed, as well as memory and more complex cognitive function impairments.[279–281] The first manifestations of poisoning by Mn are usually subjective.[282]

Biomarkers should provide information about neurotoxic effects-induced by Mn, as the preliminary early neurotoxic effects are subtle,[141] and usually precede the emergence of more serious adverse effects. Neurophysiological assessment relies on sensitive tools to assess neurophysiological functions and neuropsychological performance; Mn exposure may lead to poorer hand-eye coordination, motor slowing, increased tremor, reduced response speed, olfactory enhancement, mood changes, and possible memory and intellectual deficits.[264,283]

Neuroimaging Biomarker: ^{1}H Proton Magnetic Resonance Spectroscopy

Recent studies with ^{1}H proton magnetic resonance spectroscopy (^{1}H MRS), a noninvasive technique used for studying brain metabolites,[260] show an increase in γ-aminobutyric acid (GABA) content in the thalamus region of smelter workers occupationally exposed to Mn.[284] Classically, Mn neurotoxicity is characterized by deregulation of glutamatergic,[214,215] GABAergic,[123,199,214,216] and DAergic[123,216] systems. Striatal GABA concentrations in rats are altered after long-low exposure to Mn.[285] Conflicting data exists as to whether Mn accumulation leads to changes in regional GABA levels.[123,199] For example, exposure to 6 mg Mn/kg/d led to a significant increase in brain Mn concentrations and significant decrease in GABA concentrations.[286] Another report showed that rats exposed to 20 mg Mn/kg/d had significantly increased brain Mn and GABA concentrations.[287] Accordingly, it appears that a relationship exists between the severity of Mn exposure and GABA concentrations, with lower Mn exposure leading to decreased GABA, and high Mn exposure leading to increased GABA concentrations.[123,199] Further research is needed to study the effect of Mn exposure on GABA content in selected populations with higher risk of developing Mn-induced neurotoxicity before applying this methodology to biomonitor PN patients.

Hematologic and Urinary Biomarkers Related to Catecholaminergic System

Research strategies in development for a biomarker of Mn-induced neurotoxicity have focused mainly on the effects of Mn on the DAergic and GABAergic systems.[288] Several studies reported alterations in homovanillic acid (HVA)[33,34] and vanillylmandelic acid (VMA)[33] levels in populations exposed to higher Mn levels (Table 8.5).

In humans, VMA is the major end product of norepinephrine and epinephrine metabolism, whereas HVA is the main end product of DA metabolism.[289,290] The high prevalence of increased HVA levels suggest an increased activity of monoamine oxidase B (MAO B).[259] However, this finding was not replicated in a separate study of 11 men randomly selected in a ferromanganese-alloy plant, where a tendency toward lower platelet MAO B activity was found in the exposed workers.[291] MAO B cannot be recommended for monitoring early biochemical events of Mn exposure as platelet MAO B activity can be modified by genetically determined individual differences,[259] such as differences at the genotype of transcription factor AP-2 beta.[292]

Mn also affects dihydropteridine reductase (DHPR) activity, an enzyme required for regeneration of the cofactor tetrahydrobiopterin (BH4). Mn is an essential cofactor in enzymes involved in aromatic amino acid hydroxylation, such as phenylalanine and tyrosine hydroxylases.[293] Altindag and coworkers found that Mn in the sulfate form, led to statistically significant decreases in DHPR activity.[294]

These results are also consistent with a previous study from our group where we noted increased tyrosine and phenylalanine levels in rat's brain exposed to Mn.[295] Mn exposure in monkeys[284] and rats[28] reduces striatal DA content. The DAergic function can also be assessed indirectly measuring prolactin levels,[32] as DA is produced by tuberoinfundibular neurons and is the major factor in controlling prolactin synthesis and release. Once taken up by the capillaries of the hypophyseal portal system, DA acts directly on pituitary and neuronal DA receptors to inhibit prolactin secretion.[296] Table 8.5 shows several studies in which prolactin levels were used to assess Mn-induced neurotoxicity.[29–32,259]

TABLE 8.5 Biochemical Biomarkers of Mn-Induced Neurotoxicity

Study	Study population	Alteration in the exposed population
Ai et al. (1998)[33]	Male welders (n = 39), control group: nonoccupationally exposed to Mn (n = 19)	Incr HVA and Incr VMA (sig)
Siqueira and Moraes (1989)[34]	Male workers (n = 40) occupationally exposed to Mn in a ferromanganese alloy plant (n = 25)	Incr HVA
Montes et al. (2008)[29]	Population living close to a mine and mineral processing plant in Mexico (n = 300)	Positive correl. prolactin and WB Mn (sig)
Alessio et al. (1989)[30]	Male workers (n = 14) employed in a ferrous-Mn foundry, control group: nonoccupationally exposed to Mn (n = 14)	Incr Prolactin (sig)
Buchet (1993)[35]	Male workers (n = 68) exposed to Mn-containing dust in a dry alkaline battery plant or an Mn oxide and salt producing plant, control group: nonoccupationally exposed to Mn (n = 35)	Positive correl. HVA and urine Mn
Roels et al. (1992)[31]	Male workers (n = 92) in a dry alkaline factory, exposed to MnO_2, control group: nonoccupationally exposed to Mn (n = 101)	Incr Prolactin
Takser et al. (2004)[32]	Pregnant women at delivery (n = 87)	Positive correl. Prolactin (sig) and Mn cord blood (sig)

correl, Correlation; Decr, decreased; incr, increased; Sig, significant.

CONCLUSIONS

Though essential trace element, high exposure may cause increased levels of metal accumulation in the basal ganglia and a Parkinsonian-like syndrome. Mn affects a myriad of processes, yet the full spectrum of its neurotoxic mechanisms has yet to be fully understood. Several neurotransmitter systems are affected by Mn and an efficient chelator for excessive Mn accumulation, especially in the CNS, has yet to be identified. Future studies could be profitably directed at addressing these timely issues, and further characterizing molecular targets for this essential metal.

Acknowledgment

Michael Aschner was supported in part by grants from the National Institute of Health, R01ES010563.

References

1. Schroeder HA, Balassa JJ, Tipton IH. Essential trace metals in man: manganese. A study in homeostasis. *J Chronic Dis*. 1966;19:545–571.
2. Saric M, Lucchini R. Manganese. In: Nordberg GF, Fowler BA, Nordberg M, Friberg LT, eds. *Handbook of Toxicology of Metals*. Burlington: Academic Press, Inc; 2007:645–674.
3. Rodier J. Manganese poisoning in Moroccan miners. *Br J Ind Med*. 1955;12:21–35.

4. Santamaria AB, Sulsky SI. Risk assessment of an essential element: manganese. *J Toxicol Environ Health A*. 2010;73:128–155.
5. Kemmerer A, Elvehjem C, Hart E. Studies on the relation of manganese to the nutrition of the mouse. *J Biol Chem*. 1931;92:623–630.
6. Hurley LS. Teratogenic aspects of manganese, zinc, and copper nutrition. *Physiol Rev*. 1981;61:249–295.
7. Greger JL. Nutrition versus toxicology of manganese in humans: evaluation of potential biomarkers. *Neurotoxicology*. 1999;20:205–212.
8. Keen CL, Ensunsa JL, Watson MH, Baly DL, Donovan SM, Monaco MH, Clegg MS. Nutritional aspects of manganese from experimental studies. *Neurotoxicology*. 1999;20:213–223.
9. Takeda A, Ishiwatari S, Okada S. In vivo stimulation-induced release of manganese in rat amygdala. *Brain Res*. 1998;811:147–151.
10. Sloot WN, Gramsbergen JB. Axonal transport of manganese and its relevance to selective neurotoxicity in the rat basal ganglia. *Brain Res*. 1994;657:124–132.
11. Aschner M, Erikson KM, Dorman DC. Manganese dosimetry: species differences and implications for neurotoxicity. *Crit Rev Toxicol*. 2005;35:1–32.
12. Levy, L, Aitken, R, Holmes, P, Hughes, J, Hurley, F, Rumsby, PC, Searl, A, Shuker, LK, Spurgeon, A, Warren, F. *Occupational Exposure Limits: Criteria Document for Manganese and Inorganic Manganese Compounds*. Leicester, UK: IEHealth web report; 2004.
13. Mirtallo J, Canada T, Johnson D, Kumpf V, Petersen C, Sacks G, Seres D, Guenter P. Safe practices for parenteral nutrition. *JPEN J Parenter Enteral Nutr*. 2004;28:S39–S70.
14. Hardy IJ, Gillanders L, Hardy G. Is manganese an essential supplement for parenteral nutrition?. *Curr Opin Clin Nutr Metab Care*. 2008;11:289–296.
15. Hardy G. Manganese in parenteral nutrition: who, when, and why should we supplement?. *Gastroenterology*. 2009;137:S29–S35.
16. Frankel D. Supplementation of trace elements in parenteral nutrition: rationale and recommendations. *Nutr Res*. 1993;13:583–596.
17. Doisy EA, Effects of deficiency in manganese upon plasma levels of clotting proteins and cholesterol in man. Hoekstra WG, Suttie JW, Ganther HE, Mertz W, eds. *Trace Element Metabolism in Animals*, vol. 2. Baltimore: University Park Press; 1974:668–670.
18. Doisy EA, Micronutrient controls on biosynthesis of clotting proteins and cholesterol. Hemphill DD, ed. *Trace Substances in Environmental Health*, vol. 6. Columbia, Mo: University of Missouri; 1973:193–199.
19. Friedman BJ, Freeland-Graves JH, Bales CW, Behmardi F, Shorey-Kutschke RL, Willis RA, Crosby JB, Trickett PC, Houston SD. Manganese balance and clinical observations in young men fed a manganese-deficient diet. *J Nutr*. 1987;117:133–143.
20. Dudrick SJ, Wilmore DW, Vars HM, Rhoads JE. Long-term total parenteral nutrition with growth, development and positive nitrogen balance. *Surgery*. 1968;64;134–142.
21. Buchman AL, Howard LJ, Guenter P, Nishikawa RA, Compher CW, Tappenden KA. Micronutrients in parenteral nutrition: too little or too much? The past, present, and recommendations for the future. *Gastroenterology*. 2009;137:S1–S6.
22. Mehta R, Reilly JJ. Manganese levels in a jaundiced long-term total parenteral nutrition patient: potentiation of haloperidol toxicity? Case report and literature review. *JPEN J Parenter Enteral Nutr*. 1990;14:428–430.
23. Zielhuis RL. Recent and potential advances applicable to the protection of workers' health—biological monitoring. In: Berlin A, Yodaiken RE, Henman BA, eds. *Assessment of Toxic Agents at the Workplace—Roles of Ambient and Biological Monitoring*. Boston: Martinus Nijhoff Publishers; 1984.
24. Mirowitz SA, Westrich TJ, Hirsch JD. Hyperintense basal ganglia on T1-weighted MR images in patients receiving parenteral nutrition. *Radiology*. 1991;181:117–120.
25. Bertinet DB, Tinivella M, Balzola FA, de Francesco A, Davini O, Rizzo L, Massarenti P, Leonardi MA, Balzola F. Brain manganese deposition and blood levels in patients undergoing home parenteral nutrition. *JPEN J Parenter Enteral Nutr*. 2000;24:223–227.
26. Ejima A, Imamura T, Nakamura S, Saito H, Matsumoto K, Momono S. Manganese intoxication during total parenteral nutrition. *Lancet*. 1992;339:426.
27. Iinuma Y, Kubota M, Uchiyama M, Yagi M, Kanada S, Yamazaki S, Murata H, Okamoto K, Suzuki M, Nitta K. Whole-blood manganese levels and brain manganese accumulation in children receiving long-term home parenteral nutrition. *Pediatr Surg Int*. 2003;19:268–272.

28. Finkelstein Y, Zhang N, Fitsanakis VA, Avison MJ, Gore JC, Aschner M. Differential deposition of manganese in the rat brain following subchronic exposure to manganese: a T1-weighted magnetic resonance imaging study. *Isr Med Assoc J*. 2008;10:793–798.
29. Montes S, Riojas-Rodriguez H, Sabido-Pedraza E, Rios C. Biomarkers of manganese exposure in a population living close to a mine and mineral processing plant in Mexico. *Environ Res*. 2008;106:89–95.
30. Alessio L, Apostoli P, Ferioli A, Lombardi S. Interference of manganese on neuroendocrinal system in exposed workers. Preliminary report. *Biol Trace Elem Res*. 1989;21:249–253.
31. Roels HA, Ghyselen P, Buchet JP, Ceulemans E, Lauwerys RR. Assessment of the permissible exposure level to manganese in workers exposed to manganese dioxide dust. *Br J Ind Med*. 1992;49:25–34.
32. Takser L, Mergler D, de Grosbois S, Smargiassi A, Lafond J. Blood manganese content at birth and cord serum prolactin levels. *Neurotoxicol Teratol*. 2004;26:811–815.
33. Ai LB, Chua LH, New AL, Lee BL, Liu YM, Chia SE, Ong CN. Urinary homovanillic acid (HVA) and vanillymandelic acid (VMA) in workers exposed to manganese dust. *Biol Trace Elem Res*. 1998;64:89–99.
34. Siqueira ME, Moraes EC. Homovanillic acid (HVA) and manganese in urine of workers exposed in a ferromanganese alloy plant. *Med Lav*. 1989;80:224–228.
35. Buchet JP, Magos C, Roels H, Ceulemans E, Lauwerys R. Urinary excretion of homovanillic acid in workers exposed to manganese. *Int Arch Occup Environ Health*. 1993;65:131–133.
36. Fitzgerald K, Mikalunas V, Rubin H, McCarthey R, Vanagunas A, Craig RM. Hypermanganesemia in patients receiving total parenteral nutrition. *JPEN J Parenter Enteral Nutr*. 1999;23:333–336.
37. Mirowitz SA, Westrich TJ. Basal ganglial signal intensity alterations: reversal after discontinuation of parenteral manganese administration. *Radiology*. 1992;185:535–536.
38. Alves G, Thiebot J, Tracqui A, Delangre T, Guedon C, Lerebours E. Neurologic disorders due to brain manganese deposition in a jaundiced patient receiving long-term parenteral nutrition. *JPEN J Parenter Enteral Nutr*. 1997;21:41–45.
39. Nagatomo S, Umehara F, Hanada K, Nobuhara Y, Takenaga S, Arimura K, Osame M. Manganese intoxication during total parenteral nutrition: report of two cases and review of the literature. *J Neurol Sci*. 1999;162:102–105.
40. Hambidge KM, Sokol RJ, Fidanza SJ, Goodall MA. Plasma manganese concentrations in infants and children receiving parenteral nutrition. *JPEN J Parenter Enteral Nutr*. 1989;13:168–171.
41. Reynolds AP, Kiely E, Meadows N. Manganese in long term paediatric parenteral nutrition. *Arch Dis Child*. 1994;71:527–528.
42. Ono J, Harada K, Kodaka R, Sakurai K, Tajiri H, Takagi Y, Nagai T, Harada T, Nihei A, Okada A, et al. Manganese deposition in the brain during long-term total parenteral nutrition. *JPEN J Parenter Enteral Nutr*. 1995;19:310–312.
43. Komaki H, Maisawa S, Sugai K, Kobayashi Y, Hashimoto T. Tremor and seizures associated with chronic manganese intoxication. *Brain Dev*. 1999;21:122–124.
44. Hsieh CT, Liang JS, Peng SS, Lee WT. Seizure associated with total parenteral nutrition-related hypermanganesemia. *Pediatr Neurol*. 2007;36:181–183.
45. Fell JM, Reynolds AP, Meadows N, Khan K, Long SG, Quaghebeur G, Taylor WJ, Milla PJ. Manganese toxicity in children receiving long-term parenteral nutrition. *Lancet*. 1996;347:1218–1221.
46. Underwood EJ. The incidence of trace element deficiency diseases. *Philos Trans R Soc Lond B Biol Sci*. 1981;294:3–8.
47. Reimund JM, Dietemann JL, Warter JM, Baumann R, Duclos B. Factors associated to hypermanganesemia in patients receiving home parenteral nutrition. *Clin Nutr*. 2000;19:343–348.
48. Malecki EA, Radzanowski GM, Radzanowski TJ, Gallaher DD, Greger JL. Biliary manganese excretion in conscious rats is affected by acute and chronic manganese intake but not by dietary fat. *J Nutr*. 1996;126:489–498.
49. Barbeau A. Manganese and extrapyramidal disorders (a critical review and tribute to Dr. George C. Cotzias). *Neurotoxicology*. 1984;5:13–35.
50. Misselwitz B, Muhler A, Weinmann HJ. A toxicologic risk for using manganese complexes? A literature survey of existing data through several medical specialties. *Invest Radiol*. 1995;30:611–620.
51. Aschner JL, Aschner M. Nutritional aspects of manganese homeostasis. *Mol Aspects Med*. 2005;26:353–362.
52. Utter MF. The biochemistry of manganese. *Med Clin North Am*. 1976;60:713–727.
53. Keen CL, Ensunsa J, Lonnerdal B, Zidenberg-Cherr S. Manganese. In: Caballero B, ed. *Guide to nutritional supplements*. Oxford: Elsevier, Ltd; 2009.
54. Burton NC, Guilarte TR. Manganese neurotoxicity: lessons learned from longitudinal studies in nonhuman primates. *Environ Health Perspect*. 2009;117:325–332.

55. D'Antonio EL, Hai Y, Christianson DW. Structure and function of non-native metal clusters in human arginase I. *Biochemistry*. 2012;51:8399–8409.
56. Ensunsa JL, Symons JD, Lanoue L, Schrader HR, Keen CL. Reducing arginase activity via dietary manganese deficiency enhances endothelium-dependent vasorelaxation of rat aorta. *Exp Biol Med (Maywood)*. 2004;229:1143–1153.
57. Jitrapakdee S, Wallace JC. Structure, function and regulation of pyruvate carboxylase. *Biochem J*. 1999;340(Pt 1):1–16.
58. Xiang S, Tong L. Crystal structures of human and Staphylococcus aureus pyruvate carboxylase and molecular insights into the carboxyltransfer reaction. *Nat Struct Mol Biol*. 2008;15:295–302.
59. Gropper S, Smith J. *Advanced Nutrition and Human Metabolism*. 6th ed. Belmont, USA: Yolanda Cossio; 2013.
60. Aschner M, Aschner JL. Manganese neurotoxicity: cellular effects and blood-brain barrier transport. *Neurosci Biobehav Rev*. 1991;15:333–340.
61. Bannister JV, Bannister WH, Rotilio G. Aspects of the structure, function, and applications of superoxide dismutase. *CRC Crit Rev Biochem*. 1987;22:111–180.
62. Zhang HJ, Yan T, Oberley TD, Oberley LW. Comparison of effects of two polymorphic variants of manganese superoxide dismutase on human breast MCF-7 cancer cell phenotype. *Cancer Res*. 1999;59:6276–6283.
63. Paynter DI. Changes in activity of the manganese superoxide dismutase enzyme in tissues of the rat with changes in dietary manganese. *J Nutr*. 1980;110:437–447.
64. Erikson KM, Thompson K, Aschner J, Aschner M. Manganese neurotoxicity: a focus on the neonate. *Pharmacol Ther*. 2007;113:369–377.
65. Norenberg MD. Distribution of glutamine synthetase in the rat central nervous system. *J Histochem Cytochem*. 1979;27:756–762.
66. Wedler FC, Denman RB. Glutamine synthetase: the major Mn(II) enzyme in mammalian brain. *Curr Top Cell Regul*. 1984;24:153–169.
67. Crossgrove J, Zheng W. Manganese toxicity upon overexposure. *NMR Biomed*. 2004;17:544–553.
68. Couper J. On the effects of black oxide of manganese when inhaled into the lungs. *Br Ann Med Pharmacol*. 1837;41:41–42.
69. Huang CC, Chu NS, Lu CS, Wang JD, Tsai JL, Tzeng JL, Wolters EC, Calne DB. Chronic manganese intoxication. *Arch Neurol*. 1989;46:1104–1106.
70. Chandra SV, Shukla GS, Srivastava RS, Singh H, Gupta VP. An exploratory study of manganese exposure to welders. *Clin Toxicol*. 1981;18:407–416.
71. Hudnell HK. Effects from environmental Mn exposures: a review of the evidence from non-occupational exposure studies. *Neurotoxicology*. 1999;20:379–397.
72. Finkelstein MM, Jerrett M. A study of the relationships between Parkinson's disease and markers of traffic-derived and environmental manganese air pollution in two Canadian cities. *Environ Res*. 2007;104:420–432.
73. Loranger S, Zayed J. Environmental contamination and human exposure to airborne total and respirable manganese in Montreal. *J Air Waste Manag Assoc*. 1997;47:983–989.
74. ATSDR, AfTSaDR. Toxicological Profile for Manganese. P.H. Service, ed., 2000. Available from: http://www.atsdr.cdc.gov/toxprofiles/tp151.html
75. Stobbaerts RF, Ieven M, Deelstra H, De Leeuw I. Mn-content of total parenteral and enteral nutrition. *Z Ernahrungswiss*. 1992;31:138–146.
76. Wisner ER, Merisko-Liversidge E, Kellar K, Katzberg RW, Karpinski PH, Amparo EG, Drake C, Griffey SM, Brock JM. Preclinical evaluation of manganese carbonate particles for magnetic resonance imaging of the liver. *Acad Radiol*. 1995;2:140–147.
77. Bernardino ME, Young SW, Lee JK, Weinreb J. Contrast-enhanced magnetic resonance imaging of the liver with Mn-DPDP for known or suspected focal hepatic disease. *Invest Radiol*. 1991;26(Suppl 1):S148–S149:discussion S150-145.
78. Kreft BP, Baba Y, Tanimoto A, Finn JP, Stark DD. Orally administered manganese chloride: enhanced detection of hepatic tumors in rats. *Radiology*. 1993;186:543–548.
79. Aschner J, Aschner M. Nutritional aspects of Mn homeostasis. *In Mol Aspects Med*. 2005;26:353-352.
80. Ysart G, Miller P, Crews H, Robb P, Baxter M, De L'Argy C, Lofthouse S, Sargent C, Harrison N. Dietary exposure estimates of 30 elements from the UK total diet study. *Food Addit Contam*. 1999;16:391–403.
81. WHO, W.H.O.Trace elements in human nutrition: manganese. In: Service TR, ed. *Report of a WHO Expert Committee*. Geneva, Switzerland: WHO; 1973:34–36.

82. Nielsen F. *Manganese, Molybdenum, Boron, Chromium, and Other Trace Elements*. 10th ed. Wiley Blackwell; 2012.
83. Bell JG, Keen CL, Lonnerdal B. Higher retention of manganese in suckling than in adult rats is not due to maturational differences in manganese uptake by rat small intestine. *J Toxicol Environ Health*. 1989;26:387–398.
84. Garcia-Aranda JA, Wapnir RA, Lifshitz F. In vivo intestinal absorption of manganese in the rat. *J Nutr*. 1983;113:2601–2607.
85. Bai SP, Lu L, Luo XG, Liu B. Kinetics of manganese absorption in ligated small intestinal segments of broilers. *Poult Sci*. 2008;87:2596–2604.
86. Borg DC, Cotzias GC. Manganese metabolism in man: rapid exchange of MN56 with tissue as demonstrated by blood clearance and liver uptake. *J Clin Invest*. 1958;37:1269–1278.
87. Rehnberg GL, Hein JF, Carter SD, Linko RS, Laskey JW. Chronic ingestion of Mn3O4 by rats: tissue accumulation and distribution of manganese in two generations. *J Toxicol Environ Health*. 1982;9:175–188.
88. Sumino K, Hayakawa K, Shibata T, Kitamura S. Heavy metals in normal Japanese tissues. Amounts of 15 heavy metals in 30 subjects. *Arch Environ Health*. 1975;30:487–494.
89. Takagi Y, Okada A, Sando K, Wasa M, Yoshida H, Hirabuki N. Evaluation of indexes of in vivo manganese status and the optimal intravenous dose for adult patients undergoing home parenteral nutrition. *Am J Clin Nutr*. 2002;75:112–118.
90. Malecki EA, Lo HC, Yang H, Davis CD, Ney DM, Greger JL. Tissue manganese concentrations and antioxidant enzyme activities in rats given total parenteral nutrition with and without supplemental manganese. *JPEN J Parenter Enteral Nutr*. 1995;19:222–226.
91. Aisen P, Aasa R, Redfield AG. The chromium, manganese, and cobalt complexes of transferrin. *J Biol Chem*. 1969;244:4628–4633.
92. Critchfield JW, Keen CL. Manganese + 2 exhibits dynamic binding to multiple ligands in human plasma. *Metabolism*. 1992;41:1087–1092.
93. Aschner M, Shanker G, Erikson K, Yang J, Mutkus LA. The uptake of manganese in brain endothelial cultures. *Neurotoxicology*. 2002;23:165–168.
94. Jefferies WA, Brandon MR, Hunt SV, Williams AF, Gatter KC, Mason DY. Transferrin receptor on endothelium of brain capillaries. *Nature*. 1984;312:162–163.
95. Davidsson L, Lonnerdal B, Sandstrom B, Kunz C, Keen CL. Identification of transferrin as the major plasma carrier protein for manganese introduced orally or intravenously or after in vitro addition in the rat. *J Nutr*. 1989;119:1461–1464.
96. Dickinson TK, Devenyi AG, Connor JR. Distribution of injected iron 59 and manganese 54 in hypotransferrinemic mice. *J Lab Clin Med*. 1996;128:270–278.
97. Davis CD, Zech L, Greger JL. Manganese metabolism in rats: an improved methodology for assessing gut endogenous losses. *Proc Soc Exp Biol Med*. 1993;202:103–108.
98. Crossgrove JS, Yokel RA. Manganese distribution across the blood-brain barrier III. The divalent metal transporter-1 is not the major mechanism mediating brain manganese uptake. *Neurotoxicology*. 2004;25:451–460.
99. Tuschl K, Clayton PT, Gospe SM, Samshad G, Ibrahim S, Singhi P, Ribeiro RT, Zaki MS, Rosario M, Dyak S, et al. The first inborn error of manganese metabolism caused by mutations in SLC30A10, a newly identified manganese transporter. *Lancet*. 2013;381:S110.
100. Bertinchamps AJ, Miller ST, Cotzias GC. Interdependence of routes excreting manganese. *Am J Physiol*. 1966;211:217–224.
101. Cotzias GC, Horiuchi K, Fuenzalida S, Mena I. Chronic manganese poisoning. Clearance of tissue manganese concentrations with persistance of the neurological picture. *Neurology*. 1968;18:376–382.
102. Pal PK, Samii A, Calne DB. Manganese neurotoxicity: a review of clinical features, imaging and pathology. *Neurotoxicology*. 1999;20:227–238.
103. Kessler KR, Wunderlich G, Hefter H, Seitz RJ. Secondary progressive chronic manganism associated with markedly decreased striatal D2 receptor density. *Mov Disord*. 2003;18:217–218.
104. Abbott NJ, Ronnback L, Hansson E. Astrocyte-endothelial interactions at the blood-brain barrier. *Nat Rev Neurosci*. 2006;7:41–53.
105. Roels H, Meiers G, Delos M, Ortega I, Lauwerys R, Buchet JP, Lison D. Influence of the route of administration and the chemical form (MnCl2, MnO2) on the absorption and cerebral distribution of manganese in rats. *Arch Toxicol*. 1997;71:223–230.
106. Aschner M. The transport of manganese across the blood-brain barrier. *Neurotoxicology*. 2006;27:311–314.

107. Roberts R, Sandra A, Siek GC, Lucas JJ, Fine RE. Studies of the mechanism of iron transport across the blood-brain barrier. *Ann Neurol*. 1992;32(Suppl):S43–S50.
108. Abbott NJ. Evidence for bulk flow of brain interstitial fluid: significance for physiology and pathology. *Neurochem Int*. 2004;45:545–552.
109. Anderson JG, Cooney PT, Erikson KM. Brain manganese accumulation is inversely related to gamma-amino butyric acid uptake in male and female rats. *Toxicol Sci*. 2007;95:188–195.
110. Au C, Benedetto A, Aschner M. Manganese transport in eukaryotes: the role of DMT1. *Neurotoxicology*. 2008;29:569–576.
111. Chua AC, Morgan EH. Manganese metabolism is impaired in the Belgrade laboratory rat. *J Comp Physiol B*. 1997;167:361–369.
112. Yokel RA, Crossgrove JS. Manganese toxicokinetics at the blood-brain barrier. *Res Rep Health Eff Inst*. 2004;119:7–58:discussion 59-73.
113. Crossgrove JS, Yokel RA. Manganese distribution across the blood-brain barrier. IV. Evidence for brain influx through store-operated calcium channels. *Neurotoxicology*. 2005;26:297–307.
114. Gunshin H, Mackenzie B, Berger UV, Gunshin Y, Romero MF, Boron WF, Nussberger S, Gollan JL, Hediger MA. Cloning and characterization of a mammalian proton-coupled metal-ion transporter. *Nature*. 1997;388:482–488.
115. He L, Girijashanker K, Dalton TP, Reed J, Li H, Soleimani M, Nebert DW. ZIP8, member of the solute-carrier-39 (SLC39) metal-transporter family: characterization of transporter properties. *Mol Pharmacol*. 2006;70:171–180.
116. Aschner M, Gannon M. Manganese (Mn) transport across the rat blood-brain barrier: saturable and transferrin-dependent transport mechanisms. *Brain Res Bull*. 1994;33:345–349.
117. Lucaciu CM, Dragu C, Copaescu L, Morariu VV. Manganese transport through human erythrocyte membranes. An EPR study. *Biochim Biophys Acta*. 1997;1328:90–98.
118. Riccio A, Mattei C, Kelsell RE, Medhurst AD, Calver AR, Randall AD, Davis JB, Benham CD, Pangalos MN. Cloning and functional expression of human short TRP7, a candidate protein for store-operated Ca2+ influx. *J Biol Chem*. 2002;277:12302–12309.
119. Kannurpatti SS, Joshi PG, Joshi NB. Calcium sequestering ability of mitochondria modulates influx of calcium through glutamate receptor channel. *Neurochem Res*. 2000;25:1527–1536.
120. Crossgrove JS, Allen DD, Bukaveckas BL, Rhineheimer SS, Yokel RA. Manganese distribution across the blood-brain barrier. I. Evidence for carrier-mediated influx of managanese citrate as well as manganese and manganese transferrin. *Neurotoxicology*. 2003;24:3–13.
121. Paxinos G, Watson C, eds. *The Rat Brain in Stereotaxic Coordinates*. London: Academic Press, Ltd; 1998.
122. Moroney R, Heida C, Geelen J. Increased bradykinesia in Parkinson's disease with increased movement complexity: elbow flexion-extension movements. *J Comput Neurosci*. 2008;25:501–519.
123. Fitsanakis VA, Au C, Erikson KM, Aschner M. The effects of manganese on glutamate, dopamine and gamma-aminobutyric acid regulation. *Neurochem Int*. 2006;48:426–433.
124. Erikson KM, John CE, Jones SR, Aschner M. Manganese accumulation in striatum of mice exposed to toxic doses is dependent upon a functional dopamine transporter. *Environ Toxicol Pharmacol*. 2005;20:390–394.
125. Anderson JG, Cooney PT, Erikson KM. Inhibition of DAT function attenuates manganese accumulation in the globus pallidus. *Environ Toxicol Pharmacol*. 2007;23:179–184.
126. Tracqui A, Tayot J, Kintz P, Alves G, Bosque MA, Mangin P. Determination of manganese in human brain samples. *Forensic Sci Int*. 1995;76:199–203.
127. Calne DB, Chu NS, Huang CC, Lu CS, Olanow W. Manganism and idiopathic parkinsonism: similarities and differences. *Neurology*. 1994;44:1583–1586.
128. Newland MC, Ceckler TL, Kordower JH, Weiss B. Visualizing manganese in the primate basal ganglia with magnetic resonance imaging. *Exp Neurol*. 1989;106:251–258.
129. Hazell AS. Astrocytes and manganese neurotoxicity. *Neurochem Int*. 2002;41:271–277.
130. Silva AC, Bock NA. Manganese-enhanced MRI: an exceptional tool in translational neuroimaging. *Schizophr Bull*. 2008;34:595–604.
131. Takeda A, Sawashita J, Okada S. Biological half-lives of zinc and manganese in rat brain. *Brain Res*. 1995;695:53–58.
132. Dorman DC, Struve MF, Marshall MW, Parkinson CU, James RA, Wong BA. Tissue manganese concentrations in young male rhesus monkeys following subchronic manganese sulfate inhalation. *Toxicol Sci*. 2006;92:201–210.
133. Newland MC, Cox C, Hamada R, Oberdorster G, Weiss B. The clearance of manganese chloride in the primate. *Fundam Appl Toxicol*. 1987;9:314–328.

134. Yokel RA, Crossgrove JS, Bukaveckas BL. Manganese distribution across the blood-brain barrier. II. Manganese efflux from the brain does not appear to be carrier mediated. *Neurotoxicology*. 2003;24:15–22.
135. Gianutsos G, Seltzer MD, Saymeh R, Wu ML, Michel RG. Brain manganese accumulation following systemic administration of different forms. *Arch Toxicol*. 1985;57:272–275.
136. Suarez N, Eriksson H. Receptor-mediated endocytosis of a manganese complex of transferrin into neuroblastoma (SHSY5Y) cells in culture. *J Neurochem*. 1993;61:127–131.
137. Quintanar L, Montiel T, Marquez M, Gonzalez A, Massieu L. Calpain activation is involved in acute manganese neurotoxicity in the rat striatum in vivo. *Exp Neurol*. 2012;233:182–192.
138. Lai JC, Minski MJ, Chan AW, Leung TK, Lim L. Manganese mineral interactions in brain. *Neurotoxicology*. 1999;20:433–444.
139. Maynard LS, Cotzias GC. The partition of manganese among organs and intracellular organelles of the rat. *J Biol Chem*. 1955;214:489–495.
140. Gavin CE, Gunter KK, Gunter TE. Mn2+ sequestration by mitochondria and inhibition of oxidative phosphorylation. *Toxicol Appl Pharmacol*. 1992;115:1–5.
141. Mergler D, Baldwin M. Early manifestations of manganese neurotoxicity in humans: an update. *Environ Res*. 1997;73:92–100.
142. Eaton D, Gilbert S. Principles of Toxicology. In: Klaassen C, ed. *Casareth and Doull's Toxicology—The Basic Science of Poisons*. Kansas City: McGraw-Hill; 2008.
143. Jensen GL, Binkley J. Clinical manifestations of nutrient deficiency. *JPEN J Parenter Enteral Nutr*. 2002;26:S29–S33.
144. Dickerson RN. Manganese intoxication and parenteral nutrition. *Nutrition*. 2001;17:689–693.
145. Cotzias GC. Manganese in health and disease. *Physiol Rev*. 1958;38:503–532.
146. Goldhaber SB. Trace element risk assessment: essentiality vs. toxicity. *Regul Toxicol Pharmacol*. 2003;38:232–242.
147. Andersen ME, Gearhart JM, Clewell 3rd HJ. Pharmacokinetic data needs to support risk assessments for inhaled and ingested manganese. *Neurotoxicology*. 1999;20:161–171.
148. Finley JW, Davis CD. Manganese deficiency and toxicity: are high or low dietary amounts of manganese cause for concern?. *Biofactors*. 1999;10:15–24.
149. Abrams E, Lassiter JW, Miller WJ, Neathery MW, Gentry RP, Scarth RD. Absorption as a factor in manganese homeostasis. *J Anim Sci*. 1976;42:630–636.
150. Takeda T, Kimura M, Yokoi K, Itokawa Y. Effect of age and dietary protein level on tissue mineral levels in female rats. *Biol Trace Elem Res*. 1996;54:55–74.
151. Collipp PJ, Chen SY, Maitinsky S. Manganese in infant formulas and learning disability. *Ann Nutr Metab*. 1983;27:488–494.
152. Zlotkin S, Buchanan B. Manganese intakes in intravenously fed infants. *Biol Trace Element Res*. 1986;9:271–280.
153. Dorner K, Dziadzka S, Hohn A, Sievers E, Oldigs HD, Schulz-Lell G, Schaub J. Longitudinal manganese and copper balances in young infants and preterm infants fed on breast-milk and adapted cows milk formulas. *Br J Nutr*. 1989;61:559–572.
154. Hurley LS, Keen CL, Lonnerdal B. Aspects of trace element interactions during development. *Fed Proc J*. 1983;42:1735–1739.
155. Dorman DC, Struve MF, Vitarella D, Byerly FL, Goetz J, Miller R. Neurotoxicity of manganese chloride in neonatal and adult CD rats following subchronic (21-day) high-dose oral exposure. *J Appl Toxicol*. 2000;20:179–187.
156. Chandra SV, Shukla GS. Manganese encephalopathy in growing rats. *Environ Res*. 1978;15:28–37.
157. Deskin R, Bursian SJ, Edens FW. Neurochemical alterations induced by manganese chloride in neonatal rats. *Neurotoxicology*. 1981;2:65–73.
158. Kristensson K, Eriksson H, Lundh B, Plantin LO, Wachtmeister L, el Azazi M, Morath C, Heilbronn E. Effects of manganese chloride on the rat developing nervous system. *Acta Pharmacol Toxicol (Copenh)*. 1986;59:345–348.
159. Finley JW, Johnson PE, Johnson LK. Sex affects manganese absorption and retention by humans from a diet adequate in manganese. *Am J Clin Nutr*. 1994;60:949–955.
160. Nance, P. Reference dose (RfD). In: *Encyclopedia of Toxycology*, 2nd ed., 633–634.
161. ECETOC. Recognition of, and differentiation between, adverse and non-adverse effects in toxicology studies. Technical Report 85, 2002, Brussels, ISSN-0773-6347-85.
162. Kawamura R, Ikuta H, Fukuzumi S, Yamada R, Tsubaki S, Kodama T, Kurata S. Intoxication by manganese in well water. *Kitasato Arch Exp Med*. 1941;18:145–169.

163. Wasserman GA, Liu X, Parvez F, Ahsan H, Levy D, Factor-Litvak P, Kline J, van Geen A, Slavkovich V, LoIacono NJ, et al. Water manganese exposure and children's intellectual function in Araihazar, Bangladesh. *Environ Health Perspect*. 2006;114:124–129.
164. Wasserman GA, Liu X, Parvez F, Factor-Litvak P, Ahsan H, Levy D, Kline J, van Geen A, Mey J, Slavkovich V, et al. Arsenic and manganese exposure and children's intellectual function. *Neurotoxicology*. 2011;32:450–457.
165. Kondakis XG, Makris N, Leotsinidis M, Prinou M, Papapetropoulos T. Possible health effects of high manganese concentration in drinking water. *Arch Environ Health*. 1989;44:175–178.
166. Banta RG, Markesbery WR. Elevated manganese levels associated with dementia and extrapyramidal signs. *Neurology*. 1977;27:213–216.
167. Hurley LS, Keen CL. Manganese. In: Underwood E, Mertz W, eds. *Trace Elements in Human Health and Animal Nutrition*. New York: Academic Press; 1987:185–223.
168. USEPA. Manganese (CASRN 7439-96-5). In: Faifax, VA, ed. *IRI System*, vol. 2013; 2007.
169. Yates AA, Schlicker SA, Suitor CW. Dietary Reference Intakes: the new basis for recommendations for calcium and related nutrients, B vitamins, and choline. *J Am Diet Assoc*. 1998;98:699–706.
170. Davidsson L, Cederblad A, Lonnerdal B, Sandstrom B. Manganese absorption from human milk, cow's milk, and infant formulas in humans. *Am J Dis Child*. 1989;143:823–827.
171. Freeland-Graves JH, Behmardi F, Bales CW, Dougherty V, Lin PH, Crosby JB, Trickett PC. Metabolic balance of manganese in young men consuming diets containing five levels of dietary manganese. *J Nutr*. 1988;118:764–773.
172. Greger JL. Dietary standards for manganese: overlap between nutritional and toxicological studies. *J Nutr*. 1998;128:368S–371S.
173. Board, IoMFaN. Dietary Reference Intakes (DRIs): Tolerable Upper Intake Levels, Vitamins.
174. AMA. Guidelines for essential trace element preparations for parenteral use. *JAMA*. 1979;241:2051–2054.
175. Greene HL, Hambidge KM, Schanler R, Tsang RC. Guidelines for the use of vitamins, trace elements, calcium, magnesium, and phosphorus in infants and children receiving total parenteral nutrition: report of the Subcommittee on Pediatric Parenteral Nutrient Requirements from the Committee on Clinical Practice Issues of the American Society for Clinical Nutrition. *Am J Clin Nutr*. 1988;48:1324–1342.
176. Koletzko B, Goulet O, Hunt J, Krohn K, Shamir R. 1. Guidelines on Paediatric Parenteral Nutrition of the European Society of Paediatric Gastroenterology, Hepatology and Nutrition (ESPGHAN) and the European Society for Clinical Nutrition and Metabolism (ESPEN), supported by the European Society of Paediatric Research (ESPR). *J Pediatr Gastroenterol Nutr*. 2005;41(Suppl 2):S1–S87.
177. Jetton MM, Sullivan JF, Burch RE. Trace element contamination of intravenous solutions. *Arch Intern Med*. 1976;136:782–784.
178. Davis CD, Ney DM, Greger JL. Manganese, iron and lipid interactions in rats. *J Nutr*. 1990;120:507–513.
179. Grant EC. Epilepsy and manganese. *Lancet*. 2004;363:572.
180. Davidson DL, Ward NI. Abnormal aluminium, cobalt, manganese, strontium and zinc concentrations in untreated epilepsy. *Epilepsy Res*. 1988;2:323–330.
181. Carl GF, Keen CL, Gallagher BB, Clegg MS, Littleton WH, Flannery DB, Hurley LS. Association of low blood manganese concentrations with epilepsy. *Neurology*. 1986;36:1584–1587.
182. Carl GF, Blackwell LK, Barnett FC, Thompson LA, Rissinger CJ, Olin KL, Critchfield JW, Keen CL, Gallagher BB. Manganese and epilepsy: brain glutamine synthetase and liver arginase activities in genetically epilepsy prone and chronically seizured rats. *Epilepsia*. 1993;34:441–446.
183. Rosenstock HA, Simons DG, Meyer JS. Chronic manganism. Neurologic and laboratory studies during treatment with levodopa. *JAMA*. 1971;217:1354–1358.
184. Verhoeven WM, Egger JI, Kuijpers HJ. Manganese and acute paranoid psychosis: a case report. *J Med Case Rep*. 2011;5:146.
185. Bowler RM, Nakagawa S, Drezgic M, Roels HA, Park RM, Diamond E, Mergler D, Bouchard M, Bowler RP, Koller W. Sequelae of fume exposure in confined space welding: a neurological and neuropsychological case series. *Neurotoxicology*. 2007;28:298–311.
186. Wretlind A. Complete intravenous nutrition. Theoretical and experimental background. *Nutr Metab*. 1972;14(Suppl):1–57.
187. Taylor S, Manara AR. Manganese toxicity in a patient with cholestasis receiving total parenteral nutrition. *Anaesthesia*. 1994;49:1013.

188. Howard L, Ashley C, Lyon D, Shenkin A. Autopsy tissue trace elements in 8 long-term parenteral nutrition patients who received the current U.S. Food and Drug Administration formulation. *JPEN J Parenter Enteral Nutr*. 2007;31:388–396.
189. Ikeda S, Yamaguchi Y, Sera Y, Ohshiro H, Uchino S, Yamashita Y, Ogawa M. Manganese deposition in the globus pallidus in patients with biliary atresia. *Transplantation*. 2000;69:2339–2343.
190. McKinney AM, Filice RW, Teksam M, Casey S, Truwit C, Clark HB, Woon C, Liu HY. Diffusion abnormalities of the globi pallidi in manganese neurotoxicity. *Neuroradiology*. 2004;46:291–295.
191. Angsten G, Finkel Y, Lucas S, Kassa AM, Paulsson M, Lilja HE. Improved outcome in neonatal short bowel syndrome using parenteral fish oil in combination with omega-6/9 lipid emulsions. *JPEN J Parenter Enteral Nutr*. 2012;36:587–595.
192. Fallon EM, Le HD, Puder M. Prevention of parenteral nutrition-associated liver disease: role of omega-3 fish oil. *Curr Opin Organ Transplant*. 2010;15:334–340.
193. Graham MF, Tavill AS, Halpin TC, Louis LN. Inhibition of bile flow in the isolated perfused rat liver by a synthetic parenteral amino acid mixture: associated net amino acid fluxes. *Hepatology*. 1984;4:69–73.
194. Shattuck KE, Grinnell CD, Rassin DK. Amino acid infusions induce reversible, dose-related decreases in bile flow in the isolated rat liver. *JPEN J Parenter Enteral Nutr*. 1993;17:171–176.
195. Pierro A, Carnielli V, Filler RM, Smith J, Heim T. Metabolism of intravenous fat emulsion in the surgical newborn. *J Pediatr Surg*. 1989;24:95–101:Discussion 101–102.
196. Jones MO, Pierro A, Hammond P, Nunn A, Lloyd DA. Glucose utilization in the surgical newborn infant receiving total parenteral nutrition. *J Pediatr Surg*. 1993;28:1121–1125.
197. Angelico M, Della Guardia P. Review article: hepatobiliary complications associated with total parenteral nutrition. *Aliment Pharmacol Ther*. 2000;14(Suppl 2):54–57.
198. Heilig E, Molina R, Donaghey T, Brain JD, Wessling-Resnick M. Pharmacokinetics of pulmonary manganese absorption: evidence for increased susceptibility to manganese loading in iron-deficient rats. *Am J Physiol Lung Cell Mol Physiol*. 2005;288:L887–L893.
199. Erikson KM, Shihabi ZK, Aschner JL, Aschner M. Manganese accumulates in iron-deficient rat brain regions in a heterogeneous fashion and is associated with neurochemical alterations. *Biol Trace Elem Res*. 2002;87:143–156.
200. Punnonen K, Irjala K, Rajamaki A. Iron-deficiency anemia is associated with high concentrations of transferrin receptor in serum. *Clin Chem*. 1994;40:774–776.
201. Kivivuori SM, Pelkonen P, Ylijoki H, Verronen P, Siimes MA. Elevated serum transferrin receptor concentration in children with juvenile chronic arthritis as evidence of iron deficiency. *Rheumatology (Oxford)*. 2000;39:193–197.
202. Bounds S. *The Toxicokinetics of Manganese and its Organic Compunds*. Raleigh: Manganese REACH Administration; 2009:160.
203. Chandra SV, Shukla GS. Role of iron deficiency in inducing susceptibility to manganese toxicity. *Arch Toxicol*. 1976;35:319–323.
204. Shukla GS, Chandra SV, Seth PK. Effect of manganese on the levels of DNA, RNA, DNase and RNase in cerebrum, cerebellum and rest of brain regions of rat. *Acta Pharmacol Toxicol (Copenh)*. 1976;39:562–569.
205. Thompson K, Molina RM, Donaghey T, Schwob JE, Brain JD, Wessling-Resnick M. Olfactory uptake of manganese requires DMT1 and is enhanced by anemia. *FASEB J*. 2007;21:223–230.
206. Gunshin H, Allerson CR, Polycarpou-Schwarz M, Rofts A, Rogers JT, Kishi F, Hentze MW, Rouault TA, Andrews NC, Hediger MA. Iron-dependent regulation of the divalent metal ion transporter. *FEBS Lett*. 2001;509:309–316.
207. Erikson KM, Aschner M. Increased manganese uptake by primary astrocyte cultures with altered iron status is mediated primarily by divalent metal transporter. *Neurotoxicology*. 2006;27:125–130.
208. Bernheimer H, Birkmayer W, Hornykiewicz O, Jellinger K, Seitelberger F. Brain dopamine and the syndromes of Parkinson and Huntington. Clinical, morphological and neurochemical correlations. *J Neurol Sci*. 1973;20:415–455.
209. Yamada M, Ohno S, Okayasu I, Okeda R, Hatakeyama S, Watanabe H, Ushio K, Tsukagoshi H. Chronic manganese poisoning: a neuropathological study with determination of manganese distribution in the brain. *Acta Neuropathol*. 1986;70:273–278.
210. Katsuragi T, Takahashi T, Shibuya K, Nagatomo H, Iwabuchi K. A patient with parkinsonism presenting hyperintensity in the globus pallidus on T1-weighted MR images: the correlation with manganese poisoning. *Rinsho Shinkeigaku*. 1996;36:780–782.
211. Bikashvili TZ, Shukakidze AA, Kiknadze GI. Changes in the ultrastructure of the rat cerebral cortex after oral doses of manganese chloride. *Neurosci Behav Physiol*. 2001;31:385–389.

212. Pentschew A, Ebner FF, Kovatch RM. Experimental Manganese Encephalopathy in Monkeys. A Preliminary Report. *J Neuropathol Exp Neurol*. 1963;22:488–499.
213. Olanow CW, Good PF, Shinotoh H, Hewitt KA, Vingerhoets F, Snow BJ, Beal MF, Calne DB, Perl DP. Manganese intoxication in the rhesus monkey: a clinical, imaging, pathologic, and biochemical study. *Neurology*. 1996;46:492–498.
214. Bagga P, Patel AB. Regional cerebral metabolism in mouse under chronic manganese exposure: implications for Manganism. *Neurochem Int*. 2012;60:177–185.
215. Garcia SJ, Gellein K, Syversen T, Aschner M. A manganese-enhanced diet alters brain metals and transporters in the developing rat. *Toxicol Sci*. 2006;92:516–525.
216. Stanwood GD, Leitch DB, Savchenko V, Wu J, Fitsanakis VA, Anderson DJ, Stankowski JN, Aschner M, McLaughlin B. Manganese exposure is cytotoxic and alters dopaminergic and GABAergic neurons within the basal ganglia. *J Neurochem*. 2009;110:378–389.
217. Zwingmann C, Leibfritz D, Hazell AS. Brain energy metabolism in a sub-acute rat model of manganese neurotoxicity: an ex vivo nuclear magnetic resonance study using [1-13C]glucose. *Neurotoxicology*. 2004;25:573–587.
218. Quintanar L. Manganese neurotoxicity: a bioinorganic chemist's perspective. *Inorganica Chimica Acta*. 2008;361:875–884.
219. Guilarte TR, Chen MK, McGlothan JL, Verina T, Wong DF, Zhou Y, Alexander M, Rohde CA, Syversen T, Decamp E, et al. Nigrostriatal dopamine system dysfunction and subtle motor deficits in manganese-exposed non-human primates. *Exp Neurol*. 2006;202:381–390.
220. Khalid M, Aoun RA, Mathews TA. Altered striatal dopamine release following a sub-acute exposure to manganese. *J Neurosci Methods*. 2011;202:182–191.
221. Desole MS, Miele M, Esposito G, Migheli R, Fresu L, De Natale G, Miele E. Dopaminergic system activity and cellular defense mechanisms in the striatum and striatal synaptosomes of the rat subchronically exposed to manganese. *Arch Toxicol*. 1994;68:566–570.
222. Sloot WN, Korf J, Koster JF, De Wit LE, Gramsbergen JB. Manganese-induced hydroxyl radical formation in rat striatum is not attenuated by dopamine depletion or iron chelation in vivo. *Exp Neurol*. 1996;138:236–245.
223. Archibald FS, Tyree C. Manganese poisoning and the attack of trivalent manganese upon catecholamines. *Arch Biochem Biophys*. 1987;256:638–650.
224. Seth PK, Chandra SV. Neurotransmitters and neurotransmitter receptors in developing and adult rats during manganese poisoning. *Neurotoxicology*. 1984;5:67–76.
225. Liccione JJ, Maines MD. Selective vulnerability of glutathione metabolism and cellular defense mechanisms in rat striatum to manganese. *J Pharmacol Exp Ther*. 1988;247:156–161.
226. Wolters EC, Huang CC, Clark C, Peppard RF, Okada J, Chu NS, Adam MJ, Ruth TJ, Li D, Calne DB. Positron emission tomography in manganese intoxication. *Ann Neurol*. 1989;26:647–651.
227. Spadoni F, Stefani A, Morello M, Lavaroni F, Giacomini P, Sancesario G. Selective vulnerability of pallidal neurons in the early phases of manganese intoxication. *Exp Brain Res*. 2000;135:544–551.
228. Liu X, Sullivan KA, Madl JE, Legare M, Tjalkens RB. Manganese-induced neurotoxicity: the role of astroglial-derived nitric oxide in striatal interneuron degeneration. *Toxicol Sci*. 2006;91:521–531.
229. Gwiazda R, Lucchini R, Smith D. Adequacy and consistency of animal studies to evaluate the neurotoxicity of chronic low-level manganese exposure in humans. *J Toxicol Environ Health A*. 2007;70:594–605.
230. Shinotoh H, Snow BJ, Chu NS, Huang CC, Lu CS, Lee C, Takahashi H, Calne DB. Presynaptic and postsynaptic striatal dopaminergic function in patients with manganese intoxication: a positron emission tomography study. *Neurology*. 1997;48:1053–1056.
231. Kim JW, Kim Y, Cheong HK, Ito K. Manganese induced parkinsonism: a case report. *J Korean Med Sci*. 1998;13:437–439.
232. Huang CC, Weng YH, Lu CS, Chu NS, Yen TC. Dopamine transporter binding in chronic manganese intoxication. *J Neurol*. 2003;250:1335–1339.
233. Lafon-Cazal M, Culcasi M, Gaven F, Pietri S, Bockaert J. Nitric oxide, superoxide and peroxynitrite: putative mediators of NMDA-induced cell death in cerebellar granule cells. *Neuropharmacology*. 1993;32:1259–1266.
234. Hexum TD, Fried R. Effects of superoxide radicals on transport (Na+K) adenosine triphosphatase and protection by superoxide dismutase. *Neurochem Res*. 1979;4:73–82.
235. Hazell AS, Norenberg MD. Manganese decreases glutamate uptake in cultured astrocytes. *Neurochem Res*. 1997;22:1443–1447.

236. Trotti D, Danbolt NC, Volterra A. Glutamate transporters are oxidant-vulnerable: a molecular link between oxidative and excitotoxic neurodegeneration?. *Trends Pharmacol Sci*. 1998;19:328–334.
237. Milatovic D, Yin Z, Gupta RC, Sidoryk M, Albrecht J, Aschner JL, Aschner M. Manganese induces oxidative impairment in cultured rat astrocytes. *Toxicol Sci*. 2007;98:198–205.
238. Rao VL, Dogan A, Todd KG, Bowen KK, Kim BT, Rothstein JD, Dempsey RJ. Antisense knockdown of the glial glutamate transporter GLT-1, but not the neuronal glutamate transporter EAAC1, exacerbates transient focal cerebral ischemia-induced neuronal damage in rat brain. *J Neurosci*. 2001;21:1876–1883.
239. Hietanen E, Kilpio J, Savolainen H. Neurochemical and biotransformational enzyme responses to manganese exposure in rats. *Arch Environ Contam Toxicol*. 1981;10:339–345.
240. Zheng W, Ren S, Graziano JH. Manganese inhibits mitochondrial aconitase: a mechanism of manganese neurotoxicity. *Brain Res*. 1998;799:334–342.
241. Galvani P, Fumagalli P, Santagostino A. Vulnerability of mitochondrial complex I in PC12 cells exposed to manganese. *Eur J Pharmacol*. 1995;293:377–383.
242. HaMai D, Campbell A, Bondy SC. Modulation of oxidative events by multivalent manganese complexes in brain tissue. *Free Radic Biol Med*. 2001;31:763–768.
243. Malecki EA. Manganese toxicity is associated with mitochondrial dysfunction and DNA fragmentation in rat primary striatal neurons. *Brain Res Bull*. 2001;55:225–228.
244. Zhang S, Zhou Z, Fu J. Effect of manganese chloride exposure on liver and brain mitochondria function in rats. *Environ Res*. 2003;93:149–157.
245. Chen JY, Tsao GC, Zhao Q, Zheng W. Differential cytotoxicity of Mn(II) and Mn(III): special reference to mitochondrial [Fe-S] containing enzymes. *Toxicol Appl Pharmacol*. 2001;175:160–168.
246. Ali SF, Duhart HM, Newport GD, Lipe GW, Slikker Jr W. Manganese-induced reactive oxygen species: comparison between Mn+2 and Mn+3. *Neurodegeneration*. 1995;4:329–334.
247. Turrens JF. Mitochondrial formation of reactive oxygen species. *J Physiol*. 2003;552:335–344.
248. Blake CI, Spitz E, Leehey M, Hoffer BJ, Boyson SJ. Platelet mitochondrial respiratory chain function in Parkinson's disease. *Mov Disord*. 1997;12:3–8.
249. Catala A. Lipid peroxidation of membrane phospholipids generates hydroxy-alkenals and oxidized phospholipids active in physiological and/or pathological conditions. *Chem Phys Lipids*. 2009;157:1–11.
250. Catala A. The ability of melatonin to counteract lipid peroxidation in biological membranes. *Curr Mol Med*. 2007;7:638–649.
251. Berlett BS, Stadtman ER. Protein oxidation in aging, disease, and oxidative stress. *J Biol Chem*. 1997;272:20313–20316.
252. WHO. Environmental Health Criteria 237. Principles for evaluating health risks in children associated with exposure to chemicals; 2006.
253. Silbergeld EK, Davis DL. Role of biomarkers in identifying and understanding environmentally induced disease. *Clin Chem*. 1994;40:1363–1367.
254. Grandjean P, Landrigan PJ. Developmental neurotoxicity of industrial chemicals. *Lancet*. 2006;368:2167–2178.
255. Amorim L. Os biomarcadores e a sua aplicação na avaliação da exposição aos agentes químicos ambientais. *Revista Brasileira de Epidemiologia*. 2003;6:158–170.
256. Costa LG. Biomarker research in neurotoxicology: the role of mechanistic studies to bridge the gap between the laboratory and epidemiological investigations. *Environ Health Perspect*. 1996;104(Suppl 1):55–67.
257. Atkinson Arthur J, DeGruttola Victor CWA, DeMets David G, Downing Gregory L, Hoth Daniel J, Oates John F, Peck Carl A, Schooley Robert C, Spilker Bert T, Woodcock Janet A, ZegerScott L. Biomarkers and surrogate endpoints: preferred definitions and conceptual framework. *Clin Pharmacol Ther*. 2001;69:89–95.
258. Gil F, Pla A. Biomarkers as biological indicators of xenobiotic exposure. *J Appl Toxicol*. 2001;21:245–255.
259. Smargiassi A, Mutti A. Peripheral biomarkers and exposure to manganese. *Neurotoxicology*. 1999;20:401–406.
260. Zheng W, Fu SX, Dydak U, Cowan DM. Biomarkers of manganese intoxication. *Neurotoxicology*. 2011;32:1–8.
261. Apostoli P, Lucchini R, Alessio L. Are current biomarkers suitable for the assessment of manganese exposure in individual workers?. *Am J Ind Med*. 2000;37:283–290.
262. Iyengar V, Woittiez J. Trace elements in human clinical specimens: evaluation of literature data to identify reference values. *Clin Chem*. 1988;34:474–481.
263. Reynolds N, Blumsohn A, Baxter JP, Houston G, Pennington CR. Manganese requirement and toxicity in patients on home parenteral nutrition. *Clin Nutr*. 1998;17:227–230.
264. Mergler D, Baldwin M, Belanger S, Larribe F, Beuter A, Bowler R, Panisset M, Edwards R, de Geoffroy A, Sassine MP, et al. Manganese neurotoxicity, a continuum of dysfunction: results from a community based study. *Neurotoxicology*. 1999;20:327–342.

265. Lauwerys R, Hoet P, eds. Manganese. In: *Industrial Chemical Exposure: Guidelines for Biological Monitoring*. Boca Raton: Lewish Publisher; 1993:71–74.
266. Minoia C, Sabbioni E, Apostoli P, Pietra R, Pozzoli L, Gallorini M, Nicolaou G, Alessio L, Capodaglio E. Trace element reference values in tissues from inhabitants of the European community. I. A study of 46 elements in urine, blood and serum of Italian subjects. *Sci Total Environ*. 1990;95:89–105.
267. Blanc P. *Poisoning and Drug Overdose*. Norwalk, California: Appleton & Lange; 1990.
268. Keen CL, Clegg MS, Lonnerdal B, Hurley LS. Whole-blood manganese as an indicator of body manganese. *N Engl J Med*. 1983;308:1230.
269. Buchet JP, Lauwerys R, Roels H, De Vos C. Determination of manganese in blood and urine by flameless atomic absorption spectrophotometry. *Clin Chim Acta*. 1976;73:481–486.
270. Hagenfeldt K, Plantin LO, Diczfalusy E. Trace elements in the human endometrium. 2. Zinc, copper and manganese levels in the endometrium, cervical mucus and plasma. *Acta Endocrinol (Copenh)*. 1973;72:115–126.
271. Milne DB, Sims RL, Ralston NV. Manganese content of the cellular components of blood. *Clin Chem*. 1990;36:450–452.
272. Greger JL, Davis CD, Suttie JW, Lyle BJ. Intake, serum concentrations, and urinary excretion of manganese by adult males. *Am J Clin Nutr*. 1990;51:457–461.
273. Davis CD, Malecki EA, Greger JL. Interactions among dietary manganese, heme iron, and nonheme iron in women. *Am J Clin Nutr*. 1992;56:926–932.
274. Lucchini R, Selis L, Folli D, Apostoli P, Mutti A, Vanoni O, Iregren A, Alessio L. Neurobehavioral effects of manganese in workers from a ferroalloy plant after temporary cessation of exposure. *Scand J Work Environ Health*. 1995;21:143–149.
275. Kim Y. High signal intensities on T1-weighted MRI as a biomarker of exposure to manganese. *Ind Health*. 2004;42:111–115.
276. Saitoh Y, Kimura S, Nezu A, Ohtsuki N, Kobayashi T, Osaka H, Uehara S. Hyperintense brain lesions on T1-weighted MRI after parenteral nutrition. *No To Hattatsu*. 1996;28:39–43.
277. Masumoto K, Suita S, Taguchi T, Yamanouchi T, Nagano M, Ogita K, Nakamura M, Mihara F. Manganese intoxication during intermittent parenteral nutrition: report of two cases. *JPEN J Parenter Enteral Nutr*. 2001;25:95–99.
278. Roels H, Lauwerys R, Genet P, Sarhan MJ, de Fays M, Hanotiau I, Buchet JP. Relationship between external and internal parameters of exposure to manganese in workers from a manganese oxide and salt producing plant. *Am J Ind Med*. 1987;11:297–305.
279. Bowler RM, Gysens S, Diamond E, Booty A, Hartney C, Roels HA. Neuropsychological sequelae of exposure to welding fumes in a group of occupationally exposed men. *Int J Hyg Environ Health*. 2003;206:517–529.
280. Laohaudomchok W, Lin X, Herrick RF, Fang SC, Cavallari JM, Shrairman R, Landau A, Christiani DC, Weisskopf MG. Neuropsychological effects of low-level manganese exposure in welders. *Neurotoxicology*. 2011;32:171–179.
281. Sinczuk-Walczak H, Jakubowski M, Matczak W. Neurological and neurophysiological examinations of workers occupationally exposed to manganese. *Int J Occup Med Environ Health*. 2001;14:329–337.
282. Emara AM, el-Ghawabi SH, Madkour OI, el-Samra GH. Chronic manganese poisoning in the dry battery industry. *Br J Ind Med*. 1971;28:78–82.
283. Iregren A. Using psychological tests for the early detection of neurotoxic effects of low level manganese exposure. *Neurotoxicology*. 1994;15:671–677.
284. Dydak U, Jiang YM, Long LL, Zhu H, Chen J, Li WM, Edden RA, Hu S, Fu X, Long Z, et al. In vivo measurement of brain GABA concentrations by magnetic resonance spectroscopy in smelters occupationally exposed to manganese. *Environ Health Perspect*. 2011;119:219–224.
285. Gwiazda RH, Lee D, Sheridan J, Smith DR. Low cumulative manganese exposure affects striatal GABA but not dopamine. *Neurotoxicology*. 2002;23:69–76.
286. Chandra SV, Malhotra KM, Shukla GS. GABAergic neurochemistry in manganese exposed rats. *Acta Pharmacol Toxicol (Copenh)*. 1982;51:456–458.
287. Lipe GW, Duhart H, Newport GD, Slikker Jr W, Ali SF. Effect of manganese on the concentration of amino acids in different regions of the rat brain. *J Environ Sci Health B*. 1999;34:119–132.
288. Calabresi P, Ammassari-Teule M, Gubellini P, Sancesario G, Morello M, Centonze D, Marfia GA, Saulle E, Passino E, Picconi B, et al. A synaptic mechanism underlying the behavioral abnormalities induced by manganese intoxication. *Neurobiol Dis*. 2001;8:419–432.

289. Kvetnansky R, Sabban EL, Palkovits M. Catecholaminergic systems in stress: structural and molecular genetic approaches. *Physiol Rev*. 2009;89:535–606.
290. Eisenhofer G, Kopin IJ, Goldstein DS. Catecholamine metabolism: a contemporary view with implications for physiology and medicine. *Pharmacol Rev*. 2004;56:331–349.
291. Smargiassi A, Mergler D, Bergamaschi E, Vettori MV, Lucchini R, Apostoli P. Peripheral markers of catecholamine metabolism among workers occupationally exposed to manganese (Mn). *Toxicol Lett*. 1995;77:329–333.
292. Pivac N, Knezevic J, Mustapic M, Dezeljin M, Muck-Seler D, Kozaric-Kovacic D, Balija M, Matijevic T, Pavelic J. The lack of association between monoamine oxidase (MAO) intron 13 polymorphism and platelet MAO-B activity among men. *Life Sci*. 2006;79:45–49.
293. Butler IJ, Koslow SH, Krumholz A, Holtzman NA, Kaufman S. A disorder of biogenic amines in dihydropteridine reductase deficiency. *Ann Neurol*. 1978;3:224–230.
294. Altindag ZZ, Baydar T, Engin AB, Sahin G. Effects of the metals on dihydropteridine reductase activity. *Toxicol In Vitro*. 2003;17:533–537.
295. Santos D, Batoreu MC, Almeida I, Ramos R, Sidoryk-Wegrzynowicz M, Aschner M, Marreilha Dos Santos AP. Manganese alters rat brain amino acids levels. *Biol Trace Elem Res*. 2012.
296. Chang A, Shin SH. Relationships between dopamine-induced changes in cytosolic free calcium concentration ([Ca2+]i) and rate of prolactin secretion. Elevated [Ca2+]i does not indicate prolactin release. *Endocrine*. 1997;7:343–349.

CHAPTER

9

Zinc in Autism

Stefanie Grabrucker, Andreas M. Grabrucker*,***

*Institute for Anatomy and Cell Biology, Ulm University, Ulm Germany

**WG Molecular Analysis of Synaptopathies, Ulm University, Ulm, Germany

OUTLINE

INTRODUCTION

Zinc is a structural and regulatory component of many proteins in the brain, but has also a major function as a signaling ion in numerous pathways during brain development and normal brain physiology. For example, on a cellular level, zinc signaling was shown to play a role in neuronal differentiation, migration, as well as synapse formation and plasticity.[1]

Synaptogenesis and control of excitatory glutamatergic terminals are heavily influenced by zinc. Zinc is released along with glutamate during synaptic activity into the synaptic cleft of so called "zincergic" synapses, where the local levels of zinc might reach high μM concentrations. Furthermore, zinc levels may increase within the postsynapse by secondary mechanisms independent of presynaptic release of zinc. Several target proteins are regulated by this zinc release. For example, zinc is able to bind to the *N*-methyl-D-aspartate (NMDA) subtype of glutamate receptor (NMDAR),[2,3] or to zinc-specific postsynaptic receptors, such as mZnR/G protein-coupled receptor 39 (GPR39),[4] and might even enter the postsynaptic cell via various channels.[5] Within the postsynaptic compartment, zinc regulates, among others, the activity of "extracellular signal-regulated protein kinase" (ERK),[6] and dynamics of "SH3 and multiple ankyrin repeat domains" (Shank)2 and Shank3 scaffold proteins.[7]

Biometals in Neurodegenerative Diseases. http://dx.doi.org/10.1016/B978-0-12-804562-6.00009-9

The imbalance of essential and putative toxic trace metals shows a strong association with autism spectrum disorders (ASD),[8] which was shown by genetic studies as well as the investigation of trace metal levels in patient tissues. Furthermore, early infantile zinc deficiency is frequently found in ASD patients,[9–12] ASD candidate genes have been identified in patient studies that are part of pathways regulating metal homeostasis or encode metal binding proteins. For example, the zinc transporter 5 [ZnT5, Solute Carrier Family 30 Member 5 (SLC30A5)], Zrt-, Irt-like protein 11 [Zip11, (SLC39A11)], and mutations or copy number variation in the metal-regulatory transcription factor 1 (MTF1) and copper metabolism (Murr1) domain containing 1 (COMMD1) have been associated with ASD,[13–17] as well as the synaptic zinc binding proteins SHANK2 and SHANK3.[18] Furthermore, several synaptic targets of zinc have been associated with ASD, such as TrkB/BDNF signaling,[19] ERK1/2,[20] and NMDAR activity.[21]

The same targets show alterations in Alzheimer's disease (AD). It is therefore likely that aberrant zinc signaling results in similar impairments that, dependent upon age, lead to different outcomes such as ASD, and cognitive impairments in AD. However, the causes leading to altered zinc signaling might have alternative origins, such as zinc sequestration by protein aggregates in AD or maternal zinc deficiency during pregnancy due to increased demand caused by the developing embryo in ASD.

During brain development, altered zinc levels might induce long lasting changes. For example, studies on mouse models for gestational zinc deficiency reported that many of the immuno-deficiencies detected after birth persisted into adulthood. This was the case even though the pups were raised with a diet that contained normal amounts of zinc,[22] suggesting that a transient time-period may exist during prenatal development where the immune system is especially susceptible. This might be true for the brain as well, as circuit formation and synaptic pruning are partially developmentally time-restricted processes. For example, while with regard to cognitive functioning, both prenatal and postnatal zinc deficient rodents show impairments in learning and memory, only prenatal zinc deficient mice show ASD-like behavior, and only postnatal acute zinc deficient animals depression like behavior.[23] Importantly, prenatal zinc deficient mice were reported to display ASD like behavior later in life without acute zinc deficiency.[24,25] Similarly, ZnT3 knockout mice were reported to show some behaviors associated with ASD.[26] However, ZnT3 knockout mice also show AD like cognitive deficits later in life.[27]

Based on these insights, it is possible that neurodegenerative disorders that manifest during aging and that are classically diagnosed in old age may also have their origin in a much earlier time point, masking the separation between neurodevelopmental disorders and neurodegenerative disorders.

Despite a contribution to the etiology of specific disorders, abnormal trace metal levels might contribute to some of the shared morbidities in ASD and AD. For example, besides synaptic dysfunction, seizures, increased anxiety, and behavioral abnormalities, such as aggressiveness, irritability, anhedonia, and apathy, also depression-like behavior and cognitive impairments are inherent both to ASD and AD, and possibly linked to zinc deficiency.[23]

Here, we will discuss recent findings on the role of zinc in ASD keeping in mind a possible relation to similar pathological processes that might occur in neurodegenerative disorders, such as AD. Among these processes, neuroinflammation and synaptic dysfunction are in the focus.

ZINC SIGNALING IN AUTISM

Zinc deficiency has been associated with many brain disorders. Among them, neurodegenerative disorders,[8] but also autism can be found frequently in reports. However, while for AD, abnormal zinc levels might occur locally, for example in close vicinity to the zinc sequestering plaques, in ASD, systemic zinc deficiencies are reported. These seem to be especially frequent during early development (0–3 years of age).[28] A metaanalysis including 11 original reports on Zn/Cu concentrations in autistic patients showed a significant correlation between the levels of these trace metals and the development of ASD.[9] In particular, numerous studies have shown a clear association of low zinc levels or increased copper concentrations with autism.[28–37] This association shows that decreased Zn/Cu ratios (below 6.5 in hair and 0.7 in plasma or serum) were proposed as a biomarker for autism and risk factor for the development of ASD.

Several human populations are at high risk for developing zinc deficiency, also in industrialized nations. Among them, pregnant women and elderly seem to be most susceptible.[29]

In animal models for aging, cognitive decline was associated with a reduction in zinc and an increase in proinflammatory cytokines.[38] Serum zinc concentrations in elderly people have been associated with impaired cognitive function.[39,40] However, similar to neurodegenerative disorders, impaired cognitive function is also a frequent symptom observed in ASD. Nevertheless, in contrast to neurodegenerative disorders, the contribution of zinc deficiency to the etiology of ASD seems to be specifically associated with a time window of early pre- and postnatal brain development. In a mouse model of zinc deficiency restricted to the phase of brain development during pregnancy, wild type mice without predisposition for autism displayed features of autism later in life.[25]

Indeed, maternal micronutrient supplementation is associated with reduced risk of ASD[41] and zinc supplementation therapy in ASD patients was reported beneficial with an increase in Zn/Cu ratio in the patients correlating to an improvement in some ASD associated features.[31] Similarly, in rodent models for ASD, prenatal zinc supplementation prevents communication impairments, and social and cognitive ASD-like behaviors[42,43] in ASD mouse models generated by prenatal exposure to lipopolysaccharide (LPS), which mimics infections by Gram-negative bacteria.

Thus, impaired zinc signaling involved in both inflammatory processes and synaptic function that can be observed in neurodegenerative disorders as well, might trigger lasting pathological processes related to ASD during brain development.

Zinc and Inflammatory Processes in Autism

In ASD, apart from genetic factors, neuroinflammatory processes mediated by microglia and astrocytes may play an important role in the pathology. For example, multiple studies show higher number of activated microglial cells and astrocytes in the brain of patients suffering from ASD.[44–51] Further, a significantly increased expression of proinflammatory cytokines, for example, tumor necrosis factor (TNF)-α, interleukin (IL)-6, and interferon (IFN)-γ in the brain and cerebrospinal fluid (CSF) of patients with ASD was found.[44,52–55] Cytokines are important mediators of neuroinflammation in various pathological conditions of the CNS. In addition, altered expression levels of the transcription factor NF-κB was observed in the orbitofrontal Cortex[56] and blood plasma[57] of autistic patients.

In addition to these neuroinflammatory mechanisms, a role of maternal infection during pregnancy may represent a risk factor in the neuropathology of ASD.[58–62] However, whether and how these inflammatory mechanisms, occurring either as primary or secondary effects, may affect neuronal and synaptic functions in autistic patients and modulate the observed pathology has yet to be determined (Fig. 9.1).

One possibility is that hypozincemia induced by increased levels of cytokines, such as IL-6 will affect synapse function and maturation during brain development via modulation of zinc-binding NMDA receptors, Tropomyosin receptor kinase B (TrkB), and/or GPR39,[12] or the autism associated NEUREXIN-NEUROLIGIN-SHANK pathway.[7,63] Hypozincemia may also facilitate neuroinflammation closing a vicious circle. The increase in cytokines might then directly affect synaptic metabotropic glutamate receptor (mGluR), and p38 MAPK (mitogen-activated protein kinase)/ERK signaling pathways. For instance, IL-1 has influence on several synaptic components mediating long-term potentiation (LTP), a molecular mechanism thought to underlie synaptic plasticity, such as NMDA and α-amino-3-hydroxy-5-methyl-4-isoxazolepropionic acid (AMPA) receptor signaling,[64,65] and glutamate release.[66] IL-18 was shown to negatively modulate NMDA receptor mediated transmission in the hippocampus.[67] Further, altered IL-6 levels affect the ERK pathway. TNF-α acts on AMPA and NMDA as well as mGluR signaling, thereby modulating the activity of activated p38 MAPK.

Similar pathological processes have been detected in neurodegenerative disorders, where the presence of amyloid beta (Aβ) in case of AD or other pathological protein deposits leads to local inflammation (Fig. 9.1). For example, Aβ increases the susceptibility of microglia to a secondary stimulus and/or promotes their activation. In AD, Aβ sustains chronic activation of primed microglia resulting, similarly to ASD, in increased levels of inflammatory cytokines and chemokines. Again, IFN-γ, TNF-α, and the interleukins IL-1, IL-6, and IL-18, may be important mediators of this neuroinflammation. Aβ triggers IL-6 production in both microglia and astrocytes.

The cytokines IL-6, and S100B have gained attention in the pathological processes involved in ASD, as well as AD. S100 proteins acting as cytokines are a family of low molecular weight, regulatory, calcium- binding, but also zinc and copper binding proteins.[68] As extracellular cytokines, they function via the RAGE (receptor for advanced glycation end-products) signaling pathway and RAGE activation increases extracellular S100 concentrations via NF-κB activation, which leads to a positive feedback cycle.[69] Most of the S100 family members are prone to form aggregates of the amyloid type under physiological conditions.[70,71] Especially S100B is regulated as a response to cell damage, proteotoxic stress and aging, and altered levels accelerate AD pathology.[72] However, a pathological deregulation of S100B is described in aging brains as well as in autistic patients. S100B has been identified as autism risk candidate gene[73] and elevated serum S100B levels have been associated with autism, with S100B levels significantly correlating with the severity of symptoms.[74] Similar to Aβ, zinc sequestration by S100B may lead to local zinc deficiency in the developing and aged brain.

IL-6 was shown to be increased in the cerebellum, plasma and serum of individuals with ASD.[75,76] In mouse models, reduction of IL-6 by application of antibodies or genetic knockout ameliorated ASD-like behavior seen in the offspring of maternal immune activation (MIA) mice.[77] Zinc deficiency enhances the inflammatory response by inducing IL-6 gene transcription.[78] However, IL-6 levels are also found increased in AD and aging. Zinc supplementation in elderly subjects normalized the increased production of IL-6 associated with senescence.[79]

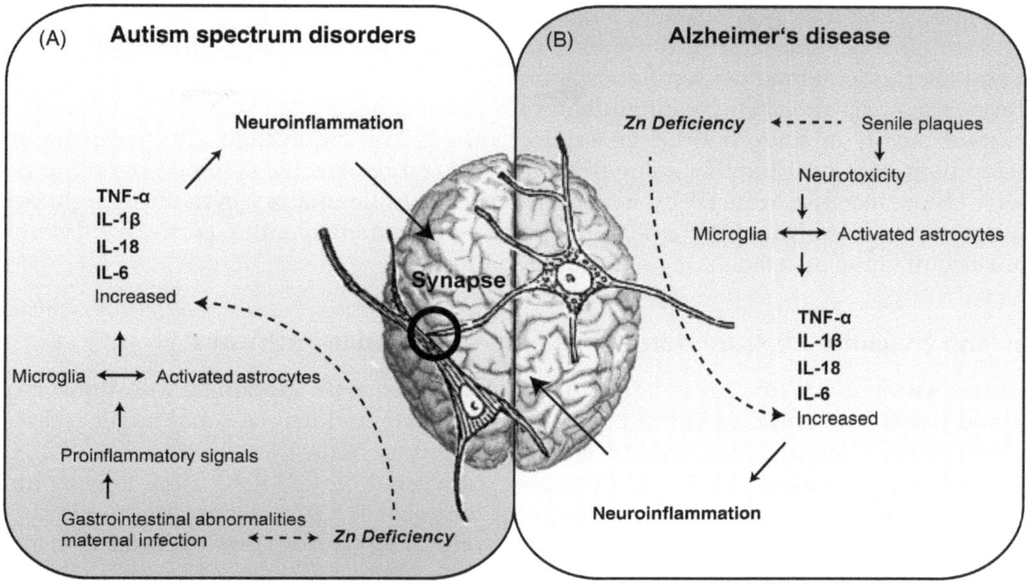

FIGURE 9.1 **Zinc and inflammatory processes in ASD.** (A) Maternal infection, or immune system activation due to gastrointestinal abnormalities (possibly facilitated by zinc deficiency) may lead to an increase in the levels of proinflammatory cytokines, such as TNF-α, IL-1β, IL-18, and IL-6 in the maternal circulation and offspring. Circulating cytokines, such as IL-6 interact with targets in the (developing) brain to induce several downstream mechanisms. Further, increased cytokine levels decrease plasma zinc levels in maternal and fetal blood via induction of metallothioneins in the liver. In the brains of the developing offspring, long-term changes can be observed, including microglial activation, increased GFAP levels, oxidative stress, zinc deficiency, and again increased cytokine levels. These alterations may affect brain development and/or long-term brain function in the offspring, for example by altering synaptic plasticity and function. (B) In AD, the presence of Aβ leads to local brain inflammation. Senile plaques recruit activated microglia and astrocytes promoting the release of cytokines and cytotoxic molecules. Further, Aβ peptides in plaques bind zinc resulting in local zinc deficiency. Similarly to ASD, increased levels of TNF-α, and the interleukins IL-1β, IL-6, and IL-18, may be important mediators of this neuroinflammation and zinc deficiency may prolong the inflammatory response. Ultimately, inflammatory processes and local zinc deficiency in AD may affect synaptic plasticity and function. Abbreviations: *GFAP*, glial fibrillary acidic protein; *IL*, interleukin; *TNF*, tumor necrosis factor; *Zn*, zinc.

A significant increase in NF-κB DNA binding activity was detected in blood samples of children with autism[57] as well as post mortem brain tissue.[56] This increase in NF-κB activity may be mediated by zinc deficiency. Zinc inhibits the I kappa B kinase (IKK) complex member IKKβ[80] and by that prevents the translocation (activation) of NF-κB into the nucleus, which leads to, among others, upregulation of IL-6.[81] Corroborating this observation, zinc transporter ZIP8 acts as a negative feedback regulator and is a transcriptional target of the NF-κB pathway. ZIP8 transporters increase intracellular zinc contents by promoting extracellular zinc uptake or release from subcellular organelles.[82] Under zinc deficient conditions, this IKK inhibition may decrease and thereby increase NF-κB activation in several tissues, resulting in prolonged or chronic inflammation. Interestingly, increased cellular NF-κB activity may also be involved in inflammatory activation in AD brains.[83] In AD, NF-κB activity is upregulated[84] and may play a role in plaque formation and cytokine signaling in AD. Again, local zinc deficiency due to sequestration of zinc in senile plaques may increase NF-κB activation and lead to sustained neuroinflammation.

Taken together, although proinflammatory cytokines have been previously identified as important factors in acute neurodegeneration, little is known on their effects during brain development. It is possible that some of their effects target specific synaptic signaling pathways.[12] Hypozincemia induced by increased levels of inflammatory cytokines might act as common factor in ASD and AD influencing zinc—dependent synaptic pathways. However, hypozincemia may also facilitate neuroinflammation.

Zinc and Synaptic Dysfunction in Autism—Molecular Pathways

Upon neuronal activity, presynaptic zinc is coreleased with glutamate into the synaptic cleft and has the potential to interact with and modulate various neuronal target receptors, ion channels and transporters, thereby shaping excitatory neurotransmission (Fig. 9.2). One of its particular targets is the NMDA receptor. Abnormal NMDAR function is both implicated in ASD as well as AD. NMDA receptors of the subtypeNR2A display high-affinity zinc binding sites. Following the stimulation of zinc containing neurons, endogenous zinc is able

FIGURE 9.2 **A model for zinc signaling at excitatory synapses in ASD and AD.** Zinc is required for various processes at synapses. Zinc binds to Shank2/3 proteins establishing and stabilizing the scaffold of the PSD. As Shank proteins are master organizers of the PSD, modulatory effects targeting Shank proteins will have profound effects on synapse formation, maturation, and stability. Synaptic activity leads to glutamate and zinc release from the presynaptic terminal. Zinc subsequently enters into the postsynaptic compartment via channels, such as NMDAR, AMPAR, or VGCC. Synaptic activity might also release intracellular zinc from MT3. Increased intracellular postsynaptic zinc can not only increase Shank2/3 platforms which provide a trans-synaptic signal via Nlgn–Nrxn complexes but also act as signal activating SRC possibly via inhibition of plasma membrane Na^+/K^+ ATPase. Activation of SRC will, among others, affect PSD95/NMDAR complexes enhancing NMDAR signaling. Additionally, the BDNF receptor TrkB shows transactivation by zinc. Activation of TrkB receptor signaling will ultimately result in a modulation of ERK1/2 and mTOR dependent signaling pathways. In addition, zinc binds to extra-synaptic neurotransmitter receptors and receptors in the synaptic cleft such NMDAR and AMPAR, modulating their activity. NMDAR are further tightly associated at the PSD with the zinc exporter ZnT1. Activation of NMDAR will similarly converge in the modulation of ERK1/2 and mTOR dependent signaling pathways. Further, specific zinc binding receptors exist at the PSD, such as GPR39. Zinc binding to GPR39 results in activation of $G\alpha_q$ stimulating phospholipase C leading to calcium influx and activation of the CamKII and finally the ERK1/2 cascade. Various components of this complex network of zinc dependent signaling pathways at synapses have been implicated in ASD but also in AD. For example, mutations in NRXN, NLGN, SHANK3, PSD95, NMDAR, HOMER1, and mTOR have been associated with ASD in genetic association studies. Further, the modulated pathways, such as AMPA, NMDA, mGluR, BDNF/ERK/mTOR signaling have been reported multiple times to be affected in ASD. For example, mutations in one of two genes, TSC1 and TSC2, as well as FMRP leading to abnormal local translation are implicated in ASD associated tuberous sclerosis and Fragile x syndrome, respectively. These zinc-dependent pathways are also targeted by inflammatory processes as they have been reported in both ASD and AD. IL-6 and TNF-α target the ERK1/2 pathway and accumulating S100B proteins may scavenge zinc. Similar mechanistic alterations have been shown at synapses in AD, where Aβ peptides sequester zinc ions leading to a loss of Shank platforms. Abbreviations: *BDNF*, Brain-derived neurotrophic factor; *Ca*, calcium; *CamKII*, Calcium/calmodulin-dependent protein kinase II; *ERK1/2*, Extracellular signal-regulated protein kinases 1 and 2; *FMRP*, fragile X mental retardation protein; *GluA1*, AMPA Receptor Subunit 1; *Glut*, Glutamate; *MT3*, Metallothionein-3; *mTOR*, mechanistic Target of Rapamycin; *NOS*, Nitric Oxide Synthase; *NO*, Nitric oxide; *NRXN*, Neurexin-1; *NLGN*, Neuroligin-3; *PSD-95*, postsynaptic density protein 95; *S6K*, S6 kinase; *SRC*, proto-oncogene tyrosine-protein kinase; *TNF*, tumor necrosis factor; *TNFR1*, Tumor necrosis factor receptor 1; *TrkB*, Tropomyosin receptor kinase B; *TSC*, tuberous sclerosis complex; *VGCC*, Voltage-gated calcium channel; *Zn*, zinc; *ZnT*, Zinc transporter.

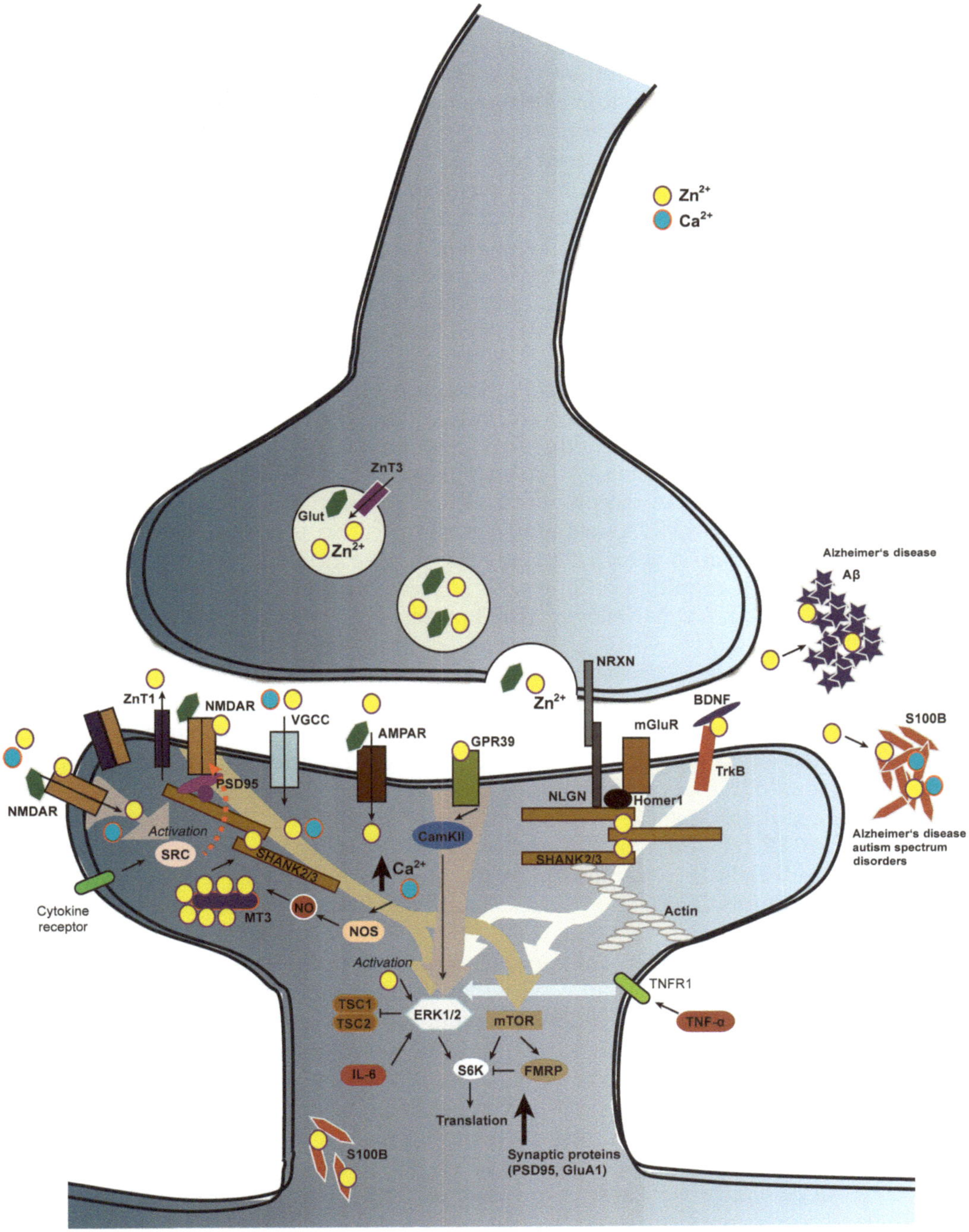
Zn2+
Ca2+
ZnT3
Glut
Zn2+
Alzheimer's disease
Aβ
NRXN
Zn2+
ZnT1
NMDAR
VGCC
AMPAR
GPR39
mGluR
BDNF
S100B
TrkB
NMDAR
PSD95
NLGN
Homer1
Activation
SRC
SHANK2/3
CamKII
Ca2+
SHANK2/3
Alzheimer's disease
autism spectrum
disorders
Cytokine
receptor
MT3
NO
NOS
Actin
Activation
TNFR1
TSC1
TSC2
ERK1/2
mTOR
TNF-α
IL-6
S6K
FMRP
Translation
S100B
Synaptic proteins
(PSD95, GluA1)

to produce both a voltage-independent reduction of NMDA receptor-gated channel opening frequency and a voltage independent flicker block of the channel.[85,86] Furthermore, upon entering the postsynaptic compartment via various ion channels, zinc is able to induce the activation of Src kinases via inhibition of plasma membrane Na^+/K^+ ATPase, thereby leading to the upregulation of NMDA receptor activity.[87] Interestingly, mutation or dysfunction of NMDA receptor function have both been reported in AD as well as ASD. ASD, for example, has been genetically associated with mutations in the NMDA receptor subunit GluN2A,[88] and GluN2B (de novo protein truncating and splice mutations).[14,89] Furthermore, disrupted NMDA-receptor mediated glutamatergic signaling has strongly been linked to ASD pathology in a number of mouse models of ASD[90–94] suggesting either an NMDA receptor hyperfunction, due to increased expression of NMDA receptors[90] or NMDA receptor hypofunction.[91–94]

Similar, in AD it was demonstrated that synthetic amyloid-β (Aβ) aggregates are able to inhibit NMDA dependent LTP formation,[95,96] affect surface expression of NMDARs,[97,98] and might lead to disrupted NMDA receptor mediated signaling by inducing either an increase[99,100] or a decrease in NMDAR conductance.[95] One proposed mechanism is that zinc upon release in the synaptic cleft and due to its high affinity to Aβ induces a rapid, aggregation of Aβ into amyloid precipitates.[101] This trapping of zinc ions by extracellular amyloid plaques might deprive NMDA receptors of zinc and so contribute to downstream cognitive loss due to disruption of NMDA mediated signaling.[102] This is in line, with previous findings in ZnT3 knock-out mice, which lack presynaptic zinc at the glutamatergic synapse and display age-dependent cognitive decline with reduced NMDAR2a and NMDAR2b protein expression, similar to an AD pathology.[27] ZnT3 protein levels are also decreased in postmortem brains of AD patients.[103]

Additionally, it has been demonstrated that synaptic released zinc is able to target AMPA receptors at the postsynaptic compartment. Upon presynaptic release, zinc was shown to inhibit synaptic AMPA currents in the hippocampus as well as dorsal cochlear nucleus.[104] AMPA—mediated excitatory synaptic dysfunctions have been reported in large number of animal models for ASD, especially Shank3 mutant mice.[105–108] Furthermore, mice lacking the transcriptional regulator MeCP2, resulting in Rett syndrome, display reduced spontaneous and evoked AMPAR transmission.[109,110] Similarly, in AD, it has been demonstrated that the presence of Aβ induced disruption of AMPA receptor function.[111] Furthermore, reduced glutamate receptor subunits GluR1 and GluR2/3 have been found in the entorhinal cortex of AD patients.[112]

Besides shaping excitatory transmission via ionotropic receptors, synaptic released zinc targets additionally metabotropic pathways within the glutamatergic postsynapse via the zinc sensing receptor GPR39 (mZnR).[4] GPR39 activation leads to an increase in Inositol trisphosphate (IP3),[113] followed by calcium release and phosphorylation of extracellular-regulated kinase (ERK) and Ca/calmodulin kinase (CAMKII).[4] Ultimately, these processes lead to activation of the cAMP response-element-driven (CREB) transcription,[114] which regulates the transcription of various genes including the neurotrophic factor BDNF.[115] Interestingly, some ASD patients display a deletion of 2q21.1q21.2 region, where the GPR39 gene is located.[116] Moreover, dysregulated downstream pathways of the GPR39 receptor activity (ERK and CAMKII) have been strongly linked to the pathophysiology of ASD[117,118] but also AD.[119–121]

Recent findings indicate that extracellular zinc targets the BDNF–TrkB pathway at the glutamatergic synapse in a further way (Fig. 9.2). BDNF belongs to the family of neutrophins and interacts with TrkB receptors. Zinc can directly promote the activation of TrkB receptor through increasing Src family kinase activity.[122] Furthermore, extracellular zinc activates metalloproteinases, which induce the release of pro-BDNF and the conversion of BDNF to mature BDNF finally resulting in TrkB activation.[123] These data are in line with the finding that chronic dietary treatment with zinc resulted in an increase of brain BDNF levels.[124,125] Interestingly, abnormalities in neutrophin expression, especially BDNF, have been implicated in the pathophysiology of ASD. A recent study reported that decreased levels of BNDF in a mouse model of ASD (Mecp2) affect disease progression.[126] A further link of disturbed BDNF signaling and ASD was found with the CADPS2 gene. CADPS2 is a gene located within the AUTS1 susceptibility locus for ASD on 7q13, and was reported aberrantly spliced in some autistic patients. CADPS2 regulates the exocytosis of dense-core vesicles, including BDNF-containing vesicles. Cadps2-knock out mice display an ASD like phenotype.[127]

Modifications of BDNF expression and its high-affinity receptor, TrkB, have also been reported in AD. Several studies have demonstrated reduced BDNF expression in postmortem brain regions of AD patients.[121,128–131]

Upon neuronal activity, some zinc ions enter the postsynaptic compartment through calcium channels, AMPAR and NMDAR[5] and regulate further target proteins and pathways implicated in ASD but also AD. One particular effector of postsynaptic zinc are Shank proteins, a family of excitatory postsynaptic scaffold proteins genetically linked to ASD[132–137] and affected in AD.[138–141] In previous studies it was shown that Shank2 and Shank3 protein levels depend on the local synaptic zinc concentration and influx.[142] Zinc binds to Shank2/Shank3 via the C-terminal sterile alpha motif (SAM) domain, thereby regulating the clustering of Shank2/Shank3 into large macromolecular platforms.[143,144] Shank platforms within the PSD function as a docking site for postsynaptic receptors (NMDAR, AMPAR, mGluR), thereby promoting postsynaptic stabilization. Additionally, it was demonstrated that zinc dependent upregulation of Shank3 proteins at the postsynapse also affects presynaptic protein levels via the trans-synaptic Neuroligin-Neurexin complex formation.[145] Reduced levels of zinc during development were shown to result in loss of immature spines along with a reduction of Shank2 and Shank3 in vitro and in vivo.[24,142] However, presence of Aβ peptides similarly reduced Shank3 levels in a zinc dependent manner.[141] As mentioned earlier, trapping of zinc ions by extracellular amyloid plaques might not only deprive the function of postsynaptic NMDA receptors. Moreover, it might deprive Shank2 and Shank3 scaffold proteins from promoting the structural stabilization of the postsynapse by binding of zinc after neuronal activity, thus contributing to the downstream cognitive and synaptic dysfunction observed in AD as well as ASD pathology.

Furthermore, zinc targets inflammatory pathways, which are both implicated in ASD[44,45,47,52,57,146] and AD.[147,148] The extracellular cytokine S100B was linked to the pathology of ASD[74] as well as AD.[147] S100B is produced primarily by astrocytes and actively participates in synaptic neurotransmission as well as binds zinc.[68,149–151] Similar to Aβ pathology, zinc sequestration by S100B may deprive the physiological targets of zinc within the glutamatergic synapse and might thereby contribute to dysfunction of excitatory neurotransmission.

Taken together, synaptic released zinc modulates many target proteins within the glutamatergic postsynapse, which are dysregulated in ASD as well as AD. Interestingly, all of these postsynaptic targets of zinc feed into downstream pathways regulating glutamatergic synapse function and homeostasis. In particular, the "mechanistic target of rapamycin" (mTOR) dependent pathway, as well as the ERK1/2 pathway, which are responsible for the regulation of translation and protein synthesis within the spine are in the focus. The mTOR pathway is activated by many factors within the postsynapse, which are modulated by zinc ions, including ionotropic and metabotropic glutamate receptors,[152,153] as well as cytokines,[154] and the neurotrophic factor BDNF/TrkB signaling.[155] It is generally accepted, that mTOR acts as a node of convergence downstream of postsynaptic receptors and several signaling pathways that include the ERK, and the phosphoinositide-3 kinase (PI3K)/Akt[154,156] pathway, which are modulated by synaptic released zinc ions. The major targets of mTOR are the components of the translational machinery within the synapse. Activated mTOR induces the initiation of protein synthesis via the phosphorylation of eukaryotic initiation factor 4b (eIF4B).[157] Additionally, activation of the ERK pathway leads to the stimulation of S6K and induces translation.[158] Among the genes locally translated are important constituents of the dendritic spine mediating synaptic plasticity. Previous studies using genetic models for ASD have placed the dysregulation of the mTOR pathway in the center of synaptic pathology.[159,160] Accordingly, both hyperactivation as well hypoactivation may lead to a synaptopathy. Similarly in AD, hyperactivation of mTOR signaling was proposed to play an important role in the pathological processes.[161]

THERAPEUTIC STRATEGIES IN AUTISM BASED ON BIOMETALS

Based on the similarities between the affected synaptic pathways in ASD and AD that are centered around zinc dependent signaling processes, it is likely that strategies developed in AD based on influencing metallostasis may also be useful in ASD. Given that zinc homeostasis is essential for proper glutamatergic synaptic function and development, the possibility of specifically altering zinc levels within the glutamatergic synapse is therefore emerging as a new target for the prevention and treatment ASD as well as AD. Here, the use of clioquinol will serve as interesting example.

Clioquinol (CQ) is considered to be a metal protein-attenuating compound (MPAC) that acts as zinc ionophore. Since 1930s, it was used as antifungal and amoebicidal drug for the treatment of skin infections as well as diarrhea. Due to its controversial association with subacute myelo-optico neuropathy it was withdrawn from the market in 1970s. CQ is able to cross the blood brain barrier after intraperitoneal injection. A phase IIa clinical trial of CQ found that CQ treatment increases plasma zinc levels.[162] Previous studies have additionally reported that CQ is able to reduce Aβ burden and restore cognitive performance in AD mouse models[163–166] and in AD patients. Analogous to CQ, its successor PBT2 showed promising features for the treatment of AD.[167]

Interestingly, CQ is also able to rescue social interaction deficits in two distinct mouse models of ASD namely, homozygous Shank2 knock-out as well as heterozygous Tbr1 knock-out mice.[168] Due to its ionophoric properties, CQ is able to mobilize zinc from presynaptic pools towards the postsynaptic compartment of the zincergic synapse, thereby increasing postsynaptic intracellular zinc concentrations. This increase of zinc was shown to activate Src kinase, thereby restoring NMDA receptor function; as described above a common characteristic observed among ASD mouse models.[21] Furthermore, increased levels of postsynaptic zinc might target additional Shank3 proteins to the PSD promoting postsynaptic stabilization[7] (Fig. 9.3).

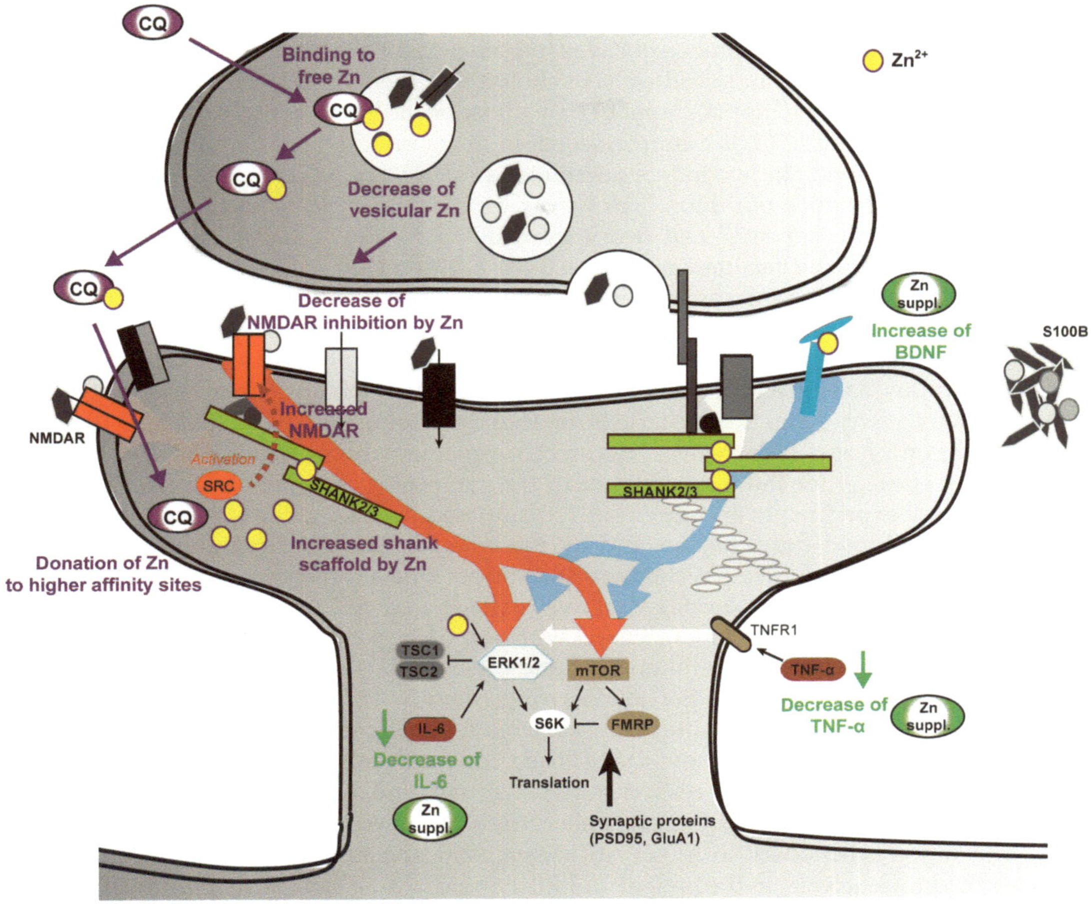

FIGURE 9.3 **Therapeutic strategies in ASD based on biometals.** Clioquinol (CQ) and zinc supplementation targeting, among others, BDNF levels have been originally proposed for the treatment of AD but may also be beneficial in ASD. CQ that was able to rescue social behavior in ASD mouse models is thought to restore abnormal NMDAR signaling due to mobilization of presynaptic free zinc and donation of zinc to postsynaptic proteins with higher affinity. The postsynaptic increase of zinc was shown to activate Src kinase and reduce inhibition of NMDAR by presynaptic released zinc, thereby restoring NMDAR receptor function. Increased levels of postsynaptic zinc may also target additional Shank3 proteins to the PSD. Zinc supplementation may lead to increased levels of BDNF as shown in an AD mouse model, thereby modulating TrkB—BDNF signaling, but also—if delivered into the brain—alter synaptic signaling, that is, via Shank. Further, it may decrease neuroinflammation and replenish zinc sequestered in aggregated proteins, ultimately restoring impaired functions in the ERK1/2 and mTOR pathway. Abbreviations: *CQ*, Clioquinol; *BDNF*, Brain-derived neurotrophic factor; *ERK1/2*, Extracellular signal-regulated protein kinases 1 and 2; *FMRP*, fragile X mental retardation protein; *mTOR*, mechanistic Target of Rapamycin; *S6K*, S6 kinase; *SRC*, protooncogene tyrosine-protein kinase; *TNF*, tumor necrosis factor; *TNFR1*, Tumor necrosis factor receptor 1; *TrkB*, Tropomyosin receptor kinase B; *TSC*, Tuberous sclerosis complex; *Zn*, zinc.

Since synaptic released zinc targets the TrkB-BDNF pathway, restoring synaptic dysfunction directly via this neurotrophic factor was hypothesized to be beneficial for the treatment of both ASD and AD. Previous studies have shown that the application of the neurotrophic factor BDNF could restore hippocampal LTP dysfunction, a shared pathology in ASD and AD in several mouse models.[169] For example, recent findings indicate that BDNF was able to rescue synaptic dysfunction in two independent mouse models of ASD namely Fmr1 knock-out mice[170] and MeCP2 knock-out mice.[171] However, exogenous applied BDNF does not readily cross the blood–brain barrier[172] and overload of BDNF has been demonstrated to increase neuronal excitability and facilitate seizure activity.[173] Interestingly, dietary zinc supplementation has been shown to increase the levels of BDNF in 3 times Tg-AD mice, a transgenic mouse model of AD. 3 times Tg-AD mice display Aβ and tau-dependent pathology and it has been demonstrated that dietary zinc supplementation reduces both Aβ and tau pathology in the hippocampus, as well as delays hippocampal-dependent memory deficits.[125]

In summary, many synaptic zinc targets are found dysregulated in AD and ASD (Fig. 9.3). Thus, alteration of zinc homeostasis by direct supplementation of zinc was also tested in the past as a strategy for the improvement of the symptoms associated with AD and ASD. However, these experiments are significantly hampered by the inability of zinc ions to passively cross the blood–brain barrier and by the many factors modifying zinc absorption. Nevertheless, several studies have shown that direct zinc supplementation had beneficial effects in the treatment of neurodegenerative diseases and ASD. For example, some studies show considerable improvement in AD with zinc therapy, both in humans and mice.[174] However, meta-analyses are mostly missing and other studies could not find such improvements. In ASD, zinc supplementation studies might have to address pregnant mothers rather than the ASD patient and surprisingly few controlled supplementation studies were done in ASD patients. The few results show that autistic children with gastro-intestinal comorbidities significantly improved with respect to hyperactivity and self-stimulatory behavior after zinc therapy.[175] Unfortunately, large controlled trials are missing. Thus, whether direct zinc supplementation is beneficial in AD or ASD remains inconclusive and might depend on the presence of zinc deficiency in the patient and further individual factors. In addition, more targeted approaches to deliver zinc across the blood–brain barrier into the brain are desired.[176]

CONCLUSIONS

Zinc biology has major influence on brain function. It is thus not surprising that altered trace metal levels on the one hand are contributing to the pathological processes of several disorders of the CNS, but on the other hand can be used as novel strategy for the treatment of brain diseases. However, despite a clear association of zinc deficiency with several neurodegenerative and neuropsychiatric disorders, the underlying molecular mechanisms are currently not well understood. The reason for this lack of understanding is mostly based on the plethora of biological processes zinc contributes to under physiological circumstances. Their dysregulation can hardly be modeled by current experimental approaches. However, some reoccurring motifs are emerging in recent years. For example, aberrant NMDAR modulation, loss of Shank2 and Shank3 proteins at the synapse and increased inflammation, all leading to altered ability of the synapse to translate synaptic activity in structural changes seem to be the cornerstone of the patho-mechanisms induced by zinc deficiency in the brain.

Today, zinc is accepted as an essential trace metal with a unique role in the CNS and the knowledge of the role of zinc has been considerably improved by more efficient detection of zinc in the brain, studies on the function of zinc as neuromodulator at the synapse, and studies on the impact of zinc on gene expression, protein levels and metabolism. In addition, important progress in the understanding of specific aspects of the neurobiology of certain neuropsychiatric and neurodegenerative disorders but also in the understanding of shared common factors between disorders has been made. Given that altered metal homeostasis is such a shared factor, targeting zinc homeostasis for the development of novel treatments is a rapidly emerging field of neuroscience research. Despite these efforts, still many fundamental issues concerning zinc biology in ASD remain unresolved.

Nevertheless, a significant progress in translational research with the aim of altering local trace metal concentrations has been made in neurodegenerative disorders. MPACs, such as CQ and PBT2 and its successors may not only be useful in the treatment of AD but also ASD. First results using CQ in ASD mouse models provide a strong experimental basis for this model. Hopefully, based on this approach, further novel treatment strategies will be developed for ASD.

References

1. Grabrucker AM. Zinc in the developing brain. In: Moran VH, Lowe N, eds. *Nutrition and the developing brain*. CRC Press; 2016:143–168.
2. Peters S, Koh J, Choi DW. Zinc selectively blocks the action of *N*-methyl-D-aspartate on cortical neurons. *Science*. 1987;236(4801):589–593.
3. Westbrook GL, Mayer ML. Micromolar concentrations of Zn^{2+} antagonize NMDA and GABA responses of hippocampal neurons. *Nature*. 1987;328(6131):640–643.
4. Besser L, Chorin E, Sekler I, Silverman WF, Atkin S, Russell JT, Hershfinkel M. Synaptically released zinc triggers metabotropic signaling via a zinc-sensing receptor in the hippocampus. *J Neurosci*. 2009;29(9):2890–2901.
5. Sensi SL, Canzoniero LM, Yu SP, Ying HS, Koh JY, Kerchner GA, Choi DW. Measurement of intracellular free zinc in living cortical neurons: routes of entry. *J Neurosci*. 1997;17(24):9554–9564.
6. Nuttall JR, Oteiza PI. Zinc and the ERK kinases in the developing brain. *Neurotox Res*. 2012;21(1):128–141.
7. Grabrucker AM. A role for synaptic zinc in ProSAP/Shank PSD scaffold malformation in autism spectrum disorders. *Dev Neurobiol*. 2014;74(2):136–146.
8. Pfaender S, Grabrucker AM. Characterization of biometal profiles in neurological disorders. *Metallomics*. 2014;6(5):960–977.
9. Sayehmiri F, Babaknejad N, Bahrami S, Sayehmiri K, Darabi M, Rezaei-Tavirani M. Zn/Cu levels in the field of autism disorders: a systematic review and meta-analysis. *Iran J Child Neurol*. 2015;9(4):1–9.
10. Yasuda H, Tsutsui T. Assessment of infantile mineral imbalances in autism spectrum disorders (ASDs). *Int J Environ Res Public Health*. 2013;10(11):6027–6043.
11. Bjorklund G. The role of zinc and copper in autism spectrum disorders. *Acta Neurobiol Exp (Wars)*. 2013;73(2):225–236.
12. Grabrucker AM. Environmental factors in autism. *Front Psychiatry*. 2012;3:118.
13. Anney R, Klei L, Pinto D, Almeida J, Bacchelli E, Baird G, Bolshakova N, Bölte S, Bolton PF, Bourgeron T, Brennan S, Brian J, Casey J, Conroy J, Correia C, Corsello C, Crawford EL, de Jonge M, Delorme R, Duketis E, Duque F, Estes A, Farrar P, Fernandez BA, Folstein SE, Fombonne E, Gilbert J, Gillberg C, Glessner JT, Green A, Green J, Guter SJ, Heron EA, Holt R, Howe JL, Hughes G, Hus V, Igliozzi R, Jacob S, Kenny GP, Kim C, Kolevzon A, Kustanovich V, Lajonchere CM, Lamb JA, Law-Smith M, Leboyer M, Le Couteur A, Leventhal BL, Liu XQ, Lombard F, Lord C, Lotspeich L, Lund SC, Magalhaes TR, Mantoulan C, McDougle CJ, Melhem NM, Merikangas A, Minshew NJ, Mirza GK, Munson J, Noakes C, Nygren G, Papanikolaou K, Pagnamenta AT, Parrini B, Paton T, Pickles A, Posey DJ, Poustka F, Ragoussis J, Regan R, Roberts W, Roeder K, Roge B, Rutter ML, Schlitt S, Shah N, Sheffield VC, Soorya L, Sousa I, Stoppioni V, Sykes N, Tancredi R, Thompson AP, Thomson S, Tryfon A, Tsiantis J, Van Engeland H, Vincent JB, Volkmar F, Vorstman JA, Wallace S, Wing K, Wittemeyer K, Wood S, Zurawiecki D, Zwaigenbaum L, Bailey AJ, Battaglia A, Cantor RM, Coon H, Cuccaro ML, Dawson G, Ennis S, Freitag CM, Geschwind DH, Haines JL, Klauck SM, McMahon WM, Maestrini E, Miller J, Monaco AP, Nelson

SF, Nurnberger JI, Oliveira G, Parr JR, Pericak-Vance MA, Piven J, Schellenberg GD, Scherer SW, Vicente AM, Wassink TH, Wijsman EM, Betancur C, Buxbaum JD, Cook EH, Gallagher L, Gill M, Hallmayer J, Paterson AD, Sutcliffe JS, Szatmari P, Vieland VJ, Hakonarson H, Devlin B. Individual common variants exert weak effects on the risk for autism spectrum disorderspi. *Hum Mol Genet*. 2012;21(21):4781–4792.
14. O'Roak BJ, Vives L, Fu W, Egertson JD, Stanaway IB, Phelps IG, Carvill G, Kumar A, Lee C, Ankenman K, Munson J, Hiatt JB, Turner EH, Levy R, O'Day DR, Krumm N, Coe BP, Martin BK, Borenstein E, Nickerson DA, Mefford HC, Doherty D, Akey JM, Bernier R, Eichler EE, Shendure J. Multiplex targeted sequencing identifies recurrently mutated genes in autism spectrum disorders. *Science*. 2012;338(6114):1619–1622.
15. Sanders SJ, Murtha MT, Gupta AR, Murdoch JD, Raubeson MJ, Willsey AJ, Ercan-Sencicek AG, DiLullo NM, Parikshak NN, Stein JL, Walker MF, Ober GT, Teran NA, Song Y, El-Fishawy P, Murtha RC, Choi M, Overton JD, Bjornson RD, Carriero NJ, Meyer KA, Bilguvar K, Mane SM, Sestan N, Lifton RP, Günel M, Roeder K, Geschwind DH, Devlin B, State MW. De novo mutations revealed by whole-exome sequencing are strongly associated with autism. *Nature*. 2012;485(7397):237–241.
16. Serajee FJ, Nabi R, Zhong H, Huq M. Polymorphisms in xenobiotic metabolism genes and autism. *J Child Neurol*. 2004;19(6):413–417.
17. Levy D, Ronemus M, Yamrom B, Lee YH, Leotta A, Kendall J, Marks S, Lakshmi B, Pai D, Ye K, Buja A, Krieger A, Yoon S, Troge J, Rodgers L, Iossifov I, Wigler M. Rare de novo and transmitted copy-number variation in autistic spectrum disorders. *Neuron*. 2011;70(5):886–897.
18. Grabrucker AM, Schmeisser MJ, Schoen M, Boeckers TM. Postsynaptic ProSAP/Shank scaffolds in the cross-hair of synaptopathies. *Trends Cell Biol*. 2011;21(10):594–603.
19. Koh JY, Lim JS, Byun HR, Yoo MH. Abnormalities in the zinc-metalloprotease-BDNF axis may contribute to megalencephaly and cortical hyperconnectivity in young autism spectrum disorder patients. *Mol Brain*. 2014;7:64.
20. Faridar A, Jones-Davis D, Rider E, Li J, Gobius I, Morcom L, Richards LJ, Sen S, Sherr EH. Mapk/Erk activation in an animal model of social deficits shows a possible link to autism. *Mol Autism*. 2014;5:57.
21. Lee EJ, Choi SY, Kim E. NMDA receptor dysfunction in autism spectrum disorders. *Curr Opin Pharmacol*. 2015;20:8–13.
22. Shankar AH, Prasad AS. Zinc and immune function: the biological basis of altered resistance to infection. *Am J Clin Nutr*. 1998;68(2 Suppl):447–463.
23. Hagmeyer S, Haderspeck JC, Grabrucker AM. Behavioral impairments in animal models for zinc deficiency. *Front Behav Neurosci*. 2014;8:443.
24. Grabrucker S, Jannetti L, Eckert M, Gaub S, Chhabra R, Pfaender S, Mangus K, Reddy PP, Rankovic V, Schmeisser MJ, Kreutz MR, Ehret G, Boeckers TM, Grabrucker AM. Zinc deficiency dysregulates the synaptic ProSAP/Shank scaffold and might contribute to autism spectrum disorders. *Brain*. 2014;137(Pt 1):137–152.
25. Grabrucker S, Boeckers TM, Grabrucker AM. Gender dependent evaluation of autism like behavior in mice exposed to prenatal zinc deficiency. *Front Behav Neurosci*. 2016;10:37.
26. Yoo M, Kim TY, Koh JY. Autism phenotype and megalencephaly in zinc transporter 3 (ZnT3) null mice: possible involvement of MMP activation and BDNF upregulation. Program No. 221.13. 2015 Neuroscience Meeting Planner. Chicago, IL: Society for Neuroscience, 2015. Online.
27. Adlard PA, Parncutt JM, Finkelstein DI, Bush AI. Cognitive loss in zinc transporter-3 knock-out mice: a phenocopy for the synaptic and memory deficits of Alzheimer's disease?. *J Neurosci*. 2010;30(5):1631–1636.
28. Yasuda H, Kobayashi M, Yasuda Y, Tsutsui T. Estimation of autistic children by metallomics analysis. *Sci Rep*. 2013;3:1199.
29. Yasuda H, Tsutsui T. Infants and elderlies are susceptible to zinc deficiency. *Sci Rep*. 2016;6:21850.
30. Lakshmi Priya MD, Geetha A. Level of trace elements (copper, zinc, magnesium and selenium) and toxic elements (lead and mercury) in the hair and nail of children with autism. *Biol Trace Elem Res*. 2011;142(2):148–158.
31. Russo AJ, Devito R. Analysis of copper and zinc plasma concentration and the efficacy of zinc therapy in individuals with Asperger's syndrome, pervasive developmental disorder not otherwise specified (PDD-NOS) and autism. *Biomark Insights*. 2011;6:127–133.
32. Russo AJ, Bazin AP, Bigega R, Carlson RS, Cole MG, Contreras DC, Galvin MB, Gaydorus SS, Holik SD, Jenkins GP, Jones BM, Languell PA, Lyman PJ, March KP, Meuer KA, Peterson SR, Piedmonte MT, Quinn MG, Smaranda NC, Steves PL, Taylor HP, Waddingham TE, Warren JS. Plasma copper and zinc concentration in individuals with autism correlate with selected symptom severity. *Nutr Metab Insights*. 2012;5:41–47.
33. Li SO, Wang JL, Bjørklund G, Zhao WN, Yin CH. Serum copper and zinc levels in individuals with autism spectrum disorders. *Neuroreport*. 2014;25(15):1216–1220.

34. Al-Farsi YM, Waly MI, Al-Sharbati MM, Al-Shafaee MA, Al-Farsi OA, Al-Khaduri MM, Gupta I, Ouhtit A, Al-Adawi S, Al-Said MF, Deth RC. Levels of heavy metals and essential minerals in hair samples of children with autism in Oman: a case-control study. *Biol Trace Elem Res*. 2013;151(2):181–186.
35. Blaurock-Busch E, Amin OR, Rabah T. Heavy metals and trace elements in hair and urine of a sample of arab children with autistic spectrum disorder. *Maedica*. 2011;6(4):247–257.
36. Faber S, Zinn GM, Kern JC, Kingston HM. The plasma zinc/serum copper ratio as a biomarker in children with autism spectrum disorders. *Biomarkers*. 2009;14(3):171–180.
37. Tabatadze T, Zhorzholiani L, Kherkheulidze M, Kandelaki E, Ivanashvili T. Hair heavy metal and essential trace element concentration in children with autism spectrum disorder. *Georgian Med News*. 2015;(248):77–82.
38. Shimada A, Hasegawa-Ishii S. Senescence-accelerated mice (SAMs) as a model for brain aging and immunosenescence. *Aging Dis*. 2011;2(5):414–435.
39. Meunier N, O'Connor JM, Maiani G, Cashman KD, Secker DL, Ferry M, Roussel AM, Coudray C. Importance of zinc in the elderly: the ZENITH study. *Eur J Clin Nutr*. 2005;59(2):1–4.
40. Ortega RM, Requejo AM, Andrés P, López-Sobaler AM, Quintas ME, Redondo MR, Navia B, Rivas T. Dietary intake and cognitive function in a group of elderly people. *Am J Clin Nutr*. 1997;66(4):803–809.
41. Nuttall JR. The plausibility of maternal toxicant exposure and nutritional status as contributing factors to the risk of autism spectrum disorders. *Nutr Neurosci*. 2015:1–10.
42. Kirsten TB, Chaves-Kirsten GP, Bernardes S, Scavone C, Sarkis JE, Bernardi MM, Felicio LF. Lipopolysaccharide Exposure Induces Maternal Hypozincemia, and Prenatal Zinc Treatment Prevents Autistic-Like Behaviors and Disturbances in the Striatal Dopaminergic and mTOR Systems of Offspring. *PLoS One*. 2015;10(7):e0134565.
43. Kirsten TB, Queiroz-Hazarbassanov N, Bernardi MM, Felicio LF. Prenatal zinc prevents communication impairments and BDNF disturbance in a rat model of autism induced by prenatal lipopolysaccharide exposure. *Life Sci*. 2015;130:12–17.
44. Vargas DL, Nascimbene C, Krishnan C, Zimmerman AW, Pardo CA. Neuroglial activation and neuroinflammation in the brain of patients with autism. *Ann Neurol*. 2005;57(1):67–81.
45. Tetreault NA, Hakeem AY, Jiang S, Williams BA, Allman E, Wold BJ, Allman JM. Microglia in the cerebral cortex in autism. *J Autism Dev Disord*. 2012;42(12):2569–2584.
46. Takano T. Role of microglia in autism: recent advances. *Dev Neurosci*. 2015;37(3):195–202.
47. Edmonson C, Ziats MN, Rennert OM. Altered glial marker expression in autistic post-mortem prefrontal cortex and cerebellum. *Mol Autism*. 2014;5(1):3.
48. Pardo CA, Vargas DL, Zimmerman AW. Immunity, neuroglia and neuroinflammation in autism. *Int Rev Psychiatry*. 2005;17(6):485–495.
49. Laurence JA, Fatemi SH. Glial fibrillary acidic protein is elevated in superior frontal, parietal and cerebellar cortices of autistic subjects. *Cerebellum*. 2005;4(3):206–210.
50. Ahlsén G, Rosengren L, Belfrage M, Palm A, Haglid K, Hamberger A, Gillberg C. Glial fibrillary acidic protein in the cerebrospinal fluid of children with autism and other neuropsychiatric disorders. *Biol Psychiatry*. 1993;33(10):734–743.
51. Fatemi SH, Folsom TD, Reutiman TJ, Lee S. Expression of astrocytic markers aquaporin 4 and connexin 43 is altered in brains of subjects with autism. *Synapse*. 2008;62(7):501–507.
52. Zimmerman AW, Jyonouchi H, Comi AM, Connors SL, Milstien S, Varsou A, Heyes MP. Cerebrospinal fluid and serum markers of inflammation in autism. *Pediatr Neurol*. 2005;33(3):195–201.
53. Chez MG, Dowling T, Patel PB, Khanna P, Kominsky M. Elevation of tumor necrosis factor-alpha in cerebrospinal fluid of autistic children. *Pediatr Neurol*. 2007;36(6):361–365.
54. Croonenberghs J, Bosmans E, Deboutte D, Kenis G, Maes M. Activation of the inflammatory response system in autism. *Neuropsychobiology*. 2002;45(1):1–6.
55. Molloy CA, Morrow AL, Meinzen-Derr J, Schleifer K, Dienger K, Manning-Courtney P, Altaye M, Wills-Karp M. Elevated cytokine levels in children with autism spectrum disorder. *J Neuroimmunol*. 2006;172(1-2):198–205.
56. Young AM, Campbell E, Lynch S, Suckling J, Powis SJ. Aberrant NF-kappaB expression in autism spectrum condition: a mechanism for neuroinflammation. *Front Psychiatry*. 2011;2:27.
57. Naik US, Gangadharan C, Abbagani K, Nagalla B, Dasari N, Manna SK. A study of nuclear transcription factor-kappa B in childhood autism. *PLoS One*. 2011;6(5):e19488.
58. Malkova NV, Yu CZ, Hsiao EY, Moore MJ, Patterson PH. Maternal immune activation yields offspring displaying mouse versions of the three core symptoms of autism. *Brain Behav Immun*. 2012;26(4):607–616.

59. Knuesel I, Chicha L, Britschgi M, Schobel SA, Bodmer M, Hellings JA, Toovey S, Prinssen EP. Maternal immune activation and abnormal brain development across CNS disorders. *Nat Rev Neurol*. 2014;10(11):643–660.
60. Shi L, Fatemi SH, Sidwell RW, Patterson PH. Maternal influenza infection causes marked behavioral and pharmacological changes in the offspring. *J Neurosci*. 2003;23(1):297–302.
61. Boksa P. Effects of prenatal infection on brain development and behavior: a review of findings from animal models. *Brain Behav Immun*. 2010;24(6):881–897.
62. Patterson PH. Maternal infection and autism. *Brain Behav Immun*. 2012;26(3):393.
63. Bourgeron T. A synaptic trek to autism. *Curr Opin Neurobiol*. 2009;19(2):231–234.
64. Coogan A, O'Connor JJ. Inhibition of NMDA receptor-mediated synaptic transmission in the rat dentate gyrus in vitro by IL-1 beta. *Neuroreport*. 1997;8(9–10):2107–2110.
65. Lai AY, Swayze RD, El-Husseini A, Song C. Interleukin-1 beta modulates AMPA receptor expression and phosphorylation in hippocampal neurons. *J Neuroimmunol*. 2006;175(1-2):97–106.
66. Murray CA, McGahon B, McBennett S, Lynch MA. Interleukin-1 beta inhibits glutamate release in hippocampus of young, but not aged, rats. *Neurobiol Aging*. 1997;18(3):343–348.
67. Curran B, O'Connor JJ. The pro-inflammatory cytokine interleukin-18 impairs long-term potentiation and NMDA receptor-mediated transmission in the rat hippocampus in vitro. *Neuroscience*. 2001;108(1):83–90.
68. Donato R, Cannon BR, Sorci G, Riuzzi F, Hsu K, Weber DJ, Geczy CL. Functions of S100 proteins. *Curr Mol Med*. 2013;13(1):24–57.
69. Leclerc E, Sturchler E, Vetter SW. The S100B/RAGE Axis in Alzheimer's Disease. *Cardiovasc Psychiatry Neurol*. 2010;2010:539581.
70. Carvalho SB, Botelho HM, Leal SS, Cardoso I, Fritz G, Gomes CM. Intrinsically disordered and aggregation prone regions underlie β-aggregation in S100 proteins. *PLoS One*. 2013;8(10):e76629.
71. Botelho HM, Leal SS, Cardoso I, Yanamandra K, Morozova-Roche LA, Fritz G, Gomes CM. S100A6 amyloid fibril formation is calcium-modulated and enhances superoxide dismutase-1 (SOD1) aggregation. *J Biol Chem*. 2012;287(50):42233–42242.
72. Mori T, Koyama N, Arendash GW, Horikoshi-Sakuraba Y, Tan J, Town T. Overexpression of human S100B exacerbates cerebral amyloidosis and gliosis in the Tg2576 mouse model of Alzheimer's disease. *Glia*. 2010;58(3):300–314.
73. Egger G, Roetzer KM, Noor A, Lionel AC, Mahmood H, Schwarzbraun T, Boright O, Mikhailov A, Marshall CR, Windpassinger C, Petek E, Scherer SW, Kaschnitz W, Vincent JB. Identification of risk genes for autism spectrum disorder through copy number variation analysis in Austrian families. *Neurogenetics*. 2014;15(2):117–127.
74. Al-Ayadhi LY, Mostafa GA. A lack of association between elevated serum levels of S100B protein and autoimmunity in autistic children. *J Neuroinflammation*. 2012;9:54.
75. Wei H, Zou H, Sheikh AM, Malik M, Dobkin C, Brown WT, Li X. IL-6 is increased in the cerebellum of autistic brain and alters neural cell adhesion, migration and synaptic formation. *J Neuroinflammation*. 2011;8:52.
76. Masi A, Quintana DS, Glozier N, Lloyd AR, Hickie IB, Guastella AJ. Cytokine aberrations in autism spectrum disorder: a systematic review and meta-analysis. *Mol Psychiatry*. 2015;20(4):440–446.
77. Smith SE, Li J, Garbett K, Mirnics K, Patterson PH. Maternal immune activation alters fetal brain development through interleukin-6. *J Neurosci*. 2007;27(40):10695–10702.
78. Wong CP, Rinaldi NA, Ho E. Zinc deficiency enhanced inflammatory response by increasing immune cell activation and inducing IL6 promoter demethylation. *Mol Nutr Food Res*. 2015;59(5):991–999.
79. Kahmann L, Uciechowski P, Warmuth S, Plümäkers B, Gressner AM, Malavolta M, Mocchegiani E, Rink L. Zinc supplementation in the elderly reduces spontaneous inflammatory cytokine release and restores T cell functions. *Rejuvenation Res*. 2008;11(1):227–237.
80. Liu MJ, Bao S, Gálvez-Peralta M, Pyle CJ, Rudawsky AC, Pavlovicz RE, Killilea DW, Li C, Nebert DW, Wewers MD, Knoell DL. ZIP8 regulates host defense through zinc-mediated inhibition of NF-κB. *Cell Rep*. 2013;3(2):386–400.
81. Libermann TA, Baltimore D. Activation of interleukin-6 gene expression through the NF-kappa B transcription factor. *Mol Cell Biol*. 1990;10(5):2327–2334.
82. Lichten LA, Cousins RJ. Mammalian zinc transporters: nutritional and physiologic regulation. *Annu Rev Nutr*. 2009;29:153–176.
83. Kitamura Y, Shimohama S, Ota T, Matsuoka Y, Nomura Y, Taniguchi T. Alteration of transcription factors NF-kappaB and STAT1 in Alzheimer's disease brains. *Neurosci Lett*. 1997;237(1):17–20.
84. Tilstra JS, Clauson CL, Niedernhofer LJ, Robbins PD. NF-κB in Aging and Disease. *Aging Dis*. 2011;2(6):449–465.

85. Mayer ML, Vyklicky L, Westbrook GL. Modulation of excitatory amino acid receptors by group IIB metal cations in cultured mouse hippocampal neurones. *J Physiol*. 1989;415:329–350.
86. Christine CW, Choi DW. Effect of zinc on NMDA receptor-mediated channel currents in cortical neurons. *J Neurosci*. 1990;10(1):108–116.
87. Manzerra P, Behrens MM, Canzoniero LM, Wang XQ, Heidinger V, Ichinose T, Yu SP, Choi DW. Zinc induces a Src family kinase-mediated up-regulation of NMDA receptor activity and excitotoxicity. *Proc Natl Acad Sci USA*. 2001;98(20):11055.
88. Barnby G, Abbott A, Sykes N, Morris A, Weeks DE, Mott R, Lamb J, Bailey AJ, Monaco AP. Candidate-gene screening and association analysis at the autism-susceptibility locus on chromosome 16p: evidence of association at GRIN2A and ABAT. *Am J Hum Genet*. 2005;76(6):950–966.
89. O'Roak BJ, Vives L, Girirajan S, Karakoc E, Krumm N, Coe BP, Levy R, Ko A, Lee C, Smith JD, Turner EH, Stanaway IB, Vernot B, Malig M, Baker C, Reilly B, Akey JM, Borenstein E, Rieder MJ, Nickerson DA, Bernier R, Shendure J, Eichler EE. Sporadic autism exomes reveal a highly interconnected protein network of de novo mutations. *Nature*. 2012;485(7397):246–250.
90. Rinaldi T, Kulangara K, Antoniello K, Markram H. Elevated NMDA receptor levels and enhanced post-synaptic long-term potentiation induced by prenatal exposure to valproic acid. *Proc Natl Acad Sci USA*. 2007;104(33):13501–13506.
91. Blundell J, Blaiss CA, Etherton MR, Espinosa F, Tabuchi K, Walz C, Bolliger MF, Südhof TC, Powell CM. Neuroligin-1 deletion results in impaired spatial memory and increased repetitive behavior. *J Neurosci*. 2010;30(6):2115–2129.
92. Eadie BD, Cushman J, Kannangara TS, Fanselow MS, Christie BR. NMDA receptor hypofunction in the dentate gyrus and impaired context discrimination in adult Fmr1 knockout mice. *Hippocampus*. 2012;22(2):241–254.
93. Won H, Lee HR, Gee HY, Mah W, Kim JI, Lee J, Ha S, Chung C, Jung ES, Cho YS, Park SG, Lee JS, Lee K, Kim D, Bae YC, Kaang BK, Lee MG, Kim E. Autistic-like social behaviour in Shank2-mutant mice improved by restoring NMDA receptor function. *Nature*. 2012;486(7402):261–265.
94. Maliszewska-Cyna E, Bawa D, Eubanks JH. Diminished prevalence but preserved synaptic distribution of N-methyl-D-aspartate receptor subunits in the methyl CpG binding protein 2(MeCP2)-null mouse brain. *Neuroscience*. 2010;168(3):624–632.
95. Chen QS, Wei WZ, Shimahara T, Xie CW. Alzheimer amyloid beta-peptide inhibits the late phase of long-term potentiation through calcineurin-dependent mechanisms in the hippocampal dentate gyrus. *Neurobiol Learn Mem*. 2002;77(3):354–371.
96. Wang Q, Rowan MJ, Anwyl R. Beta-amyloid-mediated inhibition of NMDA receptor-dependent long-term potentiation induction involves activation of microglia and stimulation of inducible nitric oxide synthase and superoxide. *J Neurosci*. 2004;24(27):6049–6056.
97. Snyder EM, Nong Y, Almeida CG, Paul S, Moran T, Choi EY, Nairn AC, Salter MW, Lombroso PJ, Gouras GK, Greengard P. Regulation of NMDA receptor trafficking by amyloid-beta. *Nat Neurosci*. 2005;8(8):1051–1058.
98. Dewachter I, Filipkowski RK, Priller C, Ris L, Neyton J, Croes S, Terwel D, Gysemans M, Devijver H, Borghgraef P, Godaux E, Kaczmarek L, Herms J, Van Leuven F. Deregulation of NMDA-receptor function and down-stream signaling in APP[V717I] transgenic mice. *Neurobiol Aging*. 2009;30(2):241–256.
99. Molnár Z, Soós K, Lengyel I, Penke B, Szegedi V, Budai D. Enhancement of NMDA responses by beta-amyloid peptides in the hippocampus in vivo. *Neuroreport*. 2004;15(10):1649–1652.
100. Wu J, Anwyl R, Rowan MJ. beta-Amyloid selectively augments NMDA receptor-mediated synaptic transmission in rat hippocampus. *Neuroreport*. 1995;6(17):2409–2413.
101. Bush AI, Pettingell WH, Multhaup G, d Paradis M, Vonsattel JP, Gusella JF, Beyreuther K, Masters CL, Tanzi RE. Rapid induction of Alzheimer A beta amyloid formation by zinc. *Science*. 1994;265(5177):1464–1467.
102. Sensi SL, Paoletti P, Koh JY, Aizenman E, Bush AI, Hershfinkel M. The neurophysiology and pathology of brain zinc. *J Neurosci*. 2011;31(45):16076–16085.
103. Beyer N, Coulson DT, Heggarty S, Ravid R, Irvine GB, Hellemans J, Johnston JA. ZnT3 mRNA levels are reduced in Alzheimer's disease post-mortem brain. *Mol Neurodegener*. 2009;4:53.
104. Kalappa BI, Anderson CT, Goldberg JM, Lippard SJ, Tzounopoulos T. AMPA receptor inhibition by synaptically released zinc. *Proc Natl Acad Sci USA*. 2015;112(51):15749–15754.
105. Peça J, Feliciano C, Ting JT, Wang W, Wells MF, Venkatraman TN, Lascola CD, Fu Z, Feng G. Shank3 mutant mice display autistic-like behaviours and striatal dysfunction. *Nature*. 2011;472(7344):437–442.
106. Lee J, Chung C, Ha S, Lee D, Kim DY, Kim H, Kim E. Shank3-mutant mice lacking exon 9 show altered excitation/inhibition balance, enhanced rearing, and spatial memory deficit. *Front Cell Neurosci*. 2015;9:94.

107. Speed HE, Kouser M, Xuan Z, Reimers JM, Ochoa CF, Gupta N, Liu S, Powell CM. Autism-Associated Insertion Mutation (InsG) of Shank3 Exon 21 Causes Impaired Synaptic Transmission and Behavioral Deficits. *J Neurosci.* 2015;35(26):9648–9665.
108. Kouser M, Speed HE, Dewey CM, Reimers JM, Widman AJ, Gupta N, Liu S, Jaramillo TC, Bangash M, Xiao B, Worley PF, Powell CM. Loss of predominant Shank3 isoforms results in hippocampus-dependent impairments in behavior and synaptic transmission. *J Neurosci.* 2013;33(47):18448–18468.
109. Nelson ED, Kavalali ET, Monteggia LM. MeCP2-dependent transcriptional repression regulates excitatory neurotransmission. *Curr Biol.* 2006;16(7):710–716.
110. Dani VS, Chang Q, Maffei A, Turrigiano GG, Jaenisch R, Nelson SB. Reduced cortical activity due to a shift in the balance between excitation and inhibition in a mouse model of Rett syndrome. *Proc Natl Acad Sci USA.* 2005;102(35):12560–12565.
111. Parameshwaran K, Dhanasekaran M, Suppiramaniam V. Amyloid beta peptides and glutamatergic synaptic dysregulation. *Exp Neurol.* 2008;210(1):7–13.
112. Yasuda RP, Ikonomovic MD, Sheffield R, Rubin RT, Wolfe BB, Armstrong DM. Reduction of AMPA-selective glutamate receptor subunits in the entorhinal cortex of patients with Alzheimer's disease pathology: a biochemical study. *Brain Res.* 1995;678(1-2):161–167.
113. Yasuda S, Miyazaki T, Munechika K, Yamashita M, Ikeda Y, Kamizono A. Isolation of Zn2+ as an endogenous agonist of GPR39 from fetal bovine serum. *J Recept Signal Transduct Res.* 2007;27(4):235–246.
114. Holst B, Holliday ND, Bach A, Elling CE, Cox HM, Schwartz TW. Common structural basis for constitutive activity of the ghrelin receptor family. *J Biol Chem.* 2004;279(51):53806–53817.
115. Silva AJ, Kogan JH, Frankland PW, Kida S. CREB and memory. *Annu Rev Neurosci.* 1998;21:127–148.
116. Gümüşlü KE, Savli H, Sünnetçi D, Çine N, Kara B, Eren Keskin S, Akkoyunlu RU. A CGH array study in nonsyndromic (primary) autism patients: deletions on 16p13.11, 16p11.2, 1q21.1, 2q21.1q21.2, and 8p23.1. *Turk J Med Sci.* 2015;45(2):313–319.
117. Kumar RA, KaraMohamed S, Sudi J, Conrad DF, Brune C, Badner JA, Gilliam TC, Nowak NJ, Cook EH, Dobyns WB, Christian SL. Recurrent 16p11.2 microdeletions in autism. *Hum Mol Genet.* 2008;17(4):628–638.
118. Moreno-De-Luca D, Mulle JG, Kaminsky EB, Sanders SJ, Myers SM, Adam MP, Pakula AT, Eisenhauer NJ, Uhas K, Weik L, Guy L, Care ME, Morel CF, Boni C, Salbert BA, Chandrareddy A, Demmer LA, Chow EW, Surti U, Aradhya S, Pickering DL, Golden DM, Sanger WG, Aston E, Brothman AR, Gliem TJ, Thorland EC, Ackley T, Iyer R, Huang S, Barber JC, Crolla JA, Warren ST, Martin CL, Ledbetter DH. Deletion 17q12 is a recurrent copy number variant that confers high risk of autism and schizophrenia. *Am J Hum Genet.* 2010;87(5):618–630.
119. Zhu X, Castellani RJ, Takeda A, Nunomura A, Atwood CS, Perry G, Smith MA. Differential activation of neuronal ERK, JNK/SAPK and p38 in Alzheimer disease: the 'two hit' hypothesis. *Mech Ageing Dev.* 2001;123(1):39–46.
120. Perry G, Roder H, Nunomura A, Takeda A, Friedlich AL, Zhu X, Raina AK, Holbrook N, Siedlak SL, Harris PL, Smith MA. Activation of neuronal extracellular receptor kinase (ERK) in Alzheimer disease links oxidative stress to abnormal phosphorylation. *Neuroreport.* 1999;10(11):2411–2415.
121. Ferrer I, Marín C, Rey MJ, Ribalta T. Brain-derived neurotrophic factor in patients with frontotemporal dementia. *Neurosci Lett.* 2000;279(1):33–36.
122. Huang YZ, Pan E, Xiong ZQ, McNamara JO. Zinc-mediated transactivation of TrkB potentiates the hippocampal mossy fiber-CA3 pyramid synapse. *Neuron.* 2008;57(4):546–558.
123. Hwang JJ, Park MH, Choi SY, Koh JY. Activation of the Trk signaling pathway by extracellular zinc. Role of metalloproteinases. *J Biol Chem.* 2005;280(12):11995–12001.
124. Nowak G, Legutko B, Szewczyk B, Papp M, Sanak M, Pilc A. Zinc treatment induces cortical brain-derived neurotrophic factor gene expression. *Eur J Pharmacol.* 2004;492(1):57–59.
125. Corona C, Masciopinto F, Silvestri E, Viscovo AD, Lattanzio R, Sorda RL, Ciavardelli D, Goglia F, Piantelli M, Canzoniero LM, Sensi SL. Dietary zinc supplementation of 3xTg-AD mice increases BDNF levels and prevents cognitive deficits as well as mitochondrial dysfunction. *Cell Death Dis.* 2010;1:e91.
126. Chang Q, Khare G, Dani V, Nelson S, Jaenisch R. The disease progression of Mecp2 mutant mice is affected by the level of BDNF expression. *Neuron.* 2006;49(3):341–348.
127. Sadakata T, Washida M, Iwayama Y, Shoji S, Sato Y, Ohkura T, Katoh-Semba R, Nakajima M, Sekine Y, Tanaka M, Nakamura K, Iwata Y, Tsuchiya KJ, Mori N, Detera-Wadleigh SD, Ichikawa H, Itohara S, Yoshikawa T, Furuichi T. Autistic-like phenotypes in Cadps2-knockout mice and aberrant CADPS2 splicing in autistic patients. *J Clin Invest.* 2007;117(4):931–943.

128. Phillips HS, Hains JM, Armanini M, Laramee GR, Johnson SA, Winslow JW. BDNF mRNA is decreased in the hippocampus of individuals with Alzheimer's disease. *Neuron*. 1991;7(5):695–702.
129. Holsinger RM, Schnarr J, Henry P, Castelo VT, Fahnestock M. Quantitation of BDNF mRNA in human parietal cortex by competitive reverse transcription-polymerase chain reaction: decreased levels in Alzheimer's disease. *Brain Res Mol Brain Res*. 2000;76(2):347–354.
130. Hock C, Heese K, Hulette C, Rosenberg C, Otten U. Region-specific neurotrophin imbalances in Alzheimer disease: decreased levels of brain-derived neurotrophic factor and increased levels of nerve growth factor in hippocampus and cortical areas. *Arch Neurol*. 2000;57(6):846–851.
131. Michalski B, Fahnestock M. Pro-brain-derived neurotrophic factor is decreased in parietal cortex in Alzheimer's disease. *Brain Res Mol Brain Res*. 2003;111(1-2):148–154.
132. Leblond CS, Heinrich J, Delorme R, Proepper C, Betancur C, Huguet G, Konyukh M, Chaste P, Ey E, Rastam M, Anckarsäter H, Nygren G, Gillberg IC, Melke J, Toro R, Regnault B, Fauchereau F, Mercati O, Lemière N, Skuse D, Poot M, Holt R, Monaco AP, Järvelä I, Kantojärvi K, Vanhala R, Curran S, Collier DA, Bolton P, Chiocchetti A, Klauck SM, Poustka F, Freitag CM, Waltes R, Kopp M, Duketis E, Bacchelli E, Minopoli F, Ruta L, Battaglia A, Mazzone L, Maestrini E, Sequeira AF, Oliveira B, Vicente A, Oliveira G, Pinto D, Scherer SW, Zelenika D, Delepine M, Lathrop M, Bonneau D, Guinchat V, Devillard F, Assouline B, Mouren MC, Leboyer M, Gillberg C, Boeckers TM, Bourgeron T. Genetic and functional analyses of SHANK2 mutations suggest a multiple hit model of autism spectrum disorders. *PLoS Genet*. 2012;8(2):e1002521.
133. Leblond CS, Nava C, Polge A, Gauthier J, Huguet G, Lumbroso S, Giuliano F, Stordeur C, Depienne C, Mouzat K, Pinto D, Howe J, Lemière N, Durand CM, Guibert J, Ey E, Toro R, Peyre H, Mathieu A, Amsellem F, Rastam M, Gillberg IC, Rappold GA, Holt R, Monaco AP, Maestrini E, Galan P, Heron D, Jacquette A, Afenjar A, Rastetter A, Brice A, Devillard F, Assouline B, Laffargue F, Lespinasse J, Chiesa J, Rivier F, Bonneau D, Regnault B, Zelenika D, Delepine M, Lathrop M, Sanlaville D, Schluth-Bolard C, Edery P, Perrin L, Tabet AC, Schmeisser MJ, Boeckers TM, Coleman M, Sato D, Szatmari P, Scherer SW, Rouleau GA, Betancur C, Leboyer M, Gillberg C, Delorme R, Bourgeron T. Meta-analysis of SHANK Mutations in Autism Spectrum Disorders: a gradient of severity in cognitive impairments. *PLoS Genet*. 2014;10(9):e1004580.
134. Berkel S, Marshall CR, Weiss B, Howe J, Roeth R, Moog U, Endris V, Roberts W, Szatmari P, Pinto D, Bonin M, Riess A, Engels H, Sprengel R, Scherer SW, Rappold GA. Mutations in the SHANK2 synaptic scaffolding gene in autism spectrum disorder and mental retardation. *Nat Genet*. 2010;42(6):489–491.
135. Durand CM, Betancur C, Boeckers TM, Bockmann J, Chaste P, Fauchereau F, Nygren G, Rastam M, Gillberg IC, Anckarsäter H, Sponheim E, Goubran-Botros H, Delorme R, Chabane N, Mouren-Simeoni MC, de Mas P, Bieth E, Rogé B, Héron D, Burglen L, Gillberg C, Leboyer M, Bourgeron T. Mutations in the gene encoding the synaptic scaffolding protein SHANK3 are associated with autism spectrum disorders. *Nat Genet*. 2007;39(1):25–27.
136. Moessner R, Marshall CR, Sutcliffe JS, Skaug J, Pinto D, Vincent J, Zwaigenbaum L, Fernandez B, Roberts W, Szatmari P, Scherer SW. Contribution of SHANK3 mutations to autism spectrum disorder. *Am J Hum Genet*. 2007;81(6):1289–1297.
137. Pinto D, Pagnamenta AT, Klei L, Anney R, Merico D, Regan R, Conroy J, Magalhaes TR, Correia C, Abrahams BS, Almeida J, Bacchelli E, Bader GD, Bailey AJ, Baird G, Battaglia A, Berney T, Bolshakova N, Bölte S, Bolton PF, Bourgeron T, Brennan S, Brian J, Bryson SE, Carson AR, Casallo G, Casey J, Chung BH, Cochrane L, Corsello C, Crawford EL, Crossett A, Cytrynbaum C, Dawson G, de Jonge M, Delorme R, Drmic I, Duketis E, Duque F, Estes A, Farrar P, Fernandez BA, Folstein SE, Fombonne E, Freitag CM, Gilbert J, Gillberg C, Glessner JT, Goldberg J, Green A, Green J, Guter SJ, Hakonarson H, Heron EA, Hill M, Holt R, Howe JL, Hughes G, Hus V, Igliozzi R, Kim C, Klauck SM, Kolevzon A, Korvatska O, Kustanovich V, Lajonchere CM, Lamb JA, Laskawiec M, Leboyer M, Le Couteur A, Leventhal BL, Lionel AC, Liu XQ, Lord C, Lotspeich L, Lund SC, Maestrini E, Mahoney W, Mantoulan C, Marshall CR, McConachie H, McDougle CJ, McGrath J, McMahon WM, Merikangas A, Migita O, Minshew NJ, Mirza GK, Munson J, Nelson SF, Noakes C, Noor A, Nygren G, Oliveira G, Papanikolaou K, Parr JR, Parrini B, Paton T, Pickles A, Pilorge M, Piven J, Ponting CP, Posey DJ, Poustka A, Poustka F, Prasad A, Ragoussis J, Renshaw K, Rickaby J, Roberts W, Roeder K, Roge B, Rutter ML, Bierut LJ, Rice JP, Salt J, Sansom K, Sato D, Segurado R, Sequeira AF, Senman L, Shah N, Sheffield VC, Soorya L, Sousa I, Stein O, Sykes N, Stoppioni V, Strawbridge C, Tancredi R, Tansey K, Thiruvahindrapduram B, Thompson AP, Thomson S, Tryfon A, Tsiantis J, Van Engeland H, Vincent JB, Volkmar F, Wallace S, Wang K, Wang Z, Wassink TH, Webber C, Weksberg R, Wing K, Wittemeyer K, Wood S, Wu J, Yaspan BL, Zurawiecki D, Zwaigenbaum L, Buxbaum JD, Cantor RM, Cook EH, Coon H, Cuccaro ML, Devlin B, Ennis S, Gallagher L, Geschwind DH, Gill M, Haines JL, Hallmayer J, Miller J, Monaco AP, Nurnberger JI, Paterson AD, Pericak-Vance MA, Schellenberg GD, Szatmari

P, Vicente AM, Vieland VJ, Wijsman EM, Scherer SW, Sutcliffe JS, Betancur C. Functional impact of global rare copy number variation in autism spectrum disorders. *Nature*. 2010;466(7304):368–372.
138. Roselli F, Hutzler P, Wegerich Y, Livrea P, Almeida OF. Disassembly of shank and homer synaptic clusters is driven by soluble beta-amyloid(1-40) through divergent NMDAR-dependent signalling pathways. *PLoS One*. 2009;4(6):e6011.
139. Pham E, Crews L, Ubhi K, Hansen L, Adame A, Cartier A, Salmon D, Galasko D, Michael S, Savas JN, Yates JR, Glabe C, Masliah E. Progressive accumulation of amyloid-beta oligomers in Alzheimer's disease and in amyloid precursor protein transgenic mice is accompanied by selective alterations in synaptic scaffold proteins. *FEBS J*. 2010;277(14):3051–3067.
140. Gong Y, Lippa CF, Zhu J, Lin Q, Rosso AL. Disruption of glutamate receptors at Shank-postsynaptic platform in Alzheimer's disease. *Brain Res*. 2009;1292:191–198.
141. Grabrucker AM, Schmeisser MJ, Udvardi PT, Arons M, Schoen M, Woodling NS, Andreasson KI, Hof PR, Buxbaum JD, Garner CC, Boeckers TM. Amyloid beta protein-induced zinc sequestration leads to synaptic loss via dysregulation of the ProSAP2/Shank3 scaffold. *Mol Neurodegener*. 2011;6:65.
142. Grabrucker AM, Knight MJ, Proepper C, Bockmann J, Joubert M, Rowan M, Nienhaus GU, Garner CC, Bowie JU, Kreutz MR, Gundelfinger ED, Boeckers TM. Concerted action of zinc and ProSAP/Shank in synaptogenesis and synapse maturation. *EMBO J*. 2011;30(3):569–581.
143. Baron MK, Boeckers TM, Vaida B, Faham S, Gingery M, Sawaya MR, Salyer D, Gundelfinger ED, Bowie JU. An architectural framework that may lie at the core of the postsynaptic density. *Science*. 2006;311(5760):531–535.
144. Qiao F, Bowie JU. The many faces of SAM. *Sci STKE*. 2005;2005(286):re7.
145. Arons MH, Thynne CJ, Grabrucker AM, Li D, Schoen M, Cheyne JE, Boeckers TM, Montgomery JM, Garner CC. Autism-associated mutations in ProSAP2/Shank3 impair synaptic transmission and neurexin-neuroligin-mediated transsynaptic signaling. *J Neurosci*. 2012;32(43):14966–14978.
146. Morgan JT, Chana G, Pardo CA, Achim C, Semendeferi K, Buckwalter J, Courchesne E, Everall IP. Microglial activation and increased microglial density observed in the dorsolateral prefrontal cortex in autism. *Biol Psychiatry*. 2010;68(4):368–376.
147. Mrak RE, Griffin WS. Interleukin-1, neuroinflammation, and Alzheimer's disease. *Neurobiol Aging*. 2001;22(6):903–908.
148. Lukiw WJ, Bazan NG. Strong nuclear factor-kappaB-DNA binding parallels cyclooxygenase-2 gene transcription in aging and in sporadic Alzheimer's disease superior temporal lobe neocortex. *J Neurosci Res*. 1998;53(5):583–592.
149. Adami C, Sorci G, Blasi E, Agneletti AL, Bistoni F, Donato R. S100B expression in and effects on microglia. *Glia*. 2001;33(2):131–142.
150. Heizmann CW, Cox JA. New perspectives on S100 proteins: a multi-functional Ca(2+)-, Zn(2+)- and Cu(2+)-binding protein family. *Biometals*. 1998;11(4):383–397.
151. Nolte C, Gore A, Sekler I, Kresse W, Hershfinkel M, Hoffmann A, Kettenmann H, Moran A. ZnT-1 expression in astroglial cells protects against zinc toxicity and slows the accumulation of intracellular zinc. *Glia*. 2004;48(2):145–155.
152. Antion MD, Hou L, Wong H, Hoeffer CA, Klann E. mGluR-dependent long-term depression is associated with increased phosphorylation of S6 and synthesis of elongation factor 1A but remains expressed in S6K-deficient mice. *Mol Cell Biol*. 2008;28(9):2996–3007.
153. Gong R, Park CS, Abbassi NR, Tang SJ. Roles of glutamate receptors and the mammalian target of rapamycin (mTOR) signaling pathway in activity-dependent dendritic protein synthesis in hippocampal neurons. *J Biol Chem*. 2006;281(27):18802–18815.
154. Hay N, Sonenberg N. Upstream and downstream of mTOR. *Genes Dev*. 2004;18(16):1926–1945.
155. Slipczuk L, Bekinschtein P, Katche C, Cammarota M, Izquierdo I, Medina JH. BDNF activates mTOR to regulate GluR1 expression required for memory formation. *PLoS One*. 2009;4(6):e6007.
156. Hoeffer CA, Klann E. mTOR signaling: at the crossroads of plasticity, memory and disease. *Trends Neurosci*. 2010;33(2):67–75.
157. Raught B, Peiretti F, Gingras AC, Livingstone M, Shahbazian D, Mayeur GL, Polakiewicz RD, Sonenberg N, Hershey JW. Phosphorylation of eucaryotic translation initiation factor 4B Ser422 is modulated by S6 kinases. *EMBO J*. 2004;23(8):1761–1769.
158. Kelleher RJ, Govindarajan A, Jung HY, Kang H, Tonegawa S. Translational control by MAPK signaling in long-term synaptic plasticity and memory. *Cell*. 2004;116(3):467–479.

159. Chano T, Okabe H, Hulette CM. RB1CC1 insufficiency causes neuronal atrophy through mTOR signaling alteration and involved in the pathology of Alzheimer's diseases. *Brain Res*. 2007;1168:97–105.
160. Wang X, Bey AL, Katz BM, Badea A, Kim N, David LK, Duffney LJ, Kumar S, Mague SD, Hulbert SW, Dutta N, Hayrapetyan V, Yu C, Gaidis E, Zhao S, Ding JD, Xu Q, Chung L, Rodriguiz RM, Wang F, Weinberg RJ, Wetsel WC, Dzirasa K, Yin H, Jiang YH. Altered mGluR5-Homer scaffolds and corticostriatal connectivity in a Shank3 complete knockout model of autism. *Nat Commun*. 2016;7:11459.
161. Wang C, Yu JT, Miao D, Wu ZC, Tan MS, Tan L. Targeting the mTOR signaling network for Alzheimer's disease therapy. *Mol Neurobiol*. 2014;49(1):120–135.
162. Ritchie CW, Bush AI, Mackinnon A, Macfarlane S, Mastwyk M, MacGregor L, Kiers L, Cherny R, Li QX, Tammer A, Carrington D, Mavros C, Volitakis I, Xilinas M, Ames D, Davis S, Beyreuther K, Tanzi RE, Masters CL. Metal-protein attenuation with iodochlorhydroxyquin (clioquinol) targeting Abeta amyloid deposition and toxicity in Alzheimer disease: a pilot phase 2 clinical trial. *Arch Neurol*. 2003;60(12):1685–1691.
163. White AR, Du T, Laughton KM, Volitakis I, Sharples RA, Xilinas ME, Hoke DE, Holsinger RM, Evin G, Cherny RA, Hill AF, Barnham KJ, Li QX, Bush AI, Masters CL. Degradation of the Alzheimer disease amyloid beta-peptide by metal-dependent up-regulation of metalloprotease activity. *J Biol Chem*. 2006;281(26):17670–17680.
164. Zhang YH, Raymick J, Sarkar S, Lahiri DK, Ray B, Holtzman D, Dumas M, Schmued LC. Efficacy and toxicity of clioquinol treatment and A-beta42 inoculation in the APP/PSI mouse model of Alzheimer's disease. *Curr Alzheimer Res*. 2013;10(5):494–506.
165. Grossi C, Francese S, Casini A, Rosi MC, Luccarini I, Fiorentini A, Gabbiani C, Messori L, Moneti G, Casamenti F. Clioquinol decreases amyloid-beta burden and reduces working memory impairment in a transgenic mouse model of Alzheimer's disease. *J Alzheimers Dis*. 2009;17(2):423–440.
166. Lei P, Ayton S, Appukuttan AT, Volitakis I, Adlard PA, Finkelstein DI, Bush AI. Clioquinol rescues Parkinsonism and dementia phenotypes of the tau knockout mouse. *Neurobiol Dis*. 2015;81:168–175.
167. Faux NG, Ritchie CW, Gunn A, Rembach A, Tsatsanis A, Bedo J, Harrison J, Lannfelt L, Blennow K, Zetterberg H, Ingelsson M, Masters CL, Tanzi RE, Cummings JL, Herd CM, Bush AI. PBT2 rapidly improves cognition in Alzheimer's disease: additional phase II analyses. *J Alzheimers Dis*. 2010;20(2):509–516.
168. Lee EJ, Lee H, Huang TN, Chung C, Shin W, Kim K, Koh JY, Hsueh YP, Kim E. Trans-synaptic zinc mobilization improves social interaction in two mouse models of autism through NMDAR activation. *Nat Commun*. 2015;6:7168.
169. Simmons DA, Rex CS, Palmer L, Pandyarajan V, Fedulov V, Gall CM, Lynch G. Up-regulating BDNF with an ampakine rescues synaptic plasticity and memory in Huntington's disease knockin mice. *Proc Natl Acad Sci USA*. 2009;106(12):4906–4911.
170. Lauterborn JC, Rex CS, Kramár E, Chen LY, Pandyarajan V, Lynch G, Gall CM. Brain-derived neurotrophic factor rescues synaptic plasticity in a mouse model of fragile X syndrome. *J Neurosci*. 2007;27(40):10685–10694.
171. Kline DD, Ogier M, Kunze DL, Katz DM. Exogenous brain-derived neurotrophic factor rescues synaptic dysfunction in Mecp2-null mice. *J Neurosci*. 2010;30(15):5303–5310.
172. Knüsel B, Beck KD, Winslow JW, Rosenthal A, Burton LE, Widmer HR, Nikolics K, Hefti F. Brain-derived neurotrophic factor administration protects basal forebrain cholinergic but not nigral dopaminergic neurons from degenerative changes after axotomy in the adult rat brain. *J Neurosci*. 1992;12(11):4391–4402.
173. Lähteinen S, Pitkänen A, Koponen E, Saarelainen T, Castrén E. Exacerbated status epilepticus and acute cell loss, but no changes in epileptogenesis, in mice with increased brain-derived neurotrophic factor signaling. *Neuroscience*. 2003;122(4):1081–1092.
174. Brewer GJ. Copper excess, zinc deficiency, and cognition loss in Alzheimer's disease. *Biofactors*. 2012;38(2):107–113.
175. Russo AJ. Increased copper in individuals with autism normalizes post zinc therapy more efficiently in individuals with concurrent GI disease. *Nutr Metab Insights*. 2011;4:49–54.
176. Grabrucker AM, Rowan M, Garner CC. Brain-delivery of zinc-ions as potential treatment for neurological diseases: mini review. *Drug Deliv Lett*. 2011;1(1):13–23.

CHAPTER

10

Metals and Motor Neuron Disease

Per M. Roos

Karolinska Institutet, Institute of Environmental Medicine, Stockholm, Sweden

OUTLINE

LIST OF ABBREVIATIONS

AD Alzheimer's disease
ALS Amyotrophic lateral sclerosis
CSF Cerebrospinal fluid
CSN Central nervous system
EMG Electromyography
MND Motor neuron disease
MT Metallothionein
PD Parkinson's disease
SOD Superoxide dismutase

Biometals in Neurodegenerative Diseases. http://dx.doi.org/10.1016/B978-0-12-804562-6.00010-5

INTRODUCTION

A paralysis of unknown origin was described in 1831 by the physician at the Birmingham Dispensary Dr John Darwall.[1] Later in the nineteenth century the French neurologist Aran presented a small case series of 11 patients with a previously not appreciated malfunction of the motor system in whom he notes a strange feature of this weakness: "instead of affecting the whole limb or part of a limb, as seen in other atrophies, it irregularly affects certain muscles, while it spares others."[2] This feature localizes the affection segmentally to the anterior horn cells of the spinal cord. Interestingly 3 out of 11 cases in the original presentation by Aran had been exposed to lead (Pb) and two of them actually had a history of Pb intoxication. In 1865, Charcot noted pathological changes in the pyramidal tracts from the brain and in the anterior spinal nerve roots and coined the term amyotrophic lateral sclerosis (ALS).[3]

Motor neuron diseases (MND) are characterized by skeletal muscle atrophy and sclerosis of motor pathways in the spinal cord. They are neurodegenerative disorders together with Alzheimer's dementia (AD) and Parkinson's disease (PD) and other conditions where nerve cell degeneration is the common denominator. Aggregations of proteins, such as amyloid beta and superoxide dismutase (SOD), are found in tissues and fluids from all of these disorders and metals seem to contribute to these aggregations.[4] Some overlaps exist between MND, AD, and PD; common features are onset in advanced age and a slow but steady progression. The most common MND is ALS, often considered a model disorder for neurodegeneration.

ALS presents with muscle weakness and atrophy of the interosseous muscles of the hand or anterior tibial muscles of the leg, or in muscles of speech and swallowing. The muscle atrophy may spread to the contralateral limb or spread from arm to leg, finally and invariably reaching the diaphragm causing progressive respiratory weakness and death from respiratory failure and pneumonia.[5]

ALS is a disorder of the corticospinal tracts and the brain (Fig. 10.1). From the motor cortex nerve action potentials travel through upper motor neurons to anterior horn cells of the spinal cord. From these cells the signals traverse lower motor neurons from the spinal cord to muscles where they pass the motor endplates to muscle cells where they cause muscle contraction and muscle growth. Anterior and lateral columns of the spinal cord are stiff and hard, that is, sclerotic, in ALS. Degeneration of these motor neurons leads to progressive muscle weakness and atrophy of skeletal muscles. The small hand muscle atrophy seen in ALS corresponds to anterior horn cell degeneration at low cervical levels. The sensory nerve system is not affected yet widespread irreversible muscle atrophy is seen in ALS. The scientific question, unanswered since more than a century, is: what is causing this spinal cord degeneration and concomitant muscle atrophy?

There is evidence for an increase in prevalence of neurodegenerative disorders in the United States[6–8] and Europe.[9–12] Viral, genetic, inflammatory, oxidative, and toxic mechanisms have been suggested to explain this increase.[13] For ALS some 150 different therapeutic substances have been tried in vain, with minor or no effect on disease progression. Combined environmental and genetic theories including epigenetic mechanisms have also been presented[14] and metal toxicity has been discussed for more than a century. There is now sufficient data[13,15,16] supporting the notion that metals with neurotoxic properties contribute to ALS. This chapter will focus on metal exposure and inorganic chemistry in ALS.

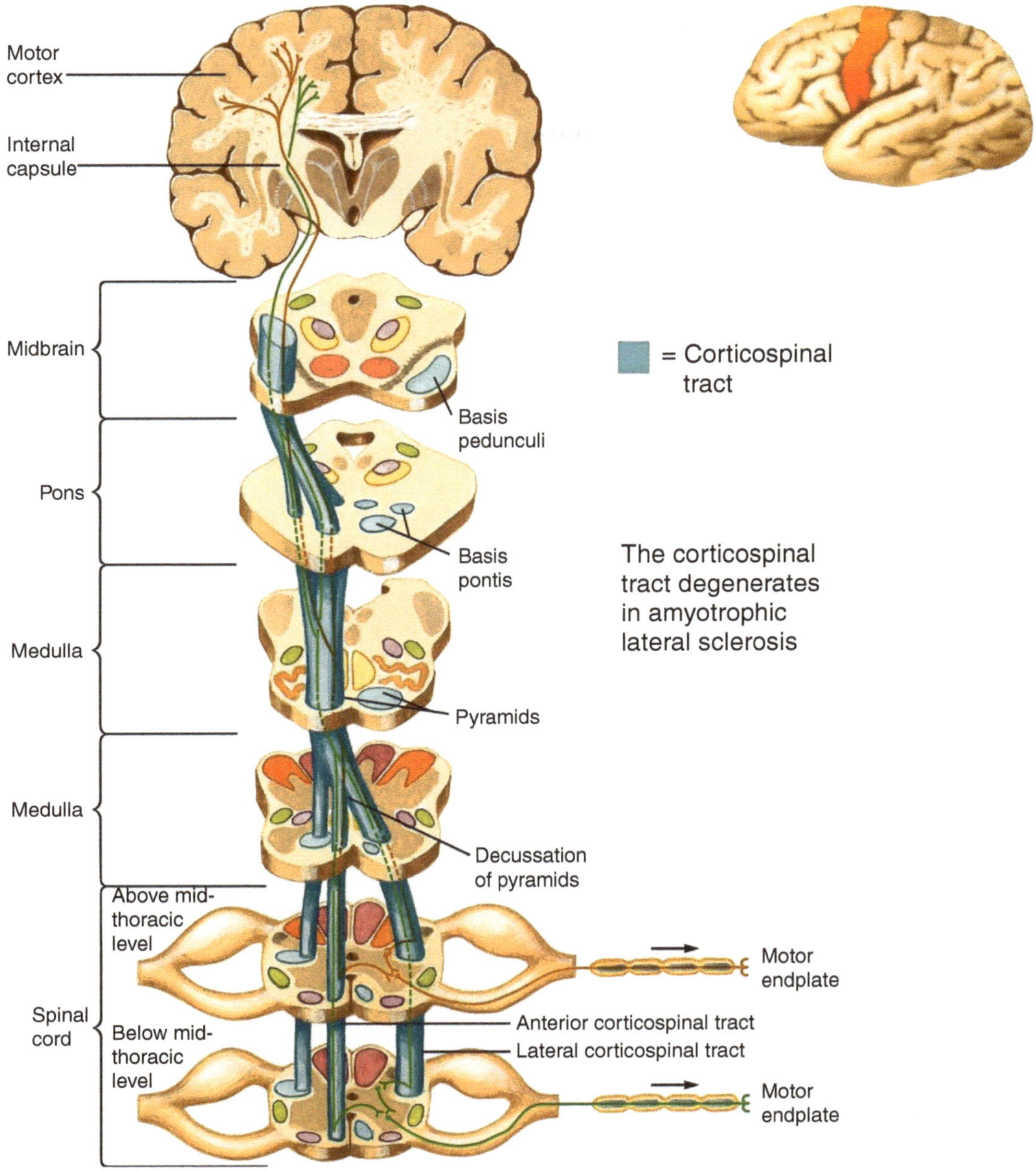

FIGURE 10.1 **The corticospinal tract *(blue)* conveys motor signals from motor cortex *(orange)* to skeletal muscles.** The corticospinal tracts degenerate in ALS leading to widespread muscle atrophy.

METAL EXPOSURE

Metals are persistent and naturally occurring in the environment, and most metals have long biological half-lives in the human body.[17] Metals considered essential to humans are chromium, cobalt (Co), copper (Cu), iron (Fe), molybdenum, selenium (Se), zinc (Zn), and manganese (Mn). In contrast to this essentiality some metals, for example, mercury (Hg), but also cadmium (Cd), arsenic (As), and Pb lack biological functions and any exposure exceeding a low background may give rise to toxicity. Both essential and nonessential metals produce toxic effects when present in excess and these effects vary considerably depending on dose, duration, exposure conditions, bioavailability, and chemical species.[17]

Metal particles and ions enter the human body through various exposure channels and can reach the nervous system via respiratory, olphactory, enteric, dermal, and intravenous routes.[13] Tissue uptake also varies between metals and organ systems. Metal exposures may be occupational or recreational or result from any repeated activity in the daily life of the patient. They form a complex web of varied and sometimes hidden and insidious exposure situations which require a thorough anamnesis and profound knowledge of inorganic chemistry and exposure mechanisms to disentangle.[18] Metal concentrations are preferably monitored by direct sampling of tissues and fluids as close to the nervous system as possible. Paired simultaneous sampling[19,20] of cerebrospinal fluid (CSF) and whole blood under ultraclean conditions is preferred in studies of metal exposures relevant to ALS.

METALS IN ALS CEREBROSPINAL FLUID

Pathological changes are found in the anterior horn cells of the spinal cord (Fig. 10.1) of ALS patients. Measurements of metal concentrations in tissues and fluids are best performed as close as possible to the structure of interest, that is, the spinal cord when metal toxicity is suspected. Studies of transverse spinal cord sections postmortem have shown elevated Mn concentrations[21] and several other direct metal measurements of ALS spinal cord tissue (summarized in Ref. [13]) have shown elevated concentrations of Mn, Al, Fe, Se, Zn, Pb, and Cu. Metal measurements in ALS CSF from living patients are scarce but an early Swedish study[22] found significantly elevated Pb concentrations in ALS, and elevated Al concentrations were found in ALS CSF in a study from India.[23] Increased selenium species were noted in CSF from Italian ALS patients,[19] and elevated concentrations of Mg, Fe, and Cu were detected in ALS CSF in a Japanese study.[24] In a detailed study[25] of paired samples, a pattern of multiple toxic metals (Table 10.1) elevated in ALS CSF but not in blood, was seen. The metals detected in significantly increased concentrations in ALS CSF were Mn, Al, Cd, Co, Cu, Zn, Pb, V, and U.[13] Most of these metals are well characterized neurotoxicants (Fig. 10.2).

METALS IN ALS

Several studies over the decades link metals and metal exposures to ALS disease and ALS-like symptoms and histopathology in humans and in animals. Some overlap with findings related to AD and PD can be found. In this section metals found[13] in tissues and fluids in ALS

TABLE 10.1 Summary of Metals Found Significantly Elevated in ALS CSF[25]

	Metal								
Identity	**Al**	**V**	**Mn**	**Co**	**Cu**	**Zn**	**Cd**	**Pb**	**U**
ALS 1									
ALS 2	▼		▼	○			▼	▼	▼
ALS 3									
ALS 4									
ALS 5	▼								
ALS 6									▼
ALS 7	▼				○				▼
ALS 8	▼	○	▼	○	○	○	▼	▼	▼
ALS 9								▼	
ALS 10									
ALS 11									▼
ALS 12								▼	▼
ALS 13					○	○	▼	▼	▼
ALS 14	▼	○	▼	○	○	○	▼		
ALS 15			▼			○	▼		▼
ALS 16			▼		○		▼		
ALS 17									
Ctrl a									
Ctrl b									
Ctrl c									
Ctrl d									
Ctrl e									
Ctrl f									
Ctrl g									
Ctrl h									
Ctrl i						○		▼	
Ctrl j									

Metals present in concentrations one standard deviation or more above the mean for the combined cases and controls for that metal are indicated by a *small circle* (○). Metals with known neurotoxic properties, also present in concentrations at or above one standard deviation, are marked with a *black triangle* (▼).

are discussed in relation to effects on the nervous system in general and specifically in relation to ALS.

Aluminum (Al) is a well-known neurotoxicant.[26] Encephalopathy from Al containing dialysis fluids has been described and nervous system symptoms from Al related medical

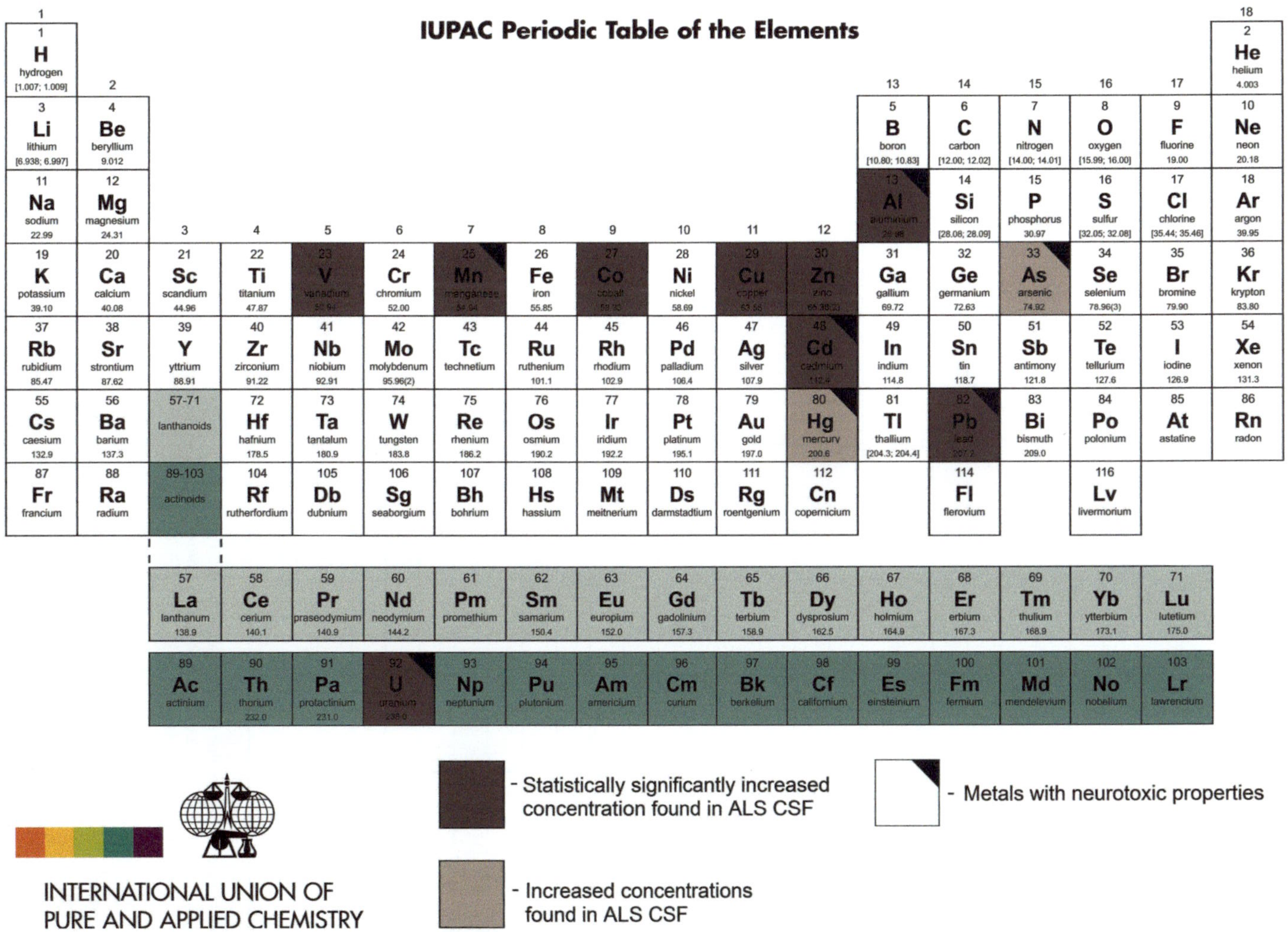

FIGURE 10.2 **Metals found in elevated concentrations in cerebrospinal fluid from patients with amyotrophic lateral sclerosis are aluminum, vanadium, manganese, cobalt, copper, zinc, cadmium, lead, and uranium.**[25] Several of these metals are well characterized neurotoxicants, indicated with a black triangle in the uppermost right corner in the IUPAC periodic table of elements.

procedures, such as bone cement, intravenous feeding, and irrigation of the urine bladder exist.[27] High Al concentrations have been noted in AD brains at autopsy,[28] but replication studies are inconsistent. Aluminum hydroxide injections in mice produces motor neuron degeneration.[29] Neurofibrillary tangle formation, chromatolysis, and abnormal localization of nuclei, resembling ALS pathology has been observed in mice after Al injection,[30] and ALS-like skin changes were noted in mice overfed with Al.[31] Monkeys receiving a low calcium high Al diet developed ALS motor neuron pathology.[32] Elevated CSF Al concentrations have been found in ALS[13,23] and an ALS-like syndrome due to Al intoxication has been described.[33]

Arsenic occurs in organic form in seafood and as inorganic As in drinking water and beverages. Arsenic is readily absorbed after ingestion and widely distributed in the body. Inorganic As causes skin lesions and skin cancer, and effects on heart, peripheral circulation, and the nervous system have been reported.[26] Other effects of As intoxication are hyperpigmentation, endocrine disruption and foetal loss. Chronic As toxicity has been described to cause hearing loss, mental retardation, encephalopathy, and polyneuropathy.[26]

To what extent As accumulates in the spinal cord is less studied, but As ingestion causes widespread neurogenic muscle atrophy and weakness as illustrated by case reports,[34–36] some systematic studies[37] and a review[38] of the effects of chronic As exposure symptoms. The motor symptoms of As intoxication are similar to the atrophy and weakness seen in ALS and most reports describe end stages of As intoxication with widespread motor impairment. In a study of 41 cases of more or less chronic As exposure,[37] severe symmetrical muscular weakness of the extremities was noted. Twenty-seven patients out of 41 showed foot-drop, 24 were unable to walk, and 16 unable to stand without assistance. Fasciculations were noted in some of these cases.[37] A large study of long time low dose exposure from groundwater As contamination in West Bengal India[39] showed muscle atrophy and weakness in 7%–10% of exposed individuals. A case of arsenicosis presenting with upper and lower motor neuron signs as in ALS has been reported from India.[40] Two detailed reports of progressive muscle weakness of all limb muscles evolving into tetraparesis and respiratory failure following As exposure are also published.[35,36]

Cadmium is not part of any normal cellular processes. It is toxic at very low exposure levels[41] and Cd exposure through tobacco smoking is a major health concern. Cadmium is transported in plasma largely bound to metallothionein (MT)[42] and Cd stimulates MT synthesis.[43] Cadmium concentrations were significantly elevated both in gray and white matter in formalin-fixed brain tissue from Guam ALS cases.[44] A patient diagnosed with ALS after 9 years of Cd exposure in a Ni-Cd battery factory has been described[45] and Cd has been found in ALS CSF[13] and in blood from some ALS patients.[46]

Cobalt is present in cooling oils, dental materials, and medical implants, such as metal hip replacements.[17,26] Cobalt exposure affects mainly the respiratory system and hematopoiesis but also the nervous system where neurotoxic effects of Co[47] have been described after release of Co to the systemic circulation in patients with orthopedic prostheses.[17] In an ALS motor neuron like cell line exposure to cobalt chloride evoked signs of oxidative toxicity associated with motor neuron death in ALS.[48]

Copper is a highly redox active metal present in water pipes, fungicides, intrauterine contraceptive devices, and dental alloys.[26] Copper concentrations are effectively regulated in the body and mutations in Cu regulatory proteins produce Menkes disease and Wilson's disease,[49] both affecting the nervous system. Inorganic Cu, as found in drinking water and in vitamin supplements is potentially toxic to the brain, possibly contributing to AD development.[50] One case of early onset ALS with elevated Cu levels has been described[51] and elevated concentrations of Cu have been detected in ALS CSF.[13] Copper is together with Zn vital for the function of the antioxidant protein SOD and mutations in the SOD gene are associated with ALS.[52] Recent findings show prolonged survival of SOD1G37R mice when Cu-deficient SOD1 was fully metallated by a Cu complexing molecule.[53]

Lead is the most extensively studied toxic metal and Pb is the metal that has been most intensely discussed over the decades as a possible causative agent for ALS. Lead causes a motor neuropathy characterized by weakness and atrophy of skeletal muscles without sensory involvement. The spinal origin of this neuropathy following chronic low dose Pb intoxications has been debated for more than a century[54–56] and the historical observations from a series of 1213 Pb intoxicated patients stating that the anterior horn of the spinal cord is the site of injury in Pb intoxication are still valid.[56] Information from early sources are necessary in evaluating long time low dose exposures to Pb as the most common exposures, such as from brass metal industry, manual paint removal work, Pb contaminated food or beverages, or even leaded gasoline, no longer exist. Worldwide however new challenges appear with the electronic industry contributing to a new increase in Pb exposure,[57] together with paint, toys, traditional remedies, smelting operations, and battery recycling as main sources.[57]

The isolated motor neuropathy seen in Pb intoxications is similar to the clinical presentation of ALS. Similarities include pure motor engagement, often normal motor conduction velocities, occurrence of fibrillation potentials[58] and slow onset. The fibrillation potentials found in Pb intoxication subjects[58] may well indicate anterior horn cell involvement. Histological evidence indicate that segmental demyelination is not present in Pb intoxication[59] and segmental demyelination is not observed in ALS. Reports of proven anterior horn cell involvement in definite Pb intoxications are however scarce[60] and further investigations using electrophysiological methods are needed to pinpoint such an involvement.

A case report of proven Pb intoxication 12 years after a Pb bullet penetrated into an intervertebral space[61] describes a patient in a lethargic state with progressive profound muscle weakness. Muscle biopsy in this case showed atrophic muscle fibers consistent with neuropathic disease and widespread weakness evolved in all muscles calling for tracheal intubation and ventilation support. A 39-year-old factory worker handling Pb oxide showed atrophy, spasticity, and fasciculations in lower extremities after excess Pb exposure and subsequently died from ALS.[62] Vesterberg used flameless atomic absorption spectrophotometry to measure Pb in blood plasma and found elevated concentrations in ALS patients.[63] Statistically significantly elevated Pb concentrations have been noted in ALS CSF.[13]

A large study conducted by the National Institute of Environmental Health Sciences observed that blood Pb levels were higher ($P < 0.0001$, age adjusted) in ALS cases than in controls.[64] Differences in bone turnover or polymorphism in Pb metabolism enzymes did not modify this distinct association. A Californian study of 165 ALS patients[65] also found a positive association between blood Pb levels and ALS, albeit not between bone Pb levels and ALS. Earlier studies have associated ALS risk with Pb elevations in blood and bone[66,67] and concluded with a potential role for Pb exposure in the etiology of ALS.

A small but significant ALS cluster has been identified next to a Pb smelter factory.[68] Of special interest is the epidemiological study conducted in possibly Pb contaminated districts in Italy[69] where elevated incidences of ALS were found. Finally, a recent meta-analysis of individuals with a history of Pb exposures[70] concluded with an almost doubled (OR = 1.81) ALS risk for the exposed.

Manganese is found in welding fumes, as a fuel additive, in alkaline battery production and in solutions for total parenteral nutrition.[26] The neurotoxic properties of Mn are well characterized.[71] Mn accumulates in the central nervous system with longer half-life within nervous tissue. Cumulative mechanisms of neurotoxicity seem to cause manganism with progressive irreversible brain impairment and similarities to PD have been discussed.[72] Muscle wasting leading to paraplegia as a result of respiratory exposure to Mn has been described.[73] Welders exposed to Mn presented dose-dependent motor impairments,[74] and reduced fine motor skills.[75] Manganese accumulation primarily in nuclei of cultured brain cells has been described.[76] Manganese concentrations were significantly higher in ALS CSF than in CSF from controls in a study of ALS CSF Mn concentrations.[20] The CSF concentrations were higher than the plasma Mn concentrations suggesting transport of Mn into the central nervous system in ALS.[20] Elevated Mn concentrations have also been reported[21] in spinal cord sections from ALS patients.

Mercury is widespread in the biosphere, both from natural and human sources, such as combustion of fossil fuels and industrial release. Mercury occurs as elemental Hg and as Hg vapor, as Hg salts, or Hg organic compounds all with different toxicological properties. Mercury has a long history of adverse reactions and CNS is the critical organ for long-term Hg exposure.[26] Effects on foetal brain development, cognitive defects, brain atrophy, and peripheral neuropathy have been described.[26] Inhaled Hg vapor can reach the spinal cord and seems to accumulate in anterior horn cells[77] of significance for ALS development. Mercury was found in spinal motor neurons of 67% of ALS patients, and in the locus coerulius in an Australian study.[78]

Several case reports or case series describe ALS development, often with a delay, after various forms of Hg exposure.[79] Accidental injection of elemental Hg from a thermometer into the hand of a nurse resulted in an ALS syndrome with a delay of 3 years.[80] A farmer noted progressive weakness in all extremities and widespread muscle atrophy, diagnosed as ALS, following respiratory exposure to ethylphenylmercury. Postmortem examination of the spinal cord showed moderate frontal lobe atrophy and almost complete absence of anterior horn cells in the spinal cord.[81] Eleven patients developed irreversible ALS after ingestion of ethylmercury-*p*-toluene sulfonanilide used as a fungicide for wheat flour used in bread.[82] Another case of Hg exposure from collecting liquid Hg from thermometers was followed 3 months later by muscle twitching, weakness, and muscle atrophy developing into an ALS-like syndrome confirmed by electromyography (EMG).[83] Two Hg oxide factory workers exposed to both Hg oxide and Hg vapor developed massive fasciculations, muscle weakness, and symptoms and signs as in ALS.[84] An elderly woman developed progressive weakness of one hand developing into ALS after dermal and/or respiratory exposure to metallic Hg.[85] Diffuse denervation of all limbs including the tongue was confirmed by EMG. From regions in India with Hg contaminated stream water elevated Hg concentrations in blood from ALS patients have been described.[86]

Selenium (Se) occurs as selenomethionine and as selenocysteine in several selenoproteins with antioxidative properties. Selenium protects against methylmercury toxicity and Se interacts with other metals, such as Cd and As attenuating their toxicity.[26] At higher doses Se seems to be toxic to the nervous system and reports from regions in China with endemically elevated (approx. 1200 μg/day) Se intake describe skin lesions, brittle hair and nails, and later on motor disturbances and paralysis.[87] Selective spinal cord anterior horn Se toxicity has been demonstrated in swine[88,89] and in regions with increased Se in soil and drinking water in South Dakota[90] and Italy[19] ALS clusters can be found. Specifically, the Se species selenite (SeO_3^{2-}), but not total Se, was elevated in these studies calling for speciation[91] when evaluating Se neurotoxicity.

Uranium (U) is mined for the ^{235}U isotope used in nuclear reactors and weapons, and depleted uranium is used in armour-piercing munitions. Uranium toxicity involves combined chemical and radiological mechanisms where chemical toxicity is the most important.[92] Human respiratory exposure to U of military origin has been documented,[93] and U in drinking water is a concern in some regions. Absorption of U is low regardless of exposure route and highly dependent on its solubility and inhaled U dust particles of low solubility can be retained for years. The main target for U toxicity is the kidney where atrophy and necrosis of glomerular walls occur. Accumulation in rat brain after respiratory U exposure is heterogeneous with the higher concentrations in the olfactory bulbs and cerebellum.[94] Rats surgically implanted with U pellets showed after 6 months presence of U in the cortex, midbrain, and cerebellum suggesting that U preferentially accumulates in specific brain regions after exposure.[95] Laboratory experiments[95] with organisms, such as *Caenorhabditis elegans* and rats have concluded with low acute neurotoxic potential of U following exposure, and a protective potential from MT. Concentrations of U in ALS CSF were generally low but all the higher U concentrations were found among the ALS cases, completely separating them from the controls in a Swedish study.[13]

Vanadium (V), used in the production of special-purpose steel also affects the nervous system.[26] Vanadium exerts neurotoxic effects in dopaminergic neuronal cells.[96] Acute V intoxication in experimental animals caused death preceded by paralysis of the hind legs. Similar hind leg paralysis was found in cattle intoxicated with V.[97] Vanadium has been found in CSF from patients with ALS.[13]

Zinc is an ubiquitous essential metal and Zn deficiency is a worldwide problem, yet excess Zn is toxic to the spinal cord.[98] Zinc is necessary for brain development and is essential for nerve conduction. Some hypotheses relate Zn deficiency to ALS.[99] Elevated ALS CSF Zn concentrations have been detected.[25] Blood Zn was however, together with Se, inversely associated with ALS severity in a recent study.[100]

PROTECTION BY METALLOTHIONEIN

Protective mechanisms against metal toxicity have evolved across species over the millennia.[101] Metallothionein is a low molecular weight cysteine rich protein with seven metals bound to it, distributed in two clusters of three and four metals, mostly Zn, Cd, Hg, and Cu.[102,103] There are several genes coding for MT and they are induced by metals and other stimuli. Astrocyte MTs seem to exert a neuroprotective role in the nervous system.[104]

After injury to the central nervous system MT expression in astrocytes is highly elevated and neuroregenerative properties of MT have been described.[105] Reduced expression of MT in ALS spinal cords has been noted.[106] A selective vulnerability of anterior horn cells to metals can be suspected in ALS.[13]

METAL DISTRIBUTION IN ALS

Metal Related ALS Clusters

Amyotrophic lateral sclerosis is unevenly distributed over the planet. The existence of geographically isolated ALS clusters[107–110] lend some support to an environmental etiology for the disease. Clusters of ALS have been described from regions with metal mining activity[111–113] and geological knowledge is important for the understanding of natural distribution of metals with neurotoxic properties. The highest ALS incidences ever described were noted in clusters of Guam, the Kii Peninsula in Japan, and Western New Guinea,[114] where ALS incidence was more than 50-fold higher than the worldwide incidence.[115] Environmental studies of soil and drinking water in these regions revealed elevated concentrations of Al and Mn, and analysis of ALS lumbar motor neurons showed high contents of Al and Mn.[116] Aluminium, Mn, and other metals, and mineral/metal imbalances, have been implicated as causative in these pacific hyperendemic ALS foci.[44,117] Uranium exposure was also present in these pacific regions at the time of the peak ALS incidences.

In southeast of Finland, significant ALS clusters have been identified by spatial-scan statistics examining both time of birth and time of death[118] and the authors discuss the possibility of clustering related to metal polluted lakes in the region. Geological conditions lowering the pH of rivers in Finland causing metal leach into the ecosystem[119] may also contribute.

The reports (summarized in Ref. [120]) on spatial clustering in ALS are varied and describe accumulations of cases in buildings, counties, proximities to lakes or rivers or war zones and several other specific but highly scattered localities. Some geographic variation may be explained by a genetic predisposition for ALS among certain ethnical groups,[121] but the variation can also be understood as an effect of a geographically uneven distribution of substances toxic to the nervous system. At the slopes of Mount Etna (Fig. 10.3) higher incidences of ALS have been noted in the direction of metal rich volcanic ash deposits.[122] Geographical covariation between ALS and the geographical occurrence of various metals is a possible scenario worth further exploration in collaborations with the geological scientific community. In summary, metal-related geomedical data lend further support to the possibility of metals contributing to ALS pathogenesis.

ALS and Occupational Exposures to Metals

An increased ALS risk has been documented for agricultural workers, athletes, cockpit occupations, electrical workers, farmers, hairdressers, laboratory technicians, leather workers, machine assemblers, medical service workers, military workers, power production plant workers, programmers, rubber workers, tobacco workers, and welders.[13] Several of these seemingly disparate occupations can in various ways be linked to metal exposures. In a meta-analysis of occupational exposures in ALS where the authors meticulously scrutinized the published studies for scientific quality before inclusion in the analysis,[123] a statistically significantly elevated risk (RR = 1.69) was noted for metal exposure.

Conjugal ALS

Two unrelated individuals living together for a long time under the same roof developing ALS within the same time span or shortly after each other provide a strong argument for

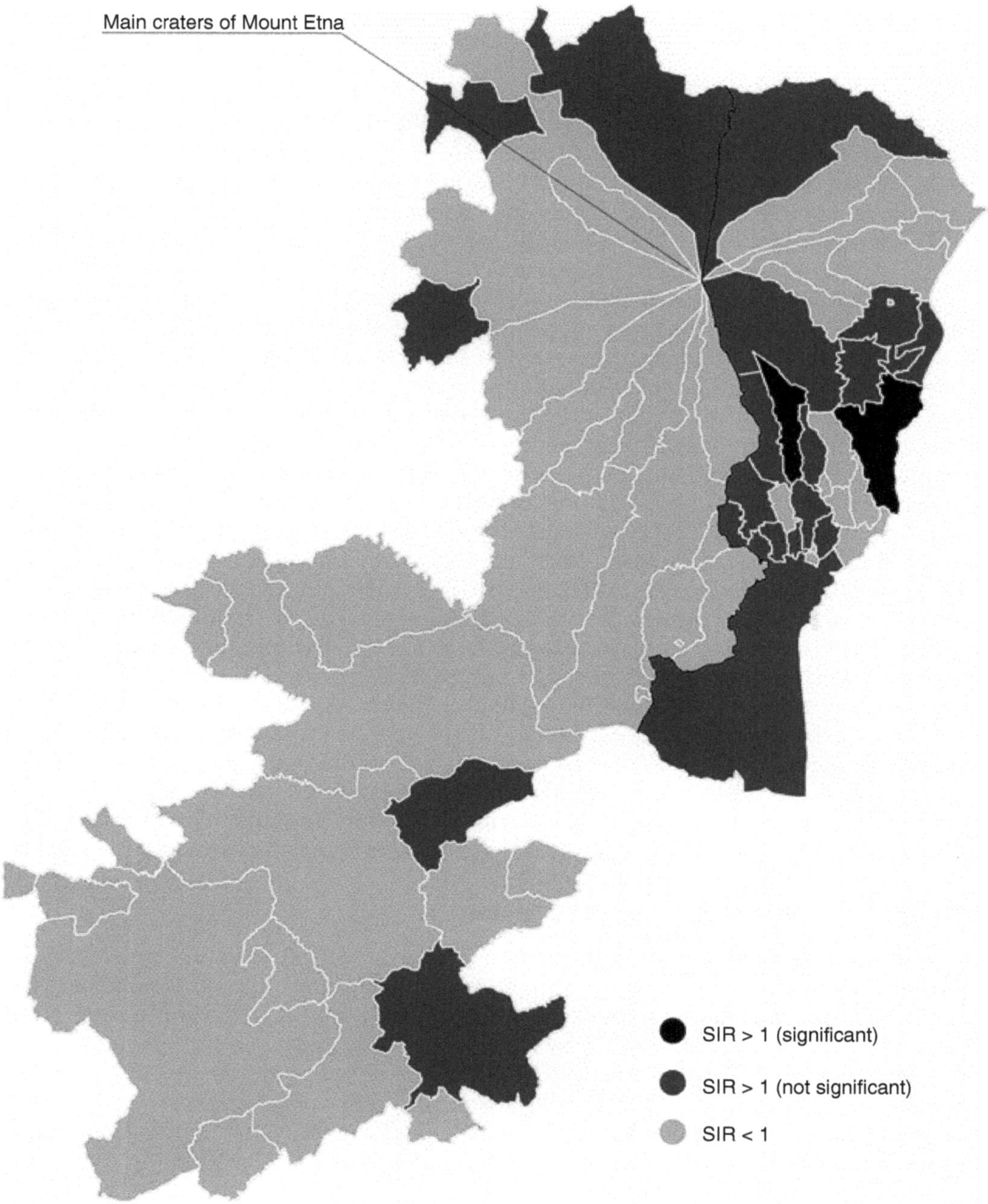

FIGURE 10.3 **Amyotrophic lateral sclerosis at the flanks of Mt.Etna Italy.**[122] Standardized incidence ratios (SIR) for each community are shown. ALS incidence was higher ($P < 0.001$) at the eastern flank possibly correlating to the geographic distribution of volcanogenic metals. *Source: Reproduced with permission from European Journal of Neurology.*

an environmental cause of the disorder. Spouses often engage in the same daily activities or work, drink the same water and eat the same food often from local sources. Several reports of such conjugal ALS exist and describe variations on this theme. Thus a shepherd couple from rural regions of Italy developed ALS shortly after each other.[124] Two conjugal cases occurred in southern France, a rural region with agricultural traditions.[125] Another clustering of nine couples in south-eastern France have been described,[126] and couples in Brazil[127] and Texas[128] can be found. Conjugal cases and clustering of ALS seems to be more common in rural areas.[129] Altogether about 20 pairs of conjugal ALS have been published,[128] and the value of conjugal cases for an understanding of the environmental influence of metals has been emphasized.[130] Clusters of conjugal ALS have been described from many different regions and countries and local environmental factors, such as metal exposure, can be suspected. The nature of such exposure may be complex and varied and differ between regions, calling for thorough chemical investigations of the local environment when couples encounter ALS within the same time frame.

GENETIC ASPECTS

Subgroups of ALS have been described according to genetic aberrations, the most valid affecting the genes *C9ORF72*, *SOD1*, and *TARDBP*. The gene *C9ORF72* is a hexanucleotide repeat at chromosome 9 that cosegregates with both ALS and frontal lobe dementia.[131–133] The superoxide dismutase (*SOD1*) gene is located at chromosome 21. The SOD1 protein binds Cu and Zn ions, and has a role in apoptosis. More than 170 mutations of *SOD1* have been identified in ALS accounting for some 20% of all familial ALS cases.[132] The *TARDBP* gene is located on chromosome 1 and codes for the DNA-binding and RNA-binding protein TDP-43 involved in transcription and transport of subcellular RNA. Mutated TDP-43 accumulates in ubiquitinated cytoplasmic inclusions in ALS motor neurons.[132,134] The exact gene products from these three genes defining subgroups of ALS are less well characterized, yet *C9ORF72* seems to be involved in endosomal trafficking and autophagy and the gene product of *SOD1* is one out of three superoxide dismutase isoenzymes responsible for the conversion of free superoxide radicals to molecular oxygen and hydrogen peroxide. Recent data indicate that both *C9ORF72* and *TARDBP* are involved in axonal transport.[135]

There is no evidence for genetic causes of sporadic ALS, which has shown a steadily increased mortality frequency throughout the century,[136] still rising.[12] This increase is of a magnitude that excludes genetic migration and has been interpreted from epidemiologic data alone to support an environmental etiology.[6] A recent very large meta-analysis[137] of genome-wide associations in ALS largely failed in associating risk gene variants with sporadic ALS. One locus at 1p34.1 modulating age of ALS onset was however identified. Considerable genetic heterogeneity seems to be present within the clinical ALS phenotype. The genetic influences on sporadic ALS can be described as weak.[137]

To what extent the specific protein functions associated with *C9ORF72*, *SOD1*, and *TARDBP* expressions interact with effects of metal exposure remains to be elucidated, and opens new and exciting avenues for future research in the intersections between genetic expression and environmental metal toxicity.

CONCLUDING REMARKS

Metal toxicity contributing to ALS pathogenesis has remained a viable hypothesis since mid-nineteenth century. Metals with neurotoxic properties have been detected in tissues and fluids from ALS patients. Disturbed metal homeostasis and various metal exposures can be suspected to contribute to ALS. Combined information from spatial clustering, occupational exposures, and conjugal cases further support this view, although precise mechanistic knowledge is still lacking. Modern analytical techniques and reliable sampling methods are needed to clarify the role of metals in ALS pathogenesis providing an incentive for preventive action.

References

1. Darwall J. Cases of a peculiar species of paralysis. *London Med Gazette*. 1831;7:231–233.
2. Aran F. Recherches sur une maladie non encore décrite du système musculaire (atrophie musculaire progressive). *Arch Gén Méd*. 1850;24(5-35):172–214.
3. Charcot J-M. Amyotrophies spinales deuteropathiques sclérose latérale amyotrophique & Sclérose latérale amyotrophique. *Bureaux du Progrès Médical*. 1874;2:234–266.
4. Ayton S, Lei P, Bush AI. Biometals and their therapeutic implications in Alzheimer's disease. *Neurotherapeutics*. 2015;12(1):109–120.
5. Kiernan MC, Vucic S, Cheah BC, et al. Amyotrophic lateral sclerosis. *Lancet*. 2011;377(9769):942–955.
6. Lilienfeld DE, Chan E, Ehland J, et al. Rising mortality from motoneuron disease in the USA, 1962-84. *Lancet*. 1989;1(8640):710–713.
7. Noonan CW, White MC, Thurman D, Wong LY. Temporal and geographic variation in United States motor neuron disease mortality, 1969-1998. *Neurology*. 2005;64(7):1215–1221.
8. Sejvar JJ, Holman RC, Bresee JS, Kochanek KD, Schonberger LB. Amyotrophic lateral sclerosis mortality in the United States, 1979-2001. *Neuroepidemiology*. 2005;25(3):144–152.
9. Chio A, Magnani C, Schiffer D. Amyotrophic lateral sclerosis mortality in Italy, 1958 to 1987: a cross-sectional and cohort study. *Neurology*. 1993;43(5):927–930.
10. Maasilta P, Jokelainen M, Loytonen M, Sabel CE, Gatrell AC. Mortality from amyotrophic lateral sclerosis in Finland, 1986-1995. *Acta Neurol Scand*. 2001;104(4):232–235.
11. Seljeseth YM, Vollset SE, Tysnes OB. Increasing mortality from amyotrophic lateral sclerosis in Norway? *Neurology*. 2000;55(9):1262–1266.
12. Fang F, Valdimarsdottir U, Bellocco R, et al. Amyotrophic lateral sclerosis in Sweden, 1991-2005. *Arch Neurol*. 2009;66(4):515–519.
13. Roos PM. *Studies on metals in motor neuron disease*. Stockholm: Institute of Environmental Medicine, Karolinska Institutet; 2013.
14. Paez-Colasante X, Figueroa-Romero C, Sakowski SA, Goutman SA, Feldman EL. Amyotrophic lateral sclerosis: mechanisms and therapeutics in the epigenomic era. *Nat Rev Neurol*. 2015;11(5):266–279.
15. Barnham KJ, Bush AI. Biological metals and metal-targeting compounds in major neurodegenerative diseases. *Chem Soc Rev*. 2014;43(19):6727–6749.
16. Bowman AB, Kwakye GF. Herrero Hernandez E, Aschner M. Role of manganese in neurodegenerative diseases. *J Trace Elem Med Biol*. 2011;25(4):191–203.
17. Nordberg M, Nordberg GF. Trace element research-historical and future aspects. *J Trace Elem Med Biol*. 2016;38:46–52.
18. McGuire V, Longstreth Jr WT, Nelson LM, et al. Occupational exposures and amyotrophic lateral sclerosis. A population-based case-control study. *Am J Epidemiol*. 1997;145(12):1076–1088.
19. Vinceti M, Solovyev N, Mandrioli J, et al. Cerebrospinal fluid of newly diagnosed amyotrophic lateral sclerosis patients exhibits abnormal levels of selenium species including elevated selenite. *Neurotoxicology*. 2013;38:25–32.
20. Roos PM, Lierhagen S, Flaten TP, Syversen T, Vesterberg O, Nordberg M. Manganese in cerebrospinal fluid and blood plasma of patients with amyotrophic lateral sclerosis. *Exp Biol Med*. 2012;237(7):803–810.

21. Miyata S, Nakamura S, Nagata H, Kameyama M. Increased manganese level in spinal cords of amyotrophic lateral sclerosis determined by radiochemical neutron activation analysis. *J Neurol Sci*. 1983;61(2):283–293.
22. Conradi S, Ronnevi LO, Vesterberg O. Abnormal tissue distribution of lead in amyotrophic lateral sclerosis. *J Neurol Sci*. 1976;29(2–4):259–265.
23. Sood K, Nag D, Chandra SV. Role of aluminium in sporadic motor neuron disease. *Indian J Med Res*. 1990;92: 9–12.
24. Hozumi I, Hasegawa T, Honda A, et al. Patterns of levels of biological metals in CSF differ among neurodegenerative diseases. *J Neurol Sci*. 2011;303(1–2):95–99.
25. Roos PM, Vesterberg O, Syversen T, Flaten TP, Nordberg M. Metal concentrations in cerebrospinal fluid and blood plasma from patients with amyotrophic lateral sclerosis. *Biol Trace Elem Res*. 2013;151(2):159–170.
26. Nordberg G, Fowler B, Nordberg M, eds. *Handbook on the Toxicology of Metals*. Amsterdam, Netherlands: Elsevier; 2014.
27. Flaten TP, Alfrey AC, Birchall JD, Savory J, Yokel RA. Status and future concerns of clinical and environmental aluminum toxicology. *J Toxicol Environ Health*. 1996;48(6):527–541.
28. Crapper DR, Krishnan SS, Dalton AJ. Brain aluminum distribution in Alzheimer's disease and experimental neurofibrillary degeneration. *Science*. 1973;180(4085):511–513.
29. Shaw CA, Petrik MS. Aluminum hydroxide injections lead to motor deficits and motor neuron degeneration. *J Inorg Biochem*. 2009;103(11):1555–1562.
30. Tanridag T, Coskun T, Hurdag C, Arbak S, Aktan S, Yegen B. Motor neuron degeneration due to aluminium deposition in the spinal cord: a light microscopical study. *Acta Histochem*. 1999;101(2):193–201.
31. Kihira T, Yoshida S, Kondo T, Yase Y, Ono S. ALS-like skin changes in mice on a chronic low-Ca/Mg high-Al diet. *J Neurol Sci*. 2004;219(1–2):7–14.
32. Garruto RM, Shankar SK, Yanagihara R, Salazar AM, Amyx HL, Gajdusek DC. Low-calcium, high-aluminum diet-induced motor neuron pathology in cynomolgus monkeys. *Acta Neuropathol*. 1989;78(2):210–219.
33. Tanndag T, Ince D, Tekin S, Nourikhalichi K, Aktan S. ALS-like syndrome due to aluminium intoxication. *Electroencephalogr Clin Neurophysiol*. 1995;97(4):S229.
34. McCutchen JJ, Utterback RA. Chronic arsenic poisoning resembling muscular dystrophy. *South Med J*. 1966;59(10):1139–1145.
35. Greenberg C, Davies S, McGowan T, Schorer A, Drage C. Acute respiratory failure following severe arsenic poisoning. *Chest*. 1979;76(5):596–598.
36. Stenehjem AE, Vahter M, Nermell B, et al. Slow recovery from severe inorganic arsenic poisoning despite treatment with DMSA (2.3-dimercaptosuccinic acid). *Clin Toxicol (Phila)*. 2007;45(4):424–428.
37. Heyman A, Pfeiffer Jr JB, Willett RW, Taylor HM. Peripheral neuropathy caused by arsenical intoxication; a study of 41 cases with observations on the effects of BAL (2, 3, dimercapto-propanol). *N Engl J Med*. 1956;254(9):401–409.
38. Hall AH. Chronic arsenic poisoning. *Toxicol Lett*. 2002;128(1–3):69–72.
39. Mukherjee SC, Rahman MM, Chowdhury UK, et al. Neuropathy in arsenic toxicity from groundwater arsenic contamination in West Bengal, India. *J Environ Sci Health A Tox Hazard Subst Environ Eng*. 2003;38(1):165–183.
40. Mazumdar S, Mukherjee P, Gowsami S, Saha B, Ahmed A, Mukhopadhyay J. Arsenicosis: unusual neurological presentation from West Bengal. *J Assoc Physicians India*. 2010;58:201–202.
41. Nordberg G, Jin T, Bernard A, et al. Low bone density and renal dysfunction following environmental cadmium exposure in China. *Ambio*. 2002;31(6):478–481.
42. Bachmeyer C, Bagur E, Lenglet T, Maier-Redelsperger M, Lecomte I. Lead poisoning mimicking amyotrophic lateral sclerosis: an adverse effect of rituals. *Am J Med*. 2012;125(6):e5–6.
43. Nordberg M, Jin T, Nordberg GF. Cadmium, metallothionein and renal tubular toxicity. *IARC Sci Publ*. 1992;(118):293–297.
44. Gellein K, Garruto RM, Syversen T, Sjobakk TE, Flaten TP. Concentrations of Cd, Co, Cu, Fe, Mn, Rb, V, and Zn in formalin-fixed brain tissue in amyotrophic lateral sclerosis and Parkinsonism-dementia complex of Guam determined by high-resolution ICP-MS. *Biol Trace Elem Res*. 2003;96(1–3):39–60.
45. Bar-Sela S, Reingold S, Richter ED. Amyotrophic lateral sclerosis in a battery-factory worker exposed to cadmium. *Int J Occup Environ Health*. 2001;7(2):109–112.
46. Vinceti M, Guidetti D, Bergomi M, et al. Lead, cadmium, and selenium in the blood of patients with sporadic amyotrophic lateral sclerosis. *Ital J Neurol Sci*. 1997;18(2):87–92.
47. Catalani S, Rizzetti MC, Padovani A, Apostoli P. Neurotoxicity of cobalt. *Hum Exp Toxicol*. 2012;31(5):421–437.

48. Xu R, Wu C, Zhang X, et al. Linking hypoxic and oxidative insults to cell death mechanisms in models of ALS. *Brain Res*. 2011;1372:133–144.
49. Dusek P, Roos PM, Litwin T, Schneider SA, Flaten TP, Aaseth J. The neurotoxicity of iron, copper and manganese in Parkinson's and Wilson's diseases. *J Trace Elem Med Biol*. 2015;31:193–203.
50. Brewer GJ. Copper toxicity in Alzheimer's disease: cognitive loss from ingestion of inorganic copper. *J Trace Elem Med Biology*. 2012;26(2–3):89–92.
51. Ibrahimagic OC, Sinanovic O, Zonic L, Hudic J. Amyotrophic lateral sclerosis in younger age associated with abnormality of copper level. *Med Arh*. 2006;60(2):108–109.
52. Wuolikainen A, Andersen PM, Moritz T, Marklund SL, Antti H. ALS patients with mutations in the SOD1 gene have an unique metabolomic profile in the cerebrospinal fluid compared with ALS patients without mutations. *Molecular Genet Metabol*. 2012;105(3):472–478.
53. Roberts BR, Lim NK, McAllum EJ, et al. Oral treatment with Cu(II)(atsm) increases mutant SOD1 in vivo but protects motor neurons and improves the phenotype of a transgenic mouse model of amyotrophic lateral sclerosis. *J Neurosci*. 2014;34(23):8021–8031.
54. Beritic T. Spinal origin of human lead neuropathy: this paper marks the 150th anniversary of Paralysie de Plomb ou Saturnine by L. Tanquerel des Planches. *Am J Ind Med*. 1989;15(6):643–656.
55. Preiskel D. Chronic lead poisoning: myopathy or neuritis. *Ann Phys Med*. 1958;4(8):293–296.
56. Planches Td. *Traités des Maladies de Plomb, ou Saturnites*. Paris: Ferra; 1839.
57. Meyer PA, Brown MJ, Falk H. Global approach to reducing lead exposure and poisoning. *Mutat Res*. 2008;659 (1–2):166–175.
58. Seppalainen AM, Hernberg S. Sensitive technique for detecting subclinical lead neuropathy. *Br J Ind Med*. 1972;29(4):443–449.
59. Buchthal F, Behse F. Electrophysiology and nerve biopsy in men exposed to lead. *Br J Ind Med*. 1979;36(2): 135–147.
60. Limonta A, Capellini A. Case of lead poisoning with polyneuritis of the upper limbs and involvement of the anterior horns of the pyramidal tract. *Med Lav*. 1976;67(1):37–42.
61. Grogan DP, Bucholz RW. Acute lead intoxication from a bullet in an intervertebral disc space. A case report. *J Bone Joint Surg Am*. 1981;63(7):1180–1182.
62. Oh SS, Kim EA, Lee SW, Kim MK, Kang SK. A case of amyotrophic lateral sclerosis in electronic parts manufacturing worker exposed to lead. *Neurotoxicology*. 2007;28(2):324–327.
63. Conradi S, Ronnevi LO, Vesterberg O. Increased plasma levels of lead in patients with amyotrophic lateral sclerosis compared with control subjects as determined by flameless atomic absorption spectrophotometry. *J Neurol Neurosurg Psychiatry*. 1978;41(5):389–393.
64. Fang F, Kwee LC, Allen KD, et al. Association between blood lead and the risk of amyotrophic lateral sclerosis. *Am J Epidemiol*. 2010;171(10):1126–1133.
65. Albers K, Nelson C, Tanner C, et al. Lead exposure and amyotrophic lateral sclerosis in a Northern California population [abstract]. *Neuroepidemiology*. 2009;33:74.
66. Kamel F, Umbach DM, Munsat TL, Shefner JM, Hu H, Sandler DP. Lead exposure and amyotrophic lateral sclerosis. *Epidemiology*. 2002;13(3):311–319.
67. Kamel F, Umbach DM, Hu H, et al. Lead exposure as a risk factor for amyotrophic lateral sclerosis. *Neurodegener Dis*. 2005;2(3–4):195–201.
68. Turabelidze G, Zhu BP, Schootman M, et al. An epidemiologic investigation of amyotrophic lateral sclerosis in Jefferson County, Missouri, 1998-2002. *Neurotoxicology*. 2008;29(1):81–86.
69. Guidetti D, Bondavalli M, Sabadini R, et al. Epidemiological survey of amyotrophic lateral sclerosis in the province of Reggio Emilia, Italy: influence of environmental exposure to lead. *Neuroepidemiology*. 1996;15(6):301–312.
70. Wang MD, Gomes J, Cashman NR, Little J, Krewski D. A meta-analysis of observational studies of the association between chronic occupational exposure to lead and amyotrophic lateral sclerosis. *J Occup Environ Med*. 2014;56(12):1235–1242.
71. Dobson AW, Erikson KM, Aschner M. Manganese neurotoxicity. *Ann N Y Acad Sci*. 2004;1012:115–128.
72. Aschner M, Erikson KM, Herrero Hernandez E, Tjalkens R. Manganese and its role in Parkinson's disease: from transport to neuropathology. *Neuromol Med*. 2009;11(4):252–266.
73. Couper J. On the effects of black oxide of manganese when inhaled into the lungs. *Br Ann Med Pharmacol*. 1837;1:41–42.

74. Sjögren B, Iregren A, Frech W, et al. Effects on the nervous system among welders exposed to aluminium and manganese. *Occup Environ Med.* 1996;53(1):32–40.
75. Ellingsen DG, Konstantinov R, Bast-Pettersen R, et al. A neurobehavioral study of current and former welders exposed to manganese. *Neurotoxicology.* 2008;29(1):48–59.
76. Kalia K, Jiang W, Zheng W. Manganese accumulates primarily in nuclei of cultured brain cells. *Neurotoxicology.* 2008;29(3):466–470.
77. Roos PM, Dencker L. Mercury in the spinal cord after inhalation of mercury. *Basic Clin Pharmacol Toxicol.* 2012;111(2):126–132.
78. Pamphlett R, Kum Jew S. Heavy metals in locus ceruleus and motor neurons in motor neuron disease. *Acta Neuropathol Commun.* 2013;1:81.
79. Johnson FO, Atchison WD. The role of environmental mercury, lead and pesticide exposure in development of amyotrophic lateral sclerosis. *Neurotoxicology.* 2009;30(5):761–765.
80. Schwarz S, Husstedt I, Bertram HP, Kuchelmeister K. Amyotrophic lateral sclerosis after accidental injection of mercury. *J Neurol Neurosurg Psychiatry.* 1996;60(6):698.
81. Brown IA. Chronic mercurialism; a cause of the clinical syndrome of amyotrophic lateral sclerosis. *AMA Arch Neurol Psychiatry.* 1954;72(6):674–681.
82. Kantarjian AD. A syndrome clinically resembling amyotrophic lateral sclerosis following chronic mercurialism. *Neurology.* 1961;11:639–644.
83. Adams CR, Ziegler DK, Lin JT. Mercury intoxication simulating amyotrophic lateral sclerosis. *JAMA.* 1983;250(5):642–643.
84. Barber TE. Inorganic mercury intoxication reminiscent of amyotrophic lateral sclerosis. *J Occup Med.* 1978;20(10): 667–669.
85. Praline J, Guennoc AM, Limousin N, Hallak H, de Toffol B, Corcia P. ALS and mercury intoxication: a relationship?. *Clin Neurol Neurosurg.* 2007;109(10):880–883.
86. Kumar A, Bhardwaj V, Tiwari JN, Patel DK, Singh DS, Singh RL, Kalita J, Misra UK, Babu GN. Mercury exposure in sporadic amyotrophic lateral sclerosis patients from Ganga plain region in India: a retrospective study. *Toxicol Environ Chem.* 2010;92(2):373–381.
87. Yang GQ, Wang SZ, Zhou RH, Sun SZ. Endemic selenium intoxication of humans in China. *Am J Clin Nutr.* 1983;37(5):872–881.
88. Raber M, Sydler T, Wolfisberg U, Geyer H, Burgi E. Feed-related selenium poisoning in swine. *Schweizer Archiv fur Tierheilkunde.* 2010;152(5):245–252.
89. Casteignau A, Fontan A, Morillo A, Oliveros JA, Segales J. Clinical, pathological and toxicological findings of a iatrogenic selenium toxicosis case in feeder pigs. *J Vet Med A.* 2006;53(6):323–326.
90. Kilness AW, Hichberg FH. Amyotrophic lateral sclerosis in a high selenium environment. *Jama.* 1977;237(26): 2843–2844.
91. Humann-Ziehank E, Ganter M, Michalke B. Selenium speciation in paired serum and cerebrospinal fluid samples of sheep. *J Trace Elem Med Biol.* 2016;33:14–20.
92. Morris KJ, Townsend KM, Batchelor AL. Studies of alveolar cell morphometry and mass clearance in the rat lung following inhalation of an enriched uranium dioxide aerosol. *Radiat Environ Biophys.* 1989;28(2):141–154.
93. Al-Shammari AM. Environmental pollutions associated to conflicts in Iraq and related health problems. *Rev Environ Health.* 2016;31(2):245–250.
94. Houpert P, Frelon S, Monleau M, Bussy C, Chazel V, Paquet F. Heterogeneous accumulation of uranium in the brain of rats. *Radiat Prot Dosimetry.* 2007;127(1–4):86–89.
95. Aschner M, Jiang GC. Toxicity studies on depleted uranium in primary rat cortical neurons and in *Caenorhabditis elegans*: what have we learned?. *J Toxicol Environ Health B Crit Rev.* 2009;12(7):525–539.
96. Afeseh Ngwa H, Kanthasamy A, Anantharam V, et al. Vanadium induces dopaminergic neurotoxicity via protein kinase Cdelta dependent oxidative signaling mechanisms: relevance to etiopathogenesis of Parkinson's disease. *Toxicol Appl Pharmacol.* 2009;240(2):273–285.
97. Frank A, Madej A, Galgan V, Petersson LR. Vanadium poisoning of cattle with basic slag. Concentrations in tissues from poisoned animals and from a reference, slaughterhouse material. *Sci Total Environ.* 1996;181(1):73–92.
98. Kumar N, Crum B, Petersen RC, Vernino SA, Ahlskog JE. Copper deficiency myelopathy. *Arch Neurol.* 2004;61(5):762–766.
99. Smith AP, Lee NM. Role of zinc in ALS. *Amyotroph Lateral Sc.* 2007;8(3):131–143.

100. Peters TL, Beard JD, Umbach DM, et al. Blood levels of trace metals and amyotrophic lateral sclerosis. *Neurotoxicology*. 2016;54:119–126.
101. Capdevila M, Atrian S. Metallothionein protein evolution: a miniassay. *J Biol Inorg Chem*. 2011;16(7):977–989.
102. Nordberg M. Metallothioneins: historical review and state of knowledge. *Talanta*. 1998;46(2):243–254.
103. Nordberg M, Nordberg GF. Toxicological aspects of metallothionein. *Cellular Mol Biol*. 2000;46(2):451–463.
104. Aschner M. Astrocyte metallothioneins (MTs) and their neuroprotective role. *Ann NY Acad Sci*. 1997;825: 334–347.
105. West AK, Hidalgo J, Eddins D, Levin ED, Aschner M. Metallothionein in the central nervous system: Roles in protection, regeneration and cognition. *Neurotoxicology*. 2008;29(3):489–503.
106. Hozumi I, Yamada M, Uchida Y, Ozawa K, Takahashi H, Inuzuka T. The expression of metallothioneins is diminished in the spinal cords of patients with sporadic ALS. *Amyotroph Lateral Sc*. 2008;9(5):294–298.
107. Melmed C, Krieger C. A cluster of amyotrophic lateral sclerosis. *Arch Neurol*. 1982;39(9):595–596.
108. Neilson S, Gunnarsson LG, Robinson I. Rising mortality from motor neurone disease in Sweden 1961–1990: the relative role of increased population life expectancy and environmental factors. *Acta Neurol Scand*. 1994;90(3):150–159.
109. Proctor SP, Feldman RG, Wolf PA, Brent B, Wartenberg D. A perceived cluster of amyotrophic lateral sclerosis cases in a Massachusetts community. *Neuroepidemiology*. 1992;11(4-6):277–281.
110. Sanders M. Clustering of amyotrophic lateral sclerosis. *Jama*. 1980;244(5):435.
111. Mitchell JD, Gatrell AC, Al-Hamad A, Davies RB, Batterby G. Geographical epidemiology of residence of patients with motor neuron disease in Lancashire and south Cumbria. *J Neurology Neurosurg Psychiatry*. 1998;65(6):842–847.
112. Mitchell JD, Gibson HN, Gatrell A. Amyotrophic lateral sclerosis in Lancashire and South Cumbria, England, 1976-1986. A geographical study. *Arch Neurology*. 1990;47(8):875–880.
113. Buckley J, Warlow C, Smith P, Hilton-Jones D, Irvine S, Tew JR. Motor neuron disease in England and Wales, 1959–1979. *J Neurol Neurosurg Psychiatry*. 1983;46(3):197–205.
114. Garruto RM, Yanagihara R. Contributions of isolated Pacific populations to understanding neurodegenerative diseases. *Folia Neuropathol*. 2009;47(2):149–170.
115. Mulder DW, Kurland LT. Motor neuron disease: epidemiologic studies. *Adv Exp Med Biol*. 1987;209:325–332.
116. Kihira T, Yoshida S, Komoto J, Wakayama I, Yase Y. Aluminum-induced model of motor neuron degeneration: subperineurial injection of aluminum in rabbits. *Neurotoxicology*. 1995;16(3):413–424.
117. Yase Y. The pathogenesis of amyotrophic lateral sclerosis. *Lancet*. 1972;2(7772):292–296.
118. Sabel CE, Boyle PJ, Loytonen M, et al. Spatial clustering of amyotrophic lateral sclerosis in Finland at place of birth and place of death. *Am J Epidemiol*. 2003;157(10):898–905.
119. Astrom M, Spiro B. Impact of isostatic uplift and ditching of sulfid sediments on the hydrochemistry of major and trace elements and sulfur isotope ratios in streams, western Finland. *Environ Sci Technol*. 2000;34:1182–1188.
120. Caller TA, Field NC, Chipman JW, Shi X, Harris BT, Stommel EW. Spatial clustering of amyotrophic lateral sclerosis and the potential role of BMAA. *Amyotroph Lateral Sc*. 2012;13(1):25–32.
121. Cronin S, Hardiman O, Traynor BJ. Ethnic variation in the incidence of ALS: a systematic review. *Neurology*. 2007;68(13):1002–1007.
122. Nicoletti A, Vasta R, Venti V, et al. The epidemiology of amyotrophic lateral sclerosis in the Mount Etna region: a possible pathogenic role of volcanogenic metals. *Eur J Neurol*. 2016;23(5):964–972.
123. Gunnarsson L-G, Bodin L. Systematiska kunskapsöversikter; 7. Epidemiologiskt påvisade samband mellan Amyotrofisk Lateral Skleros (ALS) och faktorer i arbetsmiljön. vol. 48. Gothenburg; 2014.
124. Poloni M, Micheli A, Facchetti D, Mai R, Ceriani F, Cattalini C. Conjugal amyotrophic lateral sclerosis: toxic clustering or change?. *Ital J Neurol Sci*. 1997;18(2):109–112.
125. Camu W, Cadilhac J, Billiard M. Conjugal amyotrophic lateral sclerosis: a report on two couples from southern France. *Neurology*. 1994;44(3 Pt 1):547–548.
126. Corcia P, Jafari-Schluep HF, Lardillier D, et al. A clustering of conjugal amyotrophic lateral sclerosis in southeastern France. *Arch Neurol*. 2003;60(4):553–557.
127. Godeiro Jr C, Oliveira AS, Felicio AC, Chieia MA, Gabbai AA. Conjugal amyotrophic lateral sclerosis in Brazil. *Arq Neuropsiquiatr*. 2009;67(4):1045–1048.
128. Dewitt JD, Kwon J, Burton R, Stroup JS. Conjugal amyotrophic lateral sclerosis. *Proc (Bayl Univ Med Cent)*. 2012;25(1):31–33.

129. Caller TA, Chipman JW, Field NC, Stommel EW. Spatial analysis of amyotrophic lateral sclerosis in Northern New England, USA, 1997–2009. *Muscle Nerve*. 2013;48(2):235–241.
130. Chio A, Herrero Hernandez E, Discalzi G, et al. Conjugal amyotrophic lateral sclerosis: suggestion for the implication of environmental factors. *Amyotroph Lateral Sc Other Motor Neuron Disord*. 2001;2(3):165–166.
131. Andersen PM. Mutation in C9orf72 changes the boundaries of ALS and FTD. *Lancet Neurol*. 2012;11(3):205–207.
132. Ingre C, Roos PM, Piehl F, Kamel F, Fang F. Risk factors for amyotrophic lateral sclerosis. *Clin Epidemiol*. 2015;7:181–193.
133. Rohrer JD, Isaacs AM, Mizielinska S, et al. C9orf72 expansions in frontotemporal dementia and amyotrophic lateral sclerosis. *Lancet Neurol*. 2015;14(3):291–301.
134. Neumann M, Sampathu DM, Kwong LK, et al. Ubiquitinated TDP-43 in frontotemporal lobar degeneration and amyotrophic lateral sclerosis. *Science*. 2006;314(5796):130–133.
135. Baldwin KR, Godena VK, Hewitt VL, Whitworth AJ. Axonal transport defects are a common phenotype in *Drosophila* models of ALS. *Hum Mol Genet*. 2016;25(12):2378–2392.
136. Kurtzke JF. Epidemiology of amyotrophic lateral sclerosis. *Adv Neurol*. 1982;36:281–302.
137. Ahmeti KB, Ajroud-Driss S, Al-Chalabi A, et al. Age of onset of amyotrophic lateral sclerosis is modulated by a locus on 1p34.1. *Neurobiol Aging*. 2013;34(1):357.

CHAPTER

11

Metals and Lysosomal Storage Disorders

Henna Konttinen, Katarína Lejavová, Tarja Malm, Katja M. Kanninen

A.I.Virtanen Institute for Molecular Sciences, University of Eastern Finland, Kuopio, Finland

OUTLINE

Biometals in Neurodegenerative Diseases. http://dx.doi.org/10.1016/B978-0-12-804562-6.00011-7

INTRODUCTION

Lysosomal storage diseases (LSDs) are a family of inherited metabolic disorders resulting in progressive accumulation of unmetabolized substrates into lysosomes.[1–4] LSDs include approximately 70 genetically distinct disorders and the combined incidence of these diseases is estimated to be approximately 1:5000 live births annually.[5,6] The majority of LSDs are caused by defects in autosomal recessive genes resulting in the loss of function of lysosomal enzymes or nonenzymatic proteins, and thus disruption of cellular homeostasis.[7,8] The age of clinical onset and manifestations among different LSDs vary depending on the gene mutation and residual function of the defective protein.[9–12] Many of the LSDs have been categorized into distinct subgroups according to the age of onset of symptoms, and the early onset LSDs are often the most aggressive in terms of the interval between diagnosis and death.[6,13,14] Altogether LSDs account for approximately 14% of all inherited metabolic diseases.

The LSDs are commonly classified into four subgroups based on the composition of the accumulating substrate. These subgroups include mucopolysaccharidoses, glycolipidoses, muclipidoses, and glycoproteinoises.[8] Despite the distinctive types of storage material in different LSDs, these disorders share many common biochemical, cellular, and clinical features. The accumulation of substrates activates a variety of pathogenic cascades including altered calcium homeostasis, oxidative stress, altered lipid trafficking, autophagy, endoplasmic reticulum stress, and inflammation.[7]

Several LSDs exhibit neuropathological manifestations even though most LSDs are characterized by inclusions in both the central nervous system (CNS) and periphery.[4] Nevertheless, since neurons are an extremely vulnerable cell type, they are particularly sensitive to intracellularly accumulated materials. Therefore neurodegeneration is a common hallmark of LSDs. This chapter will provide a brief overview of the common pathological features of LSDs and focus on aspects of three LSDs with prominent CNS manifestations and imbalance of biometals, namely Gaucher Disease (GD), Niemann Pick C (NPC), and the group of Neuronal Ceroid Lipofuscinoses (NCL) (Fig. 11.1).

COMMON PATHOLOGICAL FEATURES OF LYSOSOMAL STORAGE DISORDERS

Lysosomes are acidic, membrane bound cell organelles that play a central role in the clearance of cellular substrates and they are responsible for macromolecule degradation.[1] Lysosomes harbor over 60 enzymes responsible for lipid and protein degradation and recycling.[8] Compared to surrounding cytosol, the conditions in lysosomes are particularly acidic as a result of high proton and calcium concentration in lysosomes. In these acidic conditions certain enzymes become functional and lysosomes are highly enriched in particular hydrolytic enzymes, including proteases, glycosidases, nucleases, phosphatases, and lipases.[15–17] There are also certain transmembrane proteins that are especially abundant in lysosomes. The efflux permeases facilitate the inside-out translocation of small molecules generated through macromolecule catabolism.[1] Furthermore, lysosomes participate in multiple other processes required for cellular homeostasis,[4,18] such as phagocytosis, autophagy, apoptosis, signal transduction, exocytosis, and inflammatory responses.[2,8]

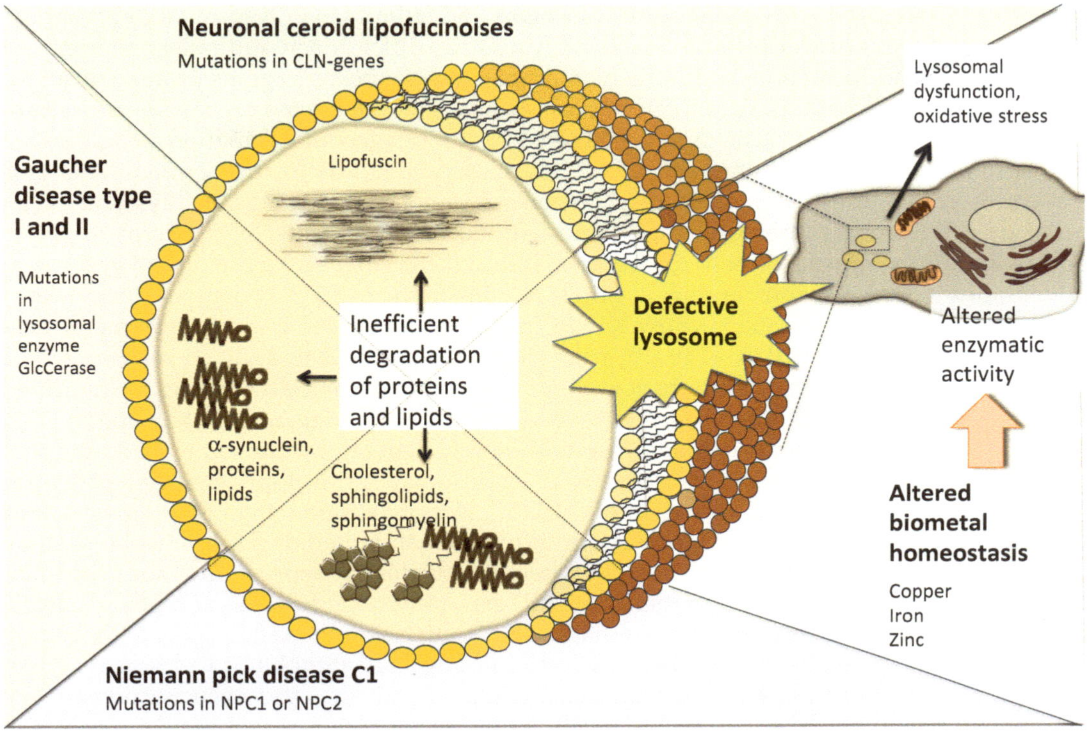

FIGURE 11.1 **Altered biometal homeostasis contributes to defects in lysosomal functions.** Lysosomal storage diseases (LSDs) are caused by mutations in genes influencing lysosomal enzymatic activity or packing of proteins, lipids, and other metabolic products into lysosomes. LSDs with clear neurodegenerative phenotype include neuronal ceroid lipofucinoises, Gaucher disease Type I and II, and Niemann Pick disease C1. Altered biometal homeostasis is implicated in all these diseases. Biometals, such as copper, iron, and zinc are required for proper lysosomal function. On the other hand, accumulation of biometals impairs lysosomal function. Both types of imbalance lead to defective lysosomes and neurodegeneration. *CLN*, ceroid lipofuscinosis; *GlcCerase*, glucosylceramidase; *Mcon1*, mucolipin1; *NPC*, Niemann Pick type C.

Endosomal–Autophagic–Lysosomal System

The lysosomal degradation of cellular material occurs in multiple locations within the endosomal–autophagic–lysosomal system.[1] Endosomes are membrane-bound compartments that are less acidic compared to lysosomes and they do not contain all the enzymes, or they have lower levels of membrane proteins, such as LAMP1 and LAMP2, that are highly abundant in lysosomes.[19] Lysosomes can be regarded as storage compartments for acidic hydrolases that enter transient fusion with late endosomes and autophagic vesicles that are called autophagosomes. After the fusion, the digestion process of endocytosed and autophagic substrates takes place primarily in endolysosomes[15,20–23] and autolysosomes[24–26] that are formed upon transient contacts or fusion with lysosomes.

Four distinct pathways of lysosomal degradation are recognized, namely macroautophagy, endosomal degradation, chaperone-mediated autophagy (CMA), and microautophagy.[1] All of these processes end with fusion with lysosomes and culminate in lysosomal degradation, albeit the pathways of substrates to reach the lysosomes differ. Macroautophagy begins with the induction and formation of double-membranes that sequester regions of the cytosol including denatured proteins, lipids, carbohydrates, and old or damaged organelles into encapsulated autophagosomes.[27] The dynamic kinetics of autophagosome formation and clearance by lysosomes is known as autophagic flux.[28,29] Endosomal degradation predominantly targets late endosomes or multivesicular bodies. Fusion between late endosomes and lysosomes can occur by full fusion or upon exchange of content via transient contact.[20–24] Microautophagy occurs without synthesis of new membranes through the direct invagination of lysosomal membranes that engulf surrounding cytosolic regions in the process known as pinocytosis.[30] CMA selectively targets proteins with a KFERQ motif for delivery to lysosomes using the heat shock cognate protein of 70 kD (Hsc-70) as its chaperone and LAMP-2A as its receptor.[31,32]

At the end of each cycle of endocytic or autophagic degradation the lysosomes are reformed from endolysosomes and autolysosomes by budding off, acidifying, and maturating to yield dense lysosomes that are available to fuse with newly generated endosomes and autophagosomes.[33] The biogenesis and functioning of endosomal and autophagosomal pathways is controlled by transcription factor EB (TFEB).[34,35] Autophagy-inducing conditions, such as deprivation of glucose or amino acids result in reduced and altered TFEB phosphorylation, leading to its translocation into the nucleus where it activates the expression of the coordinated lysosomal expression and regulation (CLEAR) gene network.[36] Recently it is being increasingly recognized that degradation is a remarkably selective process with respect to the nature of substrates degraded.[9] Accordingly, the selective endosomal–autophagic–lysosomal system is capable of sequestering specific organelles, oxidized proteins, and even portions of the cytosol by specific processes referred to as ERphagy,[37] mitophagy,[38] ribophagy[39] pexophagy,[40] and lipophagy,[41,42] respectively.

Lysosomal Dysfunction in LSDs

In LSDs numerous endolysosomes and autolysosomes are formed, and they contain excessive levels of undegraded macromolecules and monomeric substrates. Undegraded macromolecules accumulate due to enzyme deficiency, whereas monomeric catabolic products are often a result of deficiency in efflux permeases.[1] The accumulating material in LSDs consists mainly of glycolipids or glycoproteins that comprise the main structural components of cell membranes.[4,43] More specifically, storage material contains heterogeneous combinations of sphingolipids, phospholipids, or galactosylceramide, as well as proteins, depending on the disease variant. Changes in membrane lipid recycling or breakdown consequently lead to disruption of lysosomal membrane integrity, resulting in increased permeability. As a result, lysosomal contents, such as metabolites, hydrolases, and cathepsins are translocated into the cytosol and can be sensed as intracellular danger-associated molecular patterns (DAMPs) that are normally released from damaged or dying cells.[44] In addition to being components of cell membranes, these glycolipids and proteins can have a role in cellular trafficking, second messenger signaling, and cell–cell communication.

Accumulating molecules can be primary metabolites of genes that are defective in LSDs, however, in many LSDs the storage material consists of secondary metabolites, such as the gangliosides GM1 and GM3 and cholesterol, which are downstream products of genetic defects.[7,45–47] The accumulation of primary and secondary substrates sets off a cascade of events that impacts not only the endosomal–autophagic–lysosomal system, but also other organelles, including mitochondria, the ER, Golgi, peroxisomes, and overall cell function, leading to disruptions in such central cellular processes as myelin production, molecular transport systems, apoptosis, and immune system activation.[8]

Neuroinflammation

Neurodegeneration and neuroinflammation are overarching themes in the majority of the LSDs and are in most cases central for the clinical progression and devastating consequences of these diseases.[4,6,48,49] Generally neuroinflammation is elicited as a protective response to CNS injury, infection, or disease via sensing pathogen-associated molecular patterns (PAMPs) or DAMPs, latter of which are released from damaged or dying cells.[44] However, intensified or chronic inflammation as seen in several LSDs can exert detrimental effects on neural cells by creating a neurotoxic environment due to elevated levels of cytokines, chemokines, and proapoptotic molecules.[4] As a result of differences in storage material, the levels of metabolites and susceptibilities between affected neuronal subtypes, the manifestations of neurodegeneration and inflammation occur in certain brain regions depending on the type of LSD.[1,7] However, even if the triggers or brain regions affected by inflammation in LSDs may be different, the activation of the innate immune system is a seemingly universal result of lysosomal storage.

The most conspicuous feature of inflammation in the CNS is the activation of specific glial cell populations, such as microglia and astrocytes that aim to swiftly remove the insult and downregulate unnecessary damage to extremely vulnerable neurons and other brain cells.[6,50] Microglia are the principal inflammatory cells in the CNS and they constantly survey the tissue for stress signals, provide trophic support for other cells, and phagocytose cellular debris.[51,52] Activated microglia are a major source of chemokines and cytokines that serve to recruit and activate peripheral immune cells.[53] Astrocytes are the most abundant cell type in the brain and they function to provide neurotrophic support and synchronize neurotransmitter metabolism.[54,55] Reactive astrocytes also produce chemokines as well as reactive oxygen/nitrogen species and various other toxic molecules. In addition, over-activated astrocytes affect disruptively to glutamate homeostasis pathways and neurotransmitter regulation.[51,56,57] In LSDs both microglia and astrocytes display an altered phenotype, yet it remains unclear whether the activation of glia is protective or detrimental during the disease progression.[6,51,58–62]

Calcium Homeostasis, ER Stress, and Oxidative Stress in LSDs

Disrupted calcium signaling has emerged as a common feature in LSDs, however, the mechanism for defective calcium homeostasis is different for each LSD.[63] For example, calcium release from the ER can be upregulated in one LSD, whereas in another disease type, calcium uptake is hightened.[64,65] Disruptions in mitochondrial calcium homeostasis and associated activation of the mitochondrial apoptotic pathway have also been implicated in some forms of LSDs.[66] Moreover, lysosomal calcium levels have been shown to be reduced in response to sphingosine accumulation, resulting in defective endocytic fusion and trafficking subsequently leading to the induction of secondary metabolite accumulation.[67]

The unfolded protein response (UPR) may also be involved in pathology of LSDs, since it is often a result of altered calcium homeostasis. Moreover, UPR can occur in response to changes in the ER environment pathway, such as depletion of ER calcium stores.[7] In healthy conditions secretory and transmembrane proteins undergo posttranslational modifications after folding into their native conformations in the ER, however, in case these functions are impaired, misfolded proteins accumulate in the ER lumen and activate the UPR, which can initiate apoptosis. Even though the activation of the UPR has been suggested to be a common mediator of apoptosis in LSDs, there are some systematic studies that found no evidence for UPR activation in certain LSD forms.[61,68–70]

Reactive oxygen species (ROS) have been suggested to play a pivotal role and to be common mediators of cell death in many LSDs.[68] Furthermore, oxidative imbalance has been detected in several LSDs and enhanced oxidative stress, elevated ROS, and lipid peroxidation are known to render the LSD cells, such as fibroblasts, microglia, macrophages, and endothelial cells, more susceptible to cell death after an acute oxidative insult.[58,71–74] In some of the LSDs key enzymes involved in oxidative stress, such as superoxide dismutase, manganese-dependent superoxide dismutase, or 4-hydroxynonenal, are increased.[70,75,76] Since oxidative stress plays a central role in integrating other cellular pathways that are closely related to primary defects in many LSDs, it is suggested that oxidative stress is most likely enhanced in LSDs as a secondary biochemical pathway. Given that oxidative stress plays a central role in other, more studied neurodegenerative conditions, with further studies it may provide real significance in delineating LSD pathology.

DESCRIPTION OF MOST COMMON NEURODEGENERATIVE LSDS ASSOCIATED WITH BIOMETAL IMBALANCE

Gaucher Disease Type II and III

Gaucher disease (GD) is the most common LSD with an incidence of 1:50,000 live births annually.[77] There are three age-dependent clinical forms, including Type I with no neurological symptoms, the extremely rare Type II with acute neuropathology and a life expectancy of 2–4 years, and Type III with similar chronic neurological abnormalities as in Type 2 but a later onset during young adolescence.[77,78] The underlying causes of all forms are mutations in the lysosomal enzyme glucosylceramidase (GlcCerase), also known as glucocerebrosidase.[79] A reduction or complete loss of enzymatic activity causes the accumulation of glucosylceramide (GlcCer) in cells, however, the relationship between GlcCer accumulation and progression of neuropathology in GD is not completely understood.[77] Furthermore, research into the mechanism of lysosomal dysfunction in GDs has been impeded due to a lack of appropriate cellular models that display the storage phenotype observed in patients.[80] Moreover, GD is a phenotypically heterogeneous disease with more than 300 known mutations and limited correlation between genotype and phenotype.

The disease pathology in Types II and III displays many common features with other LSDs and these characteristics have been seen in GD patients as well as in transgenic animal models in vivo and in patient-specific induced pluripotent stem cells (iPSCs) in vitro.[29,81–83] The common pathologies include neuronal death and increased amount of lysosomal inclusions accompanied by accumulation of lipids, protein aggregates, insoluble α-synuclein, and autophagic substrates, such as p62. In addition, TFEB, the master regulator of lysosomal genes, is downregulated and there is reduction in lysosomal gene expression and in activity of the lysosomal enzymes cathepsins B and D. These pathologies are associated with defective mitophagy in neurons and astrocytes, a block in autophagic flux and impaired autophagosome maturation in neuronal cells, as well as enhanced cytokine production in microglia.

Enzyme replacement therapy (ERT) using recombinant versions of GlcCerase have been the base of treatment of GC patients suffering from type I for more than 20 years.[84–87] There are no treatments available for Gaucher disease type II. Recombinant human acid β-glycosidase (imiglucerase) has been shown to revert many of the disease phenotypes.[88] Two recent 36-month follow up studies report that taliglucerase alfa (Elelyso) treatment improves disease parameters, such as reduction in the volume of spleen and liver and chitotrosidase activity in Gaucher disease patients with no safety concerns.[89,90] Taliglucerase alfa is commercially known as Elelyso and is a recombinant glucocerebrosidase developed by Protalix and Pfizer. Also, a similar recombinant enzyme called velaglucerase alfa has been tested in clinical trials.[91] As an alternative to ERT, promising results have been achieved with the substrate reduction therapy in phase 1 and 2 clinical trials by blocking the activity of glucosylceramide synthase, the enzyme which catalyzes the production of glucosylceramide.[92,93] ERT is extremely expensive and recombinant GlcCerase versions are enable to cross the blood–brain barrier.[94] Thus, new therapies are urgently needed.

Niemann Pick Type C1

NPC disease is an autosomal recessive neurodegenerative LSD occurring at a frequency of 1:120,000 live births.[4,14,67] Characteristic symptoms are cerebellar ataxia caused by selective loss of Purkinje neurons, dementia associated with neurofibrillary tangles and Lewy bodies, cognitive decline, epilepsy, vertical gaze palsy, respiratory dysfunction, and premature death.[95] There are four age-dependent variants including infantile, late infantile, juvenile, and adult variants.[14]

NPC disease is caused by either a mutation in the *NPC1* (95% incidence), or the *NPC2* (5% incidence) gene, and mutations in both genes lead to an identical disease phenotype characterized by lysosomal accumulation of multiple lipids, namely sphingosine, glycosphingolipids, cholesterol, and sphingomyelin.[96] *NPC1* encodes a lysosomal/endosomal transmembrane protein the function of which is unknown.[97–99] In turn, *NPC2* encodes a soluble mannose-6-phosphorylated lysosomal transport protein that is capable of transporting cholesterol.[100] Both NPC1 and NPC2 are essential for the intracellular trafficking and processing of cholesterol and other lipids.[59,101] Because the proportion of cholesterol is clearly highest of the storage materials, NPC disease has been termed a cholesterol storage disease.[102] Still interestingly, in the brain the sphingolipids are the major storage lipid of this neurodegenerative disease.[99] Accumulation of multiple lipid substrates may be explained by a block in recycling and transport of lipids out of the endolysosomal system,[103] since a profound block in endocytosis and vesicular fusion between late endosomes and lysosomes is a classical feature of NPC disease cells.[17] Even though some functions of mutated genes are known, the pathogenic mechanisms responsible for NPC disease remain to be identified.

There are no curable therapies for NPCs. A partial and reversible inhibitor of glucosylceramide synthase, an early enzyme in the glycosphingolipid pathway called Miglustat, is approved for the treatment of NPC.[104] Although Miglustat has a capacity to modestly delay the progression of NPC in a subpopulation of patients, it fails to prevent the intracellular cholesterol accumulation.[105]

Neuronal Ceroid Lipofuscinosis or Batten Disease

NCL is a diverse group of genetically distinct neurodegenerative LSDs caused by a mutation in one of 14 different ceroid lipofuscinosis (CLN) genes.[62,106] Even though the specific sequence of the symptoms varies between the variants, all the forms share similar symptoms that include visual deterioration, neurocognitive and physical retardation, seizures, dementia, and premature death.[107–111] Previously NCLs were classified according to the age of onset to early infantile (INCL, Santavuori-Haltia disease), late infantile (LINCL, Jansky-Bielschowsky), juvenile (JNCL, Batten disease), and adult (Kufs disease) forms, but the new classification is based on gene mutations that are mostly autosomal recessively inherited.[112,113] NCLs have been estimated to occur in 1 out of every 100,000 of live births per year.[107,114]

NCLs exhibit abnormal accumulation of lysosomal storage material that consist mostly of autofluorescent lipofuscin, lipopigments made up of fats and proteins.[62,108] However, also other molecules, such as sphingolipids and mitochondrial ATP synthase subunit c are present, suggesting defective mitochondrial turnover.[115] Some of the proteins encoded by CLN genes are known, for example, CLN1 and CLN2 encode for the lysosomal enzymes PPT-1 and TPP-1, and the most common form of NCL is caused by mutations in CLN3 gene encoding an endosomal-lysosomal membrane protein called battenin.[116–118] Nevertheless, other variants caused by mutations in genes, such as CLN5 and CLN6 remain elusive. In any case, many of the NCL-related mutations result in either a loss in lysosomal enzymes, lysosomal transmembrane proteins, or synaptic vesicle-associated proteins.[62]

There is currently no cure for any of the NCLs and treatments are based on alleviating clinical symptoms caused by neurodegeneration. A recent study showed beneficial effects of anti-inflammatory treatments, suggesting that neuroinflammation plays a prominent role in NCL pathogenesis.[119,120] Gene replacement therapy has also been demonstrated in CLN2 animal models, but in clinical trials the improvement has not been significant.[121,122] Interestingly, the abnormal accumulation of mitochondrial ATP synthase subunit C and lipofuscin were shown to be reduced in CLN3 cell models by treatment of autophagy enhancers, such as lithium and inositol monophophatase inhibitors.[123] These findings point out the urgent need for a deeper understanding of the defective lysosomal mechanisms and therapeutic applications in NCLs.

FUNCTION AND REGULATION OF BIOMETALS

The first row transition metals copper, zinc, and iron, have critical roles in multiple cellular functions that are crucial for development and survival. The body utilizes biometals for general metabolic as well as more specific functions. Biometals act as cofactors for thousands of proteins and through transcription factor activity are involved in central biochemical processes, such as regulation of gene expression, cell cycle, apoptosis, antioxidative protection, and immunoregulation.[124] Furthermore, biometals also serve a structural role in a number of important proteins.

In physiological conditions, biometal levels are tightly regulated. Control of cellular uptake, storage, and export of biometals are tightly regulated not only to ensure sufficient biometal supply, but also to prevent metal-induced toxicity and oxidative stress. Because biometals are impermeable through diffusion at the cell membrane, maintaining stable biometal levels occurs at several levels through the action of metal transporter and metal storage/buffering proteins. Specific transporter proteins regulate biometal movement across the cell membrane, while others are essential for transport in and out of organelles. For example, there are two major zinc transporter families: the ZIP/SLC39 family of transporters are predominantly present on the cell membrane and control the movement of zinc into the cytoplasm, while the ZnT/SLC30 family members act in the efflux of zinc ions from the cell and are also involved in intracellular organelle zinc uptake.[125,126] Certain transporters, such as ZIP8, exist on the lysosomal membrane and are involved in the movement of metals in and out of the lysosome.[127] In the cytoplasm, metal ions are often bound to buffering proteins, such as the metallothioneins,[126] other ligands of low molecular mass, such as glutathione, or chaperones, such as the copper chaperone for superoxide dismutase (CCS).[128]

Biometals in CNS

Biometals can enter the brain via two routes, through the brain-cerebrospinal fluid barrier, or the blood-brain barrier (BBB). Biometals transverse the BBB as free ions, through specific transporters, or in complex with amino acids, such as cysteine.[129,130] In the brain, the metals are predominantly distributed in membrane-bound metalloproteins, and in synaptic vesicles.[131] Typically their concentrations vary by brain region[132] and subcellular localization.

In the brain astrocytes are considered as an important cell type regulating homeostasis of biometals.[128,133,134] It is believed that astrocytes are central for brain biometal regulation because of their location: they are the first cell type to contact biometals upon their entry through the BBB. Astrocytes also contain high levels of metal binding proteins, such as the metallothioneins and glutathione, endowing them with the ability to store metals and prevent their potential toxicity. Astrocytes are also reported to take up copper more efficiently than cultured neurons.[135]

The importance of biometals and stringent control of their homeostasis have been extensively documented. For example, proper brain development requires rigorous control of copper homeostasis,[136] as its deficiency leads to brain abnormalities and defects in development. The roles of copper and zinc in neurotransmission have also been the subject of intensive research. Increasing evidence points to a role of these biometals as CNS signaling molecules.[137] Furthermore, biometals affect both long term potentiation and receptor pharmacology at synapses.[138] As described later in this chapter, disturbances of biometal homeostasis are implicated in various disorders affecting the CNS.

Biometals in Lysosomes

The lysosome contains biometals including iron and copper, which are liberated by autophagic degradation of metalloproteins, such as the iron-containing ferritin or copper-containing superoxide dismutase. In addition, several classes of metal transporters, which export and import biometals in the lysosomes, traverse the lysosomal membrane, and are essential in maintaining both lysosomal and cellular biometal homeostasis.

The accumulation of biometals in lysosomes has been shown to lead to pathological events including lysosomal membrane permeabilization (LMP), release of lysosomal enzymes into the cytoplasm, and cell death.[139,140] However, biometals also have a physiological role in the lysosomes. For example, some lysosomal proteins, such as the lysosomal enzyme lysosomal acid sphingomyelinase, require metals in order to gain full functionality.[141] Furthermore, lysosomes have been proposed to act as biometal sinks, which absorb metals from the cytoplasm. This is exemplified by a recent report demonstrating that the absorption of zinc into lysosomes, followed by its secretion, is an important and beneficial cellular detoxification mechanism.[142]

The acidic environment of the lysosome keeps iron in a reduced, redox-active form, thereby allowing its reaction with hydrogen peroxide and subsequent generation of intralysosomal Fenton reactions. These reactions may result in the formation of lipofuscin, which is commonly observed in NCL and during aging.[143] Lipofuscin accumulation compromises the capacity of autophagic degradation, which may lead to deleterious consequences for the cell. Because lysosomal damage can be induced by iron-dependent oxidative stress, keeping the lysosomal redox-active iron levels as low as possible is thought to be important for cellular survival.[144] Conversely, lysosomal damage is also induced by iron depletion, demonstrating that a delicate balance exists between the levels of biometals in the lysosomes.

In contrast to iron, lysosomal copper is not redox active due to complex formation with thiol-containing molecules, such as glutathione. Recently the copper transport protein ATP7B was reported to play a critical part in cellular copper homeostasis in the liver.[145] An increased copper concentration induces the trafficking of this transporter from the trans Golgi network to a subset of lysosomes, in which ATP7B imports copper for lysosomal storage, activates lysosomal exocytosis and stimulates the excretion of copper into the bile. Therefore, ATP7B-containing lysosomes are a key component of copper homeostasis. Furthermore, the neuroprotective copper delivery agent CuII(atsm) is targeted to lysosomes, suggesting that the lysosome is a central organelle that also mediates the beneficial effects of metal homeostasis maintaining complexes.[146,147]

A growing amount of evidence supports the importance of zinc in the proper functioning of lysosomes.[148] Zinc regulates both basal and induced autophagy positively through a mechanism that is not yet fully understood, but the ERK1/2 signaling pathway and certain microRNAs appear to be involved. Under basal conditions the levels of lysosomal zinc are low, but these rise rapidly in response to various stressors, such as hydrogen peroxide.[149] A proportion of the zinc-laden lysosomes undergo membrane disintegration, resulting in intracellular release of lysosomal contents and eventual cell death. As is the case with iron, a reduced zinc level is harmful for the cell. Zinc deficiency results in the accumulation of lysosomal lipofuscin[150] and disrupts the integrity of the organelle.[151] Recent evidence demonstrates that lysosome disruption caused by intracellular zinc depletion occurs independently of ROS generation.[152]

Loss of Biometal Homeostasis is Connected to Disease

Aberrant biometal metabolism is a key feature of several diseases. When homeostatic control of biometal metabolism fails during aging or disease, the biometal mislocalization or altered homeostasis can drive a vast variety of pathological changes. Stringent regulation is critical to prevent both biometal deficiency and metal-induced toxicity.

The best-described examples of pathological conditions with a connection to impaired biometal homeostasis involve copper. Menkes disease is a rare inherited disorder of intestinal copper absorption leading to copper deficiency that has a severe neurodegenerative component.[153] Wilson's disease is an inherited copper-accumulating disorder caused by defects in a copper transporter protein that is also associated with neurological symptoms and pathology.[154–156] As highlighted by these inherited diseases involving copper dyshomeostasis, the altered function, caused by mutations or expression changes, of metal transporter proteins are implicated in several diseases. Transporter deficiency causes an imbalance in the trafficking, influx or export of biometals, ultimately leading to either an overload or deficiency in cellular biometal concentrations.

Cellular biometal dyshomeostasis is also linked to several human pathologies, for which a biometal-related genetic component has yet to be identified. These include developmental abnormalities, diabetes, gastrointestinal diseases, cardiovascular diseases, anemia, cancer, liver diseases, and diseases associated with impaired immune function.[157–159] Alterations of biometal homeostasis are also associated with neurodegenerative diseases, such as Alzheimer's, Huntington's, and Parkinson's diseases,[160] yet the exact causes and consequences of these alterations remain incompletely understood. As described later in this chapter, emerging evidence demonstrates the contribution of biometal alterations to LSDs.

ROLE OF BIOMETALS AND BIOMETAL BINDING PROTEINS IN LSDS

As it was mentioned earlier, biometals, such as iron, copper, and zinc play a pivotal role in mammalian metabolism. Several studies indicate that dysregulation of biometal homeostasis and lysosomal dysfunction lead to the development of neurodegenerative disorders, yet the role of biometals in LSDs has only recently started to become unraveled.[161]

LSDs and Iron Homeostasis

Iron is a crucial metal for the correct running of metabolic processes in cells. Iron homeostasis is tightly coordinated by two regulatory mechanisms. On the hormonal level it is regulated by hormone hepcidin and on cellular level via iron-regulatory proteins, which are involved in transport, influx, and storage in tissues.[162] Disruption of these two mechanisms leads to either iron overload or iron deficiency. Current experimental evidence for iron imbalance in LSDs is limited. Altered iron homeostasis has, however, been described in three types of LSDs with different pathology, including GD[163] and NPC disease.[164]

Accumulation of iron in redox-active form in lysosomes and hyperferritinemia are implicated in pathogenesis of GD. Ferritin is an iron-binding protein that protects cells from iron-mediated oxidative stress [164a]. Serum ferritin is reported to be elevated in GD patients.[165] The main reason for ferritin overload is the pathological abundant concentration of glucosylceramide in macrophages. This triggers constant, mild inflammation, which results in ferritin sequestering and thus iron accumulation in macrophages.[166] Increased levels of inflammatory cytokines force upregulation of hepcidin transcription, which in turn contributes to intracellular iron trapping.[167] All these mechanisms facilitate disruption of iron homeostasis that can lead to development of pathologies frequently associated with GD.

Altered iron homeostasis has been reported in both patients and the murine model of NPC disease, the NPC1-/- mice. A mutation in the *Npc1* gene, which encodes lysosomal transmembrane protein leads to liver dysfunction and progressive neurodegeneration in 95% of NPC cases.[104,168–170] Patient fibroblasts have increased expression of metalloproteins involved in iron metabolism,[72] ferritin immunoreactivity is reduced in several tissues of human patients,[171] and the CSF of patients is deficient in iron.[172] A recent report by Hung and coworkers[172] demonstrated that iron levels were reduced in the livers and spleens of NPC1-/- mice. This finding of reduced liver iron content has also been demonstrated previously.[173] Interestingly, the iron in the brains of NPC1-/- mice is moderately increased.[172] Taken together, these results indicate a critical role for NPC1 in the regulation of iron metabolism.

The NCLs are a group of fatal diseases with mutations in at least 14 genes causing various forms of the disease.[174] Little information exists on the role of iron in NCLs. Early reports have described changes to iron levels in blood cells of NCL patients.[175] However, we recently reported significant accumulation of iron in the brain and spinal cords of both murine and sheep NCL animal models.[176,177] Importantly, biometal accumulation preceded significant neurodegeneration in the NCL mice, indicating that biometal accumulation does not occur as a result of neurodegenerative processes, but occurs early in the disease progression.

LSDs and Copper Homeostasis

Copper is an essential cofactor of various enzymes important in neurological functions.[178] However, copper homeostasis has to be tightly regulated, because increased levels may generate free radicals and contribute to oxidative stress.[179] Liver is the primary organ for storage, distribution, and excretion of copper in mammalians. In cells, copper homeostasis is regulated by copper transporting ATPases (ATP7A and ATP7B), which mediate incorporation of copper into ferroxidase enzyme ceruloplasmin (major plasmatic copper carrying protein).[180] Ceruloplasmin is also involved in iron metabolism.[181] Another important protein in copper homeostasis is the copper transport protein CTR1.[182]

Regarding the LSDs on which this chapter focuses, copper dyshomeostasis has mainly been described in NPC disease and in NCLs, although serum copper levels are reported to be reduced in GD patients.[183] Increased serum free copper with low ceruloplasmin has been reported in NPC patients,[184] while the CSF of patients is deficient in copper.[172] In addition, high copper levels are observed in the livers and plasma of NPC1-/- mice.[185] These findings are in line with increased ceruloplasmin, metallothionein 1, and transferring receptor gene expression and, reduced gene expression of Commd1, ferritin-light chain, and ferroportin in the livers of these mice.[173] Recently it was shown that the brains of NPC1-/- mice are actually deficient in copper.[172] Interestingly, copper trafficking is altered due to impaired function of ATP7B in NPC hepatic cells. Disruption of the late endosome to the trans-Golgi network leads to impaired copper excretion in NPC hepatic cells suggesting that correct function of ATP7B depends on NPC1 function.[186] Therefore, NPC1 has an important role in copper metabolism and this biometal may be implicated in the pathophysiology of NPC disease.[173]

Copper homeostasis has been studied in various animal models of NCLs. Increased copper concentrations are found in the brain and liver in CLN6-deficient sheep.[177] The expression levels of some biometal transporters were also altered between the control group and the CLN6 sheep. As mentioned earlier, metallothionein was upregulated in the CLN6-deficient sheep at the age of 14 months.[177] Moreover, we have reported similar copper accumulation in CLN6-deficient mouse brains[176] and in a further three NCL mouse models representing CLN1, CLN3, and CLN5 variants. Based on these experimental evidences, copper dyshomeostasis is an important pathological hallmark manifesting in at least four forms of NCLs.

LSDs and Zinc Homeostasis

Zinc is an essential micronutrient in mammals and its dyshomeostasis leads to a number of pathological changes in the human body.[142] Zinc alterations have been reported in the NCLs and in NPC disease, yet little is known about zinc homeostasis in GD. Zinc serum levels have been shown to be reduced in the serum of GD patients,[183] but it remains unknown whether the tissue levels of this biometal are altered during the disease.

Skin fibroblast cells of NPC disease patients have upregulated expression of the zinc transporter Zip2.[72] In the NPC1-/- mouse model, the concentration of zinc is increased in the brain and reduced in the liver and lung.[172] Plasma zinc levels were elevated in presymptomatic mice. Interestingly, brain zinc concentrations were also significantly increased in patients while the CSF and plasma samples were deficient in zinc. These results suggest the failure of zinc homeostasis in both the mouse model and in patients suffering from NPC disease.

Both blood and tissue zinc concentrations are altered in NCLs. Zinc levels are changed in patient blood cells.[175] Elevations in zinc concentration are observed in the CLN6 ovine brain at the age of symptom onset.[176] The expression of the metal-binding protein metallothionein is also robustly increased in the brains of these animals. Zinc accumulation also occurs in the CNS and peripheral tissues of CLN6-deficient mice,[176] and the brain and plasma of preclinical CLN6-deficient sheep.[177] The biometal alterations are related to loss of the metal transporter Zip7, which triggers metal accumulation in CLN6 disease.

TARGETING METALS TO TREAT DISEASE

Various therapeutic approaches for modulating biometal homeostasis have been described.[160] Therapeutic compounds can either target cellular metal deficiency, sequestration, or changes in metal distribution. Metal chelators are perhaps the most well described therapeutics that have been used to counteract increased metal levels in diseases associated with biometal overload, such as Wilson's disease.[156] An important issue to keep in mind is that the chelators remove metal from the cell. Given the importance of biometals in central cellular processes, total removal of metal can have detrimental effects. With this view in mind, metal complexes, which redistribute mislocalized metals have been developed and shown to be effective in several disorders affecting the CNS.[160]

Metal modulating compounds are promising therapeutics for CNS diseases of aberrant biometal metabolism. Metal protein attenuating compounds like clioquinol and PBT2 are blood brain barrier permeant, can bind metals attached to protein aggregates, and redistribute metals to other compartments. These compounds are beneficial in preclinical models through various mechanisms of action, including induction of neuroprotective signaling pathways.[187] We, and others, have also shown that delivery of bioavailable copper with bis(thiosemicarbazone) complexes (in the absence of chelation) is protective in multiple preclinical models of neurodegeneration.[188,189]

Understanding the exact ways in which biometal homeostasis is perturbed in each disorder of interest is the key to discovering novel therapeutics. It is also immensely important to understand the functions of specific cell types in biometal homeostasis to target new therapies to the correct location. This knowledge will hopefully in the future lead to more effective therapies for disorders of biometal mismetabolism.

References

1. Platt FM, Boland B, van der Spoel AC. The cell biology of disease: lysosomal storage disorders: the cellular impact of lysosomal dysfunction. *J Cell Biol*. 2012;199(5):723–734.
2. Boustany RM. Lysosomal storage diseases—the horizon expands. *Nat Rev Neurol*. 2013;9(10):583–598.
3. Platt FM. Sphingolipid lysosomal storage disorders. *Nature*. 2014;510(7503):68–75.
4. Bosch ME, Kielian T. Neuroinflammatory paradigms in lysosomal storage diseases. *Front Neurosci*. 2015;9:417.
5. Fuller M, Meikle PJ, Hopwood JJ. Epidemiology of lysosomal storage diseases: an overview. In: Mehta A, Beck M, Sunder-Plassmann G, eds. *Fabry Disease: Perspectives from 5 years of FOS*. Oxford: Oxford PharmaGenesis; 2006:NBK11603 [bookaccession].
6. Vitner EB, Futerman AH, Platt N. Innate immune responses in the brain of sphingolipid lysosomal storage diseases. *Biol Chem*. 2015;396(6–7):659–667.
7. Vitner EB, Platt FM, Futerman AH. Common and uncommon pathogenic cascades in lysosomal storage diseases. *J Biol Chem*. 2010;285(27):20423–20427.
8. Alroy J, Garganta C, Wiederschain G. Secondary biochemical and morphological consequences in lysosomal storage diseases. *Biochemistry*. 2014;79(7):619–636.
9. Ward C, Martinez-Lopez N, Otten EG, et al. Autophagy, lipophagy and lysosomal lipid storage disorders. *Biochim Biophys Acta*. 2016;1861(4):269–284.
10. Spada M, Pagliardini S, Yasuda M, et al. High incidence of later-onset fabry disease revealed by newborn screening. *Am J Hum Genet*. 2006;79(1):31–40.
11. Nixon RA, Yang DS, Lee JH. Neurodegenerative lysosomal disorders: a continuum from development to late age. *Autophagy*. 2008;4(5):590–599.
12. Shapiro BE, Logigian EL, Kolodny EH, Pastores GM. Late-onset tay-sachs disease: the spectrum of peripheral neuropathy in 30 affected patients. *Muscle Nerve*. 2008;38(2):1012–1015.
13. Dolisca SB, Mehta M, Pearce DA, Mink JW, Maria BL. Batten disease: clinical aspects, molecular mechanisms, translational science, and future directions. *J Child Neurol*. 2013;28(9):1074–1100.
14. Alobaidy H. Recent advances in the diagnosis and treatment of Niemann-Pick disease type C in children: a guide to early diagnosis for the general pediatrician. *Int J Pediatr*. 2015;2015:816593.
15. Luzio JP, Pryor PR, Bright NA. Lysosomes: fusion and function. *Nat Rev Mol Cell Biol*. 2007;8(8):622–632.
16. Saftig P, Klumperman J. Lysosome biogenesis and lysosomal membrane proteins: trafficking meets function. *Nat Rev Mol Cell Biol*. 2009;10(9):623–635.
17. Morgan AJ, Platt FM, Lloyd-Evans E, Galione A. Molecular mechanisms of endolysosomal Ca2+ signalling in health and disease. *Biochem J*. 2011;439(3):349–374.
18. Appelqvist H, Waster P, Kagedal K, Ollinger K. The lysosome: from waste bag to potential therapeutic target. *J Mol Cell Biol*. 2013;5(4):214–226.
19. De Duve C, Wattiaux R. Functions of lysosomes. *Annu Rev Physiol*. 1966;28:435–492.
20. Tjelle TE, Brech A, Juvet LK, Griffiths G, Berg T. Isolation and characterization of early endosomes, late endosomes and terminal lysosomes: their role in protein degradation. *J Cell Sci*. 1996;109(Pt 12):2905–2914.
21. Bright NA, Reaves BJ, Mullock BM, Luzio JP. Dense core lysosomes can fuse with late endosomes and are reformed from the resultant hybrid organelles. *J Cell Sci*. 1997;110(Pt 17):2027–2040.
22. Bright NA, Gratian MJ, Luzio JP. Endocytic delivery to lysosomes mediated by concurrent fusion and kissing events in living cells. *Curr Biol*. 2005;15(4):360–365.

23. Mullock BM, Bright NA, Fearon CW, Gray SR, Luzio JP. Fusion of lysosomes with late endosomes produces a hybrid organelle of intermediate density and is NSF dependent. *J Cell Biol*. 1998;140(3):591–601.
24. Jahreiss L, Menzies FM, Rubinsztein DC. The itinerary of autophagosomes: from peripheral formation to kiss-and-run fusion with lysosomes. *Traffic*. 2008;9(4):574–587.
25. Fader CM, Colombo MI. Autophagy and multivesicular bodies: two closely related partners. *Cell Death Differ*. 2009;16(1):70–78.
26. Orsi A, Polson HE, Tooze SA. Membrane trafficking events that partake in autophagy. *Curr Opin Cell Biol*. 2010;22(2):150–156.
27. Mizushima N, Komatsu M. Autophagy: renovation of cells and tissues. *Cell*. 2011;147(4):728–741.
28. Ballabio A, Gieselmann V. Lysosomal disorders: from storage to cellular damage. *Biochim Biophys Acta*. 2009;1793(4):684–696.
29. Raben N, Shea L, Hill V, Plotz P. Monitoring autophagy in lysosomal storage disorders. *Methods Enzymol*. 2009;453:417–449.
30. Sahu R, Kaushik S, Clement CC, et al. Microautophagy of cytosolic proteins by late endosomes. *Dev Cell*. 2011;20(1):131–139.
31. Dice JF, Terlecky SR, Chiang HL, et al. A selective pathway for degradation of cytosolic proteins by lysosomes. *Semin Cell Biol*. 1990;1(6):449–455.
32. Venugopal B, Mesires NT, Kennedy JC, et al. Chaperone-mediated autophagy is defective in mucolipidosis type IV. *J Cell Physiol*. 2009;219(2):344–353.
33. Yu L, McPhee CK, Zheng L, et al. Termination of autophagy and reformation of lysosomes regulated by mTOR. *Nature*. 2010;465(7300):942–946.
34. Sardiello M, Palmieri M, di Ronza A, et al. A gene network regulating lysosomal biogenesis and function. *Science*. 2009;325(5939):473–477.
35. Palmieri M, Impey S, Kang H, et al. Characterization of the CLEAR network reveals an integrated control of cellular clearance pathways. *Hum Mol Genet*. 2011;20(19):3852–3866.
36. Pena-Llopis S, Vega-Rubin-de-Celis S, Schwartz JC, et al. Regulation of TFEB and V-ATPases by mTORC1. *EMBO J*. 2011;30(16):3242–3258.
37. Khaminets A, Heinrich T, Mari M, et al. Regulation of endoplasmic reticulum turnover by selective autophagy. *Nature*. 2015;522(7556):354–358.
38. Kim I, Rodriguez-Enriquez S, Lemasters JJ. Selective degradation of mitochondria by mitophagy. *Arch Biochem Biophys*. 2007;462(2):245–253.
39. Kraft C, Deplazes A, Sohrmann M, Peter M. Mature ribosomes are selectively degraded upon starvation by an autophagy pathway requiring the Ubp3p/Bre5p ubiquitin protease. *Nat Cell Biol*. 2008;10(5):602–610.
40. Hutchins MU, Veenhuis M, Klionsky DJ. Peroxisome degradation in saccharomyces cerevisiae is dependent on machinery of macroautophagy and the cvt pathway. *J Cell Sci*. 1999;112(Pt 22):4079–4087.
41. Singh R, Kaushik S, Wang Y, et al. Autophagy regulates lipid metabolism. *Nature*. 2009;458(7242):1131–1135.
42. Weidberg H, Shvets E, Elazar Z. Lipophagy: selective catabolism designed for lipids. *Dev Cell*. 2009;16(5): 628–630.
43. Farooqui AA. Lipid mediators in the neural cell nucleus: their metabolism, signaling, and association with neurological disorders. *Neuroscientist*. 2009;15(4):392–407.
44. Thundyil J, Lim KL. DAMPs and neurodegeneration. *Ageing Res Rev*. 2015;24(Pt A):17–28.
45. Walkley SU, Vanier MT. Secondary lipid accumulation in lysosomal disease. *Biochim Biophys Acta*. 2009;1793(4):726–736.
46. Lamanna WC, Lawrence R, Sarrazin S, Esko JD. Secondary storage of dermatan sulfate in sanfilippo disease. *J Biol Chem*. 2011;286(9):6955–6962.
47. Prinetti A, Prioni S, Chiricozzi E, Schuchman EH, Chigorno V, Sonnino S. Secondary alterations of sphingolipid metabolism in lysosomal storage diseases. *Neurochem Res*. 2011;36(9):1654–1668.
48. Bellettato CM, Scarpa M. Pathophysiology of neuropathic lysosomal storage disorders. *J Inherit Metab Dis*. 2010;33(4):347–362.
49. Rama Rao KV, Kielian T. Astrocytes and lysosomal storage diseases. *Neuroscience*. 2016;323:195–206.
50. Lyman M, Lloyd DG, Ji X, Vizcaychipi MP, Ma D. Neuroinflammation: the role and consequences. *Neurosci Res*. 2014;79:1–12.
51. Heneka MT, Carson MJ, El Khoury J, et al. Neuroinflammation in alzheimer's disease. *Lancet Neurol*. 2015;14(4):388–405.

52. Rock RB, Gekker G, Hu S, et al. Role of microglia in central nervous system infections. *Clin Microbiol Rev*. 2004;17(4):942–964.
53. Amor S, Peferoen LA, Vogel DY, et al. Inflammation in neurodegenerative diseases—an update. *Immunology*. 2014;142(2):151–166.
54. Haydon PG, Nedergaard M. How do astrocytes participate in neural plasticity?. *Cold Spring Harb Perspect Biol*. 2014;7(3):a020438.
55. Verkhratsky A, Zorec R, Rodriguez JJ, Parpura V. Pathobiology of neurodegeneration: the role for astroglia. *Opera Med Physiol*. 2016;1:13–22.
56. Karpuk N, Burkovetskaya M, Fritz T, Angle A, Kielian T. Neuroinflammation leads to region-dependent alterations in astrocyte gap junction communication and hemichannel activity. *J Neurosci*. 2011;31(2):414–425.
57. Orellana JA, Shoji KF, Abudara V, et al. Amyloid beta-induced death in neurons involves glial and neuronal hemichannels. *J Neurosci*. 2011;31(13):4962–4977.
58. Jeyakumar M, Thomas R, Elliot-Smith E, et al. Central nervous system inflammation is a hallmark of pathogenesis in mouse models of GM1 and GM2 gangliosidosis. *Brain*. 2003;126(Pt 4):974–987.
59. Baudry M, Yao Y, Simmons D, Liu J, Bi X. Postnatal development of inflammation in a murine model of niemann-pick type C disease: Immunohistochemical observations of microglia and astroglia. *Exp Neurol*. 2003;184(2):887–903.
60. Wilkinson FL, Holley RJ, Langford-Smith KJ, et al. Neuropathology in mouse models of mucopolysaccharidosis type I, IIIA and IIIB. *PLoS One*. 2012;7(4):e35787.
61. Farfel-Becker T, Vitner E, Dekel H, et al. No evidence for activation of the unfolded protein response in neuronopathic models of gaucher disease. *Hum Mol Genet*. 2009;18(8):1482–1488.
62. Kollmann K, Uusi-Rauva K, Scifo E, Tyynela J, Jalanko A, Braulke T. Cell biology and function of neuronal ceroid lipofuscinosis-related proteins. *Biochim Biophys Acta*. 2013;1832(11):1866–1881.
63. Lloyd-Evans E, Platt FM. Lysosomal ca(2+) homeostasis: role in pathogenesis of lysosomal storage diseases. *Cell Calcium*. 2011;50(2):200–205.
64. Korkotian E, Schwarz A, Pelled D, Schwarzmann G, Segal M, Futerman AH. Elevation of intracellular glucosylceramide levels results in an increase in endoplasmic reticulum density and in functional calcium stores in cultured neurons. *J Biol Chem*. 1999;274(31):21673–21678.
65. Ginzburg L, Futerman AH. Defective calcium homeostasis in the cerebellum in a mouse model of niemann-pick A disease. *J Neurochem*. 2005;95(6):1619–1628.
66. Jennings Jr JJ, Zhu JH, Rbaibi Y, Luo X, Chu CT, Kiselyov K. Mitochondrial aberrations in mucolipidosis type IV. *J Biol Chem*. 2006;281(51):39041–39050.
67. Lloyd-Evans E, Morgan AJ, He X, et al. Niemann-pick disease type C1 is a sphingosine storage disease that causes deregulation of lysosomal calcium. *Nat Med*. 2008;14(11):1247–1255.
68. Wei H, Kim SJ, Zhang Z, Tsai PC, Wisniewski KE, Mukherjee AB. ER and oxidative stresses are common mediators of apoptosis in both neurodegenerative and non-neurodegenerative lysosomal storage disorders and are alleviated by chemical chaperones. *Hum Mol Genet*. 2008;17(4):469–477.
69. Tessitore A, del P, Martin M, Sano R, et al. GM1-ganglioside-mediated activation of the unfolded protein response causes neuronal death in a neurodegenerative gangliosidosis. *Mol Cell*. 2004;15(5):753–766.
70. Kim SJ, Zhang Z, Hitomi E, Lee YC, Mukherjee AB. Endoplasmic reticulum stress-induced caspase-4 activation mediates apoptosis and neurodegeneration in INCL. *Hum Mol Genet*. 2006;15(11):1826–1834.
71. Shen JS, Meng XL, Moore DF, et al. Globotriaosylceramide induces oxidative stress and up-regulates cell adhesion molecule expression in fabry disease endothelial cells. *Mol Genet Metab*. 2008;95(3):163–168.
72. Reddy JV, Ganley IG, Pfeffer SR. Clues to neuro-degeneration in niemann-pick type C disease from global gene expression profiling. *PLoS One*. 2006;1:e19.
73. Zampieri S, Mellon SH, Butters TD, et al. Oxidative stress in NPC1 deficient cells: Protective effect of allopregnanolone. *J Cell Mol Med*. 2009;13(9B):3786–3796.
74. Villani GR, Di Domenico C, Musella A, Cecere F, Di Napoli D, Di Natale P. Mucopolysaccharidosis IIIB: oxidative damage and cytotoxic cell involvement in the neuronal pathogenesis. *Brain Res*. 2009;1279:99–108.
75. Hachiya Y, Hayashi M, Kumada S, Uchiyama A, Tsuchiya K, Kurata K. Mechanisms of neurodegeneration in neuronal ceroid-lipofuscinoses. *Acta Neuropathol*. 2006;111(2):168–177.
76. Heine C, Tyynela J, Cooper JD, et al. Enhanced expression of manganese-dependent superoxide dismutase in human and sheep CLN6 tissues. *Biochem J*. 2003;376(Pt 2):369–376.
77. Vitner EB, Futerman AH. Neuronal forms of Gaucher disease. *Handb Exp Pharmacol*. 2013;(216):405–419.

78. Sidransky E, Fartasch M, Lee RE, et al. Epidermal abnormalities may distinguish type 2 from type 1 and type 3 of Gaucher disease. *Pediatr Res*. 1996;39(1):134–141.
79. Hruska KS, LaMarca ME, Scott CR, Sidransky E. Gaucher disease: mutation and polymorphism spectrum in the glucocerebrosidase gene (GBA). *Hum Mutat*. 2008;29(5):567–583.
80. Aflaki E, Moaven N, Borger DK, et al. Lysosomal storage and impaired autophagy lead to inflammasome activation in Gaucher macrophages. *Aging Cell*. 2016;15(1):77–88.
81. Farfel-Becker T, Vitner EB, Kelly SL, et al. Neuronal accumulation of glucosylceramide in a mouse model of neuronopathic Gaucher disease leads to neurodegeneration. *Hum Mol Genet*. 2014;23(4):843–854.
82. Sun Y, Liou B, Ran H, et al. Neuronopathic gaucher disease in the mouse: viable combined selective saposin C deficiency and mutant glucocerebrosidase (V394L) mice with glucosylsphingosine and glucosylceramide accumulation and progressive neurological deficits. *Hum Mol Genet*. 2010;19(6):1088–1097.
83. Panicker LM, Miller D, Awad O, et al. Gaucher iPSC-derived macrophages produce elevated levels of inflammatory mediators and serve as a new platform for therapeutic development. *Stem Cells*. 2014;32(9):2338–2349.
84. Cox TM. Gaucher disease: clinical profile and therapeutic developments. *Biologics*. 2010;4:299–313.
85. Bennett LL, Mohan D. Gaucher disease and its treatment options. *Ann Pharmacother*. 2013;47(9):1182–1193.
86. Aerts JM, Yasothan U, Kirkpatrick P. Velaglucerase alfa. *Nat Rev Drug Discov*. 2010;9(11):837–838.
87. Hollak CE. An evidence-based review of the potential benefits of taliglucerase alfa in the treatment of patients with Gaucher disease. *Core Evid*. 2012;7:15–20.
88. Balwani M, Burrow TA, Charrow J, et al. Recommendations for the use of eliglustat in the treatment of adults with Gaucher disease type 1 in the united states. *Mol Genet Metab*. 2016;117(2):95–103.
89. Pastores GM, Shankar SP, Petakov M, et al. Enzyme replacement therapy with taliglucerase alfa: 36-month safety and efficacy results in adult patients with Gaucher disease previously treated with imiglucerase. *Am J Hematol*. 2016;91(7):661–665.
90. Zimran A, Duran G, Mehta A, et al. Long-term efficacy and safety results of taliglucerase alfa up to 36 months in adult treatment-naive patients with Gaucher disease. *Am J Hematol*. 2016;91(7):656–660.
91. Ida H, Tanaka A, Matsubayashi T, et al. A multicenter, open-label extension study of velaglucerase alfa in Japanese patients with Gaucher disease: results after a cumulative treatment period of 24 months. *Blood Cells Mol Dis*. 2016;59:140–147.
92. Lukina E, Watman N, Arreguin EA, et al. Improvement in hematological, visceral, and skeletal manifestations of gaucher disease type 1 with oral eliglustat tartrate (genz-112638) treatment: 2-year results of a phase 2 study. *Blood*. 2010;116(20):4095–4098.
93. Peterschmitt MJ, Burke A, Blankstein L, et al. Safety, tolerability, and pharmacokinetics of eliglustat tartrate (genz-112638) after single doses, multiple doses, and food in healthy volunteers. *J Clin Pharmacol*. 2011;51(5):695–705.
94. Connock M, Burls A, Frew E, et al. The clinical effectiveness and cost-effectiveness of enzyme replacement therapy for Gaucher's disease: a systematic review. *Health Technol Assess*. 2006;10(24):iii-iv, ix-136.
95. Vanier MT. Niemann-Pick C disease: history, current research topics, biological and molecular diagnosis. *Arch Pediatr*. 2010;17(Suppl 2):S41–S44.
96. Rosenbaum AI, Maxfield FR. Niemann-Pick type C disease: molecular mechanisms and potential therapeutic approaches. *J Neurochem*. 2011;116(5):789–795.
97. Carstea ED, Morris JA, Coleman KG, et al. Niemann-Pick C1 disease gene: homology to mediators of cholesterol homeostasis. *Science*. 1997;277(5323):228–231.
98. Kwon HJ, Abi-Mosleh L, Wang ML, et al. Structure of N-terminal domain of NPC1 reveals distinct subdomains for binding and transfer of cholesterol. *Cell*. 2009;137(7):1213–1224.
99. Naureckiene S, Sleat DE, Lackland H, et al. Identification of HE1 as the second gene of Niemann-Pick C disease. *Science*. 2000;290(5500):2298–2301.
100. Williams IM, Wallom KL, Smith DA, Al Eisa N, Smith C, Platt FM. Improved neuroprotection using miglustat, curcumin and ibuprofen as a triple combination therapy in Niemann-Pick disease type C1 mice. *Neurobiol Dis*. 2014;67:9–17.
101. Gallala HD, Breiden B, Sandhoff K. Regulation of the NPC2 protein-mediated cholesterol trafficking by membrane lipids. *J Neurochem*. 2011;116(5):702–707.
102. Lloyd-Evans E, Platt FM. Lipids on trial: the search for the offending metabolite in Niemann-Pick type C disease. *Traffic*. 2010;11(4):419–428.
103. Ko DC, Gordon MD, Jin JY, Scott MP. Dynamic movements of organelles containing Niemann-Pick C1 protein: NPC1 involvement in late endocytic events. *Mol Biol Cell*. 2001;12(3):601–614.

104. Patterson MC, Hendriksz CJ, Walterfang M, et al. Recommendations for the diagnosis and management of Niemann-Pick disease type C: an update. *Mol Genet Metab*. 2012;106(3):330–344.
105. Ottinger EA, Kao ML, Carrillo-Carrasco N, et al. Collaborative development of 2-hydroxypropyl-beta-cyclodextrin for the treatment of Niemann-Pick type C1 disease. *Curr Top Med Chem*. 2014;14(3):330–339.
106. Mole SE, Cotman SL. Genetics of the neuronal ceroid lipofuscinoses (batten disease). *Biochim Biophys Acta*. 2015;1852(10 Pt B):2237–2241.
107. Santavuori P. Neuronal ceroid-lipofuscinoses in childhood. *Brain Dev*. 1988;10(2):80–83.
108. Haltia M. The neuronal ceroid-lipofuscinoses: from past to present. *Biochim Biophys Acta*. 2006;1762(10):850–856.
109. Mitchison HM, Lim MJ, Cooper JD. Selectivity and types of cell death in the neuronal ceroid lipofuscinoses. *Brain Pathol*. 2004;14(1):86–96.
110. Anderson GW, Goebel HH, Simonati A. Human pathology in NCL. *Biochim Biophys Acta*. 2013;1832(11): 1807–1826.
111. Cotman SL, Karaa A, Staropoli JF, Sims KB. Neuronal ceroid lipofuscinosis: impact of recent genetic advances and expansion of the clinicopathologic spectrum. *Curr Neurol Neurosci Rep*. 2013;13(8):366.
112. Cooper JD, Tarczyluk MA, Nelvagal HR. Towards a new understanding of NCL pathogenesis. *Biochim Biophys Acta*. 2015;1852(10 Pt B):2256–2261.
113. Simonati A, Pezzini F, Moro F, Santorelli FM. Neuronal ceroid lipofuscinosis: the increasing spectrum of an old disease. *Curr Mol Med*. 2014;14:1043–1051.
114. Jalanko A, Braulke T. Neuronal ceroid lipofuscinoses. *Biochim Biophys Acta*. 2009;1793(4):697–709.
115. Koike M, Shibata M, Waguri S, et al. Participation of autophagy in storage of lysosomes in neurons from mouse models of neuronal ceroid-lipofuscinoses (batten disease). *Am J Pathol*. 2005;167(6):1713–1728.
116. Cao Y, Espinola JA, Fossale E, et al. Autophagy is disrupted in a knock-in mouse model of juvenile neuronal ceroid lipofuscinosis. *J Biol Chem*. 2006;281(29):20483–20493.
117. Lojewski X, Staropoli JF, Biswas-Legrand S, et al. Human iPSC models of neuronal ceroid lipofuscinosis capture distinct effects of TPP1 and CLN3 mutations on the endocytic pathway. *Hum Mol Genet*. 2014;23(8):2005–2022.
118. Cotman SL, Vrbanac V, Lebel LA, et al. Cln3(Deltaex7/8) knock-in mice with the common JNCL mutation exhibit progressive neurologic disease that begins before birth. *Hum Mol Genet*. 2002;11(22):2709–2721.
119. Macauley SL, Pekny M, Sands MS. The role of attenuated astrocyte activation in infantile neuronal ceroid lipofuscinosis. *J Neurosci*. 2011;31(43):15575–15585.
120. Macauley SL, Wong AM, Shyng C, et al. An anti-neuroinflammatory that targets dysregulated glia enhances the efficacy of CNS-directed gene therapy in murine infantile neuronal ceroid lipofuscinosis. *J Neurosci*. 2014;34(39):13077–13082.
121. Sondhi D, Peterson DA, Edelstein AM, del Fierro K, Hackett NR, Crystal RG. Survival advantage of neonatal CNS gene transfer for late infantile neuronal ceroid lipofuscinosis. *Exp Neurol*. 2008;213(1):18–27.
122. Worgall S, Sondhi D, Hackett NR, et al. Treatment of late infantile neuronal ceroid lipofuscinosis by CNS administration of a serotype 2 adeno-associated virus expressing CLN2 cDNA. *Hum Gene Ther*. 2008;19(5):463–474.
123. Chang JW, Choi H, Cotman SL, Jung YK. Lithium rescues the impaired autophagy process in CbCln3(Deltaex7/8/Deltaex7/8) cerebellar cells and reduces neuronal vulnerability to cell death via IMPase inhibition. *J Neurochem*. 2011;116(4):659–668.
124. Tyszka-Czochara M, Grzywacz A, Gdula-Argasinska J, Librowski T, Wilinski B, Opoka W. The role of zinc in the pathogenesis and treatment of central nervous system (CNS) diseases. implications of zinc homeostasis for proper CNS function. *Acta Pol Pharm*. 2014;71(3):369–377.
125. Jeong J, Eide DJ. The SLC39 family of zinc transporters. *Mol Aspects Med*. 2013;34(2–3):612–619.
126. Kimura T, Kambe T. The functions of metallothionein and ZIP and ZnT transporters: an overview and perspective. *Int J Mol Sci*. 2016;17(3):336.
127. Aydemir TB, Liuzzi JP, McClellan S, Cousins RJ. Zinc transporter ZIP8 (SLC39A8) and zinc influence IFN-gamma expression in activated human T cells. *J Leukoc Biol*. 2009;86(2):337–348.
128. Scheiber IF, Mercer JF, Dringen R. Metabolism and functions of copper in brain. *Prog Neurobiol*. 2014;116:33–57.
129. Yokel RA. Blood-brain barrier flux of aluminum, manganese, iron and other metals suspected to contribute to metal-induced neurodegeneration. *J Alzheimers Dis*. 2006;10(2–3):223–253.
130. Choi BS, Zheng W. Copper transport to the brain by the blood-brain barrier and blood-CSF barrier. *Brain Res*. 2009;1248:14–21.
131. Ximenes-da-Silva A. Metal ion toxins and brain aquaporin-4 expression: an overview. *Front Neurosci*. 2016;10:233.

132. Kozma M, Ferke A. Trace element localization and changes in zinc and copper concentrations during postnatal development of the rat CNS. *Acta Histochem*. 1979;65(2):219–227.
133. Dringen R, Bishop GM, Koeppe M, Dang TN, Robinson SR. The pivotal role of astrocytes in the metabolism of iron in the brain. *Neurochem Res*. 2007;32(11):1884–1890.
134. Tiffany-Castiglioni E, Hong S, Qian Y. Copper handling by astrocytes: insights into neurodegenerative diseases. *Int J Dev Neurosci*. 2011;29(8):811–818.
135. Brown DR. Role of the prion protein in copper turnover in astrocytes. *Neurobiol Dis*. 2004;15(3):534–543.
136. Hatori Y, Yan Y, Schmidt K, et al. Neuronal differentiation is associated with a redox-regulated increase of copper flow to the secretory pathway. *Nat Commun*. 2016;7:10640.
137. Mathie A, Sutton GL, Clarke CE, Veale EL. Zinc and copper: pharmacological probes and endogenous modulators of neuronal excitability. *Pharmacol Ther*. 2006;111(3):567–583.
138. Opazo CM, Greenough MA, Bush AI. Copper: from neurotransmission to neuroproteostasis. *Front Aging Neurosci*. 2014;6:143.
139. Li Y, Chen M, Xu Y, et al. Iron-mediated lysosomal membrane permeabilization in ethanol-induced hepatic oxidative damage and apoptosis: Protective effects of quercetin. *Oxid Med Cell Longev*. 2016;2016:4147610.
140. Ullio C, Brunk UT, Urani C, et al. Autophagy of metallothioneins prevents TNF-induced oxidative stress and toxicity in hepatoma cells. *Autophagy*. 2015;11(12):2184–2198.
141. Schissel SL, Schuchman EH, Williams KJ, Tabas I. Zn2+-stimulated sphingomyelinase is secreted by many cell types and is a product of the acid sphingomyelinase gene. *J Biol Chem*. 1996;271(31):18431–18436.
142. Kukic I, Kelleher SL, Kiselyov K. Zn2+ efflux through lysosomal exocytosis prevents Zn2+-induced toxicity. *J Cell Sci*. 2014;127(Pt 14):3094–3103.
143. Kurz T, Eaton JW, Brunk UT. Redox activity within the lysosomal compartment: Implications for aging and apoptosis. *Antioxid Redox Signal*. 2010;13(4):511–523.
144. Kurz T, Terman A, Gustafsson B, Brunk UT. Lysosomes in iron metabolism, ageing and apoptosis. *Histochem Cell Biol*. 2008;129(4):389–406.
145. Polishchuk EV, Concilli M, Iacobacci S, et al. Wilson disease protein ATP7B utilizes lysosomal exocytosis to maintain copper homeostasis. *Dev Cell*. 2014;29(6):686–700.
146. Price KA, Crouch PJ, Lim S, et al. Subcellular localization of a fluorescent derivative of CuII(atsm) offers insight into the neuroprotective action of CuII(atsm). *Metallomics*. 2011;3(12):1280–1290.
147. Hickey JL, James JL, Henderson CA, et al. Intracellular distribution of fluorescent copper and zinc bis(thiosemicarbazonato) complexes measured with fluorescence lifetime spectroscopy. *Inorg Chem*. 2015;54(19):9556–9567.
148. Liuzzi JP, Guo L, Yoo C, Stewart TS. Zinc and autophagy. *Biometals*. 2014;27(6):1087–1096.
149. Hwang JJ, Lee SJ, Kim TY, Cho JH, Koh JY. Zinc and 4-hydroxy-2-nonenal mediate lysosomal membrane permeabilization induced by H2O2 in cultured hippocampal neurons. *J Neurosci*. 2008;28(12):3114–3122.
150. Julien S, Biesemeier A, Kokkinou D, Eibl O, Schraermeyer U. Zinc deficiency leads to lipofuscin accumulation in the retinal pigment epithelium of pigmented rats. *PLoS One*. 2011;6(12):e29245.
151. Summersgill H, England H, Lopez-Castejon G, et al. Zinc depletion regulates the processing and secretion of IL-1beta. *Cell Death Dis*. 2014;5:e1040.
152. Matias AC, Manieri TM, Cerchiaro G. Zinc chelation mediates the lysosomal disruption without intracellular ROS generation. *Oxid Med Cell Longev*. 2016;2016:6724585.
153. Kodama H, Fujisawa C, Bhadhprasit W. Pathology, clinical features and treatments of congenital copper metabolic disorders—focus on neurologic aspects. *Brain Dev*. 2011;33(3):243–251.
154. Wu F, Wang J, Pu C, Qiao L, Jiang C. Wilson's disease: a comprehensive review of the molecular mechanisms. *Int J Mol Sci*. 2015;16(3):6419–6431.
155. Bandmann O, Weiss KH, Kaler SG. Wilson's disease and other neurological copper disorders. *Lancet Neurol*. 2015;14(1):103–113.
156. Purchase R. The treatment of wilson's disease, a rare genetic disorder of copper metabolism. *Sci Prog*. 2013;96(Pt 1): 19–32.
157. Gozzelino R, Arosio P. Iron homeostasis in health and disease. *Int J Mol Sci*. 2016;17(1):doi: 10.3390/ijms17010130.
158. Turski ML, Thiele DJ. New roles for copper metabolism in cell proliferation, signaling, and disease. *J Biol Chem*. 2009;284(2):717–721.
159. Maret W. Zinc and human disease. *Met Ions Life Sci*. 2013;13:389–414.

160. Barnham KJ, Bush AI. Biological metals and metal-targeting compounds in major neurodegenerative diseases. *Chem Soc Rev*. 2014;43(19):6727–6749.
161. Fraldi A, Klein AD, Medina DL, Settembre C. Brain disorders due to lysomal dysfunction. *Annu Rev Neurosci*. 2016;39:277–295.
162. Hentze MW, Muckenthaler MU, Galy B, Camaschella C. Two to tango: regulation of mammalian iron metabolism. *Cell*. 2010;142(1):24–38.
163. Stein P, Yu H, Jain D, Mistry PK. Hyperferritinemia and iron overload in type 1 Gaucher disease. *Am J Hematol*. 2010;85(7):472–476.
164. Christomanou H, Vanier MT, Santambrogio P, Arosio P, Kleijer WJ, Harzer K. Deficient ferritin immunoreactivity in tissues from Niemann-Pick type C patients: extension of findings to fetal tissues, H and L ferritin isoforms, but also one case of the rare Niemann-Pick C2 complementation group. *Mol Genet Metab*. 2000;70(3):196–202.
164a. Orino K, Lehman L, Tsuji Y, Ayaki H, Torti SV, Torti FM. Ferritin and the response to oxidative stress. *Biochem J*. 2001;357(Pt 1):241–247.
165. Mekinian A, Stirnemann J, Belmatoug N, et al. Ferritinemia during type 1 Gaucher disease: mechanisms and progression under treatment. *Blood Cells Mol Dis*. 2012;49(1):53–57.
166. Medrano-Engay B, Irun P, Gervas-Arruga J, et al. Iron homeostasis and inflammatory biomarker analysis in patients with type 1 Gaucher disease. *Blood Cells Mol Dis*. 2014;53(4):171–175.
167. Regenboog M, van Kuilenburg AB, Verheij J, Swinkels DW, Hollak CE. Hyperferritinemia and iron metabolism in Gaucher disease: potential pathophysiological implications. *Blood Rev*. 2016;30(6):431–437.
168. Wraith JE, Vecchio D, Jacklin E, et al. Miglustat in adult and juvenile patients with Niemann-Pick disease type C: long-term data from a clinical trial. *Mol Genet Metab*. 2010;99(4):351–357.
169. Sun X, Marks DL, Park WD, et al. Niemann-Pick C variant detection by altered sphingolipid trafficking and correlation with mutations within a specific domain of NPC1. *Am J Hum Genet*. 2001;68(6):1361–1372.
170. Wraith JE, Baumgartner MR, NP-C Guidelines Working Groupet al. Recommendations on the diagnosis and management of Niemann-Pick disease type C. *Mol Genet Metab*. 2009;98(1–2):152–165.
171. Christomanou H, Harzer K. Ouchterlony double immunodiffusion method demonstrates absence of ferritin immunoreactivity in visceral organs from nine patients with Niemann-Pick disease type C. *Biochem Mol Med*. 1996;58(2):176–183.
172. Hung YH, Faux NG, Killilea DW, et al. Altered transition metal homeostasis in Niemann-Pick disease, type C1. *Metallomics*. 2014;6(3):542–553.
173. Arguello G, Martinez P, Pena J, et al. Hepatic metabolic response to restricted copper intake in a Niemann-Pick C murine model. *Metallomics*. 2014;6(8):1527–1539.
174. Geraets RD, Koh S, Hastings ML, Kielian T, Pearce DA, Weimer JM. Moving towards effective therapeutic strategies for neuronal ceroid lipofuscinosis. *Orphanet J Rare Dis*. 2016;11:40.
175. Johansson E, Lindh U, Westermarck T, Heiskala H, Santavuori P. Altered elemental profiles in neuronal ceroid lipofuscinosis. *J Trace Elem Electrolytes Health Dis*. 1990;4(3):139–142.
176. Kanninen KM, Grubman A, Caragounis A, et al. Altered biometal homeostasis is associated with CLN6 mRNA loss in mouse neuronal ceroid lipofuscinosis. *Biol Open*. 2013;2(6):635–646.
177. Grubman A, Pollari E, Duncan C, et al. Deregulation of biometal homeostasis: the missing link for neuronal ceroid lipofuscinoses?. *Metallomics*. 2014;6(4):932–943.
178. Lutsenko S, Gupta A, Burkhead JL, Zuzel V. Cellular multitasking: the dual role of human cu-ATPases in cofactor delivery and intracellular copper balance. *Arch Biochem Biophys*. 2008;476(1):22–32.
179. Butterworth RF. Metal toxicity, liver disease and neurodegeneration. *Neurotox Res*. 2010;18(1):100–105.
180. Hellman NE, Kono S, Mancini GM, Hoogeboom AJ, De Jong GJ, Gitlin JD. Mechanisms of copper incorporation into human ceruloplasmin. *J Biol Chem*. 2002;277(48):46632–46638.
181. Gambling L, Andersen HS, McArdle HJ. Iron and copper, and their interactions during development. *Biochem Soc Trans*. 2008;36(Pt 6):1258–1261.
182. Davies KM, Hare DJ, Cottam V, et al. Localization of copper and copper transporters in the human brain. *Metallomics*. 2013;5(1):43–51.
183. Zahran AM, Elsayh KI, El-Deek SE, El-Baz MA. Oxidative stress, trace elements, and circulating microparticles in patients with Gaucher disease before and after enzyme replacement therapy. *Clin Appl Thromb Hemost*. 2015;21(1):58–65.
184. Connemann BJ, Gahr M, Schmid M, Runz H, Freudenmann RW. Low ceruloplasmin in a patient with Niemann-Pick type C disease. *J Clin Neurosci*. 2012;19(4):620–621.

185. Vazquez MC, Martinez P, Alvarez AR, Gonzalez M, Zanlungo S. Increased copper levels in in vitro and in vivo models of Niemann-Pick C disease. *Biometals*. 2012;25(4):777–786.
186. Yanagimoto C, Harada M, Kumemura H, et al. Copper incorporation into ceruloplasmin is regulated by Niemann-Pick C1 protein. *Hepatol Res*. 2011;41(5):484–491.
187. Filiz G, Caragounis A, Bica L, et al. Clioquinol inhibits peroxide-mediated toxicity through up-regulation of phosphoinositol-3-kinase and inhibition of p53 activity. *Int J Biochem Cell Biol*. 2008;40(5):1030–1042.
188. Roberts BR, Lim NK, McAllum EJ, et al. Oral treatment with cu(II)(atsm) increases mutant SOD1 in vivo but protects motor neurons and improves the phenotype of a transgenic mouse model of amyotrophic lateral sclerosis. *J Neurosci*. 2014;34(23):8021–8031.
189. Hung LW, Villemagne VL, Cheng L, et al. The hypoxia imaging agent CuII(atsm) is neuroprotective and improves motor and cognitive functions in multiple animal models of Parkinson's disease. *J Exp Med*. 2012;209(4):837–854.

CHAPTER

12

Developmental Exposure to Metals and its Contribution to Age-Related Neurodegeneration

*Lucio G. Costa**,**

*University of Washington, Seattle, WA, United States

**University of Parma, Parma, Italy

OUTLINE

INTRODUCTION

Neurodegenerative diseases, such as Alzheimer's disease (AD) or Parkinson's disease (PD) are increasing worldwide, mostly because of the aging of the populations.[1,2] Indeed, the sporadic forms of such diseases are usually seen in individuals >65 years old, with the incidence increasing for every decade of life. Both AD and PD also present early onset cases (at the age of 40–50 years), and these are usually associated with specific genetic mutations, and represent a small number of the overall prevalence of neurodegenerative diseases. The etiology of sporadic AD and PD is still unknown, and current view is that both genetic and environmental factors may contribute.[3–5] In PD, loss of dopaminergic neurons causes depletion of the neurotransmitter dopamine which in turn results in several motor symptoms.

Biometals in Neurodegenerative Diseases. http://dx.doi.org/10.1016/B978-0-12-804562-6.00012-9

Lewy bodies in brain are a hallmark of PD, and alpha-synuclein is their major component; measurements of alpha-synuclein in brain and in biofluids are considered useful markers of PD.[6,7] AD is the main cause of dementia worldwide, and is characterized primarily by cognitive deficits, particularly loss of recent memory and executive dysfunction.[5] Accumulation of abnormally folded amyloid beta (Aβ) and tau proteins in amyloid plaques and neuronal tangles are causally related to neurodegeneration. Measurements of total and/or phosphorylated tau, of Aβ levels, and of levels of APP (the precursor of Aβ peptides) are useful markers of AD pathology.[8,9]

The role of metals in the etiology of neurodegenerative diseases is the topic of this volume. The present chapter focuses on some studies on selected metals (namely lead and arsenic) for which initial evidence exist that developmental exposure may be associated, later in life, with the development of AD. Thus, in addition to their known neurodevelopmental effects, exposure to these metals may also have late-life effects.

DEVELOPMENTAL EXPOSURE TO TOXICANTS AND LATE EFFECTS

A great body of experimental and epidemiological evidence is indicating that exposure to toxicants during early life can be associated with significantly increased risk of disease later in life, during adulthood and/or aging. First proposed by Barker[10] with reference to fetal undernutrition and the risk for cardiovascular disease, this hypothesis forms the basis for the general concept of developmental origins of health and disease, which includes a variety of fetal-early life environmental conditions, and numerous adult and age-related diseases,[11,12] including neurodegenerative diseases.[13] A classic example is represented by diethylstilbestrol, as in utero exposure to this drug leads to an increase in vaginal adenocarcinoma at the time of puberty.[14]

In general, the existence of a large time interval between the initial damage and the appearance of clinical manifestations of toxicity is a common and recognized phenomenon in oncology, but is less recognized in neurotoxicology. Usually, neurotoxicological endpoints are measured at the end of exposure or during exposure in case of repeated treatments. However, some exceptions are known. For example, the polyneuropathy caused by some organophosphorus compounds is delayed, but only a few weeks, from the time of exposure.[15] In the case of the Parkinsonism-dementia known as Guam's disease, latencies of decades have been reported between alleged exposures and clinical signs.[16] Bovine spongiform encephalopathy (mad cow disease), a prion disease associated in humans to a variant of Creutzfeld-Jakob disease, has been shown to have an incubation period (latency) of decades.[17]

The hypothesis of a developmental origin of adult disease implies that the period between exposure and toxic insult and appearance of the disease would consist of years or decades. Even before Barker formulated his hypothesis, the problem of "silent damage," as index of delayed expression of neurotoxicity was introduced by Reuhl.[18] Such delay between exposure and clinical expression of injury may be explained by at least two models. In one model, toxic exposure results in lethal injury to a subpopulation of neuronal cells, but surviving cells and the brain's plasticity assure that the functions are not immediately compromised. The deficit would be unmasked by exogenous influences (e.g., stress, disease, exposure to a pharmacological agent), and this will result in loss of function.[19] Similarly, the process of aging, which slowly reduces the number of surviving neurons, would lead to a subfunctional state because of the previous toxic insult. For example, in case of PD (but extendable to other neurodegenerative diseases) an 80% loss of dopaminergic neurons is needed for clinical manifestations of the disease to be apparent.[20] The aging process causes a gradual loss of dopaminergic neurons, which is estimated to reach the threshold at about 100–120 years of age. In the case of exposure to a toxicant which destroys a certain number of dopaminergic neurons, the superimposing aging process would lead to an 80% loss at an early age (e.g., 65 years) with the individual developing signs of PD.[21] A second model proposes that toxic exposure would cause a sublethal injury to brain cells which result in progressive, incremental loss of function.[18] This injury may involve genetic, epigenetic or biochemical effects that with time will lead to full neuronal dysfunction or premature death. At the basis of this model is also the concept of "event threshold" (as discussed earlier for PD), in which clinical decompensation occurs when a certain number of neurons is lost.

The extension of such reasoning to developmental origins of neurodegenerative diseases follows the same logic, with the initial toxic exposure(s) occurring in utero or early in childhood, and the functional loss evidenced by clinical signs evident only later in life. An excellent example is represented by perinatal exposure to the Gram negative bacteriotoxin lipopolysaccharide (LPS), which damages dopaminergic neurons and increases the risk for dopaminergic disorders, such as PD. In utero exposure of mice to LPS causes a 30% loss of tyrosine hydroxylase-positive neurons in the postnatal midbrain of rats.[22] Similarly, early postnatal exposure to LPS caused long-term loss of tyrosine hydroxylase neurons in the substantia nigra and sustained inflammation.[23] These results would suggest that in humans prenatal infections occurring at the appropriate gestational age would result in birth of an individual with fewer dopaminergic neurons. This in turn would be inconsequential early in life, but may predispose an individual to developing PD at a progressive age.[24] Such model of developmental origin of PD has been verified with other chemical exposure (e.g., the organochlorine dieldrin or the drug cocaine[25,26]), and has been discussed in various reviews.[27–29]

A number of studies have also found associations between early-life environments and the development of AD, though less is known with regard to potential toxic chemical exposures.[30–34] Suggested risk factors include obesity, certain infections, and inflammation,[35–37] in addition to exposure to lead and arsenic which are the focus of this review (see following sections).

DEVELOPMENTAL LEAD EXPOSURE AND ALZHEIMER'S DISEASE

Exposure to lead (Pb) is ubiquitous and known since ancient times. While the effects of high acute, and of occupational exposures to Pb have been known for centuries,[29] the adverse health effects at much lower levels of exposures, seen mostly in children, have been identified only in the 1970s.[38] This has resulted in the removal of tetraethyl lead from gasoline and from removal of this metal from paints, with the consequence of reducing blood Pb levels in the general US population from about 10–15 μg/dL to <3 μg/dL. Nevertheless, exposure to Pb continues nowadays through plumbing pipes and solders containing Pb, the ingestion of leaded paint chips, and living near sites with heavy Pb contamination (e.g., lead mine or smelters, battery recycling sites etc.).

Blood Pb levels are associated with recent exposures, as Pb half-life in blood is approximately 30 days. In contrast, circulating Pb is deposited in bones, where it has a half-life of the order of years to decades, and levels of Pb in bones are an excellent biomarker of long-term cumulative exposures.[39] Occupational exposure to Pb has been associated with cognitive decline with aging. For example, cumulative Pb exposure in a large group of US workers age 60–75 years with blood Pb levels of only approximately 5 μg/dL, but bone lead of 19–36 μg/g (patella) and 13–28 μg/g (tibia) had significantly worse cognitive performance over time.[40] In another study, a group of workers exposed to Pb for about 8 years and with tibia Pb levels of 10–48 μg/g, when tested an average of 16 year after the last exposure, showed significant behavioral deficits, particularly if they carried the *ApoE-ε4* gene, a known, most relevant susceptibility factor for AD.[5,41] There is also some evidence in humans of an association between cumulative lifetime exposure to Pb and PD,[42,43] however, only limited information is available on early developmental Pb exposure and risk of PD. As said, Pb is an established neurotoxicant in children, as even at very low blood concentrations (<10 μg/dL) behavioral alterations and diminished IQ have been reported.[44]

An increasing number of in vivo studies in different animal species have associated developmental exposure to Pb with markers of AD (Table 12.1). While many come from a single laboratory (that of Dr. Nasser Zawia at the University of Rhode Island), supporting evidence has been provided by other groups of investigators. More than a decade ago, Basha and coworkers[45] reported that exposure of Long Evans rats to Pb (0.2% in drinking water) from birth to postnatal day (PND) 20 caused a significant increase in the levels of the amyloid precursor protein (APP) and of Aβ in cerebral cortex at PND 600 (20 months). Blood Pb levels were 46 μg/dL at the end of exposure (PND 20), but were <2 μg/dL at time of sacrifice. Similarly, brain Pb levels were elevated on PND 20 (0.41 mg/g) but did not differ from control on PND 600.[45] Interestingly, APP levels increased shortly after exposure to Pb (PND 20 and 50), returned to basal levels at 1 year, and then increased at 20 months of age. Specific protein 1 (Sp1), a transcription factor involved in the regulation of the APP gene, was also increased in older rats developmentally exposed to Pb.[45] Of much relevance in the context of the effects of developmental exposure to Pb are the findings that late exposure to this metal [0.2% from 18 to 20 months of age, yielding blood and brain Pb levels of 60 and 0.3 μg/dL (g), respectively] did not cause any alteration in levels of APP mRNA and protein, Aβ, and Sp1-DNA binding.[45] This suggests that exposure during brain development (PND1-20 in rats corresponds to the third trimester of pregnancy in humans) "primes" the brain to express biomarkers of AD later in life.

A follow-up study by the same group[46] showed that the same developmental exposure to Pb in rats also caused a late increase (on PND 600) of oxidative DNA damage, assessed by measuring levels of 8-hydroxy-2′-deoxyguanosine (oxo^{8}dG). Such damage was observed in the absence of any change in levels of reduced glutathione (GSH), or activities of copper/zinc- and manganese-superoxide dismutase, and was not seen when Pb exposure only occurred late in life.[46] A different group of investigators exposed Wistar rats to Pb acetate, dissolved in water, daily by gavage from gestational day (GD) 5 to PND 21.[57] On PND 90, levels of APP, $A\beta_{1\text{-}42}$, $A\beta_{1\text{-}40}$, and BACE1 (β site APP cleaving enzyme 1, the enzyme that plays a major role in the cleavage of APP) proteins were increased in cerebral cortex and hippocampus (by 30%–80%). Levels of presenilin 1 and 2 (also involved in APP processing) were also increased, as were markers of neuroinflammation, such as interleukin-1α and 1β.[57]

TABLE 12.1 Developmental Exposure to Pb and Late Effects Relevant for AD

Animal species	Exposure period	Pb dose/blood levels	Effect (age)	References
Rat (Long Evans)	PND 1–20	0.2% in drinking water; 46 μg/dL on PND 20, <2 μg/dL on PND 600	Increased APP and Aβ levels (PND 600)	Basha et al.[45]
Rat (Long Evans)	PND 1–20	0.2% in drinking water	Increased oxidative DNA damage (PND 600)	Bolin et al.[46]
Monkey (*Macaca fascicularis*)	PND 1–400	1.5 mg/kg/day in infant formula, then vehicle; 19–26 μg/dL at PND 400, 3–6 μg/dl at sacrifice (23 years)	Decreased DNA methylation. Increased oxidative DNA damage; Increased APP, Aβ, Sp1, BACE (Year 23)	Wu et al.[47]
Mouse	GD 0—PND 21	0.1%, 0. 5%, 1.0% in drinking water	Increased phospho-tau, Aβ in hippocampus. Decreased performance in Morris maze (PND 22)	Li et al.[48]
Monkey (*Macaca fascicularis*)	PND 1–400	1.5 mg/kg/day	Increased APP. Decreased DNA methylation, decreased acetylated histones (Year 23)	Bihaqi et al.[49]
Mouse (C57BL6)	GD 13—PND 20	0.2% in drinking water; 46 μg/dL on PND 20, < 2 μg/dL on PND 700	Decreased expression of genes related to immune response, metal-binding, metabolism, transcription/ transduction coupling	Dosunmu et al.[50]
Mouse (C57BL6 and Tg-SWDI)	PND 28–70	29 mg/kg once a week for 6 weeks	Increased Aβ in CSF and hippocampus. Increased number of amyloid plaques (PND 70)	Gu et al.[51]
Mouse (C57BL6)	GD 0—PND 10	27, 55, or 109 ppm in drinking water; <10, 25, and 40 μg/dL on PND 10; <1 μg/dL at PND 365	Increased body weight (PND 365)	Fox et al.[52]
Human	In utero and up to 10 years	Blood Pb levels 6–10 μg/dL	Decreased plasma Aβ, altered gene expression as adults	Mazumdar et al.[53]
Zebrafish	From 6 to 120 hours post fertilization	0.025, 0.05 mg/L	Impaired learning and memory as adults	Chen et al.[54]

(*Continued*)

TABLE 12.1 Developmental Exposure to Pb and Late Effects Relevant for AD (*cont.*)

Animal species	Exposure period	Pb dose/blood levels	Effect (age)	References
Monkey (*Macaca fascicularis*)	PND 1–400	1.5 mg/kg/day	Increased tau protein and mRNA. Increased Sp1, Sp3 (Year 23)	Bihaqi and Zawia,[55]
Mouse (C57BL6)	PND 1–20	0.2% in drinking water	Increased tau protein and mRNA. Increased tau phosphorylation, CDK5 levels (PND 700)	Bihaqi et al.[50]
Mouse (C57BL6)	PND 1–20	0.2% in drinking water	Decreased learning and memory (Morris, Y, elevated plus mazes) (PND 540–700)	Bihaqi et al.[56]
Rat (Wistar)	GD 5—PND 21	2.22 ppm by gavage	Increased Aβ (PND 90)	Ashok et al.[57]
Mouse (C57BL6)	PND 1–20	0.2% in drinking water	Altered miRNA expression (miR-106b, miR-29b, miR-124, miR-132) (PND 180 and 700)	Masoud et al.[58]
Human	0–78 months	Max blood Pb = 18 μg/dL (30 months)	Decreased methylation of Imprinted gene regulatory elements (24–36 years)	Li et al.[59]

These findings in rats were extended in following years in nonhuman primates.[47,49,55] The investigators took advantage of a cohort of female monkeys (*Macaca fascicularis*) which had been treated with 1.5 mg/kg Pb acetate from birth until 400 days of age via infant formula and vehicle after weaning, and later underwent behavioral testing.[60] Blood Pb levels in these animals at PND 400 were 19–26 μg/dL,[60] but had decreased to the levels of controls (3–6 μg/dL) at the time of behavioral testing. Monkeys were then transferred at NIH, and sacrificed at the age of 23 years, and tissues were collected and made available to other investigators. Brain (cerebral cortex) Pb levels at this time point were determined to be <0.1 μg/g.[47] Levels of APP, $A\beta_{1\text{-}40}$, and $A\beta_{1\text{-}42}$ mRNA were increased by 50%, 50%, and 100%, respectively, compared to controls.[47,49] Levels of mRNA of BACE1 and of Sp1 were also increased.[47,55] Levels of tau protein and mRNA, and of phosphorylated tau, together with Sp1 and Sp3, were also found to be increased.[55] Levels of oxo^{8}dG were also increased by developmental Pb exposure. In addition, DNA methyltransferase 1 (DNMT1) was decreased by 20%.[47,49] Gene expression, evaluated in the same tissue by microarray analysis, indicated that only 22 genes were modified by developmental Pb exposure, with most genes belonging to the neurotransmitter and growth receptors and signal transduction pathways.[49] Most genes were repressed and only a few were upregulated. Early life Pb exposure also decreased the expression of a number of acetylated histones, such as H3K9ac, H4K8ac, H4K12ac, and H3K4me2.[49]

Findings of effects of developmental Pb exposure in older animals seem to hold across species, as similar results were also seen in mice. Li and coworkers[48] reported that administration of Pb acetate in drinking water (0.1%, 0.5%, or 1.0%, from GD 0 to PND 21) increased the expression of phosphorylated tau and of Aβ in the hippocampus shortly after the end of the exposure. Performance in the Morris water maze was significantly impaired in the two higher exposure groups. Unfortunately, no biochemical or behavioral measurements were done at later time points. In C57BL6 mice exposed to 0.2% Pb in drinking water from GD 13 to PND 20, genome-wide expression and methylation profiles were determined in frontal cortex on PND 20 (right after exposure) and on PND 700 (23 months of age).[50] Blood Pb levels were 46 μg/dL on PND 20 and <2 μg/dL on PND 700. Developmental exposure to Pb caused a repression of genes related to immune response, metal-binding, metabolism, and transcription/transduction coupling. In particular, subsets of 150 genes were upregulated in normal aging, and this upregulation was inhibited by early Pb exposure.[50] Such gene repression may have been associated to altered DNA methylation.[50] Three studies in mice utilizing the same exposure paradigm (0.2% Pb acetate in drinking water, from PND 1 to PND 20) have provided a series of additional biochemical, behavioral, and molecular findings.[56,58,61] In a first study, mice were sacrificed at PND 20, 180, 270, 540, and 700.[56] Levels of tau protein and mRNA, and of phosphorylated tau (at different serine and threonine sites) were increased in frontal cortex on PND 700; however, an adult Pb exposure [0.2% in drinking water for 3 months (7–10) did not cause any effect[56]]. Performance in the Morris water maze was impaired on PND 540 and 700. Alterations were also found in the Y maze and in the elevated plus maze, supporting the finding of changes in spatial learning and memory due to developmental Pb exposure.[61] This latter study also confirmed increases of APP, Sp1, $A\beta_{1\text{-}40}$, and BACE1 protein and mRNA levels on PND 700.[61] Masoud et al.[58] examined the expression of a number of miRNAs on PND 20, 180, and 700 following early life Pb exposure. They found that Pb altered early and late expression of selected miRNAs. For example, Pb transiently increased the expression of miR-106b (which binds to AβPP mRNA), of miR-29b (which targets the mRNA for the transcription factor Sp1), and of miR-132 (which inhibits translation of proteins involved in promoter methylation.[58] These findings support the hypothesis of a central role for epigenetic mechanisms involved in the developmental effects of Pb.[62,63] In another study, Tg-SWDI APP transgenic mice (which overexpress human Swedish, Dutch, and Iowa triple-mutant APP in the brain and develop amyloid plaques at an early age[64]) were exposed to Pb acetate (50 mg/kg/day, equivalent to 29 mg/kg/day Pb, by oral gavage) from PND 28 to PND 70.[51] This treatment yielded Pb blood and brain levels of 29 μg/dL and 0.3 μg/g, respectively, measured at time of sacrifice (PND 71). Pb-treated mice had an increased expression of $A\beta_{1\text{-}40}$ and $A\beta_{1\text{-}42}$ in the hippocampus and the cerebrospinal fluid, an increased number of amyloid plaques, and a decreased performance in the Morris water maze.[51] Finally, an interesting observation derives from a study in which mice were exposed to Pb in drinking water from GD 0 to PND 10 at concentrations of 27, 55, or 109 ppm, to yield Pb blood levels of <10, ~25, and ~40 μg/dL, respectively.[52] When body weights were measured at 1 year of age, male, but not female mice, weighed more than controls (by 13%–26%). These animals also displayed less locomotor activity.[52] These observations are of interest as obesity has been identified as a risk factor for AD.[35] However, when body weight was measured in other studies, no differences between controls and Pb-exposed animals were reported.[45]

On opposite sides of the spectrum of animal species are a few studies in zebrafish and humans. Zebrafish has been suggested as a model for investigating developmental Pb exposure as a risk factor in adult neurodegenerative diseases.[65] In particular, a study by Chen and coworkers[54] showed that exposure of zebrafish embryos to low concentrations of Pb acetate (0.025–0.05 mg/L) caused significant deficits in learning and memory when zebrafish were tested as adults.[54] In humans, a study by Mazumdar et al.[53] has shown that adults exposed to Pb in utero (cord blood Pb >10 μg/dL) had lower levels of Aβ in plasma compared to individuals with lower early Pb exposure. A decreased level of Aβ in plasma has been reported in AD patients, though some contradictory findings exist.[66] Early-life Pb exposure also caused the repression of a number of genes whose products are believed to affect Aβ production and deposition in the brain.[53] A recent study by Li et al.[59] reported that a group of adults exposed in utero and early postnatally to Pb (blood Pb levels ~14 μg/dL) had altered methylation of a number of genes, giving additional support that Pb may act through epigenetic mechanisms.

The exact molecular mechanisms that may underlie the effects of early-life exposure to Pb and the late development of AD and AD-related biochemical and pathological abnormalities, are not known. However, as indicated in the studies earlier, and as pointed out in various commentaries,[62,63,67] the current consensus is that Pb may act through epigenetic mechanisms. Evidence exists that Pb can be an epigenetic modifier, as shown by its ability to affect DNA methylation, histone acetylation, and expression of miRNAs in animals and in humans,[47,49,55,58,59,68] leading to long-term changes in gene expression.[47,50,53] This remains an important area for further investigations.

DEVELOPMENTAL ARSENIC EXPOSURE AND ALZHEIMER'S DISEASE

Arsenic (As) is ubiquitous in the environment. Over the centuries it has been used as a pesticide, in traditional medicine and in cosmetic products, yet its "fame" is due to its toxicity. This metal is indeed known as the "king of poisons and the poison of kings," and has been used in several cases with homicidal intentions.[69] Nowadays, chronic human exposure occurs primarily via drinking water or foods (e.g., fish, rice). Arsenic exists primarily in the inorganic forms, as arsenite (As^{III}) and arsenate (As^{V}), with a redox reaction reducing the pentavalent As to its more toxic trivalent state.[69] Once absorbed, As undergoes hepatic biomethylation to form monomethyl As (MMA) and dimethyl As (DMA); these are seen mainly as detoxication reactions, though methylated As species are not devoid of significant toxicity (e.g., genotoxicity).

As is neurotoxic; adults chronically exposed to As experience cognitive deficits, loss of concentration, and also more generalized encephalopathy, with oxidative stress and neuroinflammation representing two important brain responses to As.[69–71] Peripheral neuropathy with decreased nerve conduction velocity is a typical and common effect of chronic As exposure.[69] As is also a developmental neurotoxicant, as evidenced by numerous epidemiological and experimental studies (reviewed by Ref. [72,73]).

The possible role of As in the etiology of AD has been suggested, based on the reported oxidative stress, neuroinflammation, and vascular toxicity induced by this metal.[71] Two additional findings that support the As–AD association are the effects of As on APP and on tau. An earlier study by Dewji and coworkers[74] showed that sodium arsenite (60–100 μM) caused a threefold increase in APP levels in NT2 (embryonal carcinoma) cells in vitro. A subsequent study reported that in Chinese hamster ovary T40 cells expressing the longest isoform of

TABLE 12.2 Effect of Developmental Exposure to Lead, Arsenic, and Cadmium on $A\beta_{1-42}$ in Rats

Metal treatment	Cerebral cortex	Hippocampus
Pb	84 ± 8**	54 ± 6**
As	1 ± 3	2 ± 5
Cd	12 ± 2	18 ± 2*
As + Pb	140 ± 15**,#	96 ± 12**,#
As + Cd	100 ± 10**	100 ± 7**
Cd + Pb	91 ± 10**	73 ± 5**,#
Pb + As + Cd	295 ± 25**	199 ± 10**

Pregnant Wistar rats were exposed by gavage in water to lead acetate (Pb; 2.22 ppm), sodium arsenite (As; 3.80 ppm), and cadmium chloride (Cd; 0.98 ppm) alone or in combination, from GD 5 to PND 21. Levels of Amyloid beta (Aβ) 1-42 were determined in cerebral cortex and hippocampus on PND 90. Results represent the mean (±SE) of 5 rats and are expressed as percent increase over control. Significantly different from control, *$P < 0.05$; **$P < 0.01$. Significantly different from Pb alone, #$P < 0.05$.
Ashok A, Rai NK, Tripathi S, Bandyopadhyay S. Exposure to As-, Cd-, and Pb-mixture induces Aβ, amyloidogenic APP processing and cognitive impairments via oxidative stress-dependent neuroinflammation in young rats. Toxicol Sci. 2015; 143: 64–80.[57]

human CNS tau, sodium arsenite (50–500 μM) caused a fourfold increase of its phosphorylation at different sites.[75] Of note is that tau phosphorylation caused by As at serine 396/404, serine 202, threonine 205, and serine 181 were very similar to those found in brain of AD patients.[75] A number of signal transduction pathways (e.g., ERK1/2, SAPK1, GSK-3) were excluded as mediators of tau phosphorylation by As, and the exact kinase(s) involved remain elusive.[75]

In addition to these in vitro studies, an in vivo study in rats investigated the effect of developmental exposure to sodium arsenite (0.38 or 3.80 ppm by gavage from GD 5 to PND 21) on expression of APP in cerebral cortex and hippocampus on PND 90. As had no effect alone, but significantly potentiated the increase of APP induced by Pb or cadmium (Table 12.2).[57] A series of studies from the laboratory of Dr. Andrea Allan at the University of New Mexico explored the long-term effects of developmental exposure to As. Mice (C57BL/6J) were provided ad libitum access to drinking water containing 50 ppb arsenic (50 μg/L) during breeding and pregnancy until weaning on PND 23–25, yielding whole brain As levels of 2.24 ppb on PND 35.[76] Tyler and Allan[77] found that developmental As exposure decreased adult neurogenesis in the hippocampus and altered expression of a number of genes involved in axonogenesis, apoptosis, Notch signaling, and AD. Impaired hippocampal neurogenesis is present in AD and may contribute to cognitive deficits.[78] Of much interest is a follow-up study[79,80] in which developmental exposure to As was found to cause epigenetic changes in adult mice. The impact of As on the epigenome has been extensively studied in relationship to cancer, but information on the brain is lacking. The genetic programs involved in the processes of adult neurogenesis are highly orchestrated by epigenetic factors.[81] As complement to previous findings,[77] developmental As exposure was found to alter histone-3K4 trimethylation, increase histone-3K9 acetylation, and decrease expression of histone deacetylase enzymes HDAC1 and HDAC2 in PND 70 mice.[79] Interestingly, the effects were sex-dependent, usually more pronounced in males.[79,80]

CONCLUSIONS AND FUTURE PERSPECTIVES

The general concept of developmental origins of health and disease, which includes a variety of fetal-early life environmental conditions and numerous adult and age-related diseases, including neurodegenerative diseases, is often referred to as "the Barker hypothesis" or "silent neurotoxicity," when specifically referring to effects on the nervous system.[10,18] The experimental studies summarized in this chapter suggest that perinatal exposure to metals, such as Pb and As may later in life, induce the expression of biomarkers typical of AD. Whether these interesting observations can hold true in humans remains to be determined. Given the very long period (several decades) between possible exposure(s) and clinical sign of the disease, these studies are most difficult to carry out. Nevertheless, the existence of several cohorts of children studied in relationship to developmental exposure to Pb (or other metals) and neurodevelopmental abnormalities may be utilized in this respect. Also of relevance would be studies investigating possible mechanisms underlying such long-term effects of metals. In addition to discussed epigenetic mechanisms,[63] possible long-term involvement of microglia dysregulation or of damage related to oxidative stress need to be considered,[82,83] particularly given the role of neuroinflammation and oxidative stress in neurodegenerative disorders.

Acknowledgment

Research by the author is supported by grants from NIEHS (ES04696, ES07033, ES022949).

References

1. Yegambaram M, Manivannan B, Beach TG, Halden RU. Role of environmental contaminants in the etiology of Alzheimer's disease: a review. *Curr Alzheimer Res*. 2015;12:116–146.
2. Chin-Chan M, Navarro-Yepes J, Quintanilla-Vega B. Environmental pollutants as risk factors for neurodegenerative disorders: Alzheimer and Parkinson diseases. *Front Cell Neurosci*. 2015;9:124.
3. Bellou V, Belbasis L, Tzoulaki I, Evangelou E, Ioannidis JPA. Environmental risk factors and Parkinson's disease: an umbrella review of meta-analyses. *Parkinson Relat Dis*. 2016;23:1–9.
4. Polito L, Greco A, Seripa D. Genetic profile, environmental exposure, and their interaction in Parkinson's disease. *Parkinson's Dis*. 2016;2016:9.
5. Schelters P, Breteler MMB, de Strooper B, Frisani GB, Salloway S, Van der Flier WM. Alzheimer's disease. *Lancet*. 2016;388(10043):505–517.
6. Atik A, Stewart T, Zhang J. Alpha-synuclein as a biomarker for Parkinson's disease. *Brain Pathol*. 2016;26:410–418.
7. Wang X, Yu S, Li F, Feng T. Detection of alpha-synuclein oligomers in red blood cells as a potential biomarker of Parkinson's disease. *Neurosci Lett*. 2015;599:115–119.
8. Khan SS, Bloom GS. Tau: the center of a signaling nexus in Alzheimer's disease. *Front Neurosci*. 2016;10:31.
9. Selkoe DJ, Hardy J. The amyloid hypothesis of Alzheimer's disease at 25 years. *EMBO Mol Med*. 2016;8(6): 595–608.
10. Barker DJP. The origins of the developmental origins theory. *J Int Med*. 2007;261:412–417.
11. Calkins K, Devaskar SU. Fetal origins of adult disease. *Curr Probl Pediatr Adolesc Health Care*. 2011;41:158–176.
12. Almond D, Currie J. Killing me softly: the fetal origins hypothesis. *J Econ Perspect*. 2011;25:153–172.
13. Tartaglione AM, Venerosi A, Calamandrei G. Early-life toxic insults and onset of sporadic neurodegenerative diseases-an overview of experimental studies. *Curr Topics Behav Neurosci*. 2016;29:231–264.
14. Godfrey KM, Barker DJ. Fetal programming and human health. *Public Health Nutr*. 2001;4:611–624.
15. Lotti M, Moretto A. Organophosphate-induced delayed polyneuropathy. *Toxicol Rev*. 2005;24:37–49.
16. Zhang ZX, Anderson DW, Lavine L, Mantel N. Patterns of acquiring Parkinsonism-dementia on Guam 1944-1985. *Arch Neurol*. 1990;32:1726–1731.

17. Macknight C. Clinical implications of bovine spongiform encephalopathy. *Clin Infect Dis*. 2001;32:1726–1731.
18. Reuhl KR. Delayed expression of neurotoxicity: the problem of silent damage. *Neurotoxicology*. 1991;12:341–346.
19. Kraft AD, Aschner M, Cory-Slechta D, Bilbo SD, Caudle WM, Makris SL. Unmasking silent neurotoxicity following developmental exposure to environmental toxicants. *Neurotoxicol Teratol*. 2016;55:38–44.
20. McGeer PL, Itagaki S, Akiyama H, McGeer EG. Comparison of neuronal loss in Parkinson's disease and aging. In: Calne DB, Crippa D, Comi G, Horowski R, Trabucchi M, eds. *Parkinsonism and Aging*. New York: Raven Press; 1989:25–34.
21. Langston JW. Predicting Parkinson's disease. *Neurology*. 1990;40(Suppl 3):70–74.
22. Ling Z, Gayle DA, Ma SY, Lipton JW, Tong CW, Hong JS, Carvey PM. In utero bacterial endotoxin exposure causes loss of tyrosine hydroxylase neurons in the postnatal rat midbrain. *Mov Disord*. 2002;17:116–124.
23. Fan LW, Tien LT, Zheng B, Pang Y, Lin RCS, Simpson KL, Ma T, Rhodes PG, Cai Z. Dopaminergic neuronal injury in the adult rat brain following neonatal exposure to lipopolysaccharide and the silent neurotoxicity. *Brain Behav Immun*. 2011;25:286–297.
24. Costa LG, Aschner M, Vitalone A, Syversen T, Soldin OP. Developmental neuropathology of environmental agents. *Annu Rev Pharmacol Toxicol*. 2004;44:87–110.
25. Richardson JR, Caudle WM, Wang M, Dean ED, Pennell KD, Miller GW. Developmental exposure to the pesticide dieldrin alters the dopamine system and increases neurotoxicity in an animal model of Parkinson's disease. *FASEB J*. 2006;20:E976–E985.
26. Lloyd SA, Faherty CJ, Smeyme RJ. Adult and in utero exposure to cocaine alters sensitivity to the parkinsonian toxin 1-methyl-4-phenyl-1,2,3,6-tetrahydropyridine. *Neuroscience*. 2006;137:905–913.
27. Barlow BK, Cory-Slechta DA, Richfield EK, Thiruchelvam M. The gestational environment and Parkinson's disease: evidence for neurodevelopmental origins of a neurodegenerative disorder. *Reprod Toxicol*. 2007;23: 457–470.
28. Miller DB, O'Callaghan JP. Do early-life insults contribute to late-life development of Parkinson and Alzheimer diseases?. *Metabolism*. 2008;57(Suppl. 2):S44–S49.
29. Giordano G, Costa LG. Developmental neurotoxicity: some old and new issues. *ISRN Toxicol*. 2012;2012:12.
30. Landrigan PJ, Sonawane B, Butler RN, Trasande L, Callan R, Droller D. Early environmental origins of neurodegenerative disease in later life. *Environ Health Perspect*. 2005;113:1230–1233.
31. Borenstein AR, Copenhaver CI, Mortimer JA. Early-life risk factors for Alzheimer's disease. *Alzheimer Dis Assoc Disord*. 2006;20:63–72.
32. Lahiri DK, Maloney B, Basha MR, Ge YW, Zawia NH. How and when environmental agents and dietary factors affect the course of Alzheimer's disease; the "LEARn" mode (latent early-life associated regulation) may explain the triggering of AD. *Curr Alzheimer Res*. 2007;4:219–228.
33. Lahiri DK, Maloney B. The "LEARn" (latent early-life associated regulation) model integrates environmental risk factors and the developmental basis of Alzheimer's disease, and proposes remedial steps. *Exp Gerontol*. 2010;45:291–296.
34. Modgil S, Lahiri DK, Sharma VL, Anand A. Role of early life exposure and environment on neurodegeneration: implications on brain disorders. *Transl Neurogener*. 2014;3:9.
35. Ross MG, Desai M, Khorram O, McKnight RA, Lane RH, Torday J. Gestational programming of offspring obesity: a potential contributor to Alzheimer's disease. *Curr Alzheimer Res*. 2007;4:213–217.
36. Kounturas J, Tsolaki M, Gavalas E, Boziki M, Zavos C, Karatzoglou P, et al. Relationship between *Helicobacter pylori* infection and Alzheimer's disease. *Neurology*. 2006;66:938–940.
37. Finch CE. Developmental origins of aging in brain and blood vessels: an overview. *Neurobiol Aging*. 2005;26: 281–291.
38. Needleman HL, Gunnoe C, Leviton A. Deficits in psychologic and classroom performance of children with elevated dentine lead levels. *New Engl J Med*. 1979;300:689–695.
39. Hu H, Rabinowitz M, Smith D. Bone lead as a biological marker in epidemiologic studies of chronic toxicity: conceptual paradigms. *Environ Health Persepct*. 1998;106:1–8.
40. Weisskopf MG, Proctor SP, Wright RO, Schwartz J, Spiro A, Sparrow D, Nie H, Hu H. Cumulative lead exposure and cognitive performance among elderly men. *Epidemiology*. 2007;18:59–66.
41. Stewart WF, Schwartz BS, Simon D, Kelsey K, Todd AC. ApoE genotype, past adult lead exposure, and neurobehavioral function. *Environ Health Perspect*. 2002;110:501–505.
42. Coon S, Stark A, Peterson E, Gloi A, Kortsha G, Pounds J, Chettle D, Gorel J. Whole-body lifetime occupational lead exposure and risk of Parkinson's disease. *Environ Health Perspect*. 2006;114:1872–1876.

43. Weisskopf MG, Weuve J, Nie H, Saint-Hilaire MH, Sudarsky L, Simon DK, Hersch B, Schwartz J, Wright RO, Hu H. Association of cumulative lead exposure with Parkinson's disease. *Environ Health Perspect*. 2010;118: 1609–1613.
44. Lanphear BP, Hornung R, Khoury J, Yolton K, Baghurst P, Bellinger DC, Canfield RL, Dietrich KN, Bornschein R, Greene T, Rothenberg SJ, Needeleman HL, Schnaas L, Wasserman G, Graziano J, Roberts R. Low-level environmental lead exposure and children's intellectual function: an international pooled analysis. *Environ Health Perspect*. 2005;113:894–899.
45. Basha MR, Wei W, Bakheet SA, Benitez N, Siddiqui HK, Ge YW, Lahiri DK. The fetal basis of amyloidogenesis: exposure to lead and latent overexpression of amyloid precursor protein and β-amyloid in the aging brain. *J Neurosci*. 2005;25:823–829.
46. Bolin CM, Basha R, Cox D, Zawia NH, Maloney B, Lahiri DK, Cardozo-Pelaez F. Exposure to lead (Pb) and the developmental origin of oxidative DNA damage in the aging brain. *FASEB J*. 2006;20:788–790.
47. Wu J, Basha MR, Brock B, Cox DP, Cardozo-Pelaez F, McPherson CA, Harry J, Rice DC, Maloney B, Chen D, Lahiri DK, Zawia NH. Alzheimer's disease (AD)-like pathology in aged monkeys after infantile exposure to environmental metal lead (Pb): evidence for a developmental origin and environmental link for AD. *J Neurosci*. 2008;28:3–9.
48. Li N, Yu ZL, Wang L, Zhang YT, Jia JX, Wang Q, Zhu MJ, Liu XL, Xia X, Li WJ. Increased tau phosphorylation and beta amyloid in the hippocampus of mouse pups by early life lead exposure. *Acta Biol Hung*. 2010;61:123–134.
49. Bihaqi SW, Huang H, Wu J, Zawia NH. Infant exposure to lead (Pb) and epigenetic modifications in the aging primate brain: implications for Alzheimer's disease. *J Alzheimer's Dis*. 2011;27:819–833.
50. Dosunmu R, Alashwal H, Zawia NH. Genome-wide expression and methylation profiling in the aged rodent brain to early-life Pb exposure and its relevance to aging. *Mech Ageing Dev*. 2012;133:435–443.
51. Gu H, Robison G, Hong L, Barrea R, Wei X, Farlow MR, Pushkar YN, Du Y, Zheng W. Increased beta-amyloid deposition in Tg-SWDI transgenic mouse brain following in vivo lead exposure. *Toxicol Lett*. 2012;213:211–219.
52. Fox DA, Grandjean P, de Groot D, Paule MG. Developmental origins of adult diseases and neurotoxicity: epidemiological and experimental studies. *Neurotoxicology*. 2012;33:810–816.
53. Mazumdar M, Xia W, Hofman O, Gregas M, Sui SH, Hide W, Yang T, Needleman HL, Bellinger DC. Prenatal lead levels, plasma amyloid β levels, and gene expression in young adulthood. *Environ Health Perspect*. 2012;120: 702–707.
54. Chen J, Chen Y, Liu W, Bai C, Liu X, Liu K, Li R, Zhu JH, Huang C. Developmental lead acetate exposure induces embryonic toxicity and memory deficit in adult zebrafish. *Neurotoxicol Teratol*. 2012;34:581–586.
55. Bihaqi SW, Zawia NH. Enhanced tauopathy and AD-like pathology in aged primate brains decades after infantile exposure to lead (Pb). *Neurotoxicology*. 2013;39:95–101.
56. Bihaqi SW, Bahmani A, Adem A, Zawia NH. Infantile postnatal exposure to lead (Pb) enhances tau expression in the cerebral cortex of aged mice: relevance to AD. *Neurotoxicology*. 2014;44:114–120.
57. Ashok A, Rai NK, Tripathi S, Bandyopadhyay S. Exposure to As-, Cd-, and Pb-mixture induces Aβ, amyloidogenic APP processing and cognitive impairments via oxidative stress-dependent neuroinflammation in young rats. *Toxicol Sci*. 2015;143:64–80.
58. Masoud AM, Bihaqi SW, Machan JT, Zawia NH, Renehan WE. Early-life exposure to lead (Pb) alters the expression of microRNA that target proteins associated with Alzheimer's disease. *J Alzheimers Dis*. 2016;51:1257–1264.
59. Li Y, Xie C, Murphy SK, Skaar D, Nye M, Vidal AC, Cecil KM, Dietrich KN, Puga A, Jirtle RL, Hoyo C. Lead exposure during early human development and DNA methylation of imprinted gene regulatory elements in adulthood. *Environ Health Perspect*. 2016;124:666–673.
60. Rice DC. Effect of lead during different developmental periods in the monkey on concurrent discrimination performance. *Neurotoxicology*. 1992;13:583–592.
61. Bihaqi SW, Bahmani A, Subaiea GM, Zawia NH. Infantile exposure to lead and late-age cognitive decline: relevance to AD. *Alzheimers Dement*. 2014;10:187–195.
62. Bakulski KM, Rozek LS, Dolinoy DC, Paulson HL, Hu H. Alzheimer's disease and environmental exposure to lead: the epidemiologic evidence and potential role of epigenetics. *Curr Alzheimer Res*. 2012;9:563–573.
63. Eid A, Zawia N. Consequences of lead exposure, and its emerging role as an epigenetic modifier in the aging brain. *Neurotoxicology*. 2016;56:254–261.
64. Davis J, Xu F, Deane R, Romanov G, Previti ML, Zeigler K, Zlokovic BV, Van Nostrand WE. Early-onset and robust cerebral microvascular accumulation of amyloid beta-protein in transgenic mice expressing low levels of a vasculotropic Dutch/Iowa mutant form of amyloid beta-protein precursor. *J Biol Chem*. 2004;279:20296–20306.

65. Lee J, Freeman JL. Zebrafish as a model for investigating developmental lead (Pb) neurotoxicity as a risk factor in adult neurodegenerative disease: a mini-review. *Neurotoxicology*. 2014;43:57–64.
66. Song F, Poljak A, Valenzuela M, Mayeux R, Smythe GA, Sachdev PS. Meta-analysis of plasma amyloid-b levels in Alzheimer's disease. *J Alzheimer Dis*. 2011;26:365–375.
67. Bihaqi SW, Schumacher A, Maloney B, Lahiri DK, Zawia NH. Do epigenetic pathways initiate late onset Alzheimer disease (LOAD): towards a new paradigm. *Curr Alzheimer Res*. 2012;9:574–588.
68. Luo M, Xu Y, Cai R, Tang Y, Ge MM, Liu ZH, Xu L, Hu F, Ruan DY, Wang HL. Epigenetic histone modifications regulates developmental lead exposure induced hyperactivity in rats. *Toxicol Lett*. 2014;225:78–85.
69. Vahidnia A, van der Voet GB, de Wolff FA. Arsenic neurotoxicity—a review. *Hum Exp Toxicol*. 2007;26:823–832.
70. Tyler CR, Allan AM. The effects of arsenic exposure on neurological and cognitive dysfunction in human and rodent studies: a review. *Curr Environ Health Rep*. 2014;1:132–147.
71. Gong G, O'Bryant SE. The arsenic exposure hypothesis for Alzheimer disease. *Alzheimers Dis Assoc Disord*. 2010;24:311–316.
72. Tolins M, Ruchirawat M, Landrigan P. The developmental neurotoxicity of arsenic: cognitive and behavioral consequences of early life exposure. *Ann Global Health*. 2014;80:303–314.
73. Rodrigues EG, Bellinger DC, Valeri L, Hasan OSI, Quamruzzaman Q, Golam M, Kile ML, Christiani DC, Wright RO, Mazumdar M. Neurodevelopmental outcomes among 2- to 3-year-old children in Bangladesh with elevated blood lead and exposure to arsenic and manganese in drinking water. *Environ Health*. 2016;15:44.
74. Dewji NN, Do C, Bayney RM. Transcriptional activation of Alzheimer's β-amyloid precursor protein gene by stress. *Mol Brain Res*. 1995;33:245–253.
75. Giasson BI, Sampathu DM, Wilson CA, Vogelsberg-Ragaglia V, Mushynski WE, Lee VMY. The environmental toxin arsenite induces tau hyperphosphorylation. *Biochemistry*. 2002;41:15376–15387.
76. Martinez-Finley EJ, Ali AMS, Allan AM. Learning deficits in C57BL/6J mice following perinatal arsenic exposure: consequence of lower corticosterone receptor levels?. *Pharmacol Biochem Behav*. 2009;94:271–277.
77. Tyler CR, Allan AM. Adult hippocampal neurogenesis and mRNA expression are altered by perinatal arsenic exposure in mice and restored by brief exposure to enrichment. *Plos One*. 2013;8:e73720.
78. Horgusluoglu E, Nudelman K, Nho K, Saykin AJ. Adult neurogenesis and neurodegenerative diseases; a systems biology perspective. *Am J Med Genet B Neuropsychiatr Genet*. 2017;174(1):93–112.
79. Tyler CR, Hafez AK, Solomon ER, Allan AM. Developmental exposure to 50 parts-per-billion arsenic influences histone modifications and associated epigenetic machinery in a region-and sex-specific manner in the adult mouse brain. *Toxicol Appl Pharmacol*. 2015;288:40–51.
80. Tyler CR, Weber JA, Labrecque M, Hessinger JM, Edwards JS, Allan AM. ChIP-Seq analysis of the adult male mouse brain after developmental exposure to arsenic. *J Data Brief*. 2015;5:248–254.
81. Covic M, Karaca E, Lie DC. Epigenetic regulation of neurogenesis in the adult hippocampus. *Heredity*. 2010;105:122–134.
82. Luo ZC, Fraser WD, Julien P, Deal CL, Audibert F, Smith GN, Xiong X, Walker M. Tracing the origins of "fetal origins" of adult diseases: programming by oxidative stress?. *Med Hyp*. 2006;66:38–44.
83. Harry GJ, Kraft AD. Microglia in the developing brain: a potential target with lifetime effects. *Neurotoxicology*. 2012;33:191–206.

CHAPTER

13

Metal Biology Associated with Huntington's Disease

Terry Jo V. Bichell,**, Timothy C. Halbesma*, K. Grace Tipps*, Aaron B. Bowman*,***

*Vanderbilt University (VU) and Vanderbilt University Medical Center (VUMC), Nashville, TN, United States

**Vanderbilt Brain Institute, Vanderbilt University Medical Center (VUMC), Nashville, TN, United States

OUTLINE

Biometals in Neurodegenerative Diseases. http://dx.doi.org/10.1016/B978-0-12-804562-6.00013-0

INTRODUCTION

Though it is well established that metal homeostasis is altered in neurodegenerative diseases, the regional metal deposition profile differs for each disorder. In Huntington's disease (HD), abnormalities have been found in the tissue or cellular deposition or handling of copper (Cu), iron (Fe), calcium (Ca), and manganese (Mn) and in their neuronal functions, which are either the result of disease processes, or the cause of pathology. In general, it is the toxicity of overexposure or excess accumulation of metals, that is associated with pathology, such as is seen with Mn or Fe intoxication in Parkinsonian conditions.[1] Recently, it has been shown that deficiency or maldistribution of metals may be just as pathological as the toxicity of overexposure. In amyotrophic lateral sclerosis, there is a reduction of Cu and zinc (Zn), while lead exposure is surprisingly protective.[2] In Alzheimer's disease (AD), a deficiency of Cu has been found in models but the Cu content of postmortem AD brain tissue did not differ from healthy controls, though the Cu stores were abnormally labile, or responsive to chelation.[3] Cell and animal models of HD have shown a surprising resistance to Mn accumulation and uptake, with downstream reductions in Mn-dependent enzyme activity and metabolism, which will be described later. In the case of HD, a subregional or subcellular maldistribution of metals may best describe the pathogenic contribution of metallostasis to HD neuropathology (Fig. 13.1).

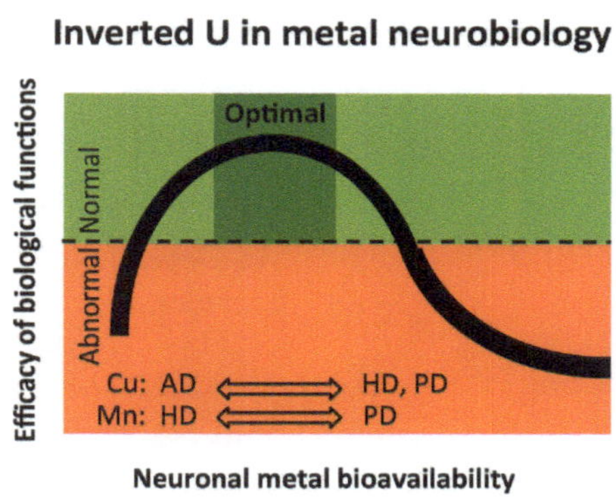

FIGURE 13.1 **The biological response to metal concentration in neuronal tissues follows an inverted U.** Low concentrations of metals, as well as high concentrations, cause damage or dysfunction, and the efficacy of biological functions is only optimal at a narrow range.

THE EPIDEMIOLOGY OF HD

HD is a relatively rare neurodegenerative disorder; the approximate worldwide prevalence is 2.71 cases per 100,000 population.[4] However, prevalence of HD around the globe ranges from 5.7 in the British Isles to only 0.40 per 100,000 in Asia.[4] While HD affects both men and women in equal numbers,[5] gender appears to play a role in disease progression and HD brain metabolism,[6] as females tend to experience more severe motor and functional symptoms along with a faster rate of disease progression.[7]

Unlike many other neurodegenerative disorders, in which there are few genetic links, HD is an autosomal dominant genetic disorder caused by a mutation in the Huntingtin gene (*HTT*) that was identified in the mid-1990s from studies of a Venezuelan community with very high incidence.[8] The causative mutation is an expanded CAG repeat in the first exon of *HTT*, which results in an extended polyglutamine (polyQ) sequence in the huntingtin protein (HTT). The *HTT* gene is highly conserved through evolution, but there is wide diversity between species in the number of CAG repeats.[9–11] In humans, between 9 and 34 CAG repeats is thought to be normal, but there are cases of symptomatic HD developing within the range of 27–34 CAG repeats,[12–14] and it appears that 35–39 CAG repeats is not fully penetrant,[15] as 1 in 400 elderly individuals from cohorts in the United Kingdom and the United States had alleles between 35 and 39 without HD symptoms.

It is still unclear whether HD pathology is caused by loss of function of the normal HTT protein or toxic gain of function from the mutant HTT protein, or a combination of both.[16–18] Transgenic mouse models with one mutant allele as well as two functioning wild-type alleles still develop symptoms of HD, suggesting that toxicity of the mutation is the root cause of pathology.[19] Conditional mouse models expressing lower levels of mutant HTT in the cortex and striatum show no behavioral deficits, and neurodegeneration of these brain regions is ameliorated.[20] Yet, overexpression of mutant HTT, as well as knockdown of wild-type HTT, alters vesicular transport, mitochondrial function, and the autophagy process in neurons, both in vitro and in vivo,[21–25] making both the loss of wild-type function and the toxic gain of mutant function important to HD pathology related to neuronal metal homeostasis.

The function of wild-type HTT protein is still not fully explained, but cellular metal dyshomeostasis is a recognized feature. HTT is known to play a part in axonal transport,[26] transcriptional regulation,[27,28] apoptosis,[29] autophagy,[30] endocytosis,[31] and as a scaffold for protein–protein interactions,[32] all of which involve metal biology. The HTT protein is huge and ubiquitously expressed, with more than 300 binding partners identified to date[16,33–35] including Cu. The expanded polyQ tract takes on a labile conformation (helix, coil, loop) that enables it to function as a regulator of multiple protein interactions.[36,37] The protein is modified posttranslationally, primarily in the same N-terminal region as the polyQ expansion, which is also the region linked to the formation of aggregates and to mitochondrial dysfunction, which are molecular hallmarks of HD pathology.[38,39]

The first symptoms of HD begin, on average, between the ages of 35 and 40,[12] with the age of onset inversely correlated to the number of polyQ repeats, though timing varies even among patients with identical CAG number. Sibling and twin studies reveal that modifier genes explain an additional 13% of the variability in age of onset in the studied patient populations, with the remainder attributed to environmental factors,[40–42] suggesting the possibility that metal toxicity or deficiency could be a factor. After the onset of motor symptoms, patients with HD typically live for 20 additional years, with aspiration pneumonia the most common cause of death.[43]

THE SYMPTOMS OF HD

Though the hallmark symptom of HD is chorea (uncontrolled movements), psychological, and cognitive changes are also common and can be equally as detrimental to quality of life.[44] The symptoms of HD appear in three phases, both in humans and mouse models. The first, premanifest phase, is without observable signs or symptoms. In the second, prodromal phase, patients demonstrate changes in cognition and personality. Families of patients often report increased apathy, anxiety, and depression.[45,46] A clinical diagnosis of adult-onset HD generally relies on the observance of chorea,[47] but as the disease progresses, dystonia, and rigidity occur. Overall, symptoms of HD and the disease progression are remarkably heterogeneous across patient populations.

Animal and cell models replicate many of the pathologies associated with HD, and include mouse, sheep, rat, zebrafish, *Drosophila* (fruit fly), *C. elegans* (worm), and *Saccharomyces cerevisiae* (yeast) models.[48,49] Mouse models include transgenics with an insertion of the 5′ region of human *HTT*, transgenic mice expressing the entire length of human *HTT*, and knock-in models where CAG repeats are inserted into the mouse *Htt* locus.[50] While mouse models effectively mimic the human disease progression, they do not develop severe motor deficits, and the age of onset is surprisingly late.[50] Animal models also lack the severe neurodegeneration that is seen in humans.[51]

THE NEUROPATHOLOGY OF HD

HTT is expressed ubiquitously across various cell types and tissues,[16] yet degeneration occurs in restricted brain regions, where it is especially marked in the striatum in the later phases of the disease. Prodromally, there is minor cortical loss, followed by massive loss of the striatal γ-aminobutyric acid transmitting (GABAergic) medium spiny neurons (MSNs), which make up 90% of the neurons in the striatum, suggesting that pathology may originate in the cortex.[52] Other brain regions, such as the hippocampus, thalamus, and globus pallidus also degenerate in HD, but not to the extent seen in the striatum,[53] so most studies focus on the neurons of the cortex and striatum.

The striatal MSNs are subcategorized by dopamine receptor expression and projection targets. Those that project to the substantia nigra and the internal segment of the globus pallidus and contain D2 dopamine receptors and substance P, form the indirect pathway, and are the first to degenerate in HD.[54] MSNs projecting to the external segment of the globus pallidus, expressing D1 receptors and met-enkaphalin, make up the direct pathway, and are spared from neurodegeneration until later in the disease course. This sequential loss of striatal MSN subtypes is partially related to metal uptake and deposition, and appears to correlate with onset of patient symptoms.[55]

Like the striatum, subtypes of cortical neurons are differentially affected by HD. Large pyramidal neurons originating in cortical layers III, V, and VI, and projecting directly to the striatum, primarily contribute to the loss of cortical volume in HD.[56,57]

BIOLOGICAL FUNCTION OF WILD-TYPE AND PATHOGENIC HTT PROTEINS

Many of the functions of wild-type HTT have been described as part of essential cellular pathways which involve metals as cofactors, for ionic gradients, and for protein stability. These include biological processes, such as axonal transport,[26] nuclear export,[27] transcriptional regulation,[58] apoptosis,[59] autophagy,[30] and the scaffolding of protein interactions.[60] The crystal structure of HTT has not been entirely elucidated, perhaps because the protein can take on many different structures.[36] The polyQ tract, which is altered by the number of CAG repeats in exon 1, forms a flexible domain that regulates intramolecular proximity and substrate specificity.[61]

Wild-type HTT is located primarily in the cytoplasm,[62,63] but plays a role in protein trafficking between nucleus and cytoplasm through transcriptional regulation of the nuclear pore protein.[27] N-terminal HTT fragments interact with the protein's translocated promoter region, and excessive polyQ expansion decreases this interaction.[27] HTT is modified post-translationally by acetylation, phosphorylation, ubiquitination, palmitoylation, and sumoylation, with each modification having effects on function and activity.[64–66] With the HD mutation, the HTT protein becomes much less soluble leading to misfolding of the extended polyQ sequences which then form a β-sheet structure, leading to abnormal post-translational modifications.[12,67,68]

Short fragments of mutant HTT form aggregates in the nucleus and cytoplasm, which may be the source of further pathology, but may also be a cellular defense process to sequester the toxic misfolded mutant HTT protein.[69] Cu interacts with the polyQ fragment of HTT and increases aggregation,[52] and Cu ions bind to HTT aggregates and induce oxidation, which increases neuronal oxidative stress,[70] potentially leading to cell death and degeneration. These aggregates can be cleared either by autophagy or by the proteasome system. A recent study indicates that macroautophagy may be more crucial to the clearance of HTT aggregates than the proteasomal process,[71] and autophagy is known to be affected by metal homeostasis.

AUTOPHAGY AND METALS IN HUNTINGTON'S DISEASE

Disturbances in macroautophagy have recently been implicated as a cause of pathology in many neurodegenerative diseases, including HD.[72] Cells transport waste products, including metalloproteins, between organelles and from within the cytoplasm to outside of the cell membrane via autophagosomes that envelope and contain toxic products, such as misfolded proteins and damaged organelles.[73] Interestingly, HTT shares structural similarity with a yeast autophagy gene, Atg11, which has similarities to both a GABA receptor and an autophagic scaffold.[30] In HD, autophagosomes are frequently devoid of cargo,[74] though their number and form is unaffected, suggesting that there is a defect in the cargo-recognition function. This abnormality may allow for the buildup of aggregates of HTT and other toxic products, especially Fe-containing proteins, which may contribute to the metal dyshomeostasis seen in HD (described later).

In a *Drosophila* model of HD, reducing wild-type HTT function disturbs macroautophagy, and conditionally knocking out HTT in adult mice also causes signs of autophagosomal dysfunction, including accumulation of p62, which is an autophagic receptor protein.[21] Selective autophagy is the process by which particular proteins are engulfed by double-membrane vesicles for transport between intracellular compartments.[75] Ochaba and coworkers, found that HTT is necessary for selective autophagy in both *Drosophila* and mouse, and that mutant HTT causes a deficit in protein clearance that is likely related to this reduction in selective autophagy.[21,76] HTT knockout in wild-type mouse brain leads to accumulation of both p62- and ubiquitin- containing aggregates, which may indicate breakdown of the selective autophagic process which disposes of these products.[21,77] Clearance of the Fe-binding protein ferritin occurs through selective autophagy, and ferritin clearance is impaired by mutant HTT in patients with HD and in mouse models.[78–80] This obstruction of ferritin processing could lead to the increased intracellular Fe-storage abnormalities seen in HD (discussed later).

One integral protein to the membrane of the autophagosome is the clathrin light chain (CLC), which is known to be regulated by Huntingtin Interacting Protein-1 (HIP1).[81] CLC forms clathrin-coated vesicles that are part of the endosomal recycling system as well as the autophagosome. This pathway is also related to Fe homeostasis, through transferrin, a protein that binds and transports Fe. The transferrin receptor is taken up by the rapid recycling endosomal G-clathrin vesicles which are mediated by CLC,[82] a pathway which links the HTT interacting proteins with both autophagy, transferrin receptor recycling and metal homeostasis.

Metal dyshomeostasis itself may be the root cause of macroautophagy alterations in HD. Zhang and coworkers found that Mn exposure increased autophagy acutely in wild-type rats postexposure, but thereafter inhibited autophagy, when measured up to 28 days later.[83] And, in cultured dopaminergic neurons, Mn nanoparticles activated autophagic cell death.[84] Furthermore, Cu exposure leads to the autophagosomal destruction of mitochondria (mitophagy) and related apoptosis when Cu is complexed with dopamine.[85] Fe also has an effect on autophagy, with some studies showing autophagic increases after Fe accumulation, and other data demonstrating Fe-induced reductions.[86] The interaction between metal homeostasis and macroautophagy has not yet been studied in the context of HD, though both pathways are clearly involved in the disease process.

Macroautophagy proteins can regulate cell cycle progression, mitosis, and selective autophagic clearance.[87–89] Other vesicular transport systems, such as microvesicles and exosomes may also connect metal homeostasis with HD. There is new interest in this interplay between metals, HTT, and macroautophagy.

EXOSOMES AND METAL IN HUNTINGTON'S DISEASE

Exosomes are very small vesicles (50 nm or less in diameter) in the extracellular space, that contain proteins and waste products, including metals.[90] These exosomes originate in the endosome and contain transferrin receptors, among other proteins, and may also play a role in intracellular metal homeostasis and metal transport between organelles. In addition to carrying metals and metal receptors, exosomes have been found to deliver toxic trinucleotide RNA's, and fragments of polyQ proteins from one cell to another, spreading these fragments in a prion-like fashion.[91] HTT has been associated with exosomal protein in several studies, suggesting that it either plays a part in exosomal regulation, or that exosomes serve to recycle or dispose of HTT.[91–93] Exosomal contents may prove to serve as a biomarker, both for metal exposure as well as for clinical treatment trials.

ENVIRONMENTAL FACTORS IMPACTING HD

Metal exposure is one environmental effect which can have an impact on a known genetic disorder, such as HD. Exercise is also an environmental exposure, albeit decidedly ameliorative, delaying the disease onset in mice.[94–98] Like cognitive enrichment, exercise increases brain derived neurotrophic factor (BDNF) levels.[99] Neurogenesis and neuronal survival are increased by BDNF binding to the tyrosine kinase B receptor (TrkB), which activates cell survival pathways,[100,101] and TrkB levels are increased with exercise along with BDNF.[102,103] In HD, BDNF protein levels are reduced in serum and brain tissue,[104,105] as is BDNF gene transcription,[106] with higher levels of BDNF linked to slowing of neurodegeneration.[107]

BDNF is not produced in the striatum, but instead must be imported via axonal transport from the cortex or substantia nigra.[24] HTT is found proximal to vesicles and endosomes[108–110] and to microtubules[109,111] and is directly associated with the plasma membrane.[112] The vesicular transport system depends upon an interaction between the HTT protein and Huntingtin-associated protein 1 (HAP1),[113] with HTT acting as a scaffold, bringing together the transport machinery, and enhancing vesicle travel speed and direction.[114] HTT is known to interact with a promoter of dynein-driven microtubule transport, dynactin subunit p150Glued, via primary interactions with HAP-1.[111,115,116] Through this protein complex, the HTT protein has been associated with both endocytic and microtubule-mediated vesicle transport, transporting substances, such as BDNF and metals into cells and organelles.[24] Overall, mutant HTT impairs vesicular transport of numerous cellular goods, including BDNF.[23]

In addition HTT also regulates transcription of BDNF through interaction with its promoter and inhibits the neuron restrictive silencer element (NRSE), which inhibits BDNF transcription.[117] Mutant HTT loses this inhibitory capability and thereby decreases BDNF transcription.[117] Increasing BDNF through gene overexpression in mouse models[118] or indirectly through exercise or enrichment[98] protects MSNs and delays degeneration. Links between BDNF and metal in HD will be discussed later.

METALS IN HD

Links between heavy metals and neurodegenerative diseases have long been described,[119,120] but the role of metal exposure in the progression and symptomology of HD is not yet well understood. Because transition (or related) metals Cu, Fe, Zn, Ca, and Mn, are essential to neurobiology, alterations in metallostasis can affect their roles as catalysts in reduction-oxidation reactions, cofactors for enzymes, and metabolism, all of which are important for neurological function.[119] Each of the transition metals plays a part in the pathology of HD.

Regional accumulation differs by metal and by concentration of exposures. Following excess exposure in wild type rats, Fe accumulates in the globus pallidus, Cu in the striatum and thalamus, and Mn in the thalamus and substantia nigra.[121] Toxic exposure to these metals has been linked to induction of oxidative stress, mitochondrial dysfunction, protein aggregation, and alterations in vesicular transport,[122–124] all of which play a part in the disease. A screen of metals [Mn^{2+}, Fe^{2+}, Cu^{2+}, Zn^{2+}, lead (Pb^{2+}), cadmium (Cd^{2+}), cobalt (Co^{2+}), and nickel (Ni^{2+})] on a striatal cell model of HD with cell survival as the outcome measure revealed a surprising interaction between mutant HTT and Mn.[125] The HD cells took up less Mn than normal controls, and HD cells were protected from Mn^{2+} exposure. This in vitro finding was recapitulated in vivo, that is, mouse models of HD accumulated less striatal Mn than wild-type after subcutaneous exposure.[125,126]

While Mn is surprisingly decreased in HD models, an increase of Fe and Cu is found in the affected brain regions (described in each section later). Interestingly, increased striatal Zn concentrations have also been noted in postmortem HD patient brain.[127] Recently, a drug targeted at an HTT-metal interaction was brought to clinical trial. Hydroxyquinoline (PBT2), a compound that reduces copper binding to the Huntingtin protein, progressed through Phase II clinical trials with 109 patients. The medication was considered safe and well received by subjects, but lack of significant improvement in cognition or function prevented the drug from continuing to Phase III trials.[128,129] Yet, the influence of environmental factors on disease progression suggests that the aberrant properties of mutant HTT can be mitigated, and exploration of these factors, such as the gene environment interaction between HTT and metals, may reveal further therapeutic targets.

IRON IN HD

HD has been associated with altered Fe homeostasis in a number of ex vivo and in vivo human studies, focusing mainly on the vulnerable basal ganglia structures. Postmortem analysis of patient brains has shown increased Fe levels in HD caudate, putamen, and globus pallidus,[127,130,131] which is consistent with the macroautophagy deficits mentioned earlier. Mice expressing mutant HTT fragments show increased Fe buildup in brain as the disease progresses.[132,133] In human patients with HD, there is also abnormal accumulation of striatal Fe and Cu as symptoms progress.[134]

MRI results point to abnormal iron deposition in HD caudate, putamen, globus pallidus, and cortex at different disease stages, including premanifest HD, suggesting a role for Fe as a biomarker for the disease and implicating Fe dysregulation in HD pathogenesis[127,135–143] (Fig. 13.2). Imaging studies correlating T2 measures with CAG repeat number and clinical features in HD patients suggest that longer CAG tracts may be associated with higher amounts of toxic forms of Fe in certain vulnerable basal ganglia structures.[139,140]

More recent magnetic resonance studies have examined the relationship between brain atrophy and Fe deposition in HD. One study reported that increased Fe accumulation in early-manifest HD basal ganglia and atrophy of those regions occurred independently of each other.[141] Another study of presymptomatic HD subjects found that both excessive Fe

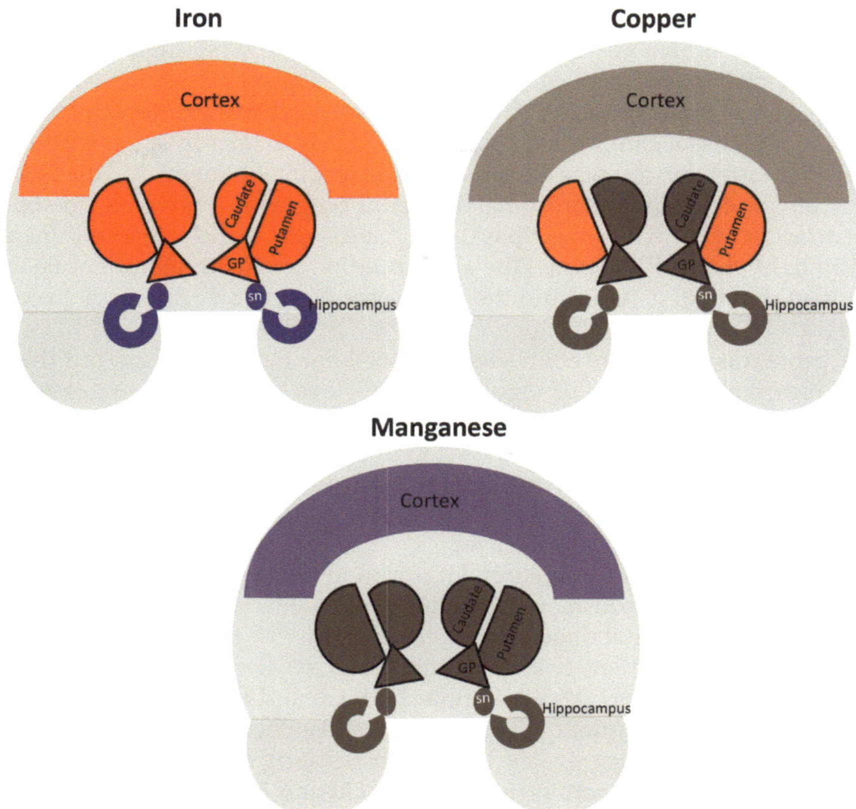

FIGURE 13.2 **Schematic representation of regional metal accumulation in HD.** Very few studies have investigated the localization of metal deposits in HD patients. *Copper*: Postmortem increases in putamen in one study,[130] no increase in another.[127] *Iron*: Postmortem studies show increased Fe in caudate, putamen and globus pallidus.[127,130,131,134] MRI confirms increased Fe in caudate nucleus, putamen and globus pallidus, and also found decreased Fe in hippocampus and substantia nigra.[135] *Manganese*: Postmortem, no differences between HD and controls.[127,130] MRI reductions in cortical subregions.[127] *Red* indicates excess deposition, *blue* indicates a deficit, *dark gray* indicates evidence of no change in regional accumulation, *light gray* indicates no or limited available data.

accumulation and volumetric losses in the basal ganglia which began at the presymptomatic disease stage intensified with disease progression and CAG repeat number.[143] A recent imaging study by van Bergen and coworkers,[135] confirmed increased Fe levels in the caudate nucleus, putamen, and globus pallidus of subjects with premanifest HD, showing significant atrophy in the caudate nucleus and putamen, which was inversely correlated with Fe levels in those regions. The investigators also reported significantly decreased Fe in hippocampus and substantia nigra of premanifest HD patients. Thus, while the role of Fe in HD neuropathology remains under investigation, the links between altered Fe homeostasis in HD brain and other clinical and biological features of the disease suggest that Fe may play a role in HD pathogenesis and/or serve as a tool for studying HD.

The mechanisms leading to Fe accumulation in HD brain are unknown, but may be related to any or all of three known Fe-related proteins: ferritin (the Fe storage protein), transferrin (a protein that binds Fe), or ferroportin (a transmembrane protein that moves Fe across membranes). Ex vivo and imaging studies have shown increased levels of ferritin, in postmortem and earlier-stage HD basal ganglia and cortex, particularly in microglia with morphologic abnormalities,[79,131] though ferritin was decreased in the serum of patients.[144] This low serum ferritin is characteristic of a similar autosomal dominant progressive movement disorder known as neuroferritinopathy, or adult-onset basal ganglia disease, which is caused by a mutation in the ferritin light chain (FTL) gene. The FTL mutation results in abnormal Fe and ferritin accumulation in the basal ganglia, and the symptoms of motor dysfunction are very similar to those of HD.[145–149]

The HTT protein is intimately connected with cellular Fe metabolism, but the exact relationship and direction of the Fe-HTT regulation, is unclear. HTT cofractionates with the transferrin receptor (TfR)[150] and some data indicates that HTT itself is an Fe-responsive protein.[151] On the other hand, reduction of HTT expression in zebrafish leads to increased TfR1 expression in hypochromic blood.[78] Upon exposure to bioavailable Fe, this phenotype is reversed, suggesting a functional role of wild-type huntingtin in making endocytosed Fe accessible, perhaps releasing Fe from endocytic vesicles.

Supplemental Fe may be detrimental in HD, even in the prodromal phases, as it has been shown in two different HD mouse models that supplementation with Fe in the neonatal period causes more severe striatal degeneration to develop.[152,153] Furthermore, HTT aggregates are increased with Fe-dependent oxidation and protected with deferoxamine, an Fe chelator.[132] Cu is also implicated in HD pathology, as both Cu and Fe exposures have been linked to increased aggregation of mutant HTT[133] and a Cu/Fe chelator, clioquinol, an antifungal drug, reduced mutant HTT aggregates while also rescuing the HD behavioral phenotype in R6/2 mice.[154] There is also a connection between Cu and Fe, in that Cu treatment induces ferroportin expression, allowing for Fe efflux from cultured macrophage cells,[155] though Cu deficiency has no impact.[156]

COPPER IN HD

The role of Cu and Cu-binding proteins in patients with HD is still under investigation. Dexter and coworkers reported increased Cu levels in postmortem HD putamen,[130] however, a more recent study by Rosas and coworkers did not find elevated Cu levels in HD brain by MRI or postmortem analysis[127] (Fig. 13.2). Indirect evidence that Cu accumulation may be high is found in analysis of gene expression data from postmortem HD patient brain tissue revealed upregulation of genes encoding Cu-binding proteins, including metallothioneins 1 and 2 (MT1 and MT2) and ceruloplasmin.[157,158] Though those studies were postmortem, another study of oxidative damage in the cerebrospinal fluid (CSF) of living patients found increased lipoperoxidation in the CSF of those with HD along with decreased Cu/Zn-dependent superoxide dismutase (SOD1) activity and decreased ceruloplasmin ferroxidase activity, which was correlated to motor assessments.[159] While these findings suggest that free Cu may be increased in HD CSF, the investigators did not report significantly higher levels of free Cu.

Rodents exposed to quinolinic acid exhibit striatal deficits that resemble those seen in HD due to neuronal death by depletion of GABA.[160] These QUIN-HD model rats accumulate excess Cu in the striatum, which may be linked to the agonistic effect of quinolinic acid on NMDA-type glutamate receptors.[161] Cu is released after activation of NMDA receptors, and their stimulation increases trafficking of a Cu-specific transporter, ATP7A, from the late Golgi into neuronal dendrites, resulting in local Cu accumulation.[162] Surprisingly, pretreatment of rats with Cu-supplemented drinking water before exposure to quinolinic acid prevents some of the HD-related symptoms.[163]

Though HTT interacts indirectly with Fe through Fe-binding proteins and transporters, the connection between HTT and Cu is direct. Experiments in vitro show that Cu^{2+} interacts with wild-type HTT, decreasing the solubility of HTT protein fragments,[52] and increasing aggregation. Previously, aggregates were thought to be inert, but it has now been shown that Cu also binds with HTT after aggregation, possibly further exacerbating their insolubility.[70] Fewer aggregates form when Cu influx transporters (DmATP7 and Ctr1B) are blocked in *Drosophila* HD models.[52,164] Furthermore, there are two residues on the HTT protein which may bind Cu (Met8 and His82), and when these sites are mutated in HD Drosophila models, the toxic effects of mutant HTT are prevented.[164] It appears that neither the Cu alone, nor the polyQ extension on HTT exon 1 alone caused HD symptoms, but the combination of the HD mutation and Cu exposure was toxic, suggesting that Cu-related treatments could be of benefit to HD patients.

CALCIUM IN HD

Ca is very important in HD, both on a regional and molecular level. Intracellular Ca^{2+} modulates many biological functions through its role as a second messenger,[165] thus it is tightly regulated by intracellular sequestration through Ca buffering proteins (such as calbindin), and by the presence of storage pools in the mitochondria and endoplasmic reticulum (ER).[166] Neuronal Ca levels were much higher in R6/2 mice (a mouse model which bears the first exon of mutant human *HTT*) than in their wild-type littermates after symptoms had begun.[167]

Optimal intracellular Ca concentration is controlled by AMPA receptors, glutamate-gated NMDA receptors, voltage-gated Ca channels, and store-operated calcium entry (SOCE) channels.[166] In cultured neurons from HD model mice, there is increased intracellular Ca response to glutamate challenge, leading to oxidative stress which can cause apoptosis.[168–172] Interestingly, it is chiefly the duration of Ca response that is altered, rather than the total Ca, implicating abnormalities in cellular Ca handling rather than influx.[166]

Subcellularly, Ca can be released from pools stored in the mitochondria or in the ER, and there is indirect evidence that HTT may be involved in the regulation of these Ca stores. The HTT protein directly binds with the mitochondrial membrane,[173] and the polyQ expansion reduces mitochondrial sequestration of Ca, suggesting a role in controlling mitochondrial Ca transport. There is also direct binding of the HTT protein with Huntington Associated Protein 1 (HAP1) and inositol triphosphate (IP3) which causes IP3 to interact with the IP3 receptor on the ER membrane.[174] The IP3 receptor is a Ca channel that is activated by IP3, allowing for the release of Ca in response to mGluR1/5 receptor activation. Mutant HTT binds to the type 1 IP3 receptor (InsP3R1), increasing its activity and reducing Ca levels in the ER.[171,175]

The store-operated calcium (SOC) release pathway is also affected in HD. Stroma Interacting Molecule 2 (STIM2) is a plasma membrane protein located in the ER that participates in SOC release as a Ca sensor.[176] When ER Ca decreases, STIM2 interacts with SOC entry channels to resupply the ER with Ca. Bezprozvanny and colleagues found that STIM2 expression is elevated in HD model mouse striatum, possibly as a compensatory mechanism to release the excess Ca accumulation caused by the abnormal sensitivity of the InsP3R1 when it is bound to mutant HTT.[177] Further, depletion of Ca from the ER activates the SOC pathway in neuronal spines in the HD mouse model, perhaps leading to the reduction in spine density found in aged HD model mice compared to wild-type. Indeed, reducing expression of either InsP3R1 or STIM2 reversed the dendritic spine abnormalities in HD mouse cortical-striatal cell cultures compared to wild-type.

Thus, the levels of Ca in neurons and within neuronal organelles contributes to HD abnormalities. Ca dyshomeostasis may also play a role in the HD associated alterations in the bioavailabilities of other metals as well. The homeostasis of both Ca and Mn are disrupted in HD, and the two metals are closely related in many biological pathways, often transported through the same channels, though sometimes moving in opposite directions.

MANGANESE IN HD

Mn exposure has long been associated with motor pathway damage, suggesting that the metal is involved in the functioning of neuronal systems that control movement. In general, it is an excess of Mn that is considered to be pathogenic. For example, chronic exposure to Mn through vocations, such as welding or smelting increases the risk of Manganism, a neurodegenerative Parkinsonian condition affecting the nigrostriatal dopaminergic pathways.[178,179] Even populations exposed to subtoxic levels of airborne Mn from nearby industries exhibit subtle, though not significant, effects on motor pathways, as measured by postural sway score.[180] In HD, it is likely the inverse. Interestingly though excess Cu and Fe are associated with the toxicity of mutant HTT, it is most likely a deficit of Mn that is associated with HD, especially in the crucial brain regions that are most susceptible to neurodegeneration in the disorder.

Confusingly, there is overlap between the symptoms of Mn toxicity and the toxicity of mutant HTT. For example, mutant HTT decreases BDNF transcription[117] and reduces BDNF transport.[181] Mn exposure decreases phosphorylation of serine 421 on HTT, which controls BDNF transport.[182] In wild-type mice, Mn exposure decreases BDNF production,[182] and Mn exposure also causes reduction in the spine density and dendritic length of MSNs.[183] These BDNF and dendritic spine alterations caused by the toxicity of Mn exposure are the same phenotypes which are seen in HD, suggesting that an inverted U-curve of dose response, may explain the relationship between Mn exposure and neuronal function.[184,185]

There is evidence that the deficiency portion of the homeostasis curve is invoked in HD. In the presence of mutant HTT, Mn bioavailability decreases: cultured striatal cell models of HD reveal a deficiency of Mn and studies of mouse models find a reduction of striatal Mn bioavailabilty.[125,186] Still, though these HD models reveal Mn dyshomeostasis, there is limited evidence of a brain regional Mn deficit in human HD patients. Postmortem analysis by Dexter and coworkers did not reveal significant alterations of Mn levels in the basal ganglia compared to normal controls,[127,130] but the sample size included only 6 females and 4 males, and the study was done before genetic confirmation of HD was possible. More recently, Rosas and coworkers reported decreased Mn in cortical regions of post mortem HD brain,[126] but not striatum. This suggests a subregional, cell-type, or even subcellular Mn dyshomeostasis.

In any case, there is substantial disagreement in the literature about the regional location of Mn in normal brain, chiefly because most methods for measuring Mn in tissues have resolution which is too low.[187] For this reason, most studies measure regional Mn deposition following excess exposure, with almost no studies of Mn localizations in conditions of a deficiency of the metal, and the distribution may be very different depending upon tissue concentration.

MANGANESE DEPOSITION: BRAIN REGIONS, CELL TYPES, AND CELLULAR ORGANELLES

Regional Deposition

Mn is paramagnetic, and therefore provides enhanced signal intensity in T1-weighted MRI,[188] allowing for imaging of Mn deposits in vivo, but the resolution of these images is not fine enough to distinguish deposits of manganese in deficiency conditions.[187] The results gathered through MRI[189] are different from those seen via other techniques, such as X-ray fluorescence,[187] atomic absorption spectroscopy,[190] or inductively coupled plasma mass spectroscopy.[191] This discrepancy may be due to the speciation of manganese (Mn^{2+} vs. Mn^{3+}) or to Mn-binding interactions.[188] MRI measurements following Mn exposure generally document elevated Mn accumulating in the hippocampus, while other methods record Mn deposits to be chiefly in the globus pallidus and substantia nigra.[189]

In normal human brain without excess Mn exposure, most studies agree that there is more Mn found in the basal ganglia than in other brain regions, particularly in the caudate and putamen,[192] which is the region of most profound degeneration in HD. In the hippocampus, Mn is most concentrated (often with Zn) in the CA2/3 region, while Fe was localized in CA1 and Dentate Gyrus, with a negative correlation between the depositions of Cu and Mn.[188]

In normal rats there are slight differences, that is the highest levels of Mn are thought to be in the globus pallidus and the striatum, followed by the hypothalamus.[190,193] After chronic Mn treatment, the globus pallidus collects the most Mn, with cortex and striatum collecting slightly less.[194] An ICP-MS study of HD patients found a slight decrease in Mn deposition in two subregions of the cortex, but not in the basal ganglia, whereas another study found no differences in Mn deposition between HD and controls[127,130] (Fig. 13.2). Robison and coworkers exposed rats to 1 month of Mn, either by injection or in the diet, and found a specific accumulation of Mn in the dopaminergic neurons of the substantia nigra pars compacta (SNc),[193] which are the neurons that degenerate in Parkinson's disease.

Aside from the difficulty in measuring Mn deposits at the subregional level, it has been even more difficult to tease out whether Mn bioavailability is altered in particular subregions or cell types in HD. The cell-type or subcellular localization under condition of Mn deficiency has not been studied.

Cell-Type Deposition

In general, it had been thought that astrocytes accounted for most of the Mn in brain, primarily because astrocytes are rich in glutamine synthetase (GS), a glia-specific enzyme that can bind as many as 4 Mn^{2+} ions per subunit, with 15 subunits in each enzyme.[195] However, GS can also bind Mg^{2+}, and other ions, as well as Mn^{2+} as a cofactor.[196] With overexposure to Mn, as when Mn is injected intracerebrally in rats, the metal collects in astrocyte-rich regions, but immunohistochemical images show that the most intense staining for astrocytes colocalizes with the lowest concentrations of Mn.[188]

Morello and coworkers, found that, under normal conditions, Mn accumulates equally in rat neurons and astrocytes.[194] Similarly, in chick embryos, Wedler found that neurons store more Mn than astrocytes[197] and Tholey and coworkers found that there is more Mn and Cu in neurons than astrocytes, but more Fe and Zn in astrocytes than neurons.[198] Robison found that sites of high Mn accumulation do not correspond to the sites where Cu accumulates, postulating that this anticorrelation suggests that astrocytes are not the storehouse for Mn under normal conditions,[188] though they may accumulate more Mn under toxic exposures. However, technical limitations have prevented robust quantitative measurements of cellular Mn levels (e.g., astrocytes versus neuron) in vivo, and the earlier studies rely on ex vivo or cultured brain cells.

Because manganese is biologically important, both as an enzymatic cofactor and in reduction of reactive oxygen species, knowing where Mn is located in cells, cell types, and brain regions is crucial to elucidating its role in HD pathology. There is no direct reporter protein for Mn, like there is for Fe (the iron storage protein ferritin), but diverse methodologies have been used to measure the metal in tissues and cell cultures, including graphite furnace, inductively-coupled mass spectroscopy (ICPMS),[194,199] energy dispersive X-ray fluorescence,[198] X-ray fluorescence,[193] synchrotron radiation X-ray and fluorescence (SRXRF).[200] As tissues and cells are prepared for assay, subcellular conditions change and may cause movement of metals between compartments, or changes in Mn levels within organelles, which might also alter measurement.

Subcellular Deposition

There is also disagreement in the literature about where Mn collects within cells. Many studies indicate that Mn preferentially accumulates in mitochondria, but other data show that Mn is found primarily in the Golgi apparatus, the ER, or the nucleus. These differences can partially be explained by the relative amounts of Mn in experimental conditions, because different biological transport and storage mechanisms may be activated when excessive Mn exposure occurs. Acute versus chronic exposure to Mn may also stimulate alternative homeostatic processes.

Several researchers agree that exposure to excess Mn results in preferential accumulation in mitochondria in both liver and brain,[191] with greatest mitochondrial accumulation in the basal ganglia.[123,201] This excess of Mn leads to mitochondrial cytochrome c release,[202,203] which activates caspase-dependent apoptotic pathways[204] leading to increased cell death.

In cases of normal Mn levels, most studies agree that Mn is not stored in mitochondria. It appears that Mn is lowest in the mitochondria, intermediate in the cytoplasm and highest in the Golgi[199,205,206] in yeast studies under normal conditions. In rats, without excess Mn exposure, Mn is highest in the nucleolus, and lowest in the mitochondria.[193,194] In chick embryos Mn is concentrated in the cytosol and microsomes,[198] rather than the mitochondria. In hippocampal CA3, Mn was distributed diffusely and localized separately from Fe, which was found in small foci.[188]

In fact, the Golgi may be the site of Mn storage under normal conditions. In cultured dopaminergic cells and in cultured pheochromocytoma cells, Mn accumulated preferentially in the Golgi apparatus.[207,208] In cultured PC12 cells, Mn was observed in the Golgi apparatus at 100 μM exposure, which was confirmed when the Golgi was ruptured with brefeldin A, redistributing Mn into the cytosol.[193]

As with excess exposure to Mn, chronic exposure to Mn also causes a shift in Mn storage, with the mitochondria of astrocytes accumulating the most Mn, followed by neuronal mitochondria, with the lowest accumulation in the nuclei of both cell types.[194,209] Because the level and duration of Mn exposure clearly affects the intracellular localization of Mn deposits, this suggests that there is tight biological regulation of Mn transport and storage pools.

MANGANESE DYSHOMEOSTASIS IN HD

As mentioned earlier, there is a significant decrease in Mn uptake and storage compared to wild-type following Mn exposure in immortalized striatal cell HD models with an expanded polyQ repeat in HTT.[186] This important finding in cell cultures was also supported by findings in HD model mice exposed to Mn. There was no detectable regional-level difference in striatal Mn levels at baseline between wild-type and mutant mice, but striatal Mn accumulation was significantly less in HD model mice after Mn exposure.[125,186] This HD associated Mn deficit was specific to the striatum, with no difference in Mn accumulation in cortex, hippocampus, or cerebellum between mutant and wild-type, at baseline or after Mn exposure.

Though a regional baseline deficit in Mn accumulation has not been detected in HD models, several downstream effects of reduced Mn bioavailability have been found (discussed below), suggesting that a subregional Mn deficit, or a defect in Mn handling may affect only a subset of neurons in the striatum. It is possible that mutant HTT interferes with neuronal Mn transporters, blocking influx or storage, or increasing efflux, but this mechanism has not been shown.

At least 15 metal transporters are known to move Mn across cell membranes,[210] usually along with other metals. Mn often travels through the same channels as Fe, including the divalent metal transporter 1 (DMT1) and the transferrin receptor. Indeed, Mn exposure causes alterations in protein expression of ferroportin-a (FPN), a cytoplasmic Fe^{2+} exporter, as well as inducing FPN to localize to the cell membrane.[211] Further evidence that Mn is moved with Fe comes from "flatiron mice: which are ferroportin deficient. Flatiron mice have both increased Mn and Fe in the olfactory bulb, and both reduced Mn and Fe in bone.[212] There is a further association between Mn and Fe in HD, through the cell stress response. Nath and coworkers established that HTT plays a role in the cell stress pathway, by observing the accumulation of HTT in the early endosomes of live cells under conditions of stress,[213] arresting recycling endosome function. During this process, HTT localized in cytosolic puncta, called Hungtingtin stress bodies (HSB's). HSBs colocalize with transferrin as well as Rab5C, a protein of the early endosome. This sequestration of transferrin in the early endosome blocks it from moving to the recycling endosome with its cargo of Fe. Though there seem to be many connections between Fe transport and Mn dyshomeostasis, Williams and coworkers found no increase in net Mn uptake even when cultured HD model cells were exposed to saturating levels of Fe.[125] The relationship between Fe transporters and Mn in HD remains enigmatic.

Mn^{2+} is also transported by the divalent metal/bicarbonate ion symporters ZIP8 and ZIP14, several Ca channels, the solute carrier-39 (SLC39) family of Zn transporters, by the Mg transporter hip14 and the transient receptor potential melastatin 7 (TRPM7) channel.[210] It is thought that Mn^{2+} is transported into the mitochondria via the Ca^{2+} uniporter.[214,215] Efflux of Mn from the mitochondria is processed through both slow and fast mechanisms (reviewed by Bowman et al.[123]) in addition to the ferroportin-1 iron transporter. Surprisingly, there were no significant alterations in gene expression for transferrin in the blood of HD patients, nor for SLC11A2 (DMT1), though there was a trend toward reduced expression in patients compared to controls,[216] and if there are mRNA expression differences in brain subregions, these might not be detectable in blood samples. In addition, the same study found no changes in expression of the transferrin receptor (TfR), nor SLC39A8 (ZIP8).

Definitive links to other neurodegenerative disorders, but not to HD, have been found between mutations in many of these metal transporters,[210,217] for example, in the case of PARK9 (also known as ATP13A2) and SLC30A1, which are both associated with forms of Parkinson's disease. Mutations in PARK9 cause a severe Parkinsonian condition, Kufor-Rakeb syndrome,[218] and mutations in SLC30A10 cause Parkinson's disease,[219] but neither are associated with HD. Two other known metal transporters, Huntington Interacting Protein-14 (HIP14) and Huntington Interacting Protein-14-Like (HIP14L) may prove to connect Mn transport issues to HD pathology because these proteins are known to palmitoylate HTT which is necessary for its proper function,[220] and mutant HTT has reduced palmytoylation.[221,222]

Many valuable studies of Mn transporters have been performed in yeast models. PARK9 is a mammalian homolog to the yeast protein, Ypk1, which was first identified in *Sacchromyces cerevisiae* as a Mn transporter on the vacuole.[223] There is evidence that another yeast protein, Spf1 (mammalian homolog is ATP13A1), located on the ER of *S. cerevisiae*, influences Mn homeostasis,[199] but it is only now being characterized.

Mtm1p is another interesting carrier protein with a mammalian homolog SLC25A39, which was first identified in yeast. Mtm1p was originally thought to be the Mn chaperone for mitochondrial Sod2 based on impaired activation of MnSOD in a genetic yeast knockout.[224,225] Mtm1p has now been shown to be involved in mitochondrial Fe homeostasis as well, in complex with pyridoxal 5′-phosphate (PLP) or vitamin B6 as the carrier substrate.[226,227] Vitamin B6 is an electrophilic catalyst, which stabilizes reactions by binding to substrates covalently. Interestingly, the harmonizome database indeed shows SLC25A39 to be reduced in HD.[228]

The *Drosophila* ortholog for SLC25A39 (shawn) is a susceptibility loci for epilepsy, and mutants display vesicle trafficking defects, as well as changes in metal homeostasis.[229] Cytosolic Mn was increased in shawn mutants while mitochondrial Ca was increased, free Fe^{2+} accumulated, and aconitase activity was decreased. Aconitase is an interesting enzyme with two distinct functions: in mitochondria it converts citrate into isocitrate with Fe/S as a cofactor, but in the cytosol, it acts as an iron regulatory protein.[230] As cytosolic Fe levels drop, aconitase unbinds from its Fe/S cofactor and binds instead to the messenger RNA for ferritin and the transferrin receptor, inhibiting the formation of ferritin so that iron can be released from storage.[231,232] Furthermore, aconitase is a transglutaminase 2 substrate, and increased transglutaminase activity in HD may incorporate aconitase into inactive polymers, causing further mitochondrial dysfunction.[233]

Though aconitase is an Fe-dependent enzyme that may impact Mn homeostasis, there are many other enzymes that are Mn-dependent, and may be impacted by metal dysregulation. Striatal Mn deficiency in HD may restrict the activity of these essential enzymatic functions.

Mn-DEPENDENT AND Mn-UTILIZING ENZYMES

Enzymes known to use Mn as a cofactor include glutamine synthetase (GS), superoxide dismutase 2 (SOD2), arginase 1 and 2 (ARG1, ARG2), ataxia telangiectasia mutated (ATM), meiotic recombination 11 (MRE-11), and Fanconi's associated nuclease 1 (FAN1).[210] A reduction of bioavailable Mn would alter the normal neuronal and glial functions of proteins that cannot function without sufficient Mn. Indeed, all manganoproteins that have been examined to date show reductions in the presence of mutant HTT, either directly or indirectly. Most eukaryotic enzymes bind to both Cu and Zn, while those from mitochondria and prokaryotes rely on Mn and Fe as cofactors, suggesting that Mn and Fe dyshomeostasis may be much more influential than that of other metals in HD, though some enzymes can substitute other transition metals as cofactors in deficiency conditions. If derangement of Mn homeostasis is one of the root causes of HD, the fact that the symptoms take so long to develop may be because so many of the Mn-utilizing enzymes can function with other metals, albeit less efficiently, or less effectively.

The following enzymes are known to incorporate Mn preferentially as a cofactor.

GS—Glutamine Synthetase

GS converts glutamate to glutamine in astrocytes, and glial dysfunction is a recognized part of the pathogenesis of HD.[234,235] A reduction in GS activity may contribute to the increased neurotoxicity in medium spiny neurons.[236] Indeed, there is reduced GS in both HD animal models and patients[237,238] and decreased activity of GS, has been reported in postmortem HD patient brain.[237] GS is reduced in HD patients even when the glial marker, GFAP, is not reduced.[237] Insufficient manganese may increase glutamate trafficking, glutamatergic signaling, and excitotoxicity,[236] leading to the increased seizure susceptibility observed in Mn-deficient individuals.[239]

A study in cultured rat astrocytes found that acute exposure to Mn reduced GS activity and increased GS protein,[240] while another 3-week exposure showed no change between exposed rats and controls,[241] and a 13-week chronic exposure reduced GS immunostaining and enzyme activity in striatum and globus pallidus, but not in motor cortex.[209] The investigators of this last study controlled for GFAP and did not see a commensurate decrease in astrocyte number, suggesting that the reduction in GS was due to enzymatic insufficiency rather than astrocytic cell death. Other studies in rats exposed to airborne Mn^{2+} for 90 days or more did not show significant changes in protein or mRNA expression of GS, even though Mn^{2+} accumulation increased.[242]

Interestingly, many other metals, such as Mg, Fe, and cobalt (Co) are able to bind with GS,[196] but at different pH levels, with Fe binding at a lower pH than the other metals. The optimal pH for GS enzymatic activity varies between 4.8 and 8.5, depending on the concentration and combination of metals present, and Ca inhibits GS activity at all pH values.[196] However, GS can also bind Mg, cadmium, and Fe as well as Mn as a cofactor, and though Mg^{2+} binds less tightly than Mn^{2+} to the enzyme, it speeds its activity, depending upon the pH.[196]

SOD2—Mn-Dependent Superoxide Dismutase

SOD2 (also known as MnSOD) acts to detoxify superoxides into hydrogen peroxide and O_2.[243] MnSOD is a mitochondrial protein that requires four Mn ions per tetramer. In HD brain tissue, a reduction in SOD2 is known to cause oxidative stress and worsen the severity of HD symptoms[244] and the expression level of MnSOD drastically changes its redox capacity.[245] Loss of Mn-SOD activity increases sensitivity to mitochondrial complex 2 inhibitors (such as 3-nitroproprionic acid), which is associated with HD-like striatal degeneration.[246,247] HD models are hypersensitive to 3-NPA and other complex II inhibitors,[245] an effect which is especially pronounced in older HD model mice.[248] These SOD2-related alterations further implicate a reduction in the bioavailability of Mn as an enzymatic cofactor, as a cause for the HD-related susceptibility to neuronal death.

Interestingly, Luk and coworkers found that Mn^{2+} can only bind to MnSOD when the peptide is newly synthesized and unfolded, and it is only the newly synthesized form of MnSOD that can enter mitochondria.[225] This suggests that Mn^{2+} associates with MnSOD as part of its import into mitochondria in an unfolded state. MnSOD is twice as active at a pH of 10 that at a pH of 7.8,[249] suggesting that gradations in acid-base balance could have an effect on efficiency of the enzyme.

ARG1 and ARG2—Arginase

The urea cycle contains three Mn^{2+}-dependent enzymes; arginase (ARG1 and ARG2; L-arginine amidinohydrolase) and agmatinase (AGMAT; agmatine ureohydrolase). AGMAT is difficult to detect in rodent brain but there is an agmatinase-like protein (ALP) that has recently been identified by Uribe and coworkers. ALP is likely to be an isoform of the protein LIM and Calponin Homology Domains 1 (LIMCH1),[250] which is ubiquitous in brain tissue, and may or may not be Mn-dependent. Arginase hydrolyzes arginine into ornithine and urea. Arginine can also be converted into the signaling molecule, nitric oxide, by nitric oxide synthase (NOS).

Recent studies have shown dysregulation of urea cycle metabolites in HD patients, both peripherally[251–253] and in postmortem brain samples.[254] In brain, one of the main functions of the urea cycle is the regulation of nitric oxide, which has been shown to be altered in HD.[255–257] An HD mouse model on a high-arginine diet exhibits earlier onset of symptoms[258] and patients with HD infused with arginine demonstrate an abnormal growth hormone response.[259]

The location of ARG1 and ARG2 in neurons and brain tissue is disputed, with some studies describing ARG1 in brain, and others ARG2, although many protein antibodies may have cross-reactivity between the two isoforms which share almost 50% homology.[260] ARG1 is cytosolic and is a marker for microglial activation in many models (though not in mice) and it is found primarily in liver, though it has been implicated in the cortical degeneration in Alzheimer's disease.[261] ARG2 is mitochondrial, and is found primarily in kidney, though ARG2 mRNA expression is upregulated in D2-containing neurons, which are the first to degenerate in HD.[262]

Arginase requires six Mn^{2+} ions per homotrimer, and except for Co^{2+}, other essential metals cannot substitute for the cofactor, as they can for most of the other Mn-dependent enzymes. The optimal pH for arginase activity is very alkaline (9.5), with activity dropping precipitously as pH drops, causing the enzyme to become relatively inactive at cytosolic pH (7.2).[263]

ATM—Ataxia Telangiectasia Mutated

A mutation in ATM causes ataxia telangiectasia (A-T), a disorder that leads to impaired immune system and motor skills, as well as cancer from DNA damage. Notably, Cu levels are significantly higher and Zn levels significantly lower in patients with A-T. The normal role of ATM is in repairing DNA damage and reacting to persistent oxidative stress.[264,265] ATM functions by phosphorylating either H2AX (which activates the DNA repair machinery) or p53 (which activates the cell death pathway), depending on the extent of DNA damage detected. In HD neuroprogenitor cell culture, a deficit of Mn-dependent activation of ATM kinase can be corrected by increasing Mn bioavailability pharmacologically.[266] This correction in ATM activation leads to normalization of the p53 signaling pathway, which has broad implications for HD pathology. Interestingly, acidic pH not only induces DNA damage, but also appears to induce ATM kinase activity as measured by H2AX phosphorylation.[267]

Improper ATM signaling could invoke the p53 response over the DNA repair response, over-inducing the cell death pathway and leading to neurodegeneration. In fact recent work shows that reducing ATM expression (in cells, flies, and mice) prevents symptoms of HD, suggesting that the Mn deficit in HD striatum might actually have a paradoxical protective effect.[268]

MRE-11—Meiotic Recombination 11, and FAN1—Fanconi's Associated Nuclease 1

Like ATM, MRE-11, and FAN1 are part of the DNA repair pathway, and both are Mn-dependent enzymes linked with DNA damage in HD. MRE-11 associates with ATM and complexes with Ras-Proximate 1 (RAP1) to maintain telomere length,[269] while FAN1 functions to remove the interstrand DNA crosslinks that impede double-stranded repair.[270,271] Pathological double-stranded DNA repair is found in HD and in other polyQ expansion diseases.[272] Recently, a genome wide association study of 1462 patients with HD and other polyQ spinocerebellar ataxias (SCAs) revealed that a single-nucleotide polymorphisms (SNP) from FAN1 was a genetic modifier for the age of onset.[273] Both Mn and Mg can serve as cofactors for FAN1,[271] but MRE-11 is not active when Mg is substituted for Mn.[274]

All of the evidence linking abnormalities in Mn-dependent enzymes to HD mentioned earlier strongly supports the data showing that there is reduced Mn bioavailability contributing to pathologies seen in the disease.

INTRACELLULAR pH AND METAL BIOLOGY IN HD

The HTT protein's involvement in so many diverse biological functions suggests that the wild-type protein serves as an overarching regulator of an aspect of neuronal biology that leads to the myriad dysfunctional processes seen in the disease. Maintenance of the acid-base balance between cells and within organelles is one such possibility, which could lead to the dysregulation of metals seen in HD. Acid–alkaline gradients partially drive intracellular metal homeostasis in many ways, including regulating the direction of metal transport as well as the binding between metal cofactors and their associated enzymes. Each of the dysregulated metals described earlier binds to enzymes that reside in specific organelles and function best within a very narrow pH range. Changes in pH can weaken or strengthen the intra- and intermolecular bonds with metal cofactors by changing the conformation of enzymes, thereby altering their enzymatic activity. For example, the ARG2 homotrimer binds tightly to six ions of Mn at a pH greater than 8, which is the normal pH within mitochondria, where ARG2 is stored (Fig. 13.3). As the pH drops, Mn disassociates from the ARG enzyme, reducing its

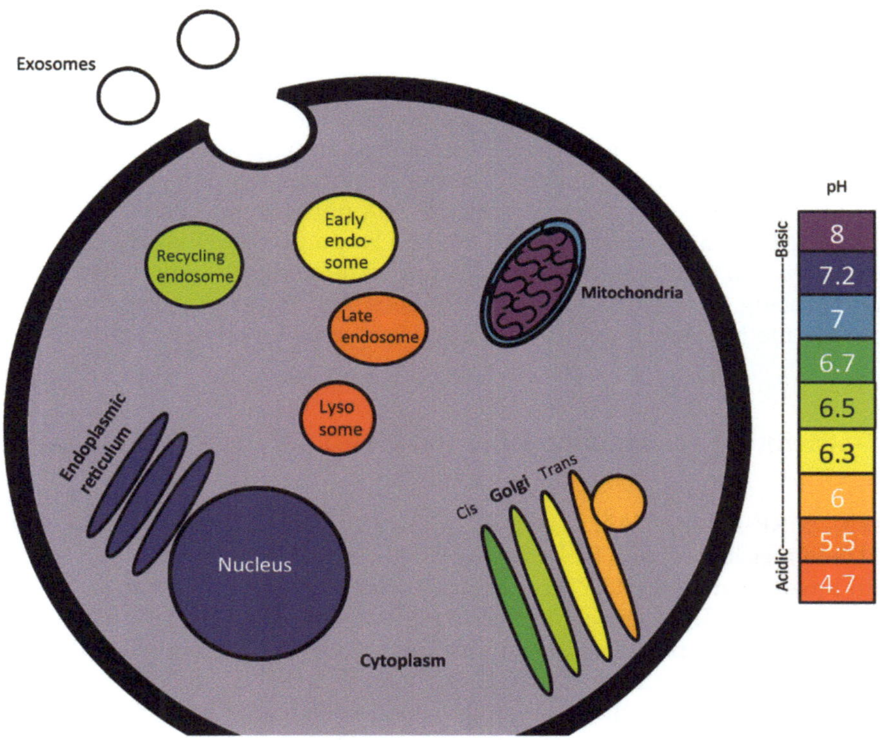

FIGURE 13.3 **Each subcellular compartment and organelle maintains a specific pH, with mitochondrial matrix being the most alkaline while lysosome being most acidic.** *Source: Adapted from Casey JR, Grinstein S, Orlowski J. Sensors and regulators of intracellular pH.* Nat Rev Mol Cell Biol. *2010;11(1):50–61.*

activity and destabilizing the protein,[275] which could lead to downstream disturbances in the urea cycle and nitric oxide signaling.

Each subcellular organelle maintains a specific pH, ranging from 4.7 in the lysosome to 8 in the mitochondria[276] (Fig. 13.3).

Several ion channels known to regulate pH are associated with the HTT protein. Chloride channels (ClC channels) exchange protons for chloride on plasma membranes, which have only recently been described in brain. ClC channels have been recently linked to epilepsy[277] as well as to Myotonia Congenita, a rare skeletal muscle disease,[278,279] and they are found to be reduced in HD in skeletal muscle.[278] In a mouse model of HD, the CLC-1 channel has reduced chloride currents in skeletal muscles.[280]

Benzamil, an amiloride-derivative that blocks epithelial sodium channels (thereby stabilizing the cytosolic pH)[281] significantly reduces HTT aggregation in vitro and had therapeutic effect in live R6/2 model mice.[282] The acid sensing ion channel (ASIC1a) is one of the subunits that forms the major acid-sensing calcium channels in neurons.[283] These ASIC channels sense extracellular H^+ ions, and maintain intercellular pH by the movement of Ca^{2+} across membranes. Blocking ASIC1a activity with RNA interference, prevents intracellular Ca overload and reduces aggregates and pathogenesis.[165]

In yeast, a pH regulator, the Golgi Ca receptor 1-dependent translation factor 1 protein (Gdt1) is a suppressor of mutant Htt toxicity,[284] suggesting that there may be a connection between intracellular pH and HD pathology, though direct links have not yet been found. The homolog for Gdt1 is Transmembrane Protein 165 (TMEM165), a novel protein involved in Golgi trafficking and pH homeostasis that has very recently been characterized.[285] Mutations in TMEM165 cause a congenital disorder of glycosylation. Experiments with the yeast ortholog demonstrate that it functions as a Ca^{2+}/H^+ antiporter, which regulates both Golgi calcium levels and pH. Mn treatment reverses the glycosylation disorder seen in the presence of high Ca concentrations in cells in which TMEM165 is knocked out. Interestingly, because lysosomal pH is altered in patients with TMEM165 mutation,[286] the counter ion for Mn^{2+} entry into the lysosome is said to be Ca^{2+} in yeast and H^+ in mammalian cells.[285]

It is possible that an abnormal ionic gradient importing Ca^{2+} into lysosomes could potentially drive Mn^{2+} export. The stability of a protein known as Golgi Phosphoprotein 4 (GPP130) is directly related to Mn concentration in Golgi,[285] that is, GPP130 degrades in the presence of Mn, and is targeted for lysosomal degradation in cultured cells exposed to excess Mn^{2+},[287] though it has no such reaction when exposed to other transition metals.[288] In HeLa cells in which TMEM165 has been knocked down with shRNA, GPP130 is insensitive to Mn^{2+} treatment. Together, these studies indicate that TMEM165, or another pH driver, may be the connection between Mn dyshomeostasis and HD pathology.

Another potential intracellular acid-base driver that may link metal homeostasis to HD is the Sodium Proton Exchanger 9 (NHE9) or Solute Carrier Family 9 (SLC9A9). NHE9 is a sodium-proton exchanger localized to recycling endosomes, that has recently been characterized as an autism susceptibility gene.[289] The function of NHE9 is to alkalinize luminal pH, which increases the uptake of transferrin as well as glutamate, and it also stabilizes the surface expression of the transferrin receptor.[289] It is found in both astrocytes and neurons. Interestingly, NHE9 interacts with HIP14 (known to be a metal transporter), as well as Vesicle Associated Membrane Protein-7 (VAMP7), two proteins which form complexes with HTT.[43]

In summary, mutations in HTT may cause alterations in the acid-base balance that is normally regulated through the movement of ions between organelles or cells, which could have downstream effects on metal homeostasis that lead to enzymatic failure and resultant HD pathology.

METAL-RELATED CLINICAL INTERVENTIONS IN HD

As mentioned earlier, one metal-related medication, PBT2, has already moved through clinical trials for HD, without significant beneficial effect. The failure of PBT2 Cu chelators may have been due in part because these chelators also alter Mn levels, maybe even more than Cu levels in the organ most vulnerable in HD. Moldovan and coworkers found that Cu chelation with cuprizone reduced Cu levels in blood and periphery, but not in brain, though it reduced Mn in striatum and cerebellum.[290] The balance of metals is exquisitely fine-tuned between brain regions, cell types, and organelles, so metal-related therapeutic approach to HD may need to be designed for cell-type specific drug delivery.

CONCLUSIONS AND FUTURE DIRECTIONS

In summary, divalent metal cations are involved in almost every aspect of HD on an anatomical and molecular level. However, exactly how the mutant HTT protein causes the derangements seen in metal homeostasis is not well understood. It is possible that metal dysregulation leads to many, if not all, of the pathological effects seen in the presence of mutant HTT, or it is possible that metal dyshomeostasis is a downstream result of the pathological disruptions caused by the HD mutation. The loss of function of wild-type HTT may contribute to some of the metal-related pathological effects, such as autophagosomal defects, at the same time that the toxic gain of function of mutant HTT may be contributing to the alterations in neuronal ionic channels. Recently, it has been shown that senescent fibroblasts in culture show increased Mn^{2+} uptake and utilization, suggesting that aging, even without disease, may require additional Mn, perhaps as a way to increase the activity of Mn-dependent enzymes to counteract aging-related increases in oxidative stress.[291]

There is, as yet, no evidence to show that metal-related treatments or exposures will ameliorate any of the symptoms of HD. However, the gene-environment interaction between mutant HTT and transition metals may help to explain the functions of the wild-type protein, and point to additional potential therapeutic targets.

References

1. Dusek P, Roos PM, Litwin T, Schneider SA, Flaten TP, Aaseth J. The neurotoxicity of iron, copper and manganese in Parkinson's and Wilson's diseases. *J Trace Elem Med Biol*. 2015;31:193–203.
2. Su FC, Goutman SA, Chernyak S, et al. Association of environmental toxins with amyotrophic lateral sclerosis. *JAMA Neurol*. 2016;73(7):803–811.
3. James SA, Volitakis I, Adlard PA, et al. Elevated labile Cu is associated with oxidative pathology in Alzheimer disease. *Free Radic Biol Med*. 2012;52(2):298–302.
4. Pringsheim T, Wiltshire K, Day L, Dykeman J, Steeves T, Jette N. The incidence and prevalence of Huntington's disease: a systematic review and meta-analysis. *Mov Disord*. 2012;27(9):1083–1091.

5. Walker FO. Huntington's disease. *Lancet*. 2007;369(9557):218–228.
6. Dorner JL, Miller BR, Barton SJ, Brock TJ, Rebec GV. Sex differences in behavior and striatal ascorbate release in the 140 CAG knock-in mouse model of Huntington's disease. *Behav Brain Res*. 2007;178(1):90–97.
7. Zielonka D, Marinus J, Roos RA, et al. The influence of gender on phenotype and disease progression in patients with Huntington's disease. *Parkinsonism Relat Disord*. 2013;19(2):192–197.
8. MacDonald ME, Christine MC, Duyao MP, Myers RH, Lin C, Srinidhi L, et al. A novel gene containing a trinucleotide repeat that is expanded and unstable on Huntington's disease chromosomes. The Huntington's Disease Collaborative Research Group. *Cell*. 1993;72(6):971–983.
9. Kremer B, Goldberg P, Andrew SE, et al. A worldwide study of the Huntington's disease mutation. The sensitivity and specificity of measuring CAG repeats. *N Engl J Med*. 1994;330(20):1401–1406.
10. Schmitt I, Bachner D, Megow D, et al. Expression of the Huntington disease gene in rodents: cloning the rat homologue and evidence for downregulation in non-neuronal tissues during development. *Hum Mol Genet*. 1995;4(7):1173–1182.
11. Barnes GT, Duyao MP, Ambrose CM, et al. Mouse Huntington's disease gene homolog (Hdh). *Somat Cell Mol Genet*. 1994;20(2):87–97.
12. Ross CA, Aylward EH, Wild EJ, et al. Huntington disease: natural history, biomarkers and prospects for therapeutics. *Nat Rev Neurol*. 2014;10(4):204–216.
13. Novak MJ, Tabrizi SJ. Huntington's disease. *BMJ*. 2010;340:c3109.
14. Squitieri F, Jankovic J. Huntington's disease: how intermediate are intermediate repeat lengths?. *Mov Disord*. 2012;27(14):1714–1717.
15. Kay C, Collins JA, Miedzybrodzka Z, et al. Huntington disease reduced penetrance alleles occur at high frequency in the general population. *Neurology*. 2016;87(3):282–288.
16. Cattaneo E, Rigamonti D, Goffredo D, Zuccato C, Squitieri F, Sipione S. Loss of normal huntingtin function: new developments in Huntington's disease research. *Trends Neurosci*. 2001;24(3):182–188.
17. Cattaneo E, Zuccato C, Tartari M. Normal huntingtin function: an alternative approach to Huntington's disease. *Nat Rev Neurosci*. 2005;6(12):919–930.
18. Nasir J, Floresco SB, O'Kusky JR, et al. Targeted disruption of the Huntington's disease gene results in embryonic lethality and behavioral and morphological changes in heterozygotes. *Cell*. 1995;81(5):811–823.
19. Zuccato C, Valenza M, Cattaneo E. Molecular mechanisms and potential therapeutical targets in Huntington's disease. *Physiol Rev*. 2010;90(3):905–981.
20. Wang N, Gray M, Lu XH, et al. Neuronal targets for reducing mutant huntingtin expression to ameliorate disease in a mouse model of Huntington's disease. *Nat Med*. 2014;20(5):536–541.
21. Ochaba J, Lukacsovich T, Csikos G, et al. Potential function for the Huntingtin protein as a scaffold for selective autophagy. *Proc Natl Acad Sci USA*. 2014;111(47):16889–16894.
22. Wong YC, Holzbaur EL. The regulation of autophagosome dynamics by huntingtin and HAP1 is disrupted by expression of mutant huntingtin, leading to defective cargo degradation. *J Neurosci*. 2014;34(4):1293–1305.
23. Trushina E, Dyer RB, Badger JD, 2nd, et al. Mutant huntingtin impairs axonal trafficking in mammalian neurons in vivo and in vitro. *Mol Cell Biol*. 2004;24(18):8195–8209.
24. Gauthier LR, Charrin BC, Borrell-Pages M, et al. Huntingtin controls neurotrophic support and survival of neurons by enhancing BDNF vesicular transport along microtubules. *Cell*. 2004;118(1):127–138.
25. Zala D, Hinckelmann MV, Saudou F. Huntingtin's function in axonal transport is conserved in Drosophila melanogaster. *PLoS One*. 2013;8(3):e60162.
26. Moughamian AJ, Osborn GE, Lazarus JE, Maday S, Holzbaur EL. Ordered recruitment of dynactin to the microtubule plus-end is required for efficient initiation of retrograde axonal transport. *J Neurosci*. 2013;33(32):13190–13203.
27. Cornett J, Cao F, Wang CE, et al. Polyglutamine expansion of huntingtin impairs its nuclear export. *Nat Genet*. 2005;37(2):198–204.
28. Valor LM. Transcription, epigenetics and ameliorative strategies in Huntington's disease: a genome-wide perspective. *Mol Neurobiol*. 2015;51(1):406–423.
29. Bae BI, Xu H, Igarashi S, et al. p53 mediates cellular dysfunction and behavioral abnormalities in Huntington's disease. *Neuron*. 2005;47(1):29–41.
30. Steffan JS. Does Huntingtin play a role in selective macroautophagy?. *Cell Cycle*. 2010;9(17):3401–3413.
31. Higgins MK, McMahon HT. Snap-shots of clathrin-mediated endocytosis. *Trends Biochem Sci*. 2002;27(5):257–263.

32. Harjes P, Wanker EE. The hunt for huntingtin function: interaction partners tell many different stories. *Trends Biochem Sci*. 2003;28(8):425–433.
33. Kaltenbach LS, Romero E, Becklin RR, et al. Huntingtin interacting proteins are genetic modifiers of neurodegeneration. *PLoS Genet*. 2007;3(5):e82.
34. Culver BP, Savas JN, Park SK, et al. Proteomic analysis of wild-type and mutant huntingtin-associated proteins in mouse brains identifies unique interactions and involvement in protein synthesis. *J Biol Chem*. 2012;287(26):21599–21614.
35. Goehler H, Lalowski M, Stelzl U, et al. A protein interaction network links GIT1, an enhancer of huntingtin aggregation, to Huntington's disease. *Mol Cell*. 2004;15(6):853–865.
36. Kim MW, Chelliah Y, Kim SW, Otwinowski Z, Bezprozvanny I. Secondary structure of Huntingtin amino-terminal region. *Structure*. 2009;17(9):1205–1212.
37. Warby SC, Doty CN, Graham RK, Shively J, Singaraja RR, Hayden MR. Phosphorylation of huntingtin reduces the accumulation of its nuclear fragments. *Mol Cell Neurosci*. 2009;40(2):121–127.
38. Squitieri F, Gellera C, Cannella M, et al. Homozygosity for CAG mutation in Huntington disease is associated with a more severe clinical course. *Brain*. 2003;126(Pt 4):946–955.
39. Mangiarini L, Sathasivam K, Seller M, et al. Exon 1 of the HD gene with an expanded CAG repeat is sufficient to cause a progressive neurological phenotype in transgenic mice. *Cell*. 1996;87(3):493–506.
40. Gusella JF, MacDonald ME. Huntington's disease: the case for genetic modifiers. *Genome Med*. 2009;1(8):80.
41. Rosenblatt A, Brinkman RR, Liang KY, et al. Familial influence on age of onset among siblings with Huntington disease. *Am J Med Genet*. 2001;105(5):399–403.
42. Friedman JH, Trieschmann ME, Myers RH, Fernandez HH. Monozygotic twins discordant for Huntington disease after 7 years. *Arch Neurol*. 2005;62(6):995–997.
43. Saudou F, Humbert S. The biology of Huntingtin. *Neuron*. 2016;89(5):910–926.
44. Ho AK, Gilbert AS, Mason SL, Goodman AO, Barker RA. Health-related quality of life in Huntington's disease: which factors matter most?. *Mov Disord*. 2009;24(4):574–578.
45. Duff K, Beglinger LJ, Theriault D, Allison J, Paulsen JS. Cognitive deficits in Huntington's disease on the repeatable battery for the assessment of neuropsychological status. *J Clin Exp Neuropsychol*. 2010;32(3):231–238.
46. Thompson JC, Harris J, Sollom AC, et al. Longitudinal evaluation of neuropsychiatric symptoms in Huntington's disease. *J Neuropsychiatry Clin Neurosci*. 2012;24(1):53–60.
47. Kirkwood SC, Su JL, Conneally P, Foroud T. Progression of symptoms in the early and middle stages of Huntington disease. *Arch Neurol*. 2001;58(2):273–278.
48. Rubinsztein DC. Lessons from animal models of Huntington's disease. *Trends Genet*. 2002;18(4):202–209.
49. Ramaswamy S, McBride JL, Kordower JH. Animal models of Huntington's disease. *ILAR J*. 2007;48(4):356–373.
50. Menalled LB, Chesselet MF. Mouse models of Huntington's disease. *Trends Pharmacol Sci*. 2002;23(1):32–39.
51. Li XJ, Li S. Influence of species differences on the neuropathology of transgenic Huntington's disease animal models. *J Genet Genomics*. 2012;39(6):239–245.
52. Fox JH, Connor T, Stiles M, et al. Cysteine oxidation within N-terminal mutant huntingtin promotes oligomerization and delays clearance of soluble protein. *J Biol Chem*. 2011;286(20):18320–18330.
53. Younes L, Ratnanather JT, Brown T, et al. Regionally selective atrophy of subcortical structures in prodromal HD as revealed by statistical shape analysis. *Hum Brain Mapp*. 2014;35(3):792–809.
54. Raymond LA, Andre VM, Cepeda C, Gladding CM, Milnerwood AJ, Levine MS. Pathophysiology of Huntington's disease: time-dependent alterations in synaptic and receptor function. *Neuroscience*. 2011;198:252–273.
55. Paulson HL, Albin RL. Huntington's disease: clinical features and routes to therapy. In: Lo DC, Hughes RE, eds. *Neurobiology of Huntington's Disease: Applications to Drug Discovery*. Boca Raton (FL): CRC Press, 2011.
56. Wagster MV, Hedreen JC, Peyser CE, Folstein SE, Ross CA. Selective loss of [3H]kainic acid and [3H]AMPA binding in layer VI of frontal cortex in Huntington's disease. *Exp Neurol*. 1994;127(1):70–75.
57. Hedreen JC, Peyser CE, Folstein SE, Ross CA. Neuronal loss in layers V and VI of cerebral cortex in Huntington's disease. *Neurosci Lett*. 1991;133(2):257–261.
58. Benn CL, Sun T, Sadri-Vakili G, et al. Huntingtin modulates transcription, occupies gene promoters in vivo, and binds directly to DNA in a polyglutamine-dependent manner. *J Neurosci*. 2008;28(42):10720–10733.
59. Saudou F, Finkbeiner S, Devys D, Greenberg ME. Huntingtin acts in the nucleus to induce apoptosis but death does not correlate with the formation of intranuclear inclusions. *Cell*. 1998;95(1):55–66.
60. Davranche A, Aviolat H, Zeder-Lutz G, et al. Huntingtin affinity for partners is not changed by polyglutamine length: aggregation itself triggers aberrant interactions. *Hum Mol Genet*. 2011;20(14):2795–2806.

61. Caron NS, Desmond CR, Xia J, Truant R. Polyglutamine domain flexibility mediates the proximity between flanking sequences in huntingtin. *Proc Natl Acad Sci USA*. 2013;110(36):14610–14615.
62. DiFiglia M, Sapp E, Chase K, et al. Huntingtin is a cytoplasmic protein associated with vesicles in human and rat brain neurons. *Neuron*. 1995;14(5):1075–1081.
63. Sharp AH, Loev SJ, Schilling G, et al. Widespread expression of Huntington's disease gene (IT15) protein product. *Neuron*. 1995;14(5):1065–1074.
64. Atwal RS, Xia J, Pinchev D, Taylor J, Epand RM, Truant R. Huntingtin has a membrane association signal that can modulate huntingtin aggregation, nuclear entry and toxicity. *Hum Mol Genet*. 2007;16(21):2600–2615.
65. Thompson LM, Aiken CT, Kaltenbach LS, et al. IKK phosphorylates Huntingtin and targets it for degradation by the proteasome and lysosome. *J Cell Biol*. 2009;187(7):1083–1099.
66. Steffan JS, Agrawal N, Pallos J, et al. SUMO modification of Huntingtin and Huntington's disease pathology. *Science*. 2004;304(5667):100–104.
67. Ehrnhoefer DE, Sutton L, Hayden MR. Small changes, big impact: posttranslational modifications and function of huntingtin in Huntington disease. *Neuroscientist*. 2011;17(5):475–492.
68. Poirier MA, Jiang H, Ross CA. A structure-based analysis of huntingtin mutant polyglutamine aggregation and toxicity: evidence for a compact beta-sheet structure. *Hum Mol Genet*. 2005;14(6):765–774.
69. Arrasate M, Finkbeiner S. Protein aggregates in Huntington's disease. *Exp Neurol*. 2012;238(1):1–11.
70. Mitomi Y, Nomura T, Kurosawa M, Nukina N, Furukawa Y. Post-aggregation oxidation of mutant huntingtin controls the interactions between aggregates. *J Biol Chem*. 2012;287(41):34764–34775.
71. Zhao T, Hong Y, Li S, Li XJ. Compartment-dependent degradation of mutant Huntingtin accounts for its preferential accumulation in neuronal processes. *J Neurosci*. 2016;36(32):8317–8328.
72. Zhang Z, Miah M, Culbreth M, Aschner M. Autophagy in neurodegenerative diseases and metal neurotoxicity. *Neurochem Res*. 2016;41(1–2):409–422.
73. Ohsumi Y. Historical landmarks of autophagy research. *Cell Res*. 2014;24(1):9–23.
74. Martinez-Vicente M, Talloczy Z, Wong E, et al. Cargo recognition failure is responsible for inefficient autophagy in Huntington's disease. *Nat Neurosci*. 2010;13(5):567–576.
75. Stolz A, Ernst A, Dikic I. Cargo recognition and trafficking in selective autophagy. *Nat Cell Biol*. 2014;16(6): 495–501.
76. Ochaba J, Monteys AM, O'Rourke JG, et al. PIAS1 regulates mutant Huntingtin accumulation and Huntington's disease-associated phenotypes in vivo. *Neuron*. 2016;90(3):507–520.
77. Lamark T, Johansen T. Aggrephagy: selective disposal of protein aggregates by macroautophagy. *Int J Cell Biol*. 2012;2012:736905.
78. Lumsden AL, Henshall TL, Dayan S, Lardelli MT, Richards RI. Huntingtin-deficient zebrafish exhibit defects in iron utilization and development. *Hum Mol Genet*. 2007;16(16):1905–1920.
79. Simmons DA, Casale M, Alcon B, Pham N, Narayan N, Lynch G. Ferritin accumulation in dystrophic microglia is an early event in the development of Huntington's disease. *Glia*. 2007;55(10):1074–1084.
80. Mancias JD, Wang X, Gygi SP, Harper JW, Kimmelman AC. Quantitative proteomics identifies NCOA4 as the cargo receptor mediating ferritinophagy. *Nature*. 2014;509(7498):105–109.
81. Legendre-Guillemin V, Metzler M, Lemaire JF, et al. Huntingtin interacting protein 1 (HIP1) regulates clathrin assembly through direct binding to the regulatory region of the clathrin light chain. *J Biol Chem*. 2005;280(7): 6101–6108.
82. Majeed SR, Vasudevan L, Chen CY, et al. Clathrin light chains are required for the gyrating-clathrin recycling pathway and thereby promote cell migration. *Nat Commun*. 2014;5:3891.
83. Zhang J, Cao R, Cai T, et al. The role of autophagy dysregulation in manganese-induced dopaminergic neurodegeneration. *Neurotox Res*. 2013;24(4):478–490.
84. Afeseh Ngwa H, Kanthasamy A, Gu Y, Fang N, Anantharam V, Kanthasamy AG. Manganese nanoparticle activates mitochondrial dependent apoptotic signaling and autophagy in dopaminergic neuronal cells. *Toxicol Appl Pharmacol*. 2011;256(3):227–240.
85. Paris I, Perez-Pastene C, Couve E, Caviedes P, Ledoux S, Segura-Aguilar J. Copper dopamine complex induces mitochondrial autophagy preceding caspase-independent apoptotic cell death. *J Biol Chem*. 2009;284(20): 13306–13315.
86. Castino R, Fiorentino I, Cagnin M, Giovia A, Isidoro C. Chelation of lysosomal iron protects dopaminergic SH-SY5Y neuroblastoma cells from hydrogen peroxide toxicity by precluding autophagy and Akt dephosphorylation. *Toxicol Sci*. 2011;123(2):523–541.

87. Dotiwala F, Eapen VV, Harrison JC, et al. DNA damage checkpoint triggers autophagy to regulate the initiation of anaphase. *Proc Natl Acad Sci USA*. 2013;110(1):E41–E49.
88. Maskey D, Yousefi S, Schmid I, et al. ATG5 is induced by DNA-damaging agents and promotes mitotic catastrophe independent of autophagy. *Nat Commun*. 2013;4:2130.
89. Pohl C, Jentsch S. Midbody ring disposal by autophagy is a post-abscission event of cytokinesis. *Nat Cell Biol*. 2009;11(1):65–70.
90. Bellingham SA, Guo B, Hill AF. The secret life of extracellular vesicles in metal homeostasis and neurodegeneration. *Biol Cell*. 2015;107(11):389–418.
91. Zhang X, Abels ER, Redzic JS, Margulis J, Finkbeiner S, Breakefield XO. Potential transfer of polyglutamine and CAG-Repeat RNA in extracellular vesicles in Huntington's disease: background and evaluation in cell culture. *Cell Mol Neurobiol*. 2016;36(3):459–470.
92. Lee M, Liu T, Im W, Kim M. Exosomes from adipose-derived stem cells ameliorate phenotype of Huntington's disease in vitro model. *Eur J Neurosci*. 2016;44(4):2114–2119.
93. Jeon I, Cicchetti F, Cisbani G, et al. Human-to-mouse prion-like propagation of mutant huntingtin protein. *Acta Neuropathol*. 2016;132(4):577–592.
94. Carter RJ, Hunt MJ, Morton AJ. Environmental stimulation increases survival in mice transgenic for exon 1 of the Huntington's disease gene. *Mov Disord*. 2000;15(5):925–937.
95. Hockly E, Cordery PM, Woodman B, et al. Environmental enrichment slows disease progression in R6/2 Huntington's disease mice. *Ann Neurol*. 2002;51(2):235–242.
96. Wood NI, Glynn D, Morton AJ. Brain training" improves cognitive performance and survival in a transgenic mouse model of Huntington's disease. *Neurobiol Dis*. 2011;42(3):427–437.
97. Turner CA, Lewis MH. Environmental enrichment: effects on stereotyped behavior and neurotrophin levels. *Physiol Behav*. 2003;80(2–3):259–266.
98. Laviola G, Hannan AJ, Macri S, Solinas M, Jaber M. Effects of enriched environment on animal models of neurodegenerative diseases and psychiatric disorders. *Neurobiol Dis*. 2008;31(2):159–168.
99. Ferris LT, Williams JS, Shen CL. The effect of acute exercise on serum brain-derived neurotrophic factor levels and cognitive function. *Med Sci Sports Exerc*. 2007;39(4):728–734.
100. Saylor AJ, McGinty JF. An intrastriatal brain-derived neurotrophic factor infusion restores striatal gene expression in Bdnf heterozygous mice. *Brain Struct Funct*. 2010;215(2):97–104.
101. Altar CA, Cai N, Bliven T, et al. Anterograde transport of brain-derived neurotrophic factor and its role in the brain. *Nature*. 1997;389(6653):856–860.
102. Molteni R, Ying Z, Gomez-Pinilla F. Differential effects of acute and chronic exercise on plasticity-related genes in the rat hippocampus revealed by microarray. *Eur J Neurosci*. 2002;16(6):1107–1116.
103. Ding Q, Ying Z, Gomez-Pinilla F. Exercise influences hippocampal plasticity by modulating brain-derived neurotrophic factor processing. *Neuroscience*. 2011;192:773–780.
104. Zuccato C, Marullo M, Conforti P, MacDonald ME, Tartari M, Cattaneo E. Systematic assessment of BDNF and its receptor levels in human cortices affected by Huntington's disease. *Brain Pathol*. 2008;18(2):225–238.
105. Spires TL, Grote HE, Varshney NK, et al. Environmental enrichment rescues protein deficits in a mouse model of Huntington's disease, indicating a possible disease mechanism. *J Neurosci*. 2004;24(9):2270–2276.
106. Ciammola A, Sassone J, Cannella M, et al. Low brain-derived neurotrophic factor (BDNF) levels in serum of Huntington's disease patients. *Am J Med Genet B Neuropsychiatr Genet*. 2007;144B(4):574–577.
107. Laske C, Stellos K, Hoffmann N, et al. Higher BDNF serum levels predict slower cognitive decline in Alzheimer's disease patients. *Int J Neuropsychopharmacol*. 2011;14(3):399–404.
108. Velier J, Kim M, Schwarz C, et al. Wild-type and mutant huntingtins function in vesicle trafficking in the secretory and endocytic pathways. *Exp Neurol*. 1998;152(1):34–40.
109. Hoffner G, Kahlem P, Djian P. Perinuclear localization of huntingtin as a consequence of its binding to microtubules through an interaction with beta-tubulin: relevance to Huntington's disease. *J Cell Sci*. 2002;115(Pt 5):941–948.
110. Kegel KB, Sapp E, Yoder J, et al. Huntingtin associates with acidic phospholipids at the plasma membrane. *J Biol Chem*. 2005;280(43):36464–36473.
111. Li SH, Gutekunst CA, Hersch SM, Li XJ. Interaction of huntingtin-associated protein with dynactin P150Glued. *J Neurosci*. 1998;18(4):1261–1269.
112. Qin ZH, Wang Y, Sapp E, et al. Huntingtin bodies sequester vesicle-associated proteins by a polyproline-dependent interaction. *J Neurosci*. 2004;24(1):269–281.

113. Shimojo M. Huntingtin regulates RE1-silencing transcription factor/neuron-restrictive silencer factor (REST/NRSF) nuclear trafficking indirectly through a complex with REST/NRSF-interacting LIM domain protein (RILP) and dynactin p150 Glued. *J Biol Chem*. 2008;283(50):34880–34886.
114. Zala D, Hinckelmann MV, Yu H, et al. Vesicular glycolysis provides on-board energy for fast axonal transport. *Cell*. 2013;152(3):479–491.
115. Lazarus JE, Moughamian AJ, Tokito MK, Holzbaur EL. Dynactin subunit p150(Glued) is a neuron-specific anti-catastrophe factor. *PLoS Biol*. 2013;11(7):e1001611.
116. Jeong H, Then F, Melia Jr TJ, et al. Acetylation targets mutant huntingtin to autophagosomes for degradation. *Cell*. 2009;137(1):60–72.
117. Zuccato C, Tartari M, Crotti A, et al. Huntingtin interacts with REST/NRSF to modulate the transcription of NRSE-controlled neuronal genes. *Nat Genet*. 2003;35(1):76–83.
118. Wu CL, Hwang CS, Chen SD, Yin JH, Yang DI. Neuroprotective mechanisms of brain-derived neurotrophic factor against 3-nitropropionic acid toxicity: therapeutic implications for Huntington's disease. *Ann N Y Acad Sci*. 2010;1201:8–12.
119. Wright RO, Baccarelli A. Metals and neurotoxicology. *J Nutr*. 2007;137(12):2809–2813.
120. Mates JM, Segura JA, Alonso FJ, Marquez J. Roles of dioxins and heavy metals in cancer and neurological diseases using ROS-mediated mechanisms. *Free Radic Biol Med*. 2010;49(9):1328–1341.
121. Brouillet E, Hantraye P, Ferrante RJ, et al. Chronic mitochondrial energy impairment produces selective striatal degeneration and abnormal choreiform movements in primates. *Proc Natl Acad Sci USA*. 1995;92(15):7105–7109.
122. Martinez-Finley EJ, Avila DS, Chakraborty S, Aschner M. Insights from Caenorhabditis elegans on the role of metals in neurodegenerative diseases. *Metallomics*. 2011;3(3):271–279.
123. Bowman AB, Kwakye GF, Herrero Hernandez E, Aschner M. Role of manganese in neurodegenerative diseases. *J Trace Elem Med Biol*. 2011;25(4):191–203.
124. Park JS, Koentjoro B, Veivers D, Mackay-Sim A, Sue CM. Parkinson's disease-associated human ATP13A2 (PARK9) deficiency causes zinc dyshomeostasis and mitochondrial dysfunction. *Hum Mol Genet*. 2014;23(11):2802–2815.
125. Williams BB, Kwakye GF, Wegrzynowicz M, et al. Altered manganese homeostasis and manganese toxicity in a Huntington's disease striatal cell model are not explained by defects in the iron transport system. *Toxicol Sci*. 2010;117(1):169–179.
126. Dodd CA, Ward DL, Klein BG. Basal Ganglia accumulation and motor assessment following manganese chloride exposure in the C57BL/6 mouse. *Int J Toxicol*. 2005;24(6):389–397.
127. Rosas HD, Chen YI, Doros G, et al. Alterations in brain transition metals in Huntington disease: an evolving and intricate story. *Arch Neurol*. 2012;69(7):887–893.
128. Huntington Study Group Reach HDISafety, tolerability, and efficacy of PBT2 in Huntington's disease: a phase 2, randomised, double-blind, placebo-controlled trial. *Lancet Neurol*. 2015;14(1):39–47.
129. Shannon KM, Fraint A. Therapeutic advances in Huntington's disease. *Mov Disord*. 2015;30(11):1539–1546.
130. Dexter DT, Carayon A, Javoy-Agid F, et al. Alterations in the levels of iron, ferritin and other trace metals in Parkinson's disease and other neurodegenerative diseases affecting the basal ganglia. *Brain*. 1991;114(Pt 4):1953–1975.
131. Chen JC, Hardy PA, Kucharczyk W, et al. MR of human postmortem brain tissue: correlative study between T2 and assays of iron and ferritin in Parkinson and Huntington disease. *AJNR Am J Neuroradiol*. 1993;14(2):275–281.
132. Chen J, Marks E, Lai B, et al. Iron accumulates in Huntington's disease neurons: protection by deferoxamine. *PLoS One*. 2013;8(10):e77023.
133. Fox JH, Kama JA, Lieberman G, et al. Mechanisms of copper ion mediated Huntington's disease progression. *PLoS One*. 2007;2(3):e334.
134. Dal-Pan A, Pifferi F, Marchal J, Picq JL, Aujard F, Consortium R. Cognitive performances are selectively enhanced during chronic caloric restriction or resveratrol supplementation in a primate. *PLoS One*. 2011;6(1):e16581.
135. van Bergen JM, Hua J, Unschuld PG, et al. Quantitative susceptibility mapping suggests altered brain iron in premanifest Huntington disease. *AJNR Am J Neuroradiol*. 2016;37(5):789–796.
136. Dominguez JF, Ng AC, Poudel G, et al. Iron accumulation in the basal ganglia in Huntington's disease: cross-sectional data from the IMAGE-HD study. *J Neurol Neurosurg Psychiatry*. 2016;87(5):545–549.
137. Bartzokis G, Cummings J, Perlman S, Hance DB, Mintz J. Increased basal ganglia iron levels in Huntington disease. *Arch Neurol*. 1999;56(5):569–574.
138. Bartzokis G, Lu PH, Tishler TA, et al. Myelin breakdown and iron changes in Huntington's disease: pathogenesis and treatment implications. *Neurochem Res*. 2007;32(10):1655–1664.

139. Vymazal J, Klempir J, Jech R, et al. MR relaxometry in Huntington's disease: correlation between imaging, genetic and clinical parameters. *J Neurol Sci*. 2007;263(1–2):20–25.
140. Jurgens CK, Jasinschi R, Ekin A, et al. MRI T2 hypointensities in basal ganglia of premanifest Huntington's disease. *PLoS Curr*. 2010;2. doi: 10.1371/currents.RRN1173.
141. Dumas EM, Versluis MJ, van den Bogaard SJ, et al. Elevated brain iron is independent from atrophy in Huntington's disease. *Neuroimage*. 2012;61(3):558–564.
142. Sanchez-Castaneda C, Cherubini A, Elifani F, et al. Seeking Huntington disease biomarkers by multimodal, cross-sectional basal ganglia imaging. *Hum Brain Mapp*. 2013;34(7):1625–1635.
143. Sanchez-Castaneda C, Squitieri F, Di Paola M, Dayan M, Petrollini M, Sabatini U. The role of iron in gray matter degeneration in Huntington's disease: a magnetic resonance imaging study. *Hum Brain Mapp*. 2015;36(1):50–66.
144. Verina T, Kiihl SF, Schneider JS, Guilarte TR. Manganese exposure induces microglia activation and dystrophy in the substantia nigra of non-human primates. *Neurotoxicology*. 2011;32(2):215–226.
145. Bonilla E, Estevez J, Suarez H, et al. Serum ferritin deficiency in Huntington's disease patients. *Neurosci Lett*. 1991;129(1):22–24.
146. Curtis AR, Fey C, Morris CM, et al. Mutation in the gene encoding ferritin light polypeptide causes dominant adult-onset basal ganglia disease. *Nat Genet*. 2001;28(4):350–354.
147. Levi S, Cozzi A, Arosio P. Neuroferritinopathy: a neurodegenerative disorder associated with L-ferritin mutation. *Best Pract Res Clin Haematol*. 2005;18(2):265–276.
148. Chinnery PF, Crompton DE, Birchall D, et al. Clinical features and natural history of neuroferritinopathy caused by the FTL1 460InsA mutation. *Brain*. 2007;130(Pt 1):110–119.
149. Martino D, Stamelou M, Bhatia KP. The differential diagnosis of Huntington's disease-like syndromes: 'red flags' for the clinician. *J Neurol Neurosurg Psychiatry*. 2013;84(6):650–656.
150. Kegel KB, Kim M, Sapp E, et al. Huntingtin expression stimulates endosomal-lysosomal activity, endosome tubulation, and autophagy. *J Neurosci*. 2000;20(19):7268–7278.
151. Hilditch-Maguire P, Trettel F, Passani LA, Auerbach A, Persichetti F, MacDonald ME. Huntingtin: an iron-regulated protein essential for normal nuclear and perinuclear organelles. *Hum Mol Genet*. 2000;9(19):2789–2797.
152. Berggren KL, Lu Z, Fox JA, Dudenhoeffer M, Agrawal S, Fox JH. Neonatal iron supplementation induces striatal atrophy in female YAC128 Huntington's disease mice. *J Huntingtons Dis*. 2016;5(1):53–63.
153. Berggren KL, Chen J, Fox J, et al. Neonatal iron supplementation potentiates oxidative stress, energetic dysfunction and neurodegeneration in the R6/2 mouse model of Huntington's disease. *Redox Biol*. 2015;4:363–374.
154. Nguyen T, Hamby A, Massa SM. Clioquinol down-regulates mutant huntingtin expression in vitro and mitigates pathology in a Huntington's disease mouse model. *Proc Natl Acad Sci USA*. 2005;102(33):11840–11845.
155. Chung J, Haile DJ, Wessling-Resnick M. Copper-induced ferroportin-1 expression in J774 macrophages is associated with increased iron efflux. *Proc Natl Acad Sci USA*. 2004;101(9):2700–2705.
156. Prohaska JR, Broderius M. Copper deficiency has minimal impact on ferroportin expression or function. *Biometals*. 2012;25(4):633–642.
157. Hodges A, Strand AD, Aragaki AK, et al. Regional and cellular gene expression changes in human Huntington's disease brain. *Hum Mol Genet*. 2006;15(6):965–977.
158. Hands SL, Mason R, Sajjad MU, Giorgini F, Wyttenbach A. Metallothioneins and copper metabolism are candidate therapeutic targets in Huntington's disease. *Biochem Soc Trans*. 2010;38(2):552–558.
159. Boll MC, Alcaraz-Zubeldia M, Montes S, Rios C. Free copper, ferroxidase and SOD1 activities, lipid peroxidation and NO(x) content in the CSF. A different marker profile in four neurodegenerative diseases. *Neurochem Res*. 2008;33(9):1717–1723.
160. Sanberg PR, Calderon SF, Giordano M, Tew JM, Norman AB. The quinolinic acid model of Huntington's disease: locomotor abnormalities. *Exp Neurol*. 1989;105(1):45–53.
161. Santamaria A, Rios C, Perez P, et al. Quinolinic acid neurotoxicity: in vivo increased copper and manganese content in rat corpus striatum after quinolinate intrastriatal injection. *Toxicol Lett*. 1996;87(2–3):113–119.
162. Schlief ML, West T, Craig AM, Holtzman DM, Gitlin JD. Role of the Menkes copper-transporting ATPase in NMDA receptor-mediated neuronal toxicity. *Proc Natl Acad Sci USA*. 2006;103(40):14919–14924.
163. Martinez-Lazcano JC, Montes S, Sanchez-Mendoza MA, et al. Sub-chronic copper pretreatment reduces oxidative damage in an experimental Huntington's disease model. *Biol Trace Elem Res*. 2014;162(1–3):211–218.
164. Xiao G, Fan Q, Wang X, Zhou B. Huntington disease arises from a combinatory toxicity of polyglutamine and copper binding. *Proc Natl Acad Sci USA*. 2013;110(37):14995–15000.
165. Zhou RP, Wu XS, Wang ZS, Xie YY, Ge JF, Chen FH. Novel insights into acid-sensing ion channels: implications for degenerative diseases. *Aging Dis*. 2016;7(4):491–501.

166. Raymond LA. Striatal synaptic dysfunction and altered calcium regulation in Huntington disease. *Biochem Biophys Res Commun*. 2016. doi: 10.1016/j.bbrc.2016.07.058.
167. Kolodziejczyk K, Raymond LA. Differential changes in thalamic and cortical excitatory synapses onto striatal spiny projection neurons in a Huntington disease mouse model. *Neurobiol Dis*. 2016;86:62–74.
168. Chen X, Wu J, Lvovskaya S, Herndon E, Supnet C, Bezprozvanny I. Dantrolene is neuroprotective in Huntington's disease transgenic mouse model. *Mol Neurodegener*. 2011;6:81.
169. Fernandes HB, Baimbridge KG, Church J, Hayden MR, Raymond LA. Mitochondrial sensitivity and altered calcium handling underlie enhanced NMDA-induced apoptosis in YAC128 model of Huntington's disease. *J Neurosci*. 2007;27(50):13614–13623.
170. Rosenstock TR, Bertoncini CR, Teles AV, Hirata H, Fernandes MJ, Smaili SS. Glutamate-induced alterations in Ca2+ signaling are modulated by mitochondrial Ca2+ handling capacity in brain slices of R6/1 transgenic mice. *Eur J Neurosci*. 2010;32(1):60–70.
171. Tang TS, Slow E, Lupu V, et al. Disturbed Ca2+ signaling and apoptosis of medium spiny neurons in Huntington's disease. *Proc Natl Acad Sci USA*. 2005;102(7):2602–2607.
172. Zhang H, Li Q, Graham RK, Slow E, Hayden MR, Bezprozvanny I. Full length mutant huntingtin is required for altered Ca2+ signaling and apoptosis of striatal neurons in the YAC mouse model of Huntington's disease. *Neurobiol Dis*. 2008;31(1):80–88.
173. Panov AV, Gutekunst CA, Leavitt BR, et al. Early mitochondrial calcium defects in Huntington's disease are a direct effect of polyglutamines. *Nat Neurosci*. 2002;5(8):731–736.
174. Parent A, Fortin M, Cote PY, Cicchetti F. Calcium-binding proteins in primate basal ganglia. *Neurosci Res*. 1996;25(4):309–334.
175. Tang TS, Tu H, Chan EY, et al. Huntingtin and huntingtin-associated protein 1 influence neuronal calcium signaling mediated by inositol-(1,4,5) triphosphate receptor type 1. *Neuron*. 2003;39(2):227–239.
176. Rana A, Yen M, Sadaghiani AM, et al. Alternative splicing converts STIM2 from an activator to an inhibitor of store-operated calcium channels. *J Cell Biol*. 2015;209(5):653–669.
177. Wu J, Ryskamp DA, Liang X, et al. Enhanced store-operated calcium entry leads to striatal synaptic loss in a Huntington's disease mouse model. *J Neurosci*. 2016;36(1):125–141.
178. Saxena S, Caroni P. Selective neuronal vulnerability in neurodegenerative diseases: from stressor thresholds to degeneration. *Neuron*. 2011;71(1):35–48.
179. Racette BA, Aschner M, Guilarte TR, Dydak U, Criswell SR, Zheng W. Pathophysiology of manganese-associated neurotoxicity. *Neurotoxicology*. 2012;33(4):881–886.
180. Kim Y, Bowler RM, Abdelouahab N, Harris M, Gocheva V, Roels HA. Motor function in adults of an Ohio community with environmental manganese exposure. *Neurotoxicology*. 2011;32(5):606–614.
181. Colin E, Zala D, Liot G, et al. Huntingtin phosphorylation acts as a molecular switch for anterograde/retrograde transport in neurons. *EMBO J*. 2008;27(15):2124–2134.
182. Stansfield KH, Bichell TJ, Bowman AB, Guilarte TR. BDNF and Huntingtin protein modifications by manganese: implications for striatal medium spiny neuron pathology in manganese neurotoxicity. *J Neurochem*. 2014;131(5):655–666.
183. Madison JL, Wegrzynowicz M, Aschner M, Bowman AB. Disease-toxicant interactions in manganese exposed Huntington disease mice: early changes in striatal neuron morphology and dopamine metabolism. *PLoS One*. 2012;7(2):e31024.
184. Calabrese EJ. Hormesis is central to toxicology, pharmacology and risk assessment. *Hum Exp Toxicol*. 2010;29(4):249–261.
185. Calabrese EJ, Baldwin LA. Hormesis: U-shaped dose responses and their centrality in toxicology. *Trends Pharmacol Sci*. 2001;22(6):285–291.
186. Williams BB, Li D, Wegrzynowicz M, et al. Disease-toxicant screen reveals a neuroprotective interaction between Huntington's disease and manganese exposure. *J Neurochem*. 2010;112(1):227–237.
187. Robison G, Zakharova T, Fu S, et al. X-ray fluorescence imaging: a new tool for studying manganese neurotoxicity. *PLoS One*. 2012;7(11):e48899.
188. Robison G, Zakharova T, Fu S, et al. X-ray fluorescence imaging of the hippocampal formation after manganese exposure. *Metallomics*. 2013;5(11):1554–1565.
189. Mok SI, Munasinghe JP, Young WS. Infusion-based manganese-enhanced MRI: a new imaging technique to visualize the mouse brain. *Brain Struct Funct*. 2012;217(1):107–114.
190. Bonilla E. Flameless atomic absorption spectrophotometric determination of manganese in rat brain and other tissues. *Clin Chem*. 1978;24(3):471–474.

191. Tarohda T, Yamamoto M, Amamo R. Regional distribution of manganese, iron, copper, and zinc in the rat brain during development. *Anal Bioanal Chem*. 2004;380(2):240–246.
192. Larsen NA, Pakkenberg H, Damsgaard E, Heydorn K. Topographical distribution of arsenic, manganese, and selenium in the normal human brain. *J Neurol Sci*. 1979;42(3):407–416.
193. Robison G, Sullivan B, Cannon JR, Pushkar Y. Identification of dopaminergic neurons of the substantia nigra pars compacta as a target of manganese accumulation. *Metallomics*. 2015;7(5):748–755.
194. Morello M, Canini A, Mattioli P, et al. Sub-cellular localization of manganese in the basal ganglia of normal and manganese-treated rats. An electron spectroscopy imaging and electron energy-loss spectroscopy study. *Neurotoxicology*. 2008;29(1):60–72.
195. Krajewski WW, Collins R, Holmberg-Schiavone L, Jones TA, Karlberg T, Mowbray SL. Crystal structures of mammalian glutamine synthetases illustrate substrate-induced conformational changes and provide opportunities for drug and herbicide design. *J Mol Biol*. 2008;375(1):217–228.
196. Monder C. Metal ion interactions and glutamine synthetase activity. *Biochemistry*. 1965;4(12):2677–2686.
197. Wedler FC. *The Role of Glia in Neurotoxicity*. Boca Raton, FL: CRC Press; 1996.
198. Tholey G, Sena AH, Ledig M. Specific insulin-mediated regulation of glutamine synthetase in cultured chick astroglial cells. *J Neurochem*. 1986;47(5):1490–1492.
199. Cohen Y, Megyeri M, Chen OC, et al. The yeast p5 type ATPase, spf1, regulates manganese transport into the endoplasmic reticulum. *PLoS One*. 2013;8(12):e85519.
200. Colvin RA, Lai B, Holmes WR, Lee D. Understanding metal homeostasis in primary cultured neurons. Studies using single neuron subcellular and quantitative metallomics. *Metallomics*. 2015;7(7):1111–1123.
201. Prohaska JR. Functions of trace elements in brain metabolism. *Physiol Rev*. 1987;67(3):858–901.
202. Prabhakaran K, Chapman GD, Gunasekar PG. BNIP3 up-regulation and mitochondrial dysfunction in manganese-induced neurotoxicity. *Neurotoxicology*. 2009;30(3):414–422.
203. Choo YS, Johnson GV, MacDonald M, Detloff PJ, Lesort M. Mutant huntingtin directly increases susceptibility of mitochondria to the calcium-induced permeability transition and cytochrome c release. *Hum Mol Genet*. 2004;13(14):1407–1420.
204. Tamm C, Sabri F, Ceccatelli S. Mitochondrial-mediated apoptosis in neural stem cells exposed to manganese. *Toxicol Sci*. 2008;101(2):310–320.
205. Garcia-Rodriguez N, Manzano-Lopez J, Munoz-Bravo M, Fernandez-Garcia E, Muniz M, Wellinger RE. Manganese redistribution by calcium-stimulated vesicle trafficking bypasses the need for P-type ATPase function. *J Biol Chem*. 2015;290(15):9335–9347.
206. Pierrel F, Cobine PA, Winge DR. Metal ion availability in mitochondria. *Biometals*. 2007;20(3-4):675–682.
207. Carmona A, Roudeau S, Perrin L, Veronesi G, Ortega R. Environmental manganese compounds accumulate as Mn(II) within the Golgi apparatus of dopamine cells: relationship between speciation, subcellular distribution, and cytotoxicity. *Metallomics*. 2014;6(4):822–832.
208. Carmona A, Deves G, Roudeau S, Cloetens P, Bohic S, Ortega R. Manganese accumulates within golgi apparatus in dopaminergic cells as revealed by synchrotron X-ray fluorescence nanoimaging. *ACS Chem Neurosci*. 2010;1(3):194–203.
209. Morello M, Zatta P, Zambenedetti P, et al. Manganese intoxication decreases the expression of manganoproteins in the rat basal ganglia: an immunohistochemical study. *Brain Res Bull*. 2007;74(6):406–415.
210. Horning KJ, Caito SW, Tipps KG, Bowman AB, Aschner M. Manganese is essential for neuronal health. *Annu Rev Nutr*. 2015;35:71–108.
211. Eller M, Williams DR. alpha-Synuclein in Parkinson disease and other neurodegenerative disorders. *Clin Chem Lab Med*. 2011;49(3):403–408.
212. Seo YA, Elkhader JA, Wessling-Resnick M. Distribution of manganese and other biometals in flatiron mice. *Biometals*. 2016;29(1):147–155.
213. Nath S, Munsie LN, Truant R. A huntingtin-mediated fast stress response halting endosomal trafficking is defective in Huntington's disease. *Hum Mol Genet*. 2015;24(2):450–462.
214. Gunter TE, Puskin JS. Manganous ion as a spin label in studies of mitochondrial uptake of manganese. *Biophys J*. 1972;12(6):625–635.
215. Liccione JJ, Maines MD. Selective vulnerability of glutathione metabolism and cellular defense mechanisms in rat striatum to manganese. *J Pharmacol Exp Ther*. 1988;247(1):156–161.
216. Szeliga M, Rozycka A, Jedrak P, et al. Expression of RNAs coding for metal transporters in blood of patients with Huntington's disease. *Neurochem Res*. 2016;41(1–2):101–106.

217. Ugolino J, Fang S, Kubisch C, Monteiro MJ. Mutant Atp13a2 proteins involved in parkinsonism are degraded by ER-associated degradation and sensitize cells to ER-stress induced cell death. *Hum Mol Genet*. 2011;20(18): 3565–3577.
218. Tan J, Zhang T, Jiang L, et al. Regulation of intracellular manganese homeostasis by Kufor-Rakeb syndrome-associated ATP13A2 protein. *J Biol Chem*. 2011;286(34):29654–29662.
219. Chen P, Bowman AB, Mukhopadhyay S, Aschner M. SLC30A10: a novel manganese transporter. *Worm*. 2015;4(3):e1042648.
220. Goytain A, Hines RM, Quamme GA. Huntingtin-interacting proteins, HIP14 and HIP14L, mediate dual functions, palmitoyl acyltransferase and Mg2+ transport. *J Biol Chem*. 2008;283(48):33365–33374.
221. Singaraja RR, Huang K, Sanders SS, et al. Altered palmitoylation and neuropathological deficits in mice lacking HIP14. *Hum Mol Genet*. 2011;20(20):3899–3909.
222. Ohyama T, Verstreken P, Ly CV, et al. Huntingtin-interacting protein 14, a palmitoyl transferase required for exocytosis and targeting of CSP to synaptic vesicles. *J Cell Biol*. 2007;179(7):1481–1496.
223. Wiederhold E, Gandhi T, Permentier HP, Breitling R, Poolman B, Slotboom DJ. The yeast vacuolar membrane proteome. *Mol Cell Proteomics*. 2009;8(2):380–392.
224. Luk E, Carroll M, Baker M, Culotta VC. Manganese activation of superoxide dismutase 2 in Saccharomyces cerevisiae requires MTM1, a member of the mitochondrial carrier family. *Proc Natl Acad Sci USA*. 2003;100(18): 10353–10357.
225. Luk E, Yang M, Jensen LT, Bourbonnais Y, Culotta VC. Manganese activation of superoxide dismutase 2 in the mitochondria of Saccharomyces cerevisiae. *J Biol Chem*. 2005;280(24):22715–22720.
226. Yang M, Cobine PA, Molik S, et al. The effects of mitochondrial iron homeostasis on cofactor specificity of superoxide dismutase 2. *EMBO J*. 2006;25(8):1775–1783.
227. Park J, McCormick SP, Chakrabarti M, Lindahl PA. Insights into the iron-ome and manganese-ome of Deltamtm1 *Saccharomyces cerevisiae* mitochondria. *Metallomics*. 2013;5(6):656–672.
228. Rouillard AD, Gundersen GW, Fernandez NF, et al. The harmonizome: a collection of processed datasets gathered to serve and mine knowledge about genes and proteins. *Database (Oxford)*. 2016;2016:1–16.
229. Slabbaert JR, Kuenen S, Swerts J, et al. Shawn, the drosophila homolog of SLC25A39/40. is a mitochondrial carrier that promotes neuronal survival. *J Neurosci*. 2016;36(6):1914–1929.
230. Artymiuk PJ, Green J. The double life of aconitase. *Structure*. 2006;14(1):2–4.
231. Jeffery CJ. Molecular mechanisms for multitasking: recent crystal structures of moonlighting proteins. *Curr Opin Struct Biol*. 2004;14(6):663–668.
232. Copley SD. Enzymes with extra talents: moonlighting functions and catalytic promiscuity. *Curr Opin Chem Biol*. 2003;7(2):265–272.
233. Kim SY, Marekov L, Bubber P, et al. Mitochondrial aconitase is a transglutaminase 2 substrate: transglutamination is a probable mechanism contributing to high-molecular-weight aggregates of aconitase and loss of aconitase activity in Huntington disease brain. *Neurochem Res*. 2005;30(10):1245–1255.
234. Lobsiger CS, Cleveland DW. Glial cells as intrinsic components of non-cell-autonomous neurodegenerative disease. *Nat Neurosci*. 2007;10(11):1355–1360.
235. Behrens PF, Franz P, Woodman B, Lindenberg KS, Landwehrmeyer GB. Impaired glutamate transport and glutamate-glutamine cycling: downstream effects of the Huntington mutation. *Brain*. 2002;125(Pt 8):1908–1922.
236. Maciejewski PK, Rothman DL. Proposed cycles for functional glutamate trafficking in synaptic neurotransmission. *Neurochem Int*. 2008;52(4-5):809–825.
237. Butterworth J. Changes in nine enzyme markers for neurons, glia, and endothelial cells in agonal state and Huntington's disease caudate nucleus. *J Neurochem*. 1986;47(2):583–587.
238. Carter CJ. Loss of glutamine synthetase activity in the brain in Huntington's disease. *Lancet*. 1981;1(8223): 782–783.
239. Eid T, Williamson A, Lee TS, Petroff OA, de Lanerolle NC. Glutamate and astrocytes—key players in human mesial temporal lobe epilepsy?. *Epilepsia*. 2008;49(Suppl 2):42–52.
240. Chen CJ, Liao SL. Oxidative stress involves in astrocytic alterations induced by manganese. *Exp Neurol*. 2002;175(1):216–225.
241. Weber S, Dorman DC, Lash LH, Erikson K, Vrana KE, Aschner M. Effects of manganese (Mn) on the developing rat brain: oxidative-stress related endpoints. *Neurotoxicology*. 2002;23(2):169–175.
242. Taylor MD, Erikson KM, Dobson AW, Fitsanakis VA, Dorman DC, Aschner M. Effects of inhaled manganese on biomarkers of oxidative stress in the rat brain. *Neurotoxicology*. 2006;27(5):788–797.

243. Zelko IN, Mariani TJ, Folz RJ. Superoxide dismutase multigene family: a comparison of the CuZn-SOD (SOD1), Mn-SOD (SOD2), and EC-SOD (SOD3) gene structures, evolution, and expression. *Free Radic Biol Med*. 2002;33(3):337–349.
244. Kim J, Moody JP, Edgerly CK, et al. Mitochondrial loss, dysfunction and altered dynamics in Huntington's disease. *Hum Mol Genet*. 2010;19(20):3919–3935.
245. Ansenberger-Fricano K, Ganini D, Mao M, et al. The peroxidase activity of mitochondrial superoxide dismutase. *Free Radic Biol Med*. 2013;54:116–124.
246. Andreassen OA, Ferrante RJ, Dedeoglu A, et al. Mice with a partial deficiency of manganese superoxide dismutase show increased vulnerability to the mitochondrial toxins malonate, 3-nitropropionic acid, and MPTP. *Exp Neurol*. 2001;167(1):189–195.
247. Bogdanov MB, Ferrante RJ, Kuemmerle S, Klivenyi P, Beal MF. Increased vulnerability to 3-nitropropionic acid in an animal model of Huntington's disease. *J Neurochem*. 1998;71(6):2642–2644.
248. Hickey MA, Morton AJ. Mice transgenic for the Huntington's disease mutation are resistant to chronic 3-nitropropionic acid-induced striatal toxicity. *J Neurochem*. 2000;75(5):2163–2171.
249. Crapo JD, McCord JM, Fridovich I. Preparation and assay of superoxide dismutases. *Methods Enzymol*. 1978;53:382–393.
250. Quinones M, Cofre J, Benitez J, et al. Insight on the interaction of an agmatinase-like protein with Mn(2+) activator ions. *J Inorg Biochem*. 2015;145:65–69.
251. Gruber B, Klaczkow G, Jaworska M, et al. Huntington' disease—imbalance of amino acid levels in plasma of patients and mutation carriers. *Ann Agric Environ Med*. 2013;20(4):779–783.
252. Chiang MC, Chen HM, Lee YH, et al. Dysregulation of C/EBPalpha by mutant Huntingtin causes the urea cycle deficiency in Huntington's disease. *Hum Mol Genet*. 2007;16(5):483–498.
253. Chiang MC, Chen HM, Lai HL, et al. The A2A adenosine receptor rescues the urea cycle deficiency of Huntington's disease by enhancing the activity of the ubiquitin-proteasome system. *Hum Mol Genet*. 2009;18(16):2929–2942.
254. Patassini S, Begley P, Reid SJ, et al. Identification of elevated urea as a severe, ubiquitous metabolic defect in the brain of patients with Huntington's disease. *Biochem Biophys Res Commun*. 2015;468(1-2):161–166.
255. Narayanan SP, Suwanpradid J, Saul A, et al. Arginase 2 deletion reduces neuro-glial injury and improves retinal function in a model of retinopathy of prematurity. *PLoS One*. 2011;6(7):e22460.
256. Wiesinger H. Arginine metabolism and the synthesis of nitric oxide in the nervous system. *Prog Neurobiol*. 2001;64(4):365–391.
257. Perez-Severiano F, Escalante B, Vergara P, Rios C, Segovia J. Age-dependent changes in nitric oxide synthase activity and protein expression in striata of mice transgenic for the Huntington's disease mutation. *Brain Res*. 2002;951(1):36–42.
258. Deckel AW, Volmer P, Weiner R, et al. Dietary arginine alters time of symptom onset in Huntington's disease transgenic mice. *Brain Res*. 2000;875(1-2):187–195.
259. Leopold NA, Podolsky S. Exaggerated growth hormone response to arginine infusion in Huntington's disease. *J Clin Endocrinol Metab*. 1975;41(1):160–163.
260. Caldwell RB, Toque HA, Narayanan SP, Caldwell RW. Arginase: an old enzyme with new tricks. *Trends Pharmacol Sci*. 2015;36(6):395–405.
261. Liu P, Fleete MS, Jing Y, et al. Altered arginine metabolism in Alzheimer's disease brains. *Neurobiol Aging*. 2014;35(9):1992–2003.
262. Doyle JP, Dougherty JD, Heiman M, et al. Application of a translational profiling approach for the comparative analysis of CNS cell types. *Cell*. 2008;135(4):749–762.
263. Stone EM, Glazer ES, Chantranupong L, et al. Replacing Mn(2+) with Co(2+) in human arginase i enhances cytotoxicity toward l-arginine auxotrophic cancer cell lines. *ACS Chem Biol*. 2010;5(3):333–342.
264. Guo Z, Deshpande R, Paull TT. ATM activation in the presence of oxidative stress. *Cell Cycle*. 2010;9(24): 4805–4811.
265. Squadrone S, Brizio P, Mancini C, et al. Blood metal levels and related antioxidant enzyme activities in patients with ataxia telangiectasia. *Neurobiol Dis*. 2015;81:162–167.
266. Tidball AM, Bryan MR, Uhouse MA, et al. A novel manganese-dependent ATM-p53 signaling pathway is selectively impaired in patient-based neuroprogenitor and murine striatal models of Huntington's disease. *Hum Mol Genet*. 2015;24(7):1929–1944.
267. Xiao H, Li TK, Yang JM, Liu LF. Acidic pH induces topoisomerase II-mediated DNA damage. *Proc Natl Acad Sci USA*. 2003;100(9):5205–5210.

268. Lu XH, Mattis VB, Wang N, et al. Targeting ATM ameliorates mutant Huntingtin toxicity in cell and animal models of Huntington's disease. *Sci Transl Med*. 2014;6(268):268ra178.
269. O'Connor MS, Safari A, Liu D, Qin J, Songyang Z. The human Rap1 protein complex and modulation of telomere length. *J Biol Chem*. 2004;279(27):28585–28591.
270. Yoshikiyo K, Kratz K, Hirota K, et al. KIAA1018/FAN1 nuclease protects cells against genomic instability induced by interstrand cross-linking agents. *Proc Natl Acad Sci USA*. 2010;107(50):21553–21557.
271. Kratz K, Schopf B, Kaden S, et al. Deficiency of FANCD2-associated nuclease KIAA1018/FAN1 sensitizes cells to interstrand crosslinking agents. *Cell*. 2010;142(1):77–88.
272. Shiwaku H, Okazawa H. Impaired DNA damage repair as a common feature of neurodegenerative diseases and psychiatric disorders. *Curr Mol Med*. 2015;15(2):119–128.
273. Bettencourt C, Hensman-Moss D, Flower M, et al. DNA repair pathways underlie a common genetic mechanism modulating onset in polyglutamine diseases. *Ann Neurol*. 2016;79(6):983–990.
274. Hopfner KP, Karcher A, Shin D, Fairley C, Tainer JA, Carney JP. Mre11 and Rad50 from *Pyrococcus furiosus*: cloning and biochemical characterization reveal an evolutionarily conserved multiprotein machine. *J Bacteriol*. 2000;182(21):6036–6041.
275. Romero PA, Stone E, Lamb C, et al. SCHEMA-designed variants of human Arginase I and II reveal sequence elements important to stability and catalysis. *ACS Synth Biol*. 2012;1(6):221–228.
276. Casey JR, Grinstein S, Orlowski J. Sensors and regulators of intracellular pH. *Nat Rev Mol Cell Biol*. 2010;11(1):50–61.
277. Chen TT, Klassen TL, Goldman AM, Marini C, Guerrini R, Noebels JL. Novel brain expression of ClC-1 chloride channels and enrichment of CLCN1 variants in epilepsy. *Neurology*. 2013;80(12):1078–1085.
278. Imbrici P, Maggi L, Mangiatordi GF, et al. ClC-1 mutations in myotonia congenita patients: insights into molecular gating mechanisms and genotype-phenotype correlation. *J Physiol*. 2015;593(18):4181–4199.
279. Liu XL, Huang XJ, Shen JY, et al. Myotonia congenita: novel mutations in CLCN1 gene. *Channels (Austin)*. 2015;9(5):292–298.
280. Waters CW, Varuzhanyan G, Talmadge RJ, Voss AA. Huntington disease skeletal muscle is hyperexcitable owing to chloride and potassium channel dysfunction. *Proc Natl Acad Sci USA*. 2013;110(22):9160–9165.
281. Shono Y, Kamouchi M, Kitazono T, et al. Change in intracellular pH causes the toxic Ca2+ entry via NCX1 in neuron- and glia-derived cells. *Cell Mol Neurobiol*. 2010;30(3):453–460.
282. Wong HK, Bauer PO, Kurosawa M, et al. Blocking acid-sensing ion channel 1 alleviates Huntington's disease pathology via an ubiquitin-proteasome system-dependent mechanism. *Hum Mol Genet*. 2008;17(20):3223–3235.
283. Chu XP, Close N, Saugstad JA, Xiong ZG. ASIC1a-specific modulation of acid-sensing ion channels in mouse cortical neurons by redox reagents. *J Neurosci*. 2006;26(20):5329–5339.
284. Mason RP, Casu M, Butler N, et al. Glutathione peroxidase activity is neuroprotective in models of Huntington's disease. *Nat Genet*. 2013;45(10):1249–1254.
285. Potelle S, Morelle W, Dulary E, et al. Glycosylation abnormalities in Gdt1p/TMEM165 deficient cells result from a defect in Golgi manganese homeostasis. *Hum Mol Genet*. 2016;25(8):1489–1500.
286. Demaegd D, Foulquier F, Colinet AS, et al. Newly characterized Golgi-localized family of proteins is involved in calcium and pH homeostasis in yeast and human cells. *Proc Natl Acad Sci USA*. 2013;110(17):6859–6864.
287. Mukhopadhyay S, Bachert C, Smith DR, Linstedt AD. Manganese-induced trafficking and turnover of the cis-Golgi glycoprotein GPP130. *Mol Biol Cell*. 2010;21(7):1282–1292.
288. Masuda M, Braun-Sommargren M, Crooks D, Smith DR. Golgi phosphoprotein 4 (GPP130) is a sensitive and selective cellular target of manganese exposure. *Synapse*. 2013;67(5):205–215.
289. Kondapalli KC, Hack A, Schushan M, Landau M, Ben-Tal N, Rao R. Functional evaluation of autism-associated mutations in NHE9. *Nat Commun*. 2013;4:2510.
290. Moldovan N, Al-Ebraheem A, Lobo L, Park R, Farquharson MJ, Bock NA. Altered transition metal homeostasis in the cuprizone model of demyelination. *Neurotoxicology*. 2015;48:1–8.
291. Ghneim HK. The kinetics of the effect of manganese supplementation on SOD2 activity in senescent human fibroblasts. *Eur Rev Med Pharmacol Sci*. 2016;20(9):1866–1880.

CHAPTER

14

Metal-Binding to Amyloid-β Peptide: Coordination, Aggregation, and Reactive Oxygen Species Production

Melisa del Barrio,**, Valentina Borghesani*,**, Christelle Hureau*,**, Peter Faller†*

*CNRS, LCC (Laboratory of Chemical Coordination), France

**University of Toulouse, Toulouse, France

†Biometals and Biological Chemistry, Institute of Chemistry, UMR 7177, University of Strasbourg, Strasbourg, France

OUTLINE

Biometals in Neurodegenerative Diseases. http://dx.doi.org/10.1016/B978-0-12-804562-6.00014-2

INTRODUCTION

Interest in Chemistry of Metal-Amyloid-β Complexes

Amyloid-β (Aβ) is a peptide of around 40–42 amino acids and is the major constituent of the amyloid plaques, a hallmark of Alzheimer's disease. The amyloid plaques also contain a high amount of metal ions, in particular Cu, Zn, and Fe.[1] Zn and Cu copurify with Aβ from brain extract[2] and Raman studies suggested that Cu and Zn ions bind directly to the Aβ in the plaques.[3] Based on these results, chemists and biophysicists became interested in the interaction of metal ions, in particular Cu and Zn with the peptide Aβ in the test tube.

The main form of Aβ is 40 amino acids long (Aβ1-40). A longer form, 42 amino acids long (Aβ1-42, 2 additional amino acids at the C-terminus), is more prone to aggregation and hence enriched in amyloid plaques (Fig. 14.1). Aβ1-42 is also the more toxic form, in line with the idea that aggregation is an important step in the toxicity of Aβ. Aβ is produced by cleavage of precursor protein APP (amyloid-precursor protein) a transmembrane protein (Fig. 14.2). Aβ is generated under healthy conditions and its role is ill defined. Also the role of APP is not clear and might be multiple.[4]

Zn and Cu metabolism is tightly controlled and they are mainly bound to metalloproteins, where they have catalytic and/or structural functions. Generally, there is little free Cu or Zn in cells due to their tight binding. Free or loosely bound Cu is dangerous due to its capacity to produce reactive oxygen species (ROS). However, there are some particular tissues, clearly established for Zn, where higher concentrations of less strongly bound Zn are available. This is the case of certain glutamatergic neurons, in which Zn is ejected into the synaptic cleft upon neuron activation and then taken up again (Fig. 14.2). Local Zn concentration in and around the synaptic cleft is estimated to rise up to hundreds of μM. This Zn pool is not strongly bound (thermodynamically and kinetically) as fluorophores that sense Zn are able to compete.[5]

It has also been suggested, although less established yet, that Cu ions can also be ejected in certain synaptic clefts by the ATPase7a. Estimations go up to 10th of μM. The oxidation state and type of complex they are present in is not known.[6]

This makes certain synapses and their surroundings a potential place where complexes between Cu/Zn and Aβ could occur. When, and under which conditions, is not known, apart from the well-established complex formation in the amyloid plaques.

With this background, chemists and biophysicists were interested in the following points among others:

1. Coordination chemistry of metal ions with Aβ: where and how do the metals bind and with what affinity.
2. What is the impact of metal-binding on the structure of Aβ and on Aβ aggregation. Latter is considered an event linked to AD.

Aβ40 (Aβ1-40): DAEFRHDSGY^{10}EVHHQKLVFF^{20}AEDVGSNKGA^{30}IIGLMVGGVV^{40}
Aβ42 (Aβ1-42): DAEFRHDSGY^{10}EVHHQKLVFF^{20}AEDVGSNKGA^{30}IIGLMVGGVV^{40}IA

FIGURE 14.1 **Amino acid sequence (1-letter code) of the two most abundant forms of Aβ, Aβ1-40, and Aβ1-42 (the color represents the amino acids involved in metal binding, with red as the main amino acids).**

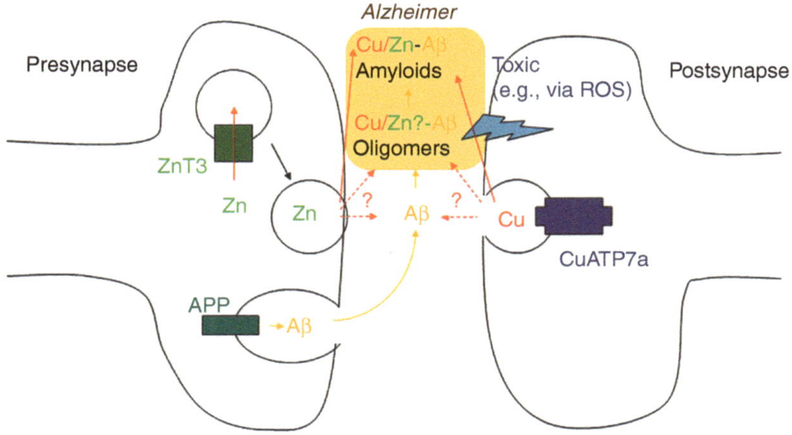

FIGURE 14.2 **Metal ions and Aβ at the synapse: Aβ is cleaved from the amyloid precursor protein (APP) under healthy conditions.** Amyloid aggregates (oligomers and plaques) are found in Alzheimer's disease. In certain synapses Zn can be released from vesicles upon excitation of the presynapses. The transporter ZnT3 is pumping Zn into these vesicles. In certain synapses, upon postsynaptic activation, Cu can be released in the synapse upon translocation of the Cu-transporter CuATP7a to the plasma membrane.

3. What is the chemical reactivity of the complex of metals with Aβ. Particular attention was paid on the catalysis of reaction that could be linked to the toxicity of Aβ, like the production of ROS in the case of Cu (and Fe).
4. Metal transfer reactions of metal-Aβ with other biological metal-binding compounds (like metalloproteins) and with synthetic chelators. Latter can be considered as a therapeutic approach, based on the idea that metals ions (or one specific) bind only to Aβ under AD conditions and have detrimental effects when they are bound to Aβ.

The present chapter deals with the first three points and reports on the current knowledge from in vitro studies.

STRUCTURE OF THE METAL-Aβ COMPLEXES

Coordination of Metal Ions Cu, Zn, and Fe to Soluble, Monomeric Amyloid-β

It is well established that for soluble, monomeric Aβ, Cu(I), Cu(II), Zn(II), and Fe(II) bind to the N-terminal domain, that is, between amino acids 1–16. This means that the main binding site is in this domain. As the metal-binding is very dynamic, this does not exclude that amino acids outside of this domain could not transiently bind to the metals, although not as major ligands. Moreover, amino acids from the 17–40/42 could also play a modulating role via second (or further) sphere interaction. In other words, the Aβ1-16 provides the main ligands and mimics well the main binding site of full length Aβ. However, the rest (17–40/2) has likely subtle influence on the metal-binding, like for instance on the affinity (see later).

Thus a lot of work on the coordination sphere of metals with Aβ used the soluble peptide Aβ1-16, which can be considered as a good (but not perfect) model of the monomeric full length Aβ (i.e., Aβ1-40/42). Aβ1-16 does not form fibrils and hence is a limited model for the aggregated Aβ.[7]

Cu(II)-β-Amyloid

The high-affinity Cu(II) binding site is located in the N-terminal residues spanning from 1 to 16.[7–9] Further binding can be observed, with a second relatively well-defined binding site. The affinity of this second site is at least two orders of magnitude weaker than the high-affinity binding site[10] and hence this second binding site might not be biologically relevant. Thus, most effort concerned the study of the complex $Cu(II)_1A\beta_1$. (noted further as Cu(II)-Aβ).

Two species of Cu(II)Aβ coexist around neutral pH, noted as components **I** (predominant at lower pH) and **II** (predominant at higher pH) (Fig. 14.3A and G). These two components have different spectroscopic signatures in EPR, CD, UV–vis, XAS, and NMR. The pH value corresponding with transition between **I** and **II** [pK_a (**I**/**II**)] is near pH 7.7 and **II** is obtained from **I** by one deprotonation of an amide of the peptide backbone upon Cu(II)-binding. In both forms the Cu(II) ion lies in a distorted square planar geometry. In particular, the species predominant at lower pH is constituted of two equivalent sets of equatorial ligands (noted **Ia** and **Ib**), where the terminal NH_2 (from Asp1), the CO from the Asp1–Ala2 peptide bond, a N atom from imidazole ring of His6 and from His13 (component **Ia**) or from His14 (component **Ib**) are involved (Fig. 14.3A). The two components (**Ia** and **Ib**) are in equilibrium in 1:1 ratio[8,11] and are thus noted component **I**.

Regarding the second component (**II**) (Fig. 14.3G), predominant at higher pH, the NH_2 terminal, the amidyl function N− from the Asp1–Ala2 peptide bond, the CO from the Ala2–Glu3 peptide bond, and one N atom from one of the three imidazole rings of His are the groups predominantly involved in equatorial Cu(II) binding.[7] Regarding the apical positions, involvement of water and carboxylate groups has been proposed in the literature.[7,11,12]

Cu(I)-β-Amyloid

The Cu(I) is bound predominantly via two His (His13–His14) residues in a linear fashion[7,13] (Fig. 14.3H). The Cu(I) environment has been revealed by XAS and IR spectroscopy.[13,14] The NMR and XAS studies also indicated that His6 is involved in the Cu(I) coordination,[7] by replacing His13 and/or His14 and keeping a diagonal geometry.

Zn(II)-β-Amyloid

The first metal-binding site for the Zn(II) ion is in the N-terminal hydrophilic region Aβ1-16 of the Aβ peptide. The most often proposed Zn(II):Aβ stoichiometry is 1:1 with a mononuclear binding site. Further Zn-binding is possible, but is likely less defined and there is no strong indication for a biological relevance.[7,15,16] The Zn(II) coordination sphere is less well known than for Cu(II) and Cu(I), as Zn is not EPR and UV-Vis active. The most involved ligands are the imidazoles of the three His residues and the carboxylate of Glu11[17] and to a lesser extent Asp1 and Glu3.[18] The most recent propositions based on a multimethod approach are shown in Fig. 14.3K (unpublished results).

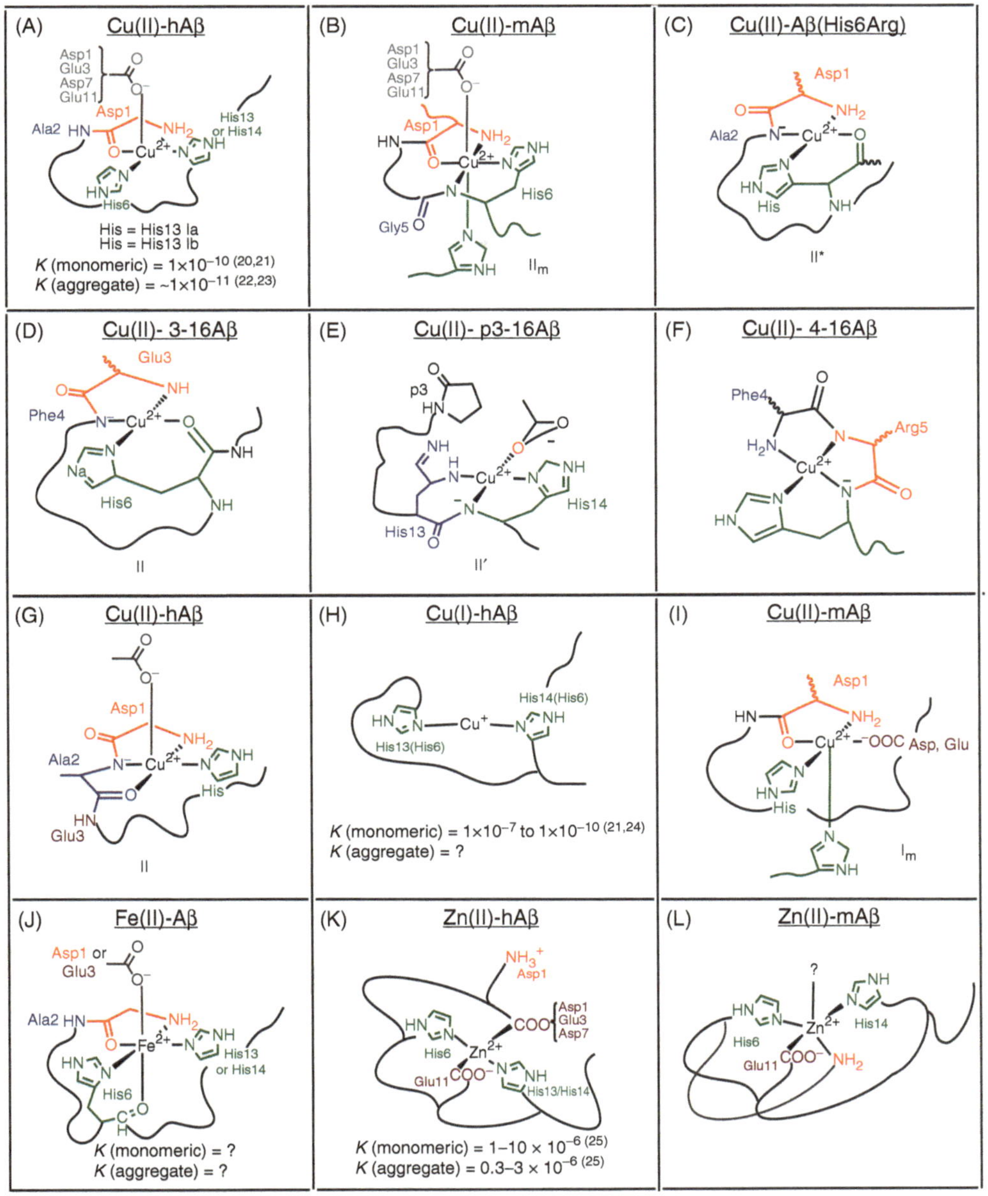

FIGURE 14.3 Proposed coordination sites of major components at physiological pH for Cu(II)-hAβ (A), Cu(I)-mAβ (B), Cu(II)-Aβ(His6Arg) (C), Cu(II)-3-16Aβ (D), Cu(II)-p3-16Aβ (E), and Cu(II)-4-16Aβ (F). The minor binding modes of Cu(II) to hAβ and mAβ are also proposed (G and I, respectively). Proposed binding modes of Cu(I) (H), Fe(II) (J), and Zn(II) (K) to human Aβ and Zn(II) to murine Aβ (L). *K* represents the apparent dissociation constant of the metal ion in monomeric Aβ form and in aggregate form at pH 7.4 with 0.1 M salt but in the absence of a competing buffer. Affinities taken from Ref. [20–26].

Fe(II)-β-Amyloid

In contrast to Cu(II) and Zn(II), Fe(II) has not been detected in Aβ brain extracts.[10] Fe(II) is air-sensitive and can oxidize into Fe(III) under aerobic conditions. Fe(II) binding to Aβ was investigated under anaerobic conditions and a coordination model was suggested (Fig. 14.3J).[9,19]

Cu(II) Coordination to Aβ With Disease Relevant Mutations or Other Derivatives

The coordination of Cu(II) to different derivatives of Aβ have been studies in the past (for recent review see reference[27]). This includes several biologically relevant mutations such as the one occurring in familial AD cases (e.g. H6R, D7N and D7H) and truncations.[9,28–30] Some examples are given in Fig. 14.3. In general, for all the Aβ modifications, the Cu(II) coordination sphere is pH dependent. Thus the binding can differ in the coordination's sphere and also in the pH dependence (at which pH one form changes into another).

It is important to notice that mutations of amino acids that are not coordinated to Cu(II) can change the first coordination sphere dramatically via second sphere interactions.[28] This is for instance the case for the mutation of Arg5 to Gly that occurs in the murine Aβ (Fig. 14.3I). In contrast, mutations of a coordinating amino acid might change less. This is for instance the case for the mutation of His14, as it can be substituted by His13.

Coordination of Metal Ions Cu and Zn to Aggregated β-Amyloid

Knowledge about the coordination chemistry of Zn and Cu ions in the aggregates might be important, because this could contribute to the explanation why the aggregates are more toxic than monomeric Aβ. The structures of Aβ fibrils derived from solid state NMR indicate that the N-terminal part (residues 1 to about 10–14) is flexible and does not take part of the rigid β-sheet structure typical for amyloids. Thus, it is possible that the metal-binding is quite similar to the monomeric Aβ.

Cu(II) Coordination to Aggregated Aβ Peptide

Comparison of EPR signature of fibers and oligomeric forms with those of corresponding soluble forms did not show significant difference in the EPR parameters. This suggests that the coordination is similar and that the same type of ligands are involved. However, if in this case the ligands come all from the same peptide as in the monomer or from different peptides is not clear yet. There are also indications that subtle differences, which might be important for activity, are present. For instance solid state NMR indicated binding of the carboxylate of the C-terminus and of Glu22.[31]

Cu(I) Coordination to Aggregated Aβ Peptide

The Cu(I)-coordination in aggregated Aβ has been little studied and is not well described. Only one study reports a tetrahedral geometry for Cu(I), thus different from the monomeric diagonal geometry.[7,32]

Zn(II) Coordination to Aggregated Aβ Peptide

Very little is known about the detailed Zn-coordination in the aggregated Aβ, but likely the same ligands are mainly involved. There are some propositions based on experimental results and more detailed models from theoretical studies. It has also been suggested that the peptide aggregates through intermolecular His(N_τ)-Zn(II)-His(N_τ) bridges.[33]

AFFINITY OF METALS TO Aβ

Affinity of Metal Ions Cu(I/II) and Zn(II) to Soluble, Monomeric Amyloid-β

There are a lot of reports on the affinity of metal ions, mostly Cu(II) to Aβ in the literature.[34] The results seem to be very divergent. However, one has to consider the different type of affinities. They can be (1) apparent, that is, at a given pH and without considering competition with buffer; (2) conditional, that is, at a given pH but with considering contribution of buffers. This reflects the affinity at a given pH (often 7.4 is used) in water at 0.1 M ionic strength; and (3) thermodynamical, (a theoretical affinity extrapolated at an infinite pH). Here we refer to the conditional dissociation constant at pH 7.4. There are also other reasons for the discrepancies.[10] However, recently, at least for Cu(II) and Zn(II) converging values have been obtained (Fig. 14.2).

Affinity of Metal Ions Cu(I/II) and Zn(II) to Aggregated β-Amyloid

The conditional affinities were only determined for Cu(II) and Zn(II), but not for Cu(I) nor Fe(II). In general, the affinities are a little stronger for both metals. For Zn(II) represents about a threefold increase.[10] In contrast, Cu(II) values of at least an order of magnitude have been proposed in some reports,[22] but not in others.[23] However, one has to keep in mind that several types and structures of aggregates are known and hence the affinities could be aggregation dependent.

Cu(II) versus Zn(II) Binding

In terms of the Kd, Cu(II) binding to Aβ is about 4–5 orders of magnitude stronger than Zn(II) binding. It is also clear that the two metal ions are at least partially bound to the same ligands. This means that Cu(II) is principally able to displace Zn(II) from its main binding-site in the Zn(Aβ) complex. In the plaque, the concentration of Aβ seems to be higher than those of Cu plus Zn, implying that the two metal ions are likely bound in their respective site. However, Aβ, Cu and Zn concentrations are not well defined elsewhere in the brain and thus the binding of the two metal ions might be of biological relevance.[35]

AGGREGATION

General Consideration for Aβ

The term amyloid is a structural definition, in which an amyloidogenic peptide or protein is in a cross β-structure (where the secondary structure is a β-sheet). Macroscopically, they often form fibrils, tubes, or ribbons. Folded proteins have first to undergo a partial unfolding,

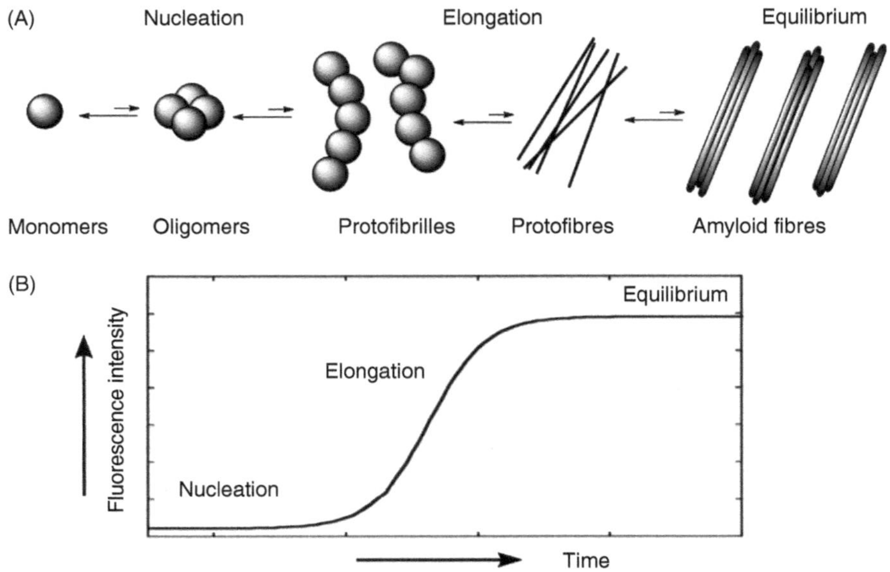

SCHEME 14.1 Schematic representation of amyloid aggregation paths of the Aβ peptide (A) and the typical sigmoid curve of fibril formation often revealed by thioflavin T (ThT) fluorescence (B). Nucleation–polymerization reaction causes a sigmoidal growth curve with a lag-phase and elongation. Fiber formation is initially very slow until nucleating seeds are generated; this initiates rapid fiber generation until equilibrium with low amounts of protein monomer is reached. *Source: Adapted from Viles JH. Metal ions and amyloid fiber formation in neurodegenerative diseases. Copper, zinc and iron in Alzheimer's, Parkinson's and prion diseases. Coord Chem Rev 2012;256(19–20):2271–2284.*[37]

before being able to convert to an amyloid. Monomeric Aβ belongs to the class of intrinsically disordered proteins, meaning that in its isolated state it does not acquire a well-defined 3D structure. No unfolding is needed to acquire the β-sheet conformation. It is proposed that aggregation of Aβ into amyloids is an autocatalytic self-assembly process, in which aggregates can serve as template to catalyze the growth of amyloids. Hence, it resembles the better known crystal growth. Although amyloids are ordered structures, they are not crystalline. Aβ can also form amorphous aggregates. There also several smaller Aβ aggregates described, but it is not clear if these are amyloid off-pathways or intermediates. Small and soluble aggregates, often called oligomers, are supposed to be the most toxic species of Aβ (and hence a prime therapeutic target). However, little is known about their exact identity, their structure, and their biological action (Scheme 14.1).[36]

Impact of Metal Ions on Aβ Aggregation

A multitude of articles report on the impact of metal ions on Aβ aggregations.[37] It is very difficult to obtain a general tendency, as the results are very divergent, like inhibiting or promoting amyloid formation, generation of amyloid or amorphous aggregates. As an autocatalytic process, the event is very sensitive to various conditions and in particular to the presence of aggregation nuclei (seeds). The latter might be responsible for the strong batch dependence observed, including batches that do not form amyloids. Considering that already aggregation results are difficult to reproduce without metal-ions, with metal ions it seems worse. Never mind, let's start with some robust results:

1. Metal ions [at least Cu(II) and Zn(II)] always impact the aggregation behavior (in terms of kinetics or obtained structure). This is not very surprising as the process is very sensitive and metal-binding can change the structure and/or charge of the peptide.
2. The impact is metal-specific: Cu(II) and Zn(II) do not impact the Aβ in the same way.

That's about all the good news there is. In a recent review,[7] we tried to distill some more tendencies from all the literature. It seems that depending on the conditions, metal-ions can promote the formation of amyloids or the formation of amorphous aggregates (could be larger or smaller including oligomeric type). What might be a crucial factor is the proneness of the system to aggregate. Under conditions where Aβ already aggregates fast into amyloids (e.g., high Aβ concentrations, longer peptide Aβ1−42, pH close to pI, etc.), Cu(II) or Zn(II) binding (in particular at high concentrations or ratios) promotes aggregation, but aggregation becomes too fast to properly align the Aβ into an ordered β-sheet structure and hence amorphous aggregates are formed. Under conditions with a low propensity to aggregate (higher pH, low concentrations of Aβ, etc.) metal ion-binding can promote amyloid-type aggregates.

In summary, in the absence of batch and research group independent results for Aβ aggregation in absence of metal ions, and so far little systematic studies on this problem, one can hardly say anything about the effect of metal ions on the aggregation behavior in the test tube.

REACTIVE OXYGEN SPECIES INDUCED OXIDATIVE STRESS

Oxidative stress, which can be defined as the consequence of an imbalance between pro-oxidants and defence systems (antioxidants, enzymes), resulting in (often irreversible) cell damage, is implicated in numerous neurodegenerative disorders, including AD. Increased levels of ROS, such as superoxide ($O_2^{\bullet-}$) and hydroxyl ($HO^{\bullet}$) radicals and hydrogen peroxide (H_2O_2) lead to oxidative stress.

There is considerable evidence of the toxicity of ROS in the context of AD. Postmortem brains from AD patients clearly show indications of ROS in affected tissues. However, it is still debated if ROS is a cause or a consequence of the disease.[38]

The toxicity of Aβ to neurons is related to the production of ROS.[39] In this sense, the addition of the H_2O_2 scavenging catalase[40–42] or synthetic catalytic free radical scavenger[43] inhibits the Aβ toxicity toward cells in culture.

Free or loosely bound Cu and Fe ions efficiently catalyze the production of ROS in the presence of a reducing agent (ascorbate, glutathione, etc.) and molecular oxygen.[44] Recently, it was shown that an increased labile Cu pool and oxidative stress markers correlated well with brain regions most affected in AD victims.[45] Given the scarce understanding of the role of Fe-Aβ in ROS production, we will uniquely concentrate here on Cu-Aβ complexes and their study of redox reactions in vitro.

Reactive Oxygen Species Production by Cu-Aβ Complexes

In terms of redox activity of Cu-Aβ, most activity in vitro was about the reaction of the production of ROS from dioxygen with physiologically relevant reducing agents. The following questions are of interest:

1. What kind of reaction can Cu-Aβ catalyze?
2. What are the mechanisms of these reactions?
3. What is the efficiency of its catalytic activity? This is an issue in order to evaluate the in vivo relevance. A low activity might be negligible due to other competing reactions in vivo, sometimes with very high efficiency (like SOD or catalase).

Cu-Aβ and ROS Production

In principle, the catalytic cycle of ROS production by Cu(II)-Aβ in the presence of a reductant and dioxygen can involve six one-electron reaction steps that successively generate O_2^-, H_2O_2 and HO• (Fig. 14.4).

In the late 1990s, it has been shown that Cu-Aβ in the presence of a reducing agent and O_2 can produce H_2O_2 and HO•. Different reductants were able to drive the production of ROS. Mostly ascorbate was studied. Other reductants were also tested, but sometimes, contradictory results were obtained, such as for dopamine and cholesterol.[46–48]

Early studies proposed that no superoxide is produced, that is, that the reaction 1b occurs, rather than reactions 2–4 (Fig. 14.4). This seemed to make sense as the reaction from O_2 to O_2^- (step 2) is an uphill process but reaction 1b [from O_2 to H_2O_2 is downhill (see redox potentials, Fig. 14.4)]. This last reaction would require the presence of two reduced metal ions in close vicinity (likely a dimeric form $Cu_2A\beta_2$). Theoretical studies supported a direct reaction from O_2 to H_2O_2 without a release of O_2^- (but O_2^- bound to Cu-Aβ was proposed as a reaction intermediate).[49,50] Thus, O_2^- would not be released during the H_2O_2 production. Recently, it has been shown that H_2O_2 production by Cu-Aβ in the presence of ascorbate occurs mainly via a

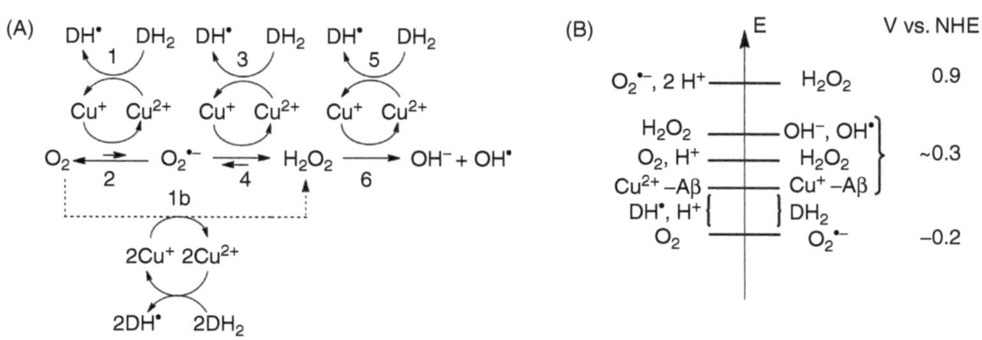

FIGURE 14.4 Scheme of potential mechanisms of ROS production by Cu-Aβ in the presence of a reductant (e.g., ascorbate) and O_2 (A) and redox potentials of the involved species (B). DH_2 represents cellular reductants, such as ascorbate, glutathione, quinol, etc., and •DH represents the single oxidized species (i.e., ascorbyl radical). *Source: From Balland V, Hureau C, Savéant J-M. Electrochemical and homogeneous electron transfers to the Alzheimer amyloid- ? copper complex follow a preorganization mechanism. Proc Natl Acad Sci USA. 2010;107(40):17113–17118.*

free O_2^- intermediate.[51] This finding could have not only mechanistic consequences, but also biological relevance. First, it has been shown that the formation of H_2O_2 (steps 1–4) requires only one Cu center to cycle between Cu(I) and Cu(II) and hence the transfer of one electron at a time. Thus, there would be no need for a dimeric Cu center and monomeric Cu-Aβ would be sufficient to catalyze these reactions.[2,38] Regarding the biological consequences, the potential role of Cu-Aβ as a catalyst in the context of oxidative stress has been extended, given that Cu-Aβ would not be only able to generate H_2O_2 and $HO^•$, but also O_2^-. Additionally, the production of O_2^- can lead to very deleterious species, in particular peroxynitrite whose role in neurodegenerative diseases has been reviewed.[52]

In summary, the in vitro experiments show that Cu-Aβ is able to catalyze the reactions 2, 4, and 6 in Fig. 14.4, that is, Cu(I)-Aβ reacts with O_2, O_2^-, and H_2O_2 to form O_2^-, H_2O_2, and $HO^•$, respectively. The next question is what is the exact reaction mechanism, that is, structure of the Cu-Aβ, substrate binding, electron transfer etc.

Redox Chemistry of Cu-Aβ Complexes by Cyclic Voltammetry

The production of ROS by Cu-Aβ species requires the redox cycling of the metallic center and thus determining the electron transfer reactivity of the Cu-Aβ complex is a key issue. Several electrochemical studies using cyclic voltammetry have been reported with divergent results.[9,39,53]

As previously described, the coordination spheres of Cu(I) and Cu(II) in Aβ differ quite a lot and, as a consequence, a large structural rearrangement in the Cu coordination environment is expected during the electron transfer.[54] This was confirmed by electrochemical studies on the model Cu-Aβ1-16.[55] Actually, the reduction or oxidation process of the Cu(II)-Aβ or Cu(I)-Aβ states (resting states) proceeds via an intermediate species ("in-between" state), which is in equilibrium with the resting states and undergoes a fast redox reaction (Fig. 14.5). This "in-between" state represents only 1/1000 of the species in solution but leads to the redox conversion of the totality of the Cu-Aβ species.[55] The standard potential of the redox couple is 0.300 V versus normal hydrogen electrode (NHE).

The identity of the "in-between" state or if there are an assembly of different states is not known yet. It is likely that the electrochemically "in-between" state is different from the redox active state(s) in the presence of a substrate, such as ascorbate and O_2, as discussed later.

Mechanism of ROS Production and the Reactive State of Cu-Aβ Complexes

THE FENTON TYPE REACTION

Information about the coordination chemistry of the reactive state of Cu-Aβ, which catalyzes the reaction of $H_2O_2 \rightarrow HO^•$, has been provided by experiments and calculations.[56,57] This reactive state has to be different from the redox-silent resting state and is only little populated. Since the highly reactive $HO^•$ obtained from the Cu-Aβ/ascorbate/O_2 or H_2O_2 systems is only produced by the "in-between" state, the resulting oxidative damages should occur predominantly on the Cu ligands. Based on this assumption, the potential ligands involved in the "in between state" have been identified: Asp1, His13, and His14. Thus, the coordination sphere differs from those of the resting states of Cu(II)-Aβ and Cu(I)-Aβ.[56] Further theoretical studies suggest that the reactive state able to form $HO^•$ from H_2O_2 consists of Cu(I) bound by two peptide ligands with an angle far from 180° (Fig. 14.6).

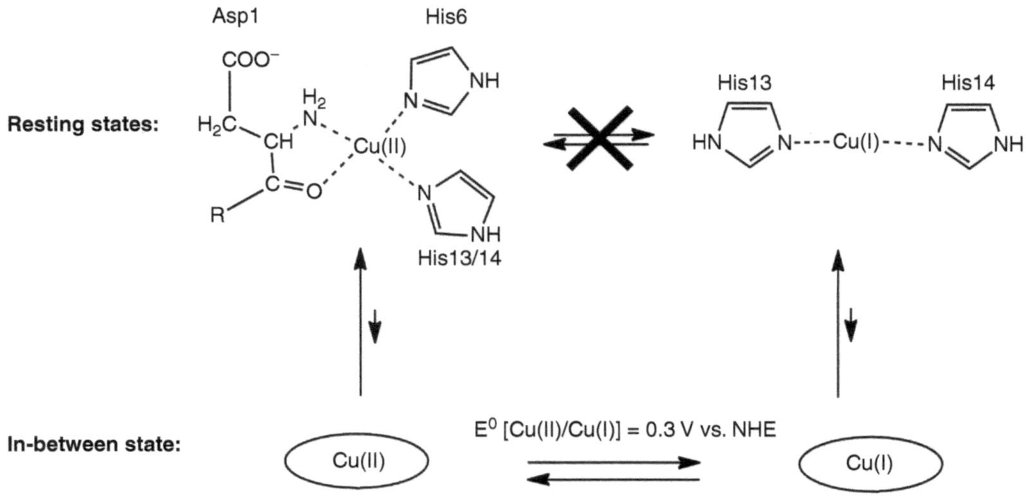

FIGURE 14.5 **Mechanism involved in Cu^{II}-Aβ/ Cu^{I}-Aβ redox process.** (A) resting states, that is, the most populated states. The redox reaction between these states is sluggish owing to a large reorganization energy. (B) ROS production through the in-between state, which can undergo fast electron transfer. *Source: Adapted from Cassagnes L-E, Hervé V, Nepveu F, Hureau C, Faller P, Collin F. The catalytically active copper-amyloid-beta state: coordination site responsible for reactive oxygen species production. Angew Chem Int Ed 2013;52(42):11110–11113.*

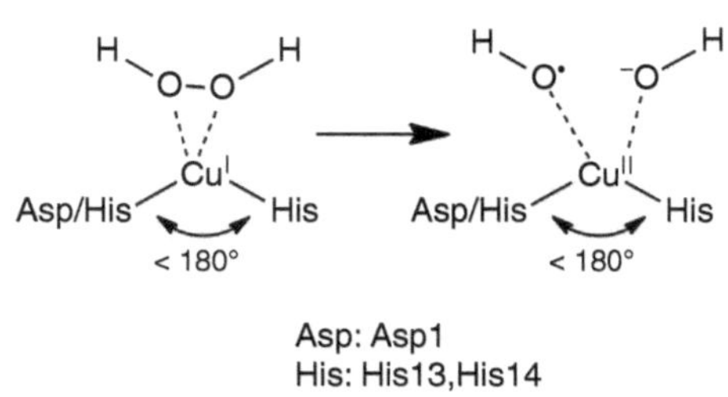

FIGURE 14.6 **Structures of the Cu states catalyzing the formation of $HO^•$ from H_2O_2.**

Dioxygen Reduction

Recently, theoretical studies investigated the reactive structures of Cu(I)-Aβ most prone to activate dioxygen to superoxide and Cu(II)-Aβ.[57] The study indicates that this active state is different from the one able to reduce H_2O_2 and likely from the state being redox-competent in electrochemistry. The active state included a tetra-coordinated Cu(I) with the substrate O_2 bound and three peptide coordination, most favorable was 1His, carboxylate, and amine from Asp1.

Efficiency and Biological Relevance of the ROS Production by Cu-Aβ Complexes

To the best of our knowledge, the rate constants of the formation of $O_2^{\bullet-}$, H_2O_2, and $HO^{\bullet}$ are still undetermined. This makes it difficult to comment on the biological relevance for each individual reaction. However, several studies measured the reaction rates of ascorbate oxidation (Fig. 14.4: reactions 1, 3, and 5) and superoxide dismutation (Fig. 14.4: reactions 2 and 4).[58,59] The rate constants determined for the reaction of $O_2^{\bullet-}$ with Cu-Aβ1-12/16/42 are $2.0/1.1/0.3 \times 10^5\ M^{-1}\ s^{-1}$, respectively. These values are in the range of spontaneous dismutation ($\sim 10^5\ M^{-1}\ s^{-1}$ at pH 7) and at least 10^3 times slower than that of superoxide dismutase, and hence likely of little biological relevance.[38]

At low ascorbate concentrations (<100 μM), the rate of ascorbate oxidation reaction by O_2 mediated by Cu-Aβ is $117\ M^{-1}\ s^{-1}$ $[Asc][Cu]_0$ and is independent of $[O_2]$. At higher ascorbate concentrations, the rate is $16\ M^{-1}\ s^{-1}$ $[Cu]_0[O_2]$.[58] It is worth pointing out that the rate of ascorbate oxidation catalyzed by the enzyme ascorbate oxidase is $1.7 \times 10^4\ M^{-1}\ s^{-1}$. Thus, the reaction rates obtained for the ascorbate oxidation by O_2 mediated by Cu-Aβ are moderately high.

In general, the activity of Cu-Aβ seems to be intermediate as the efficiency is below enzymes that catalyze ascorbate oxidation[58] or H_2O_2 production,[59] but Cu-Aβ produces more than biologically relevant Cu-peptides/proteins tested, such as metallothionein and human serum albumin.[38,60] Nevertheless, antioxidant properties were also proposed for the monomeric form of Aβ,[61] as well as dual role.[62]

In vitro studies support the prooxidant role of Cu-Aβ complex. H_2O_2, which seems to be the major ROS observed, was generated in the (necessary) presence of a reductant,[47] and the production of $HO^{\bullet}$ in presence of ascorbate was described by several groups.[59,63–66] The argument that Aβ is an antioxidant since Cu-Aβ produces less H_2O_2 and/or $HO^{\bullet}$ than free Cu ions might be not valid, as free Cu does not exist in a biological environment (its metabolism is tightly controlled and Cu is always bound to a ligand). If Cu binding is involved in AD by catalyzing ROS production, Cu-Aβ should generate more ROS than Cu bound to other physiologically relevant peptides/proteins under normal (healthy) conditions, and it generally occurs indeed (see earlier).

Thus, taking into account the time scale in AD development, the contribution of ROS produced by Cu-Aβ might be significant. If aggregates are more or less active in ROS production is not clear, and might depend on the type of ROS and/or type of aggregate.[38,63,67] However, this does not exclude that Aβ may have antioxidant activity via other mechanisms or through an indirect interaction with Cu.

CONCLUSIONS

In conclusion, the interaction of the metal ions Cu and Zn with Aβ is very versatile and dynamic. On the one side this is a very interesting feature for a chemist, as the versatility is also mirrored in the structure (indeed several structures are present in fast equilibrium) and in the reactivity. On the other side, it makes the system difficult to study, as one has to consider always a multitude of structures and reactions. At least for Cu-Aβ one could also wonder if such a versatile and difficult to control reactivity, can be physiologically useful or if Cu-Aβ is not rather a potential danger.

Acknowledgments

The authors gratefully acknowledge the support from ERC aLzINK—Contract no. 638712 and of the University of Strasbourg Institute for Advanced Study (USIAS).

References

1. Miller LM, Wang Q, Telivala TP, Smith RJ, Lanzirotti A, Miklossy J. Synchrotron-based infrared and X-ray imaging shows focalized accumulation of Cu and Zn co-localized with beta-amyloid deposits in Alzheimer's disease. *J Struct Biol*. 2006;155(1):30–37.
2. Smith DG, Cappai R, Barnham KJ. The redox chemistry of the Alzheimer's disease amyloid β peptide. *Biochim Biophys Acta*. 2007;1768(8):1976–1990.
3. Dong J, Atwood CS, Anderson VE, Siedlak SL, Smith MA, Perry G, Carey PR. Metal binding and oxidation of amyloid-beta within isolated senile plaque cores: Raman microscopic evidence. *Biochemistry*. 2003;42(10):2768–2773.
4. Haass C, Selkoe DJ. Soluble protein oligomers in neurodegeneration: lessons from the Alzheimer's amyloid beta-peptide. *Nat Rev Mol Cell Biol*. 2007;8(2):101–112.
5. Sensi SL, Paoletti P, Bush AI, Sekler I. Zinc in the physiology and pathology of the CNS. *Nat Rev Neurosci*. 2009;10(11):780–791.
6. Scheiber IF, Mercer JF, Dringen R. Metabolism and functions of copper in brain. *Prog Neurobiol*. 2014;116: 33–57.
7. Faller P, Hureau C, Berthoumieu O. Role of metal ions in the self-assembly of the Alzheimer's amyloid-β peptide. *Inorg Chem*. 2013;52(21):12193–12206.
8. Drew SC, Noble CJ, Masters CL, Hanson GR, Barnham KJ. Pleomorphic copper coordination by Alzheimer's disease amyloid-beta peptide. *J Am Chem Soc*. 2009;131(3):1195–1207.
9. Hureau C. Coordination of redox active metal ions to the amyloid precursor protein and to amyloid-β peptides involved in Alzheimer disease. Part 1: an overview. *Coord Chem Rev*. 2012;256(19–20):2164–2174.
10. Faller P, Hureau C. Bioinorganic chemistry of copper and zinc ions coordinated to amyloid-beta peptide. *Dalton Trans*. 2009;(7):1080–1094.
11. Dorlet P, Gambarelli S, Faller P, Hureau C. Pulse EPR spectroscopy reveals the coordination sphere of copper(II) ions in the 1-16 amyloid-beta peptide: a key role of the first two N-terminus residues. *Angew Chem Int Ed Engl*. 2009;48(49):9273–9276.
12. Hureau C, Coppel Y, Dorlet P, Solari PL, Sayen S, Guillon E, Sabater L, Faller P. Deprotonation of the Asp1-Ala2 peptide bond induces modification of the dynamic copper(II) environment in the amyloid-beta peptide near physiological pH. *Angew Chem Int Ed Engl*. 2009;48(50):9522–9525.
13. Himes RA, Park GY, Siluvai GS, Blackburn NJ, Karlin KD. Structural studies of copper(I) complexes of amyloid-beta peptide fragments: formation of two-coordinate bis(histidine) complexes. *Angew Chem Int Ed Engl*. 2008;47(47):9084–9087.
14. Shearer J, Szalai VA. The amyloid-β peptide of Alzheimer's disease binds Cu(I) in a linear bis-His coordination environment: insight into a possible neuroprotective mechanism for the amyloid-β peptide. *JACS*. 2008;130(52):17826–17835.
15. Bush AI, Masters CL, Tanzi RE. Copper, β-amyloid, and Alzheimer's disease: tapping a sensitive connection. *Proc Natl Acad Sci USA*. 2003;100(20):11193–11194.
16. Donnelly PS, Xiao Z, Wedd AG. Copper and Alzheimer's disease. *Curr Opin Chem Biol*. 2007;11(2):128–133.
17. Noel S, Bustos Rodriguez S, Sayen S, Guillon E, Faller P, Hureau C. Use of a new water-soluble Zn sensor to determine Zn affinity for the amyloid-beta peptide and relevant mutants. *Metallomics*. 2014;6(7):1220–1222.
18. Zirah S, Kozin SA, Mazur AK, Blond A, Cheminant M, Segalas-Milazzo I, Debey P, Rebuffat S. Structural changes of region 1-16 of the Alzheimer disease amyloid beta-peptide upon zinc binding and in vitro aging. *J Biol Chem*. 2006;281(4):2151–2161.
19. Bousejra-ElGarah F, Bijani C, Coppel Y, Faller P, Hureau C. Iron(II) binding to amyloid-beta, the Alzheimer's peptide. *Inorg Chem*. 2011;50(18):9024–9030.
20. Alies B, Renaglia E, Rózga M, Bal W, Faller P, Hureau C. Cu(II) affinity for the Alzheimer's Peptide: tyrosine fluorescence studies revisited. *Anal Chem*. 2013;85(3):1501–1508.

21. Xiao Z, Gottschlich L, van der Meulen R, Udagedara SR, Wedd AG. Evaluation of quantitative probes for weaker Cu(i) binding sites completes a set of four capable of detecting Cu(i) affinities from nanomolar to attomolar. *Metallomics*. 2013;5(5):501–513.
22. Jiang D, Zhang L, Grant GP, Dudzik CG, Chen S, Patel S, Hao Y, Millhauser GL, Zhou F. The elevated copper binding strength of amyloid-beta aggregates allows the sequestration of copper from albumin: a pathway to accumulation of copper in senile plaques. *Biochemistry*. 2013;52(3):547–556.
23. Sarell CJ, Syme CD, Rigby SE, Viles JH. Copper(II) binding to amyloid-beta fibrils of Alzheimer's disease reveals a picomolar affinity: stoichiometry and coordination geometry are independent of Abeta oligomeric form. *Biochemistry*. 2009;48(20):4388–4402.
24. Alies B, Badei B, Faller P, Hureau C. Reevaluation of copper(I) affinity for amyloid-beta peptides by competition with ferrozine--an unusual copper(I) indicator. *Chem Eur J*. 2012;18(4):1161–1167.
25. Talmard C, Bouzan A, Faller P. Zinc binding to amyloid-beta: isothermal titration calorimetry and Zn competition experiments with Zn sensors. *Biochemistry*. 2007;46(47):13658–13666.
26. Eury H, Bijani C, Faller P, Hureau C. Copper(II) coordination to amyloid beta: murine versus human peptide. *Angew Chem Int Ed Engl*. 2011;50(4):901–905.
27. Hureau C, Dorlet P. Coordination of redox active metal ions to the amyloid precursor protein and to amyloid-β peptides involved in Alzheimer disease. Part 2: dependence of Cu(II) binding sites with Aβ sequences. *Coord Chem Rev*. 2012;256(19-20):2175–2187.
28. Alies B, Bijani C, Sayen S, Guillon E, Faller P, Hureau C. Copper coordination to native N-terminally modified versus full-length amyloid-beta: second-sphere effects determine the species present at physiological pH. *Inorg Chem*. 2012;51(23):12988–13000.
29. Alies B, Eury H, Bijani C, Rechignat L, Faller P, Hureau C. pH-Dependent Cu(II) coordination to amyloid-beta peptide: impact of sequence alterations, including the H6R and D7N familial mutations. *Inorg Chem*. 2011;50(21):11192–11201.
30. Mital M, Wezynfeld NE, Fraczyk T, Wiloch MZ, Wawrzyniak UE, Bonna A, Tumpach C, Barnham KJ, Haigh CL, Bal W, Drew SC. A functional role for Abeta in metal homeostasis? N-truncation and high-affinity copper binding. *Angew Chem Int Ed Engl*. 2015;54(36):10460–10464.
31. Parthasarathy S, Long F, Miller Y, Xiao Y, McElheny D, Thurber K, Ma B, Nussinov R, Ishii Y. Molecular-level examination of Cu2+ binding structure for amyloid fibrils of 40-residue Alzheimer's β by solid-state NMR spectroscopy. *JACS*. 2011;133(10):3390–3400.
32. Shearer J, Callan PE, Tran T, Szalai VA. Cu K-edge X-ray absorption spectroscopy reveals differential copper coordination within amyloid-beta oligomers compared to amyloid-beta monomers. *Chem Commun (Camb)*. 2010;46(48):9137–9139.
33. Miller Y, Ma B, Nussinov R. Metal binding sites in amyloid oligomers: complexes and mechanisms. *Coord Chem Rev*. 2012;256(19–20):2245–2252.
34. Zawisza I, Rózga M, Bal W. Affinity of copper and zinc ions to proteins and peptides related to neurodegenerative conditions (Aβ, APP, α-synuclein, PrP). *Coord Chem Rev*. 2012;256(19–20):2297–2307.
35. Alies B, Sasaki I, Proux O, Sayen S, Guillon E, Faller P, Hureau C. Zn impacts Cu coordination to amyloid-beta, the Alzheimer's peptide, but not the ROS production and the associated cell toxicity. *Chem Commun*. 2013;49(12):1214–1216.
36. Knowles TP, Vendruscolo M, Dobson CM. The amyloid state and its association with protein misfolding diseases. *Nat Rev Mol Cell Biol*. 2014;15(6):384–396.
37. Viles JH. Metal ions and amyloid fiber formation in neurodegenerative diseases. Copper, zinc and iron in Alzheimer's, Parkinson's and prion diseases. *Coord Chem Rev*. 2012;256(19–20):2271–2284.
38. Chassaing S, Collin F, Dorlet P, Gout J, Hureau C, Faller P. Copper and heme-mediated Abeta toxicity: redox chemistry. Abeta oxidations and anti-ROS compounds. *Curr Top Med Chem*. 2012;12(22):2573–2595.
39. Hureau C, Faller P. Abeta-mediated ROS production by Cu ions: structural insights, mechanisms and relevance to Alzheimer's disease. *Biochimie*. 2009;91(10):1212–1217.
40. Behl C, Davis JB, Lesley R, Schubert D. Hydrogen peroxide mediates amyloid beta protein toxicity. *Cell*. 1994;77(6):817–827.
41. Barnham KJ, Ciccotosto GD, Tickler AK, Ali FE, Smith DG, Williamson NA, Lam YH, Carrington D, Tew D, Kocak G, Volitakis I, Separovic F, Barrow CJ, Wade JD, Masters CL, Cherny RA, Curtain CC, Bush AI, Cappai R. Neurotoxic, redox-competent Alzheimer's beta-amyloid is released from lipid membrane by methionine oxidation. *J Biol Chem*. 2003;278(44):42959–42965.

42. Huang X, Cuajungco MP, Atwood CS, Hartshorn MA, Tyndall JD, Hanson GR, Stokes KC, Leopold M, Multhaup G, Goldstein LE, Scarpa RC, Saunders AJ, Lim J, Moir RD, Glabe C, Bowden EF, Masters CL, Fairlie DP, Tanzi RE, Bush AI. Cu(II) potentiation of alzheimer abeta neurotoxicity. Correlation with cell-free hydrogen peroxide production and metal reduction. *J Biol Chem*. 1999;274(52):37111–37116.
43. Bruce AJ, Malfroy B, Baudry M. beta-Amyloid toxicity in organotypic hippocampal cultures: protection by EUK-8, a synthetic catalytic free radical scavenger. *Proc Natl Acad Sci USA*. 1996;93(6):2312–2316.
44. Halliwell B. Oxidative stress and neurodegeneration: where are we now?. *J Neurochem*. 2006;97(6):1634–1658.
45. James SA, Volitakis I, Adlard PA, Duce JA, Masters CL, Cherny RA, Bush AI. Elevated labile Cu is associated with oxidative pathology in Alzheimer disease. *Free Radic Biol Med*. 2012;52(2):298–302.
46. da Silva GFZ, Ming L-J. Metallo-ROS in Alzheimer's disease: oxidation of neurotransmitters by CuII-β-amyloid and neuropathology of the disease. *Angew Chem Int Ed*. 2007;46(18):3337–3341.
47. Opazo C, Huang X, Cherny RA, Moir RD, Roher AE, White AR, Cappai R, Masters CL, Tanzi RE, Inestrosa NC, Bush AI. Metalloenzyme-like activity of Alzheimer's disease beta-amyloid. Cu-dependent catalytic conversion of dopamine, cholesterol, and biological reducing agents to neurotoxic H(2)O(2). *J Biol Chem*. 2002;277(43):40302–40308.
48. Streltsov VA, Varghese JN. Substrate mediated reduction of copper-amyloid-beta complex in Alzheimer's disease. *Chem Commun (Camb)*. 2008;(27):3169–3171.
49. Hewitt N, Rauk A. Mechanism of hydrogen peroxide production by copper-bound amyloid beta peptide: a theoretical study. *J Phys Chem B*. 2009;113(4):1202–1209.
50. Mirats A, Ali-Torres J, Rodriguez-Santiago L, Sodupe M, La Penna G. Dioxygen activation in the Cu-amyloid [small beta] complex. *PCCP*. 2015;17(41):27270–27274.
51. Reybier K, Ayala S, Alies B, Rodrigues JV, Bustos Rodriguez S, La Penna G, Collin F, Gomes CM, Hureau C, Faller P. Free superoxide is an intermediate in the production of H_2O_2 by Copper(I)-Abeta peptide and O. *Angew Chem Int Ed Engl*. 2015;55(3):1085–1089.
52. Torreilles F, Salman-Tabcheh S, Guerin M, Torreilles J. Neurodegenerative disorders: the role of peroxynitrite. *Brain Res Brain Res Rev*. 1999;30(2):153–163.
53. Faller P, Hureau C, Dorlet P, Hellwig P, Coppel Y, Collin F, Alies B. Methods and techniques to study the bioinorganic chemistry of metal–peptide complexes linked to neurodegenerative diseases. *Coord Chem Rev*. 2012;256(19-20):2381–2396.
54. Furlan S, Hureau C, Faller P, La Penna G. Modeling copper binding to the amyloid-β peptide at different pH: toward a molecular mechanism for Cu reduction. *J Phys Chem B*. 2012;116(39):11899–11910.
55. Balland V, Hureau C, Savéant J-M. Electrochemical and homogeneous electron transfers to the Alzheimer amyloid-β copper complex follow a preorganization mechanism. *Proc Natl Acad Sci USA*. 2010;107(40):17113–17118.
56. Cassagnes L-E, Hervé V, Nepveu F, Hureau C, Faller P, Collin F. The catalytically active copper-amyloid-beta state: coordination site responsible for reactive oxygen species production. *Angew Chem Int Ed*. 2013;52(42):11110–11113.
57. La Penna G, Hureau C, Andreussi O, Faller P. Identifying, by first-principles simulations, Cu[amyloid-beta] species making Fenton-type reactions in Alzheimer's disease. *J Phys Chem B*. 2013;117(51):16455–16467.
58. Jiang D, Li X, Liu L, Yagnik GB, Zhou F. Reaction rates and mechanism of the ascorbic acid oxidation by molecular oxygen facilitated by Cu(II)-containing amyloid-beta complexes and aggregates. *J Phys Chem B*. 2010;114(14):4896–4903.
59. Nakamura M, Shishido N, Nunomura A, Smith MA, Perry G, Hayashi Y, Nakayama K, Hayashi T. Three histidine residues of amyloid-β peptide control the redox activity of copper and iron. *Biochemistry*. 2007;46(44):12737–12743.
60. Meloni G, Sonois V, Delaine T, Guilloreau L, Gillet A, Teissie J, Faller P, Vasak M. Metal swap between Zn7-metallothionein-3 and amyloid-beta-Cu protects against amyloid-beta toxicity. *Nat Chem Biol*. 2008;4(6):366–372.
61. Zou K, Gong JS, Yanagisawa K, Michikawa M. A novel function of monomeric amyloid beta-protein serving as an antioxidant molecule against metal-induced oxidative damage. *J Neurosci*. 2002;22(12):4833–4841.
62. Atwood CS, Obrenovich ME, Liu T, Chan H, Perry G, Smith MA, Martins RN. Amyloid-beta: a chameleon walking in two worlds: a review of the trophic and toxic properties of amyloid-beta. *Brain Res Brain Res Rev*. 2003;43(1):1–16.
63. Nadal RC, Rigby SE, Viles JH. Amyloid beta-Cu^{2+} complexes in both monomeric and fibrillar forms do not generate H_2O_2 catalytically but quench hydroxyl radicals. *Biochemistry*. 2008;47(44):11653–11664.

64. Guilloreau L, Combalbert S, Sournia-Saquet A, Mazarguil H, Faller P. Redox chemistry of copper-amyloid-beta: the generation of hydroxyl radical in the presence of ascorbate is linked to redox-potentials and aggregation state. *Chembiochem*. 2007;8(11):1317–1325.
65. Dikalov SI, Vitek MP, Mason RP. Cupric-amyloid beta peptide complex stimulates oxidation of ascorbate and generation of hydroxyl radical. *Free Radic Biol Med*. 2004;36(3):340–347.
66. Baruch-Suchodolsky R, Fischer B. Soluble amyloid beta1-28-copper(I)/copper(II)/Iron(II) complexes are potent antioxidants in cell-free systems. *Biochemistry*. 2008;47(30):7796–7806.
67. Pedersen JT, Chen SW, Borg CB, Ness S, Bahl JM, Heegaard NH, Dobson CM, Hemmingsen L, Cremades N, Teilum K. Amyloid-beta and alpha-Synuclein decrease the level of metal-catalyzed reactive oxygen species by radical scavenging and redox silencing. *J Am Chem Soc*. 2016;138(12):3966–3969.

CHAPTER

15

Metals and Mitochondria in Neurodegeneration

Germán Plascencia-Villa, Miguel José-Yacamán, George Perry
The University of Texas at San Antonio (UTSA), San Antonio, TX, United States

OUTLINE

INTRODUCTION

Neurodegeneration is a general term that involves progressive loss of brain cells, especially neurons. Neurodegenerative diseases are very diverse, but most of them result in dementia. The general term dementia indicates a decline in mental functions with a wide range of symptoms, including memory loss, impaired communication, altered ability to focus and reasoning, and even altered visual perception. Most neurodegenerative diseases classified as dementia show a progressive and gradual pattern of damage to brain cells in specific particular regions or in specialized neuronal cells. The most common neurodegenerative disorders include Alzheimer's, Parkinson's, Huntington's, multiple sclerosis, amyotrophic lateral sclerosis, dementia with Lewy bodies, Creutzfeldt–Jakob, spinocerebellar ataxia, spinal muscular atrophy, and motor neuron diseases. Development of these neurodegenerative pathologies have been associated to predisposition with genetic mutations, aging processes, traumatic brain injuries, and altered neurotransmitters. Despite the diversity in these neuropathologies, some common features have emerged in these diseases, including presence of aggregates of misfolded proteins, severe mitochondrial dysfunction, and altered biometals

Biometals in Neurodegenerative Diseases. http://dx.doi.org/10.1016/B978-0-12-804562-6.00015-4

in the affected neurons. The events that trigger dysregulation of brain biometals are not yet completely understood, but data points to a correlation with the formation of protein aggregates, increased oxidative stress, and generation of mitochondrial dysfunction in neurons. Presence of abnormal protein isoforms with high tendency to form fibrils and aggregates in or outside the neurons has been the key and common pathological feature of many neurodegenerative diseases; unfortunately in most cases it indicates that the disease has spread to advanced stages, particularly in elderly patients. Examples of amyloidogenic proteins are amyloid-β a tau, α-synuclein, and prion protein, present in Alzheimer's, Parkinson's, and Creutzfeldt–Jakob, respectively. Detailed pathways or mechanisms that trigger the processing of normally expressed neuronal proteins into highly active and toxic precursors with self-assembly capacity are not completely understood, but key clues have emerged trying to elucidate and understand the metabolic context and circumstances in the brain that permit the aggregation. Metal sensing, internalization, and trafficking are highly regulated processes in multicellular eukaryotes and particularly critical in the nervous system. Regulation involves specific receptors and endocytic pathways for each biometal that responds to maintain cellular homeostasis (Fig. 15.1).

Here, we discuss data that correlate the close interplay between altered brain biometals and mitochondrial dysfunction in age-related neurodegenerative diseases, particularly showing molecular events correlating their interactions with neuronal amyloidogenic proteins to promote or direct the formation of fibrils and ultimately the formation of intricate aggregates in the brain that cause irreversible neuronal degeneration.

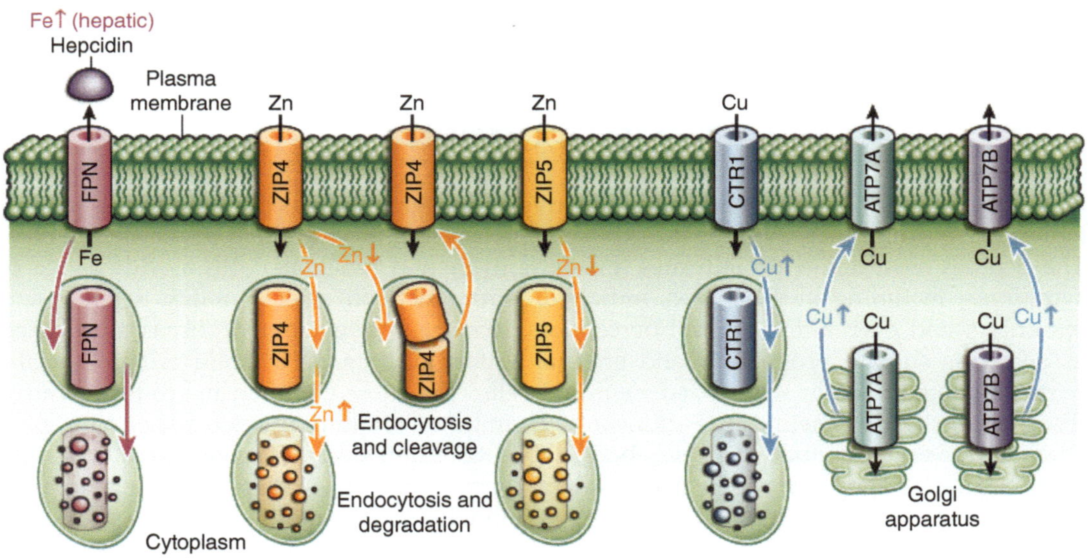

FIGURE 15.1 **Biometal eukaryotic cell transporters.** Metal transporters in mammalian cells indicating internalization and transport of Fe, Zn and Cu. *Source: Reproduced with permission Waldron KJ, Rutherford JC, Ford D, Robinson NJ. Metalloproteins and metal sensing.* Nature. *2009;460:823–830. Copyright 2009, Nature Publishing.*

IRON DYSHOMEOSTASIS

Iron functions essentially as a cofactor, especially in the mitochondrial respiratory chain complexes where its ability for electron transport between ferric (Fe^{3+}) and ferrous (Fe^{2+}) forms is efficiently exploited in ATP generation. Among the biometals, iron is the most abundant transition metal in the human body. Transport of iron to the brain occurs by transferrin (Tf) complexed with Fe^{3+}.[2,3] Intracellularly, ferric ions remain stored inside ferritin cages forming insoluble crystalline oxides with up to 4500 Fe^{3+} ions combined with phosphate and OH^- [4] (Fig. 15.2).

In 1906, Alois Alzheimer described a peculiar psychiatric case with morphological changes in the brain tissue of a 51 year-old female, published in *"A peculiar disease of the cerebral cortex"* (English translation from original paper published in *Allgemeine Zeitschrift für Psychiatrie und Psychisch-Gerichtliche Medizin*).[5] Today, more than 100 years later, we still do not completely understand this complex disease, even though some genetic mutations linked to less than 1% of the AD cases have been identified. The majority of cases are sporadic AD, mostly observed in patients over 60 years of age. Metabolic alterations related to the aging process are providing clues to the understanding of this neurodegenerative disease.

AD patients show a drastic dyshomeostasis of iron metabolism, particularly with accumulation over time showing significant elevated levels in cortical, subcortical, white matter areas, and hippocampus,[6,7] as observed in late onset AD patients 60 years and older. Elevated Fe levels have been associated with amyloid-β plaque core (AβPC) formation. Synthetic $A\beta_{1-42}$ (DAEFRHDSGYEVHHQKLVFFAEDVGSNKGAIIGLMVGGVVIA) self-assemble into stable but poorly ordered filaments. Cryo-EM revealed that Aβ filaments are formed by two

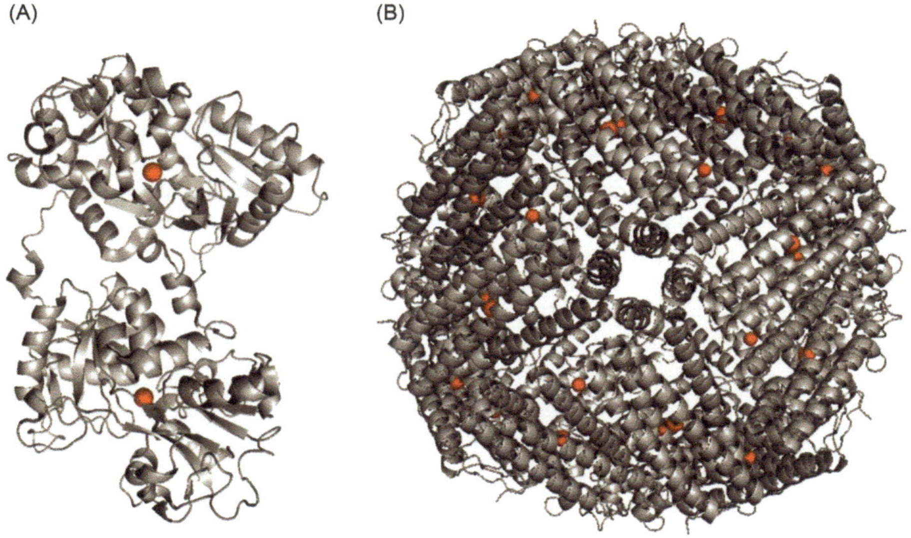

FIGURE 15.2 **Proteins involved in iron transportation and storage.** (A) Transferrin (PDB: 3V83).[3] (B) Ferritin (PBD: 1FHA).[4] Fe ions as red spheres. Molecular modeling with UCSF Chimera v1.10 and PyMOL v1.5 (Schrödinger).

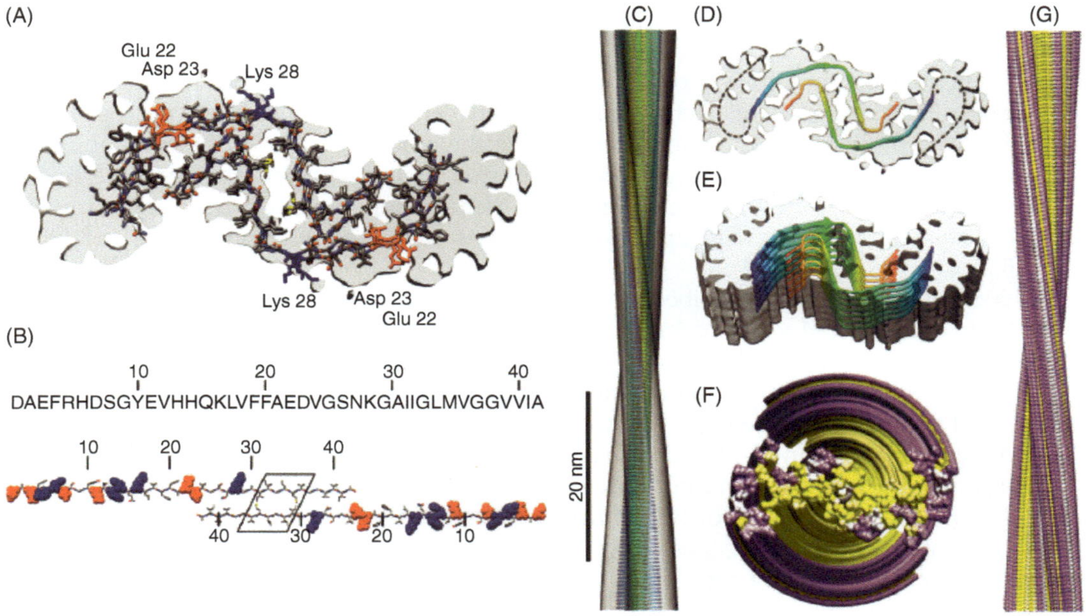

FIGURE 15.3 **Amyloid-β aggregation.** Structure of $A\beta_{1-42}$ fibrils. (A) Density maps. (B) Electrostatic interactions between $A\beta_{1-42}$ fibrils. (C) Side view of the fibril density maps. (D–F) Fibril cross-section, of a dimer, seven dimers, and top view, respectively. (G) Side view of the fibril density maps, showing charged residues. *Source: Reproduced with permission. Schmidt M, Rohou A, Lasker K, et al. Peptide dimer structure in an Abeta(1–42) fibril visualized with cryo-EM.* Proc Natl Acad Sci USA. *2015;112(38):11858–11863.*[14] *Copyright 2015, HighWire Press.*

juxtaposed strands with a hollow core (~20 Å radius) (Fig. 15.3); both strands interact electrostatically via the N-terminus of one unit with the loop region of the opposite strand.[8,9] The flexible N-terminus ($A\beta_{1-16}$) locates on the external surface of the fibrils and available to interact with external media, ultimately the morphology and assembly of these protofilaments depend on physicochemical parameters, such as pH, temperature, and importantly, presence of metal ions (Fe^{2+}, Fe^{3+}, Cu^{2+}, Zn^{2+}).[10] At the structural level, the location of metal binding sited on $A\beta_{1-16}$ is unclear as to whether it is on the external or internal lumen of the Aβ fibers (Fig. 15.3). During the aging process the brain levels of key biometals increase (especially Fe), even though the imbalance between Fe^{3+}/Fe^{2+} species could be more important than the net amount of iron in neurons since Fe^{3+}/Fe^{2+} are linked to oxidative damage and over-production of reactive oxygen species (ROS), but specific mechanisms that lead to brain misregulation of metal ions are still largely unknown.[11,12] Amyloid-β protein precursor (AβPP) shows ferroxidase activity, specifically by a sequence similar to H-ferritin that oxidases Fe^{2+} to Fe^{3+}.[13] In vitro studies showed that ΔAβPP neuronal cells accumulated iron with impact in extracellular Zn^{2+} accumulation within Aβ aggregates.

Histochemical analysis showed that redox active iron is significantly elevated in AD compared to control tissue sections, these Fe(II/III) complexes were associated with senile plaques and neurofibrillary tangles[15] (Fig. 15.4). Importantly, iron accumulation was also related to increased oxidative damage of neurons. The association of metal ions with Aβ

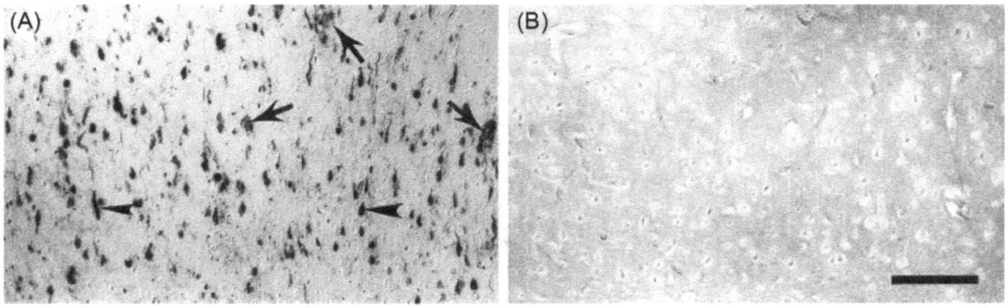

FIGURE 15.4 **Brain section with Fe staining.** (A) Histochemical detection of iron in AD compared with control case (B). *Arrows* and *arrow heads* indicate presence of plaques and tangles, respectively. Scale bar 200 μm. *Source: Reproduced with permission Smith MA, Harris PL, Sayre LM, Perry G, Iron accumulation in Alzheimer disease is a source of redox-generated free radicals.* Proc Natl Acad Sci USA. *1997;94(18):9866–9868.*[15] *Copyright 1997, HighWire Press.*

occur by coordination through His residues, as observed by significant increment of characteristic Raman scattering peaks of amine (N_τ and N_π) residues upon interaction with metal ions.[16] Iron ions (Fe^{2+} and Fe^{3+}) are highly redox active compounds that may cause metabolic alterations or damage of biomolecules in the cellular environment. The chemical forms of iron associated with AD neurodegeneration are not completely understood. Valence state of iron is of extreme importance, particularly for the potential to generate free radicals and alterations of biochemical pathways.[17] The elevated quantities of Fe have been linked with the formation of inorganic aggregates of different iron oxides present in the human brain: ferrihydrite $[(Fe^{3+})_2O_3 \bullet 0.5H_2O]$, haematite ($Fe_2O_3$), magnetite ($Fe_3O_4$), maghemite ($\gamma$-$Fe_2O_3$), wüstite ($FeO$), and goethite [$\alpha$-$FeO(OH)$].[18] Among these, magnetite stands as the only stable iron oxide containing Fe^{2+}.[18–20] Magnetite-maghemite particles were found in the human brain from extracts of solubilized brain tissues and showed high-field saturation effects through ultrasensitive superconducting magnetometry.[21] TEM and diffraction of the extracted particles showed a mixture of magnetite and maghemite phases of iron oxide, with variable sizes of up to 200 nm. Similarly, AD samples evaluated by a highly sensitive superconducting interference device (SQUID) showed a magnetic response, due to the high concentration of iron oxide particles in the AD tissues from 1.0 ± 0.4 to 7.0 ± 0.3 μg/g,[19] whereas control tissues showed a much lower or even absent presence of magnetite-like aggregates. AD biopsies revealed that more than 90% of the iron oxide particles are smaller than 20 nm in diameter, and that the amount of magnetite is significantly higher in AD female than in AD male.[17] Due to the size range of magnetite particles in brain, it was hypothesized that the origin of iron oxide is from the store protein ferritin that possesses an internal diameter of 8 nm, in association with aging and abnormal iron metabolism in neurons. Larger particles may be the result of aggregation or coalescence of several small particles, or also by continuous growth of small particles by reduction of available free Fe(II/III) ions on their highly active surfaces. More sensitive techniques, such as high-resolution X-ray fluorescence mapping (XRF), X-ray absorption near edge spectroscopy (XANES), high field magnetic resonance microscopy and synchrotron X-ray absorption microscopy showed a mapping of Fe in brain sections, identifying aggregates in frontal-lobe tissue areas of the brain, as well as observing the characteristic X-ray Fe peaks at 711 eV and 6950–7750 eV confirming chemical identity of inorganic aggregates of ferritin, ferrihydrite, and magnetite.[22–24] In vitro interactions between synthetic

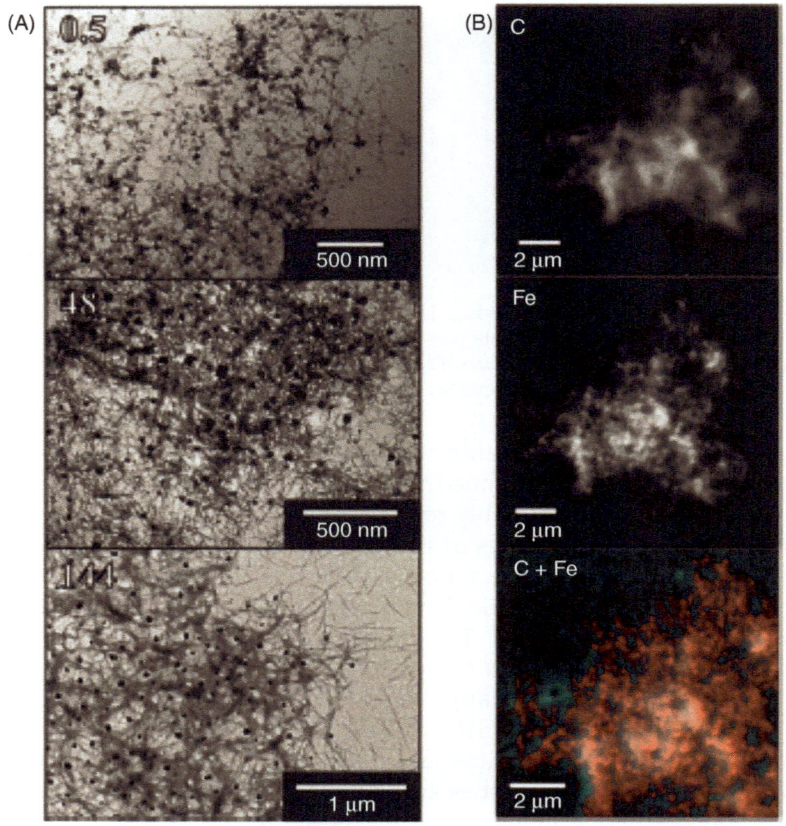

FIGURE 15.5 **Amyloid-β aggregation with iron oxide nanoparticles.** Time lapse at 0.5, 48, and 144 h interaction Aβ with ferrihydrite. (A) Bright field TEM. (B) Scanning transmission X-ray microscopy (STXM). *Source: Reproduced with permission Everett J, Cespedes E, Shelford LR, et al. Evidence of redox-active iron formation following aggregation of ferrihydrite and the Alzheimer's disease peptide beta-amyloid.* Inorg Chem. *2014;53(6):2803–2809.*[26] *Copyright 2014, ACS Publications.*

$A\beta_{1-42}$, ferrihydrite particles or Fe^{3+} revealed spontaneous formation of hybrid aggregates[25,26] (Fig. 15.5). Upon interaction the final form of iron was similar to magnetite, showing activity of Aβ peptides to reduce ionic precursors, as demonstrated by X-ray absorption and X-ray magnetic circular dichroism spectroscopy, and direct observations by electron microscopy and diffraction. These iron oxide aggregates were identified in isolated AβPC from postmortem AD tissues as a mixture of magnetite/maghemite, tomographic projections showed that the inorganic particles were mostly located on the periphery of AβPC.[27] Most of the Fe-based particles were between 5 and 15 nm, but larger particles of up to 35–40 nm were identified by electron microscopy techniques, including high-resolution imaging and diffraction patterns. Even though there is strong evidence of presence of iron oxide particles in AD brain, the association with AβPC or other neuronal proteins, such as tau, remains to be clarified. Proteomics of postmortem AD patients revealed that APC contained a diverse variety of proteins; besides Aβ the major component (~80%), different proteins, such as tau, ATPase, collagen, fibrinogen, clathrin were identified.[28,29] Remarkably proteins from iron transport, serotransferrin and ferritin were identified in APC isolated by laser capture microdissection from AD brain tissue.

Importantly, another question is the physiological and metabolic implications of the presence of iron oxide particles within or outside neurons and their possible interference with electrical and chemical signals, synapses, microglial activation, and overall brain function. Cultured neurons show neurotoxic effects and neurophysiological alterations caused by oligomeric and fibrillary Aβ.[30,31] Clustered neural networks derived from cortical rat neurons show alterations in functional connectivity and cellular damage when dosed with synthetic magnetite-$A\beta_{1-42}$.[20] Surprisingly, pure magnetite or $A\beta_{1-42}$ showed minor changes, concluding that neuronal damage may occur by a synergistic effect between magnetite particles and Aβ peptides. Alternatively, Aβ related magnetite might represent the redox stabilized form of iron much as performed by ferritin. Tau protein is also involved in this complex iron–Aβ interaction, since it promoted iron export related to AβPP trafficking in neurons and tau knock-out showed no iron accumulation.[32] The coaggregation of Aβ with metals and many other cellular proteins could lead to a general misbalance with a toxic environment, in combination with limited regenerative potential of neurons, and result in neuronal failure and death. It is speculated that interaction of Aβ with Fe species is a neuronal protective mechanism to cope with highly redox-active ions, the question still remains if the formation of iron oxide particles is the cause or consequence for the formation of complex AβPC aggregates. Electron holography and advanced analytical imaging demonstrated that Fe in AβPC is present as iron oxide (Fe_3O_4) magnetite (8–50 nm), highly organized crystalline nanostructures with a characteristic of superparamagnetic response.[33]

Recent reports have raised concerns of human-to-human transmissibility of AD, Particularly in groups of patients that developed Creutzfeld–Jakob disease many years after administration of human-derived growth hormone or surgical grafts of dura mater contaminated with prions.[34,35] Pathology studies found Aβ deposits similar to AD that did not colocalize with prion deposits, suggesting a iatrogenic transmission of active Aβ deposits which served as seeds to develop AD.

Parkinson's disease (PD) is the second most common progressive neurodegenerative disorder, also related to formation of amyloidogenic aggregates. Neuropathological evidence of PD stands by the presence of insoluble abnormal filamentous aggregates of misfolded α-synuclein (α-Syn). Principally intracytoplasmic accumulated in neurons of the substantia nigra forming Lewy bodies and Lewy neurites that exert neurotoxic effects.[36]

Similar to AD, alterations in iron metabolism have been related with progress ion of PD, with overexpression of iron uptake proteins (DMT1, TfR) and underexpression of iron exporters (ferroportin) producing Fe accumulation, in combination with other factors, such as mitochondrial dysfunction, oxidative stress, and autophagy.[37] PD patients showed a 31%–35% increment in brain iron, this change was localized in the substantia nigra in regions with decreased or lacking neuromelanin aggregates, related to formation of oxygen radicals and dopamine cell death, iron levels decreased in the globus pallidus.[38–41] Interestingly, elevated levels of ferritin were immunodetected, and other metals, such as Cu, Zn, Mg, and Mn that also suffered important alterations. Presence of Lewy bodies in neurodegeneration with brain iron accumulation type 1 (NBIA1, Hallervorden–Spatz syndrome) showed immunostaining for α-Syn indicating a relationship between iron misbalance and its aggregation.[42,43] Remarkably, iron species present in α-Syn aggregates in LB, where redox-active Fe generated OH^- radicals.[44] Even though in mild PD the total content of Fe is not significantly altered, but is however focused in substantia nigra. Importantly, there is a shift in Fe^{2+}/Fe^{3+} to Fe^{3+} correlated with increased ferritin levels that bind Fe^{3+} ions and a lower glutathione content.[45] Binding of divalent metal ions (Fe^{2+}, Cu^{2+}, Mn^{2+}, Co^{2+}, and Ni^{2+}) directly impact the aggregation of α-Syn, through interaction at the C-terminus whereas N-terminus binds preferentially copper.[46–48] Dependency of α-Syn for divalent ions to attain fine structure was demonstrated with presence of fibril morphologies by electron microscopy. In initial steps, Fe^{3+} ions are involved in formation of α-Syn oligomers, then triggering aggregation.[48] Structural changes in oligomerization and α-Syn protofibril formation are linked to metal-catalyzed oxidation of peptides by an increased amount of ROS.[49] Recent reports present the idea of synergistic neurotoxic effects of α-Syn–Fe complex in a dose- and time-dependent manner (at least in in vitro models) that lead to aggregation, simultaneously ferrous ions cause downregulation of nuclear factor E2-related factor 2 (Nrf2) and heme oxygenase-1 (HO-1).[50] Dopamine metabolism is drastically altered by metals, since the 3,4-dihydroxyphenylacetaldehyde (DOPAL) intermediate of dopamine can cause oligomerization with α-Syn in PC12 cells, especially in the presence of divalent ions Cu^{2+}, Fe^{2+}, and Mn^{2+}, but not with Cu^{1+} or Fe^{3+}.[51] The combination and interdependency of dopamine depletion, metal misbalance and protein aggregation forming LB lead to neuronal toxicity in PD.

Human prion disorder or Creutzfeld-Jakob disease is characterized by a conformational change of prion protein PrP (isoform of a normal cell-surface glycoprotein, PrP^C to PrP^{Sc}) and its accumulation in brain parenchyma. Recent reports have identified links between PrP and iron metabolism and their interrelation with pathogenesis. PrP aggregates have sequestered iron, usually colocalized with ferritin.[52,53] This is accompanied by upregulated Tf levels directly related to disease progression. Human neuroblastoma cells expressing PrP under exposure to inorganic iron (Fe^{2+}) showed that PrP binds iron forming aggregates also associated with ferritin cages, whereas iron depletion treatment reduced significantly the propagation of prions.[54]

The interaction of PrP with ferritin may cause an iron deficiency status in affected neurons, forming complex protein aggregates and increased oxidative stress by formation of ROS (H_2O_2) leading to detriment of cell viability in vitro.[54–56] PrP is a hemin (iron photoporphyrin IX, Fe^{3+}) binding protein though the N-terminal third of PrP, as a consequence the complex suffers aggregation and clathrin-mediated internalization in N2a5E4E cells with direct implication in iron homeostasis.[57] The C-terminal PrP fragment implicated in prion disease transmission was co-purified and co-transported with ferritin, forming a complex in in vitro and mice models, suggesting that iron-transport mechanisms including receptors may facilitate uptake of PrP.[53,58] As observed in cell models, PrP affected human, hamster and mouse brains showed increased levels of Fe^{2+} and also upregulated Tf and transferrin receptor (TfR) especially in advanced stages.[59] Iron imbalance seems to be highly related with progression of prion disease, causing neuronal iron deficiency despite overall increased iron levels, mainly related to aggregation of PrP–ferritin complexes. Interestingly, PrP showed ferriductase activity resulting in iron imbalance with the presence of insoluble iron aggregates; mutant PrP (present in familial prion disorder) shows higher ferriductase activity.[60] The physiological role of PrP^C is not clear, but this normal cell-surface glycoprotein has been proposed in diverse functions, including:

protection from apoptosis and oxidative stress, cellular uptake or binding of iron and copper, signaling, synapses, and adhesion to extracellular matrix.[61] PrP clearly plays a critical role in brain iron imbalance, particularly forming protein aggregates of PrP-ferritin.

COPPER DISLOCATION

In the brain, copper ions (Cu^{2+} and Cu^{+} oxidation states) are essential for development and normal functioning of neurons, especially as cofactor of growth factors, respiration, neurotransmitter synthesis, activation of neuropeptides and hormones, redox activity, myelination, and pigmentation. Copper dysregulation has been observed in neurodegenerative disorders, such as Alzheimer's, Parkinson's, Huntington's, motor neuron, and prion diseases; but also some uncommon genetic disorders, such as Menkes disease, occipital horn syndrome, and Wilson disease. Our current understanding of the mechanisms of action and regulation of Cu in neurodegeneration is still limited, but recent research has provided additional insights to elucidate the complexity of neuronal damage related to dysregulation of biometals.

In the first place, copper enters the brain via the blood–brain barrier and the blood–cerebrospinal fluid barrier, and regulated by copper transporters CTR1 and P-type ATPases: ATP7A, and ATP7B (copper-ATPases) as part of the Cu-regulatory pathway localized at the *trans*-Golgi network. These proteins are especially involved in copper translocation across cellular membranes and removal of excessive Cu preventing toxicity. Cu^{2+} ions are reduced to Cu^{+} by metalloreductases then transported by CTR1.[62] ATP7A plays an important role in Cu delivery from astrocytes to neurons and is preferentially expressed in cerebellum and substantia nigra, whereas ATP7B supplies copper to cuproenzymes in the secretory pathway including ceruloplasmin (the copper-transporting protein)(Fig. 15.6A).[63] Mutations in ATP7B

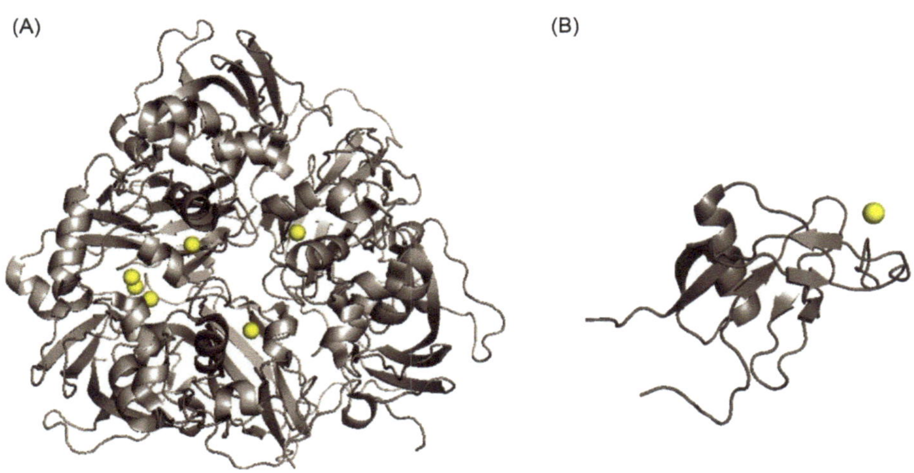

FIGURE 15.6 **Proteins in copper transportation and modulation.** (A) Ceruloplasmin (PDB: 4ENZ), Cu^{2+} ions shown in *yellow*. (B) Growth factor-like domain of the amyloid-β precursor protein bound to copper (PDB: 4JFN). Molecular modeling with UCSF Chimera v1.10 and PyMOL v1.5 (Schrödinger)

gene result in Cu imbalance and possibly relate to sporadic hereditary AD.[64] AD patients and age-matched controls displayed similar levels of ceruloplasmin in neurons, but only AD cases showed significant increase in neuropil ceruloplasmin levels.[65] Elevated copper concentration in peripheral serum and ceruloplasmin was found in patients with AD in comparison with healthy controls.[66,67] The brain areas with significantly increased ceruloplasmin were hippocampus, entorhinal cortex, frontal cortex, and putamen. Remarkably, AD patients showed a significant amount of apo-ceruloplasmin (lacking Cu ions) compared to normal individuals, indicating that ceruloplasmin and other copper enzymes could be defective. Also, in PD patients there is a correlation between low concentration and activity of ceruloplasmin, associated with high iron levels.[68]

In addition to P-type ATPases and ceruloplasmin, AβPP is involved in maintaining copper homeostasis in the brain through the copper efflux pathway, with a Cu-binding site located in the growth factor-like domain (Fig. 15.6B). Cu modulates expression and processing of AβPP. An increase in copper leads to overexpression of AβPP and nonamyloidogenic processing pathway of AβPP, whereas a decrease of copper in neurons causes underexpression of AβPP.

Copper binds strongly with Aβ aggregates, AβPP will remove Cu^{2+} from serum albumin leading to accumulation in APC. Binding strength of Aβ for copper through His residues depends on aggregation state, being more elevated in the fibrillary arrangements than in monomers.[69] The source of Cu seems to be ceruloplasmin, since the net amount of free Cu^{2+} and apoceruloplasmin (protein lacking Cu ions) were significantly elevated in AD,[70] possibly related to alterations in ceruloplasmin activity.

Copper dislocation in AD might be related to a combination of many factors including alterations in its transport and cellular distribution carried out by ceruloplasmin and P-type ATPases. Sporadic reports have even proposed a link of AD susceptibility with increased levels of dietary copper. In clinical studies of mild to moderate AD, 87% of patients showed serum levels of copper between normal range, only with minor reductions in Cu and ceruloplasmin levels that were determined in cerebrospinal fluid (CSF) and compared with healthy individuals.[71,72] CSF and serum levels of copper in several clinical studies showed overall no statistical differences.[70,73–75] Even though the peripheral total content of Cu seems normal, the free or ionic Cu suffered an increment which was related to presence of defective ceruloplasmin.[76–78] Also, this tendency was correlated with Apolipoprotein E-4 (APOE4) gene carriers, that overall showed higher copper and free copper levels than controls. Importantly, over time this dislocation of Cu in the AD brain may cause copper deficiency in neighboring neurons, which compromises activities of Cu-dependent enzymes: cytochrome *c*-oxidase and Cu/Zn-superoxide dismutase (SOD1), both important in cell respiration and as antioxidants.[68,79]

Dysregulation of brain biometals correlates with stages of AD development and also with specific affected areas. Copper, iron, and zinc levels were significantly elevated in AD in an age-dependent mode in cortex and hippocampus areas, synchrotron radiation micro beam X-ray fluorescence (SR-μXRF), and X-ray absorption near edge spectroscopy revealed presence of a mixture of Cu^{+} and Cu^{2+} oxidation states in hippocampus and midbrain areas.[80] Early studies suggested that Cu accelerates aggregation of Aβ, the increased amount of biometals colocalized with AβPC in AD patients.[81] More recent analysis found that Cu and Zn effectively accumulate with AβPC with a strong spatial correlation, observed as hot spots with high biometals contents through synchrotron X-ray fluorescence and scanning transmission

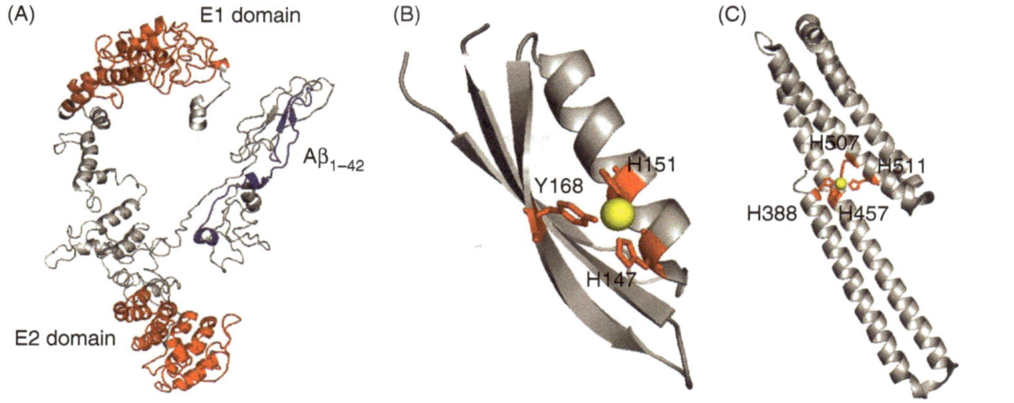

FIGURE 15.7 **Cu-binding sites in AβPP.** (A) Model of complete APP_{770}, showing E1 and E2 domains *(red)*, and $A\beta_{1\text{-}42}$ peptide *(blue)*. (B) E1 domain (PDB: 2FK1),[85] Cu^{2+} ion *(shown in yellow)* coordinated by H147-H168-Y168. (C) E2 domain (PDB: 3UMK),[86] Cu^{2+} ion *(shown in yellow)* coordinated by H388-H457-H507-H511. Molecular modeling with UCSF Chimera v1.10 and PyMOL v1.5 (Schrödinger).

ion microscopy coupled with particle induce X-ray emission and Rutherford backscattering spectrometry.[82,83]

Structurally, AβPP possesses two copper-binding subdomains: E1 (18-203) and E2 (376-554).[62,84–87] AβPP E1-domain binds Cu^{2+} through His147-His151-Tyr168, with partial reduction to Cu^{+}. In AβPP E2 domain coordinates another Cu ion by four-coordinate residues (His388-His457-His507-His511).[85–87] The $A\beta_{1\text{-}42}$ peptide that aggregates to form AβPC is located at transmembrane domain close to C-terminal of AβPP, that after processing by secretases will be excised (Fig. 15.7). AβPP possesses ferroxidase activity similar to ceruloplasmin, with presence of consensus sequence–REXXE- similar to the H-ferritin domain.[13]

Excised Aβ peptides coordinate Cu^{2+}, this molecular interaction occurred by imidazole rings of His residues at positions 6, 13, and 14 with high affinity.[88] Formation of fibrillary structures was confirmed by TEM and AFM, but also with presence of amorphous aggregates. Electro spin echo envelope modulation spectroscopy indicated the possibility of a second Cu-binding site in Aβ in a proton-rich environment exposed to water.[89] Solute pH is of great significance in Cu-Aβ binding, since at physiological conditions Cu-Aβ lead to formation of heterogeneous aggregates. Under acidic conditions (pH 6.0), His 6 was the main binding site, but above pH 7.4 His14 and His13 contributed in metal binding.[90] Importantly, data showed simultaneous coordination of imidazole rings which may form intermolecular bridges sharing His13 and two Cu^{2+}.

Aβ-Cu^{2+} complexes reduced with ascorbate indicated that His13 and His14 were oxidized, leading to Aβ-Cu^{+} and generation of ROS (H_2O_2) in a redox-cycle,[91] consequently oxidative damage to Aβ inhibits Cu-binding promoting oxidative stress in neurons. It was suggested that upon multiple rounds of redox-cycles of AβCu^{2}-AβCu^{+} promoted aggregation and occurrence of crosslinking, which finally results in formation of AβPC. In AD, interaction of $A\beta_{1\text{-}42}$ peptides with copper promotes oligomerization and formation of protein aggregates, also the reduction of Cu and Fe ions generate ROS leading to elevated oxidative stress in neurons.

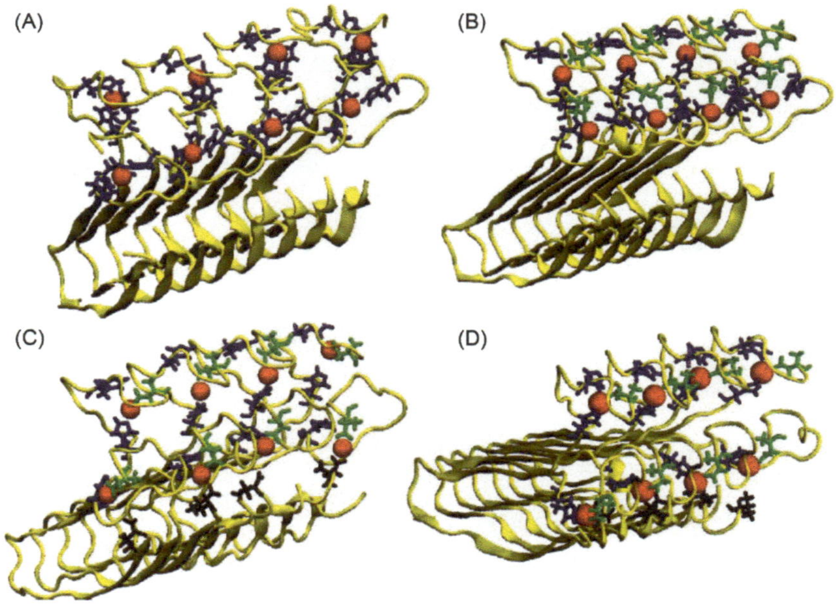

FIGURE 15.8 **Interactions of Cu-Amyloidβ.** (A) Conformer 1, Cu ion coordinated by His6, His 13, and His14. (B) Conformer 2, Cu ion coordinated by Asp1, His6, and His14. (C) Conformer 3, Cu ion coordinated by Asp1, His6, and His14, second Cu ion coordinated by Asp1, His14, and Val49. (D) Conformed 4, Cu ion coordinated by Asp1, His6, and His14, second Cu ion coordinated by Asp1, His13, and Val40. *Source: Reproduced with permission Parthasarathy S, Long F, Miller Y, et al. Molecular-level examination of Cu^{2+} binding structure for amyloid fibrils of 40-residue Alzheimer's beta by solid-state NMR spectroscopy.* J Am. Chem Soc. *2011;133(10):3390–3400.*[10] *Copyright 2011, ACS Publications.*

It was also proposed that interactions of Aβ-Cu may have some neuroprotective functions. Since Aβ–Cu^+ are stable under presence of O_2 whereas AβCu^{2+} reacted forming ROS, so the potential damage of highly active free Cu^{2+}/Cu^+ ions will be abolished in the presence of Aβ that will reduce its availability to react, preventing neuronal death caused by transition metal-induced oxidative damage.[91,92]

The molecular interaction of Aβ with Cu^{2+} ions leads to production of ROS (H_2O_2) and highly toxic radicals OH^- by redox cycling, in particular this redox reaction occurred by a selective quenching coordinated by two His residues (His13 and His14), and –COO^- groups (Val40, Glu3, Glu11, and Glu22).[10] Besides these multistep conformational changes of Aβ during interaction with Cu^{2+} causing oxidation of Met35, generation of H_2O_2, and OH^- radicals by a Fenton process also occur simultaneously in the presence of O_2 and other reducing agents (i.e., ascorbate) contributing to neuronal oxidative stress.[10,93,94] Fig. 15.8 shows the different conformations that Aβ may adopt upon interaction with Cu^{2+}, but the high mobility of the N-terminus opened the possibility for different intra- and intermolecular contacts, and even the capacity for binding two equivalents of Cu^{2+} per Aβ peptide.[95] Affinity of amyloid peptides for copper is up to 3x higher than serum albumin, consequently Cu^{2+} (and other metal ions like zinc and iron) influenced amyloid fiber formation by stabilizing cross-linked oligomers and longer fibers.[96–98]

Tau protein aggregated into neurofibrillary tangles which are aggregates of bundles of paired helical filaments (PHF) also have capacity to bind copper. The residues 287–304 and 318–335 of tau demonstrate conformational changes in the presence of Cu^{2+} and may promote its aggregation.[99,100] Importantly, binding tau-Cu is pH-dependent, equimolar, and coordinated by His residues in the -HVPGGG- sequence and other amine-residues forming stable complexes.[101,102] Upon interaction with tau, copper modulates the in vitro aggregation into PHF.[103] During the molecular interaction, tau (peptide 287–304) showed reductive activity to convert Cu^{2+} to Cu^{+} generating H_2O_2 in a redox-cycle manner, and as a consequence forming S-S linked tau dimers.[104]

Patients with PD, Huntington's and progressive supranuclear palsy showed increased levels of ceruloplasmin, especially in hippocampus, frontal, temporal, and parietal cortex and substantia nigra.[67] Brain tissue samples in PD showed a drastic reduction of 34%–45% of total Cu in the substantia nigra, whereas other areas showed no alterations.[38,39] These significant changes observed in neurodegenerative diseases were explained as an acute phase-type and compensatory responses to oxidative stress. Isotope measurements of Cu absorption revealed that PD patients had a less controlled metabolism in comparison with healthy controls. In particular with abnormally large accumulation in plasma (albumin and ceruloplasmin) and tissue cells (muscle), but similar levels in liver and gut.[105] If we focus on the brain, copper concentration in CSF was significantly higher in idiopathic PD (0.5–0.6 μmol/L, compared to controls 0.2 μmol/L).[106,107] But similar clinical studies showed no significant differences in Cu related to PD even under L-DOPA therapy.[108,109] Total content of copper, as well as copper transport proteins (CTR1, ATOX1, ATP7A, and ATP7B) were at least 2x higher in substantia nigra than in other brain areas (visual cortex, anterior cortex, putamen, and cerebellum).[110,111] Ceruloplasmin activity (measured as ferroxidase activity) was ~80% lower in subtantia nigra of PD, whereas ceruloplasmin knock-out mice developed PD-like symptoms,[112] concluding that failure in ceruloplasmin functionality may contribute to high amounts of free Cu ions and could be involved in the development of parkinsonism. When the different proteins related to Cu-internalization and transport are compromised, specifically in substantia nigra and locus coeruleus there is a higher vulnerability to develop PD with Lewy bodies. As confirmed by analysis of brain regions affected with α-Syn aggregation, which displayed vulnerability and neuronal death that correlated with alterations in copper metabolism.[113] Aggregation of α-Syn showed a close dependency with its Cu-binding capacity, with a decrease in cellular available copper and reduction in the formation of oligomers and intracellular aggregates.[114] In contrast, when copper was restored in SH-SY5Y cells the capacity of aggregation of α-Syn was reestablished, whereas iron ions showed no impact in its aggregation. Binding sites of α-Syn are distributed in three domains: N-terminus (residues 1–9), His50, and C-terminal (residues 119–126), triggering its aggregation.[114] Met residues in α-Syn N-terminus (Met1 and Met5) effectively bind Cu^{+}, importantly Met5 coordinates Cu^{2+} and Cu^{+} displaying susceptibility to oxidative damage with ROS generation by redox cycling of copper under physiological conditions.[115] The other site at His50 also binds Cu^{+} with no major impact in overall structure, but similarly displayed copper catalyzed oxidation of residues.[116] Physicochemical conditions, particularly pH and Cu/α-Syn ratio control metal binding properties, under acidic pH, Cu^{2+} binds to N-terminal amine and Asp2, at pH 7.4 binding occurred at His50, the later one with important promotion of aggregation.[117] Posttranslational modification of α-Syn, particularly acetylation at its N-terminal is important for stabilization/restriction of local structures and

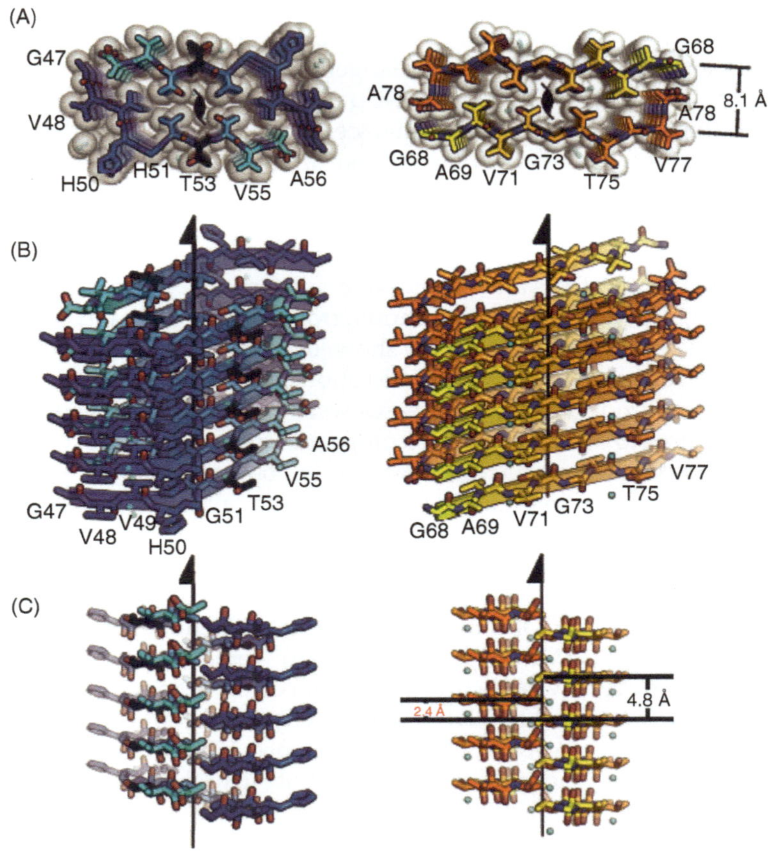

FIGURE 15.9 **Structure of α-synuclein amyloid core (Parkinsons and Lewy bodies).** (A) Crystal structure α-Syn. (Band C) Fibrillar assemblies of α-Syn. *Source: Reproduced with permission Rodriguez JA, Ivanova MI, Sawaya MR, et al. Structure of the toxic core of alpha-synuclein from invisible crystals.* Nature. *2015;525(7570):486–490.*[123] *Copyright 2015, Nature Publishing.*

interaction with Cu^{+}.[118] Coordination of α-Syn and Aβ with Cu^{2+}/Cu^{+} (but also for Fe^{3+}, Co^{2+}, Mn^{2+}, Zn^{2+}) resulted from the high affinity of residues promoting metal-catalyzed oxidation, triggering structural transformations and formation of heterodimers, aggregation, and fibrillation, with simultaneous production of ROS.[119–122] Recently the structure of an 11-residue α-Syn core fragment that forms highly organized protofibrils in a face-to-face β-sheets arrangements was resolved.[123] Even though the structure obtained from cryo-EM did not contain Cu ions and lacks the C-terminus, it provided important information regarding the formation and arrangement of α-Syn aggregates present in PD. (Fig. 15.9). Crystallization and structure-resolving of amyloid proteins have proved to be an extremely challenging task, and involvement of metal ions, oxidation/reduction of residues, cross-linking and posttranslational modifications complicate even more the scenario.

Alterations in copper metabolism have been effectively linked to prion disease pathogenesis. Physiological functions of PrP^C is not completely understood, but reports proposed the involvement in copper metabolism in nervous system and brain. Particularly, a high concentrations of copper and zinc (but not Mn^{2+}) promote endocytosis of PrP^C in cultured cells.[57,124] Conversely, at physiological levels, free Cu promoted regulation of PrP^C gene transcription and increased its exocytosis in GN11 neurons.[125] The repeated consensus sequence PHGG(G/S)WGQ located at the N-terminal in PrP^C specifically bind Cu^{2+} ions, in particular His residues control metal coordination and structural binding.[126,127] Additionally, PrP exerts regulation of iron acting as a ferrireductase in a copper-dependent mode.[60] Consequently, in the presence of PrP^C the activity of NMDA receptors is altered in a copper-dependent mode with alterations in Ca^{2+} excess and potential cytotoxicity.[128] Ultimately, Cu^{2+} and Zn^{2+} binding by residues His111-Met109-Met 112 of PrP (peptides 106–126) exacerbate aggregation into fibril structures leading to neurotoxicity. Removing of divalent ions prevented formation of aggregates.[129] Binding of Cu ions affect structure of PrP^C to a misfolded form of PrP^{Sc} which will form oligomers though oxidative reactions finally forming amyloid fibrils.[130]

Interestingly, free Cu^{2+} showed important effects on ubiquitin stability and aggregation, forming large aggregates and altering tertiary structure into a beta-sheet exposed conformer.[131] These structural changes and aggregation of ubiquitin seem to be a secondary reaction by the presence of high amounts of free redox active ions (Cu^{2+}, Fe^{2+}, Fe^{3+}), occurring when cells try to ubiquitinate toxic substrates for processing or modulation of cell responses, such as in the case of neurodegenerative amyloidogenic peptides. Consequently, impeding a proper processing that may lead to its accumulation over the time and progression of neurodegeneration. Proteomics of APC from AD patients revealed that ubiquitin and ubiquitin-processing proteins are present in plaques by coaggregation with Aβ as the main component.[28,29]

ZINC DEFICIENCY

Zinc, the second most abundant biometal, is widely present in enzymes as cofactor and as structure stabilizing agent in bioassemblies. In brain, zinc is involved in oxidative stress, apoptosis, aging, synaptic transmission, and as a neuromodulator.[132] In neurons, zinc is bound to proteins or present as free ions of Zn^{2+} (cytoplasmic or extracellular), particularly within synaptic vesicles at glutaminergic neurons and highly involved in neuronal synapses. Homeostasis of zinc occurs by transporters (ZnT and ZIP), and metallothioneins (MT1, MT2, MT3, MT4) participating in the uptake, transport, and regulation of zinc.[132,133]

Zinc deficiencies have been associated with neurodegenerative diseases. It was observed that zinc is related with dementia, particularly by age-associated low availability of zinc.[134] CSF and serum levels of zinc did not differ in AD and healthy patients or was only reduced slightly (12.3–10.9 μmol/L). Interestingly AD may be accompanied with lower body and body mass index indicating a dietary deficiency of Zn.[73,74,135] Quantification of Zn in brain tissues from AD revealed its deficiency in hippocampus (31.4–57.9 μg/g) with important differences in contrast with controls (37.3–87.1 μg/g).[136,137] The imbalance of zinc in hippocampus and amygdala was related to a displacement phenomenon by other biometals, possibly iron, copper, but also aluminum and silicon.[138,139] The brain areas that presented major signs of biometals alterations correlated with areas known to be affected by AD. Zinc was importantly elevated in cortex; the amount of zinc showed a close correlation with location and the amount of AβPC levels of severe AD cases.[16,81,82,140,141] Location of different zinc transporters (ZnT) matched with cortex areas with plaques of AD tissues, as confirmed by immunofluorescence and recently by proteomics of AβPC.[28,142] Synaptic zinc contributed with accumulation of Aβ aggregates and plaque formation in transgenic mice, whereas animals lacking ZnT3 transporter even under overexpression of Aβ had reduced amounts of amyloid aggregates.[143] Other genetic factors, such as mutant AβPP, presenilin-1 and tau proteins also showed influence in zinc mobilization and accumulation in transgenic mice.[144]

More data concerning the close interactions of Zn with Aβ-peptides was obtained on in vitro studies confirming that Zn^{2+} binds with $A\beta_{1-40}$ peptides inducing formation of aggregates, importantly the metal binding showed pH-dependency mediated by three His residues.[145,146] Presence of Zn ions interfere in formation of Aβ-Aβ intermediates and promote further aggregation into fibers.[98] Coordination of Zn^{2+} by Aβ peptide is not completely understood.[147] Imidazole rings from His6-His13-His14 in conjunction with Glu11 and N-terminal of Asp1 are the proposed metal binding sites for zinc.[148] All these amino acids correspond to the same binding sites for copper ions of Aβ, but with a lower binding affinity for Zn. Another interesting idea is that metal ions (Zn and Cu) induce aggregation of amyloid proteins by creating a bridge between two peptides, that repeatedly spread, inducing aggregation or even reducing the charge of Aβ.[149,150] This interfiber binding coordinates by Cu and Zn is a dynamic process and will have different coordination sites depending on pH (acidic, neutral, or basic) and stoichiometric availability of ions.

Levels of zinc measured in Parkinson's disease patients showed an important increment of 50%–54% in contrast with age-matched controls, but not only substantia nigra areas showed accumulation, the caudate nucleus and lateral putamen also presented 18%–35% higher zinc levels.[38,39] PD patients presented a significant decrease in serum zinc levels even on L-DOPA treatment, this deficiency showed a correlation with the worsening conditions of PD.[109] Some reports linked occupational exposure to metals (including Mn, Pb, Fe, Hg, Al, and Zn) with PD, with significant elevated tendency to develop parkinsonism. The presence of metal ions directly accelerate the fibrillation and aggregation of α-Syn, by inducing conformational changes into a partially folded intermediate.[151] Influence of biometals was evident by formation of spherical oligomers (5–8nm) of alpha synuclein in the presence of Mg, Cd, and Zn, even though Co and Ca produced larger oligomers (up to 90 nm).[152] The metal binding capacity of α-Syn comes from the C-terminal amino acid sequence DPDNEA (residues 119–124), with similar arrangement to a calcium-binding domain involving Asp and Glu residues, and also His50 at N-terminus.[46,153,154] The α-Syn-metal ion complexes appear to be formed by a complex coordination between several subunits, which eventually suffer cross-linking and aggregation into protofibers that are proposed to grow forming LB.

Aggregation of α-Syn in dopaminergic neurons of the substantia nigra is inhibited by oxidation of Met residues; but in the presence of zinc, the oxidation of methionine residues was inhibited, maintaining α-Syn fibrinogenic function.[155,156]

Other proteins from the homeostasis machinery of zinc are involved in α-Syn aggregation and trafficking, particularly, Zn-metallothionein-3 (ZnT3) participates in oxidase activity of α-Syn-Cu^{2+} to the more stable α-Syn-Cu+ intermediate inhibiting aggregation, so its failure or unavailability will result in production of OH- and oligomerization of α-Syn-Cu^{2+} into toxic aggregates.[157] Also, the release of aggregated, misfolded, and oxidized α-Syn from compromised dopaminergic neurons was regulated by ion channels and zinc pump PARK9/ATP13A2.[158,159] Free zinc ions and several proteins from the zinc transport/regulation system exert multiple and complex functions in PD, from a direct influence in oligomerization and aggregation of α-Syn, ROS production, oxidation, and release of protein aggregates from affected dopaminergic neurons.

Prion protein (PrP) coordinates zinc and copper ions through the N-terminus octapeptide causing conformational changes to its infectious form. PrP activities in neurons might be related to zinc homeostasis: transport and sensor.[124,160] Furthermore, mice PrP showed superoxide dismutase (SOD) activity related to cellular resistance to oxidative stress. Formation of the active structure requires metal ions.[161,162] The flexible N-terminus of PrP undergoes conformational changes into a more structured conformation in the presence of divalent cations (Cu^{2+}, Zn^{2+}, Mn^{2+}) and coordinated by His111-Met109-Met112, modeling the aggregation and ability to form fibrils with neurotoxic effects.[129,163,164] Upon interaction with cations, other regions of PrP suffered structural modifications with eventual formation of electrostatic and hydrogen bonds between Trp65-Trp73 and Gln67-Gln75 promoting oligomerization and aggregation of prion peptides.[165] PrP showed three distinct divalent ion coordination modes, mostly though His residues, where zinc competes with copper for the coordination sites under physiological conditions.[148,166] Presence of both divalent ions, Cu^{2+} and Zn^{2+}, promoted the interactions between prions by 117% and 300%, respectively, forming PrP–PrP intermediates that aggregate to form fibrils and aggregates, responsive to neuronal levels of these cations.[167,168] Moreover, zinc and copper stimulate trafficking and redistribution of PrP into Tf-contained endosomes. PrP possesses high affinity for Cu^{2+} (4×10^{-14} M), with other metals like Zn^{2+} demonstrating a three or more orders of magnitude lower affinity.[169]

Finally, the failure in Zn^{2+} metabolism through the activation/deactivation of pathways in neurodegenerative diseases may eventually cause dyshomeostasis and neuronal death. This is an extremely complex scenario, where ATP depletion, alteration of NAD^{+}, generation of ROS and NO, ion channel inhibition, mitochondrial damage, DNA damage, and alterations in neurotransmitters and enzymes exist, merging with aberrant forms of normal neuronal proteins that form cross-linked oligomers and amyloidogenic deposits leading to apoptotic, necrotic, or autophagic neuronal death[170] (Fig. 15.10).

MITOCHONDRIAL DYSFUNCTION

Dyshomeostasis of biometals in neurodegenerative disorders is closely related with mitochondrial dysfunction.[171] The principal role of mitochondria is bioenergetics by the synthesis of ATP via the electron transport chain, but mitochondria also are key participants in regulating iron homeostasis (import, utilization, storage, and export), consequently their failure in neurons leads to a global dysfunction and eventually to cell death. ATP production in mitochondria generates important amounts of ROS. Dissolved oxygen captures electrons forming superoxide (O_2^-), then mitochondrial superoxide dismutase (SOD1) forms H_2O_2 and O_2.[172] Consequently, oxidative stress in neurons increases. The iron-sulfur clusters (ISCs) and heme-prosthetic groups (HPGs) in mitochondria intervene importantly in keeping iron homeostasis, which is present in highly active ionic forms (Fe^{3+}/Fe^{2+}) in the cellular environment and generate important amounts of ROS via Fenton chemistry with potential deleterious consequences for the neurons.[173] Iron (as Fe^{3+}) enters to the cells anchored to Tf via TfR1, endosome-processing and delivery to mitochondria as Fe^{2+} to be used for ISCs and HPGs, or stored in mitochondrial ferritin (FtMt, similar to cytosolic ferritin), which is highly expressed in

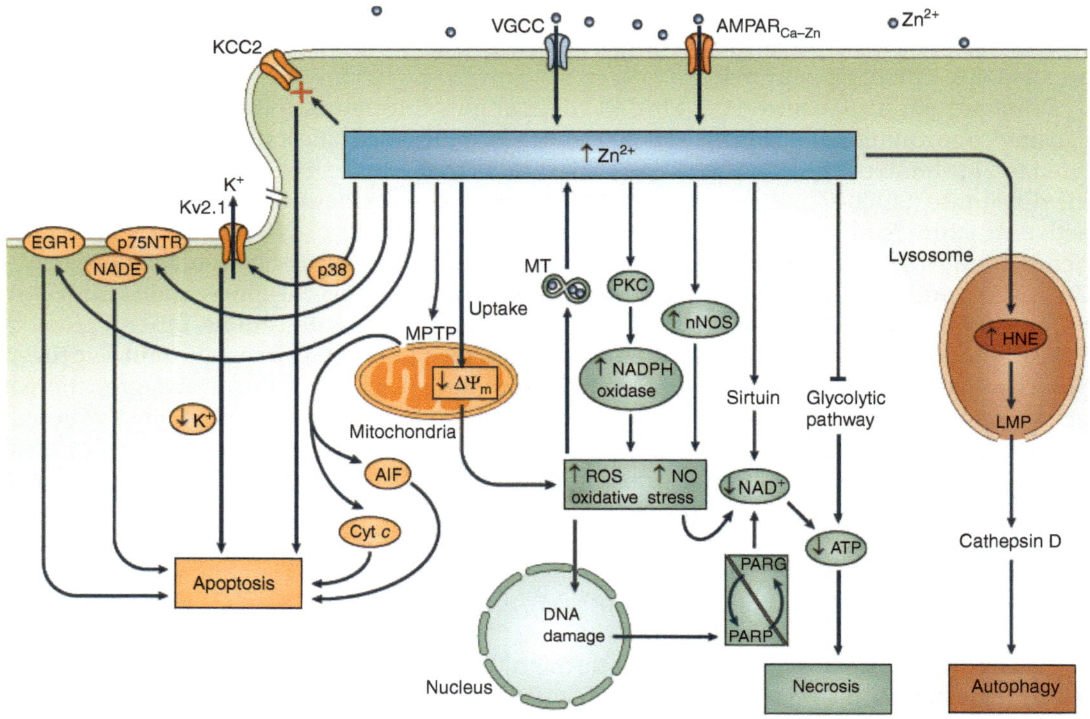

FIGURE 15.10 **Zinc dyshomeostasis impacts in neuronal death.** Illustration of neuronal death pathways activated by Zn^{2+}, leading to necrotic, apoptotic and autophagic neuronal death, ATP depletion, decreasing NAD^+ levels, mitochondrial depolarization, and generation of ROS. *Source: Reproduced with permission Sensi SL, Paoletti P, Bush AI, Sekler I. Zinc in the physiology and pathology of the CNS.* Nat Rev Neurosci. *2009;10(11):780–791.*[170] *Copyright 2015, Nature Publishing.*

neurons.[174] Mitochondrial iron homeostasis is altered in neurodegenerative pathologies. The question regarding whether iron dysregulation promotes neurodegeneration or occurs as a consequence of neurodegeneration is still unanswered. Due to the complex interconnections, it is probable that both situations occur simultaneously.

Free Fe^{2+}, non-Tf bound, has the capacity to directly permeate cells and reach mitochondria in a nonlabile form resulting eventually in oxidative stress and ensuing damage.[175] FtMt may be a neuroprotective, since ΔMtFt mice showed an overexpression of Aβ and neurotoxic effects, related to dysregulated iron, enhanced oxidative stress, and apoptosis, whereas overexpression of FtMt clearly inhibited Aβ, and reduced oxidative damage through Erk/p38 MAPK kinase (implicated in cell proliferation, stress, and survival).[176,177] Another pool of Fe^{2+} is delivered to mitochondria by endosomes containing Tf-Fe^{3+}, avoiding cytosolic oxygen.[178] SOD1 mutation caused overexpression of mitoferrin 1 and 2 (mitochondrial inner membrane iron transporters), ISCs and TfR1; with increased iron content in mitochondria in cell models of the neurodegenerative disorder amyotrophic lateral sclerosis.[179]

Aβ may exhibit a protective antioxidant function, since Aβ aggregates prevented protein and lipid oxidation, and formation of ROS by Fe^{2+} on rat brain mitochondria, whereas pure

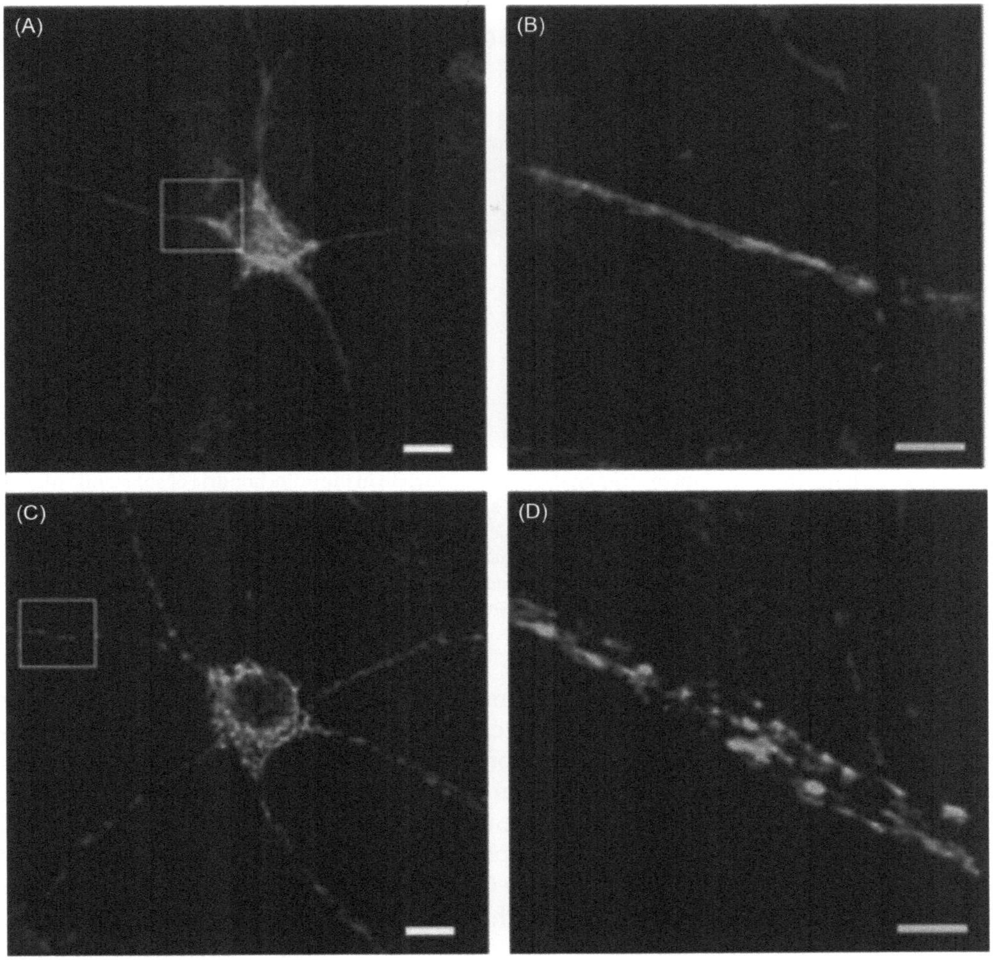

FIGURE 15.11 **Fragmentation of mitochondrial network caused by iron.** (A) Hsp-70 (green) to label mitochondrial network. (B) Detail of area in A. (C) Hsp-70 in a neuron cultured with 30 μM Fe-NTA for 24h. (D) Detail of area in C. Scale bar of 10 μm in (A) and (C). Scale bar of 5 μm in (B) and (D). *Source: Reproduced with permission Sanmartin CD, Paula-Lima AC, Garcia A, et al. Ryanodine receptor-mediated Ca(2+) release underlies iron-induced mitochondrial fission and stimulates mitochondrial Ca(2+) uptake in primary hippocampal neurons.* Front Mol Neurosci. *2014;7:13.*[182] *Copyright 2014, Frontiers Media.*

Aβ aggregates caused mitochondrial impairment with membrane depolarization and loss of phosphorylation activity, but not ROS.[180] In the same direction, Aβ aggregates promoted mitochondrial network disruption in hippocampal neurons by inhibition of ryanodine receptors (RyR) and Ca^{2+} release; similarly mitochondrial network fragmentation was broadly observed with iron treatments (30 μM for 24 h), related to redox-sensitive RyR-mediated Ca^{2+} release in primary rat hippocampal cultures[181,182] (Fig. 15.11).

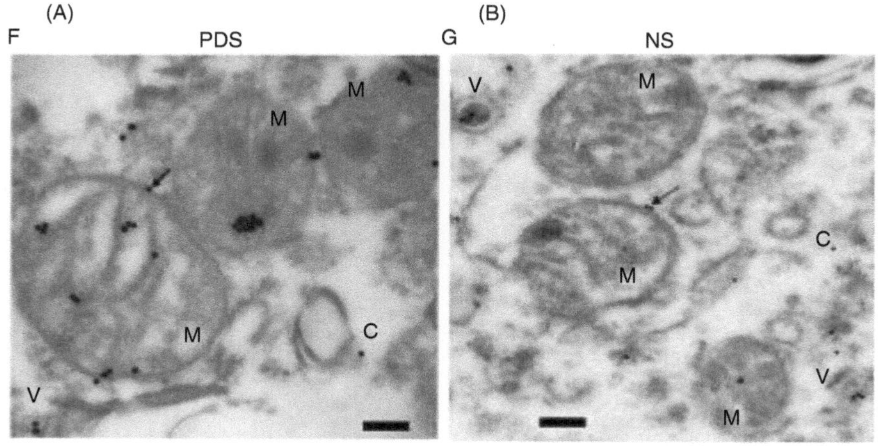

FIGURE 15.12 **Immunoelectron microscopy analysis of α-synuclein in the mitochondria of substantia nigra of PD.** Immuno-electron microscopy of mitochondria in Parkinson's disease (A) and normal (B). Secondary antibody conjugated to 10–20 nm gold particles. Labels: mitochondria *(M)*, vesicle *(V)*, cytosol *(C)*. Scale bar of 100 nm. *Source: Reproduced with permission Devi L, Raghavendran V, Prabhu BM, Avadhani NG, Anandatheerthavarada HK. Mitochondrial import and accumulation of alpha-synuclein impair complex I in human dopaminergic neuronal cultures and Parkinson disease brain.* J Biol Chem. *2008;283(14):9089–9100.*[183] *Copyright 2008, American Society for Biochemistry and Molecular Biology.*

Similarly, Parkinson's disease is accompanied by mitochondrial dysfunction, oxidative damage.[148] α-Syn aggregates in dopaminergic neurons were imported to mitochondria by the N-terminal domain that served as mitochondrial targeting domain. This accumulation of α-Syn oligomers with the inner mitochondrial membrane caused disrupted functionality of the mitochondrial Complex I of the electron transport chain, with increased free radical ROS production and eventual mitochondrial autophagy[37,183,184] (Fig. 15.12). As a cascade reaction of mitochondrial internalization of α-Syn, the Complex I inhibition disrupts normal activity of ISCs then inhibition of GRX2 causes glutathione depletion in dopaminergic neurons.[185,186] Overexpression of α-Syn caused mitochondria dysfunction with altered morphology, with increased O_2^- and favored phosphorylation of α-Syn. But in the presence of Fe^{2+}, the amount of ROS, O_2^-, α-Syn phosphorylation, and mitochondrial depolarization was enhanced, leading to overall functional degeneration in PD.[187] Mitochondrial damage and dysfunction was observed in PrP^C, with induced oxidative stress and neuronal damage.[188] Similarly to other neurodegenerative diseases, this resulted in ROS mediated damage, accumulation, alterations in respiratory chain, and apoptosis.

Copper also enters the mitochondria, but the exact mechanism is not understood. Cu constitutes an essential component of mitochondrial inner membrane complexes IV (CuA, CuB) and in distinct mitochondrial proteins: SCO1, SCO2, COX17, CCS, Zn-Cu SOD1, among others.[189] Under normal conditions, most of Cu is bound to proteins or glutathione; presence of high amounts of free copper will be related to cellular dysfunctions. Mutant Cu-Zn SOD1 develop mitochondrial dysfunctionalities related to neurodegenerative disorders, affecting upper and lower motor neurons.[190] SOD is one of the primary antioxidant defenses against ROS, its failure will result in oxidative stress. Mitochondrial functions in neurons are also closely modulated by intracellular zinc. Besides of Zn^{2+} pool at synaptic vesicles, neurons contain a distinct Zn^{2+} mitochondrial pool that is mobilized independently of each other. In neurons, under low levels of Zn^{2+}, membrane depolarization occurs, with increased O_2 consumption and decreased ROS, but at high Zn^{2+} levels, there is decreased O_2 consumption and increased amount of ROS.[191]

CONCLUSIONS

Neurogenegenerative diseases are complex and multifactorial. Even through the great efforts to elucidate their mechanisms at genetic, metabolic, protein, regulatory, signaling, immune, cellular, and age-related levels, the data suggest that neurodegeneration is multifaceted through combinatorial factors that trigger failure of neuronal functions and death.

Importantly, amyloid proteins are dynamic and intrinsically disordered with high affinity to bind different transition metal ions, and the key pathology hallmarks of Alzheimer's, Parkinson's, Prion, and other neurodegenerative disorders. Upon coordination of biometals (Fe^{2+}/Fe^{3+}, Cu^{2+}/Cu^{+}, Zn^{2+}, and others) the structure reorganizes, oligomerizes, fibrillizes, and maturates to form amyloid peptides of large deposits critical to the aging processes. Detailed information of interactions of biometals with specific available residues have revealed that oxidation, chemical modifications and posttranslational modifications of amino acid residues, including cross-linking may occur and producing ROS (H_2O_2 and OH^-) as by-products and metal ions promote their cellular trafficking. The combination of these factors causes mitochondrial dysfunctions, increased oxidative stress and cyto-toxic effects in neurons. It is necessary to continue the research to fully understand the relationship between dysregulation of key biometals in neurodegenerative disorders. Importantly, by incorporation of novel analytical techniques, including advanced imaging and sensitive biochemical and genetic tools, it will be possible to elucidate the molecular and neuronal mechanisms that converge in specific brain areas for early diagnostics and treatments of neurodegeneration.

Acknowledgments

This work was supported by Semmes Foundation and NIH Research Centers in Minority Institutions (RCMI) Program (5G12RR013646-12 and G12MD007591): NIH RCMI Nanotechnology and Human Health Core and NIH RCMI Biophotonics Core at UTSA.

References

1. Waldron KJ, Rutherford JC, Ford D, Robinson NJ. Metalloproteins and metal sensing. *Nature*. 2009;460(7257):823–830.
2. Mills E, Dong X-p, Wang F, Xu H. Mechanisms of brain iron transport: insight into neurodegeneration and CNS disorders. *Future Med Chem*. 2010;2(1):51–151.
3. Noinaj N, Easley NC, Oke M, et al. Structural basis for iron piracy by pathogenic Neisseria. *Nature*. 2012;483(7387):53–58.
4. Lawson DM, Artymiuk PJ, Yewdall SJ, et al. Solving the structure of human H ferritin by genetically engineering intermolecular crystal contacts. *Nature*. 1991;349(6309):541–544.
5. Strassnig M, Ganguli M. About a peculiar disease of the cerebral cortex: Alzheimer's original case revisited. *Psychiatry*. 2005;2(9):30–33.

6. Peters DG, Connor JR, Meadowcroft MD. The relationship between iron dyshomeostasis and amyloidogenesis in Alzheimer's disease: two sides of the same coin. *Neurobiol Dis*. 2015;81:49–65.
7. Goodman L. Alzheimer's disease: a clinico-pathologic analysis of twenty-three cases with a theory on pathogenesis. *J Nerv Ment Dis*. 1953;118(2):97–130.
8. Xiao Y, Ma B, McElheny D, et al. Abeta(1–42) fibril structure illuminates self-recognition and replication of amyloid in Alzheimer's disease. *Nat Struct Mol Biol*. 2015;22(6):499–505.
9. Zhang R, Hu X, Khant H, et al. Interprotofilament interactions between Alzheimer's Abeta1-42 peptides in amyloid fibrils revealed by cryoEM. *Proc Natl Acad Sci USA*. 2009;106(12):4653–4658.
10. Parthasarathy S, Long F, Miller Y, et al. Molecular-level examination of Cu2+ binding structure for amyloid fibrils of 40-residue Alzheimer's beta by solid-state NMR spectroscopy. *J Am Chem Soc*. 2011;133(10):3390–3400.
11. Pal A, Siotto M, Prasad R, Squitti R. Towards a unified vision of copper involvement in Alzheimer's disease: a review connecting basic, experimental, and clinical research. *J Alzheimers Dis*. 2015;44(2):343–354.
12. Roberts BR, Ryan TM, Bush AI, Masters CL, Duce JA. The role of metallobiology and amyloid-beta peptides in Alzheimer's disease. *J Neurochem*. 2012;120:149–166.
13. Duce JA, Tsatsanis A, Cater MA, et al. An iron-export ferroxidase activity of β-amyloid protein precursor is inhibited by zinc in Alzheimer's Disease. *Cell*. 2010;142(6):857–867.
14. Schmidt M, Rohou A, Lasker K, et al. Peptide dimer structure in an Abeta(1–42) fibril visualized with cryo-EM. *Proc Natl Acad Sci USA*. 2015;112(38):11858–11863.
15. Smith MA, Harris PL, Sayre LM, Perry G. Iron accumulation in Alzheimer disease is a source of redox-generated free radicals. *Proc Natl Acad Sci USA*. 1997;94(18):9866–9868.
16. Dong J, Atwood CS, Anderson VE, et al. Metal binding and oxidation of amyloid-beta within isolated senile plaque cores: Raman microscopic evidence. *Biochemistry*. 2003;42(10):2768–2773.
17. Pankhurst Q, Hautot D, Khan N, Dobson J. Increased levels of magnetic iron compounds in Alzheimer's disease. *J Alzheimers Dis*. 2008;13(1):49–52.
18. Collingwood JF, Telling ND. Iron oxides in the human brain. In: Faivre D, ed. *Iron Oxides: From Nature to Applications*. Weinheim, Germany: Wiley-VCH Verlag GmbH & Co. KGaA; 2016.
19. Hautot D, Pankhurst QA, Khan N, Dobson J. Preliminary evaluation of nanoscale biogenic magnetite in Alzheimer's disease brain tissue. *Proc Biol Sci*. 2003;270:S62–S64.
20. Teller S, Tahirbegi IB, Mir M, Samitier J, Soriano J. Magnetite-Amyloid-beta deteriorates activity and functional organization in an in vitro model for Alzheimer's disease. *Sci Rep*. 2015;5:17261.
21. Kirschvink JL, Kobayashi-Kirschvink A, Woodford BJ. Magnetite biomineralization in the human brain. *Proc Natl Acad Sci USA*. 1992;89(16):7683–7687.
22. Collingwood J, Dobson J. Mapping and characterization of iron compounds in Alzheimer's tissue. *J Alzheimers Dis*. 2006;10(2–3):215–222.
23. Collingwood JF, Mikhaylova A, Davidson M, et al. In situ characterization and mapping of iron compounds in Alzheimer's disease tissue. *J Alzheimers Dis*. 2005;7(4):267–272.
24. Antharam V, Collingwood JF, Bullivant J-P, et al. High field magnetic resonance microscopy of the human hippocampus in Alzheimer's disease: quantitative imaging and correlation with iron. *NeuroImage*. 2012;59(2):1249–1260.
25. Everett J, Cespedes E, Shelford LR, et al. Ferrous iron formation following the co-aggregation of ferric iron and the Alzheimer's disease peptide beta-amyloid (1-42). *J R Soc Interface*. 2014;11(95):20140165.
26. Everett J, Cespedes E, Shelford LR, et al. Evidence of redox-active iron formation following aggregation of ferrihydrite and the Alzheimer's disease peptide beta-amyloid. *Inorg Chem*. 2014;53(6):2803–2809.
27. Collingwood JF, Chong RK, Kasama T, et al. Three-dimensional tomographic imaging and characterization of iron compounds within Alzheimer's plaque core material. *J Alzheimers Dis*. 2008;14(2):235–245.
28. Drummond ES, Nayak S, Ueberheide B, Wisniewski T. Proteomic analysis of neurons microdissected from formalin-fixed, paraffin-embedded Alzheimer's disease brain tissue. *Sci Rep*. 2015;5:15456.
29. Liao L, Cheng D, Wang J, et al. Proteomic characterization of postmortem amyloid plaques isolated by laser capture microdissection. *J Biol Chem*. 2004;279(35):37061–37068.
30. Dahlgren KN, Manelli AM, Stine Jr WB, Baker LK, Krafft GA, LaDu MJ. Oligomeric and fibrillar species of amyloid-beta peptides differentially affect neuronal viability. *J Biol Chem*. 2002;277(35):32046–32053.
31. Hartley DM, Walsh DM, Ye CP, et al. Protofibrillar intermediates of amyloid beta-protein induce acute electrophysiological changes and progressive neurotoxicity in cortical neurons. *J Neurosci*. 1999;19(20):8876–8884.

32. Li X, Lei P, Tuo Q, et al. Enduring elevations of hippocampal amyloid precursor protein and iron are features of beta-amyloid toxicity and are mediated by tau. *Neurotherapeutics*. 2015;12(4):862–873.
33. Plascencia-Villa G, Ponce A, Collingwood JF, Arellano-Jiménez MJ, Zhu X, Rogers JT, Betancourt I, José-Yacamán M, Perry G. High-resolution analytical imaging and electron holography of magnetite particles in amyloid cores of Alzheimer's disease. *Sci Rep*. 2016;6:24873.
34. Jaunmuktane Z, Mead S, Ellis M, et al. Evidence for human transmission of amyloid-β pathology and cerebral amyloid angiopathy. *Nature*. 2015;525(7568):247–250.
35. Frontzek K, Lutz MI, Aguzzi A, Kovacs GG, Budka H. Amyloid-beta pathology and cerebral amyloid angiopathy are frequent in iatrogenic Creutzfeldt–Jakob disease after dural grafting. *Swiss Med Weekly*. 2016;146:w14287.
36. Shults CW. Lewy bodies. *Proc Natl Acad Sci USA*. 2006;103(6):1661–1668.
37. Singh N, Haldar S, Tripathi AK, McElwee MK, Horback K, Beserra A. Iron in neurodegenerative disorders of protein misfolding: a case of prion disorders and Parkinson's disease. *Antioxid Redox Signal*. 2014;21(3):471–484.
38. Dexter DT, Wells FR, Lees AJ, et al. Increased nigral iron content and alterations in other metal ions occurring in brain in Parkinson's disease. *J Neurochem*. 1989;52(6):1830–1836.
39. Dexter DT, Carayon A, Javoy-Agid F, et al. Alterations in the levels of iron, ferritin and other trace metals in Parkinson's disease and other neurodegenerative diseases affecting the basal ganglia. *Brain*. 1991;114(Pt 4):1953–1975.
40. Hirsch EC, Brandel JP, Galle P, Javoy-Agid F, Agid Y. Iron and aluminum increase in the substantia nigra of patients with Parkinson's disease: an X-ray microanalysis. *J Neurochem*. 1991;56(2):446–451.
41. Galvin JE, Giasson B, Hurtig HI, Lee VM, Trojanowski JQ. Neurodegeneration with brain iron accumulation, type 1 is characterized by alpha-, beta-, and gamma-synuclein neuropathology. *Am J Path*. 2000;157(2):361–368.
42. Arawaka S, Saito Y, Murayama S, Mori H. Lewy body in neurodegeneration with brain iron accumulation type 1 is immunoreactive for alpha-synuclein. *Neurology*. 1998;51(3):887–889.
43. Neumann M, Adler S, Schluter O, Kremmer E, Benecke R, Kretzschmar HA. Alpha-synuclein accumulation in a case of neurodegeneration with brain iron accumulation type 1 (NBIA-1, formerly Hallervorden-Spatz syndrome) with widespread cortical and brainstem-type Lewy bodies. *Acta Neuropath*. 2000;100(5):568–574.
44. Castellani RJ, Siedlak SL, Perry G, Smith MA. Sequestration of iron by Lewy bodies in Parkinson's disease. *Acta Neuropath*. 2000;100(2):111–114.
45. Riederer P, Sofic E, Rausch WD, et al. Transition metals, ferritin, glutathione, and ascorbic acid in parkinsonian brains. *J Neurochem*. 1989;52(2):515–520.
46. Binolfi A, Rasia RM, Bertoncini CW, et al. Interaction of alpha-synuclein with divalent metal ions reveals key differences: a link between structure, binding specificity and fibrillation enhancement. *J Am Chem Soc*. 2006;128(30):9893–9901.
47. Bharathi, Indi SS, Rao KS. Copper- and iron-induced differential fibril formation in alpha-synuclein: TEM study. *Neurosci Lett*. 2007;424(2):78–82.
48. Kostka M, Hogen T, Danzer KM, et al. Single particle characterization of iron-induced pore-forming alpha-synuclein oligomers. *J Biol Chem*. 2008;283(16):10992–11003.
49. Cole NB, Murphy DD, Lebowitz J, Di Noto L, Levine RL, Nussbaum RL. Metal-catalyzed oxidation of alpha-synuclein: helping to define the relationship between oligomers, protofibrils, and filaments. *J Biol Chem*. 2005;280(10):9678–9690.
50. He Q, Song N, Jia F, et al. Role of alpha-synuclein aggregation and the nuclear factor E2-related factor 2/heme oxygenase-1 pathway in iron-induced neurotoxicity. *Inter J Biochem Cell Biol*. 2013;45(6):1019–1030.
51. Jinsmaa Y, Sullivan P, Gross D, Cooney A, Sharabi Y, Goldstein DS. Divalent metal ions enhance DOPAL-induced oligomerization of alpha-synuclein. *Neurosci Lett*. 2014;569:27–32.
52. Singh A, Qing L, Kong Q, Singh N. Change in the characteristics of ferritin induces iron imbalance in prion disease affected brains. *Neurobiol Dis*. 2012;45(3):930–938.
53. Mishra RS, Basu S, Gu Y, et al. Protease-resistant human prion protein and ferritin are cotransported across Caco-2 epithelial cells: implications for species barrier in prion uptake from the intestine. *J Neurosci*. 2004;24(50):11280–11290.
54. Basu S, Mohan ML, Luo X, Kundu B, Kong Q, Singh N. Modulation of proteinase K-resistant prion protein in cells and infectious brain homogenate by redox iron: implications for prion replication and disease pathogenesis. *Mol Biol Cell*. 2007;18(9):3302–3312.
55. Fernaeus S, Land T. Increased iron-induced oxidative stress and toxicity in scrapie-infected neuroblastoma cells. *Neurosci Lett*. 2005;382(3):217–220.

56. Fernaeus S, Reis K, Bedecs K, Land T. Increased susceptibility to oxidative stress in scrapie-infected neuroblastoma cells is associated with intracellular iron status. *Neurosci Lett*. 2005;389(3):133–136.
57. Lee KS, Raymond LD, Schoen B, et al. Hemin interactions and alterations of the subcellular localization of prion protein. *J Biol Chem*. 2007;282(50):36525–36533.
58. Moore RA, Timmes A, Wilmarth PA, Priola SA. Comparative profiling of highly enriched 22L and Chandler mouse scrapie prion protein preparations. *Proteomics*. 2010;10(15):2858–2869.
59. Singh A, Isaac AO, Luo X, et al. Abnormal brain iron homeostasis in human and animal prion disorders. *PLoS Pathog*. 2009;5(3):e1000336.
60. Singh A, Haldar S, Horback K, et al. Prion protein regulates iron transport by functioning as a ferrireductase. *J Alzheimers Dis*. 2013;35(3):541–552.
61. Westergard L, Christensen HM, Harris DA. The cellular prion protein (PrP(C)): its physiological function and role in disease. *Biochim Biophys Acta*. 2007;1772(6):629–644.
62. Eskici G, Axelsen PH. Copper and oxidative stress in the pathogenesis of Alzheimer's disease. *Biochemistry*. 2012;51(32):6289–6311.
63. Telianidis J, Hung YH, Materia S, Fontaine SL. Role of the P-Type ATPases, ATP7A and ATP7B in brain copper homeostasis. *Front Aging Neurosci*. 2013;5:44.
64. Squitti R, Polimanti R. Copper hypothesis in the missing hereditability of sporadic Alzheimer's disease: ATP7B gene as potential harbor of rare variants. *J Alzheimers Dis*. 2012;29(3):493–501.
65. Castellani RJ, Smith MA, Nunomura A, Harris PLR, Perry G. Is increased redox-active iron in Alzheimer disease a failure of the copper-binding protein ceruloplasmin?. *Free Rad Biol Med*. 1999;26(11-12):1508–1512.
66. Park JH, Lee DW, Park KS. Elevated serum copper and ceruloplasmin levels in Alzheimer's disease. *Asia-Pac Psychiatry*. 2014;6(1):38–45.
67. Loeffler DA, LeWitt PA, Juneau PL, et al. Increased regional brain concentrations of ceruloplasmin in neurodegenerative disorders. *Brain Res*. 1996;738(2):265–274.
68. Kristinsson J, Snaedal J, Torsdottir G, Johannesson T. Ceruloplasmin and iron in Alzheimer's disease and Parkinson's disease: a synopsis of recent studies. *Neuropsychiatry Dis Treat*. 2012;8:515–521.
69. Jiang D, Zhang L, Grant GP, et al. The elevated copper binding strength of amyloid-beta aggregates allows the sequestration of copper from albumin: a pathway to accumulation of copper in senile plaques. *Biochemistry*. 2013;52(3):547–556.
70. Brewer GJ, Kanzer SH, Zimmerman EA, Celmins DF, Heckman SM, Dick R. Copper and ceruloplasmin abnormalities in Alzheimer's disease. *Am J Alzheimers Dis Other Demen*. 2010;25(6):490–497.
71. Pajonk FG, Kessler H, Supprian T, et al. Cognitive decline correlates with low plasma concentrations of copper in patients with mild to moderate Alzheimer's disease. *J Alzheimers Dis*. 2005;8(1):23–27.
72. Kessler H, Pajonk FG, Meisser P, et al. Cerebrospinal fluid diagnostic markers correlate with lower plasma copper and ceruloplasmin in patients with Alzheimer's disease. *J Neural Transm*. 2006;113(11):1763–1769.
73. Molina JA, Jimenez-Jimenez FJ, Aguilar MV, et al. Cerebrospinal fluid levels of transition metals in patients with Alzheimer's disease. *J Neural Transm*. 1998;105(4-5):479–488.
74. Baum L, Chan IH, Cheung SK, et al. Serum zinc is decreased in Alzheimer's disease and serum arsenic correlates positively with cognitive ability. *Biometals*. 2010;23(1):173–179.
75. Mueller C, Schrag M, Crofton A, et al. Altered serum iron and copper homeostasis predicts cognitive decline in mild cognitive impairment. *J Alzheimers Dis*. 2012;29(2):341–350.
76. Squitti R, Lupoi D, Pasqualetti P, et al. Elevation of serum copper levels in Alzheimer's disease. *Neurology*. 2002;59(8):1153–1161.
77. Squitti R, Pasqualetti P, Dal Forno G, et al. Excess of serum copper not related to ceruloplasmin in Alzheimer disease. *Neurology*. 2005;64(6):1040–1046.
78. Squitti R, Ventriglia M, Barbati G, et al. 'Free' copper in serum of Alzheimer's disease patients correlates with markers of liver function. *J Neural Transm*. 2007;114(12):1589–1594.
79. Acevedo KM, Hung YH, Dalziel AH, et al. Copper promotes the trafficking of the amyloid precursor protein. *J Biol Chem*. 2011;286(10):8252–8262.
80. Wang H, Wang M, Wang B, et al. The distribution profile and oxidation states of biometals in APP transgenic mouse brain: dyshomeostasis with age and as a function of the development of Alzheimer's disease. *Metallomics*. 2012;4(3):289–296.
81. Lovell MA, Robertson JD, Teesdale WJ, Campbell JL, Markesbery WR. Copper, iron and zinc in Alzheimer's disease senile plaques. *J Neurol Sci*. 1998;158(1):47–52.

82. Miller LM, Wang Q, Telivala TP, Smith RJ, Lanzirotti A, Miklossy J. Synchrotron-based infrared and X-ray imaging shows focalized accumulation of Cu and Zn co-localized with beta-amyloid deposits in Alzheimer's disease. *J Struct Biol*. 2006;155(1):30–37.
83. Rajendran R, Minqin R, Ynsa MD, et al. A novel approach to the identification and quantitative elemental analysis of amyloid deposits—Insights into the pathology of Alzheimer's disease. *Biochem Biophys Res Commun*. 2009;382(1):91–95.
84. Reinhard C, Hebert SS, De Strooper B. The amyloid-beta precursor protein: integrating structure with biological function. *EMBO J*. 2005;24(23):3996–4006.
85. Kong GK, Adams JJ, Harris HH, et al. Structural studies of the Alzheimer's amyloid precursor protein copper-binding domain reveal how it binds copper ions. *J Mol Biol*. 2007;367(1):148–161.
86. Dahms SO, Konnig I, Roeser D, et al. Metal binding dictates conformation and function of the amyloid precursor protein (APP) E2 domain. *J Mol Biol*. 2012;416(3):438–452.
87. Dawkins E, Small DH. Insights into the physiological function of the beta-amyloid precursor protein: beyond Alzheimer's disease. *J Neurochem*. 2014;129(5):756–769.
88. Shin BK, Saxena S. Direct evidence that all three histidine residues coordinate to Cu(II) in amyloid-beta1-16. *Biochemistry*. 2008;47(35):9117–9123.
89. Jun S, Gillespie JR, Shin BK, Saxena S. The second Cu(II)-binding site in a proton-rich environment interferes with the aggregation of amyloid-beta(1-40) into amyloid fibrils. *Biochemistry*. 2009;48(45):10724–10732.
90. Shin BK, Saxena S. Substantial contribution of the two imidazole rings of the His13-His14 dyad to Cu(II) binding in amyloid-beta(1-16) at physiological pH and its significance. *J Phys Chem*. 2011;115(34):9590–9602.
91. Shearer J, Szalai VA. The amyloid-beta peptide of Alzheimer's disease binds Cu(I) in a linear bis-his coordination environment: insight into a possible neuroprotective mechanism for the amyloid-beta peptide. *J Am Chem Soc*. 2008;130(52):17826–17835.
92. Zou K, Gong JS, Yanagisawa K, Michikawa M. A novel function of monomeric amyloid beta-protein serving as an antioxidant molecule against metal-induced oxidative damage. *J Neurosci*. 2002;22(12):4833–4841.
93. Prosdocimi T, De Gioia L, Zampella G, Bertini L. On the generation of OH radical species from HO by Cu(I) amyloid beta peptide model complexes: a DFT investigation. *J Biol Inorg Chem*. 2015;21(2):197–212.
94. Reybier K, Ayala S, Alies B, et al. Free superoxide is an intermediate in the production of H2O2 by copper(I)-abeta peptide and O2. *Angew Chem Int Ed Engl*. 2016;55(3):1085–1089.
95. Ginotra YP, Ramteke SN, Walke GR, Rapole S, Kulkarni PP. Histidine availability is decisive in ROS-mediated cytotoxicity of copper complexes of Abeta1-16 peptide. *Free Radic Res*. 2016;:1–9.
96. Barritt JD, Viles JH. Truncated amyloid-beta(11-40/42) from Alzheimer disease binds Cu^{2+} with a femtomolar affinity and influences fiber assembly. *J Biol Chem*. 2015;290(46):27791–27802.
97. Williams TL, Serpell LC, Urbanc B. Stabilization of native amyloid beta-protein oligomers by copper and hydrogen peroxide induced cross-linking of unmodified proteins (CHICUP). *Biochim Biophys Acta*. 2016;1864(3):249–259.
98. Hane FT, Hayes R, Lee BY, Leonenko Z. Effect of copper and zinc on the single molecule self-affinity of Alzheimer's amyloid-beta peptides. *PloS one*. 2016;11(1):e0147488.
99. Ma QF, Li YM, Du JT, et al. Binding of copper (II) ion to an Alzheimer's tau peptide as revealed by MALDI-TOF MS, CD, and NMR. *Biopolymers*. 2005;79(2):74–85.
100. Ma Q, Li Y, Du J, et al. Copper binding properties of a tau peptide associated with Alzheimer's disease studied by CD, NMR, and MALDI-TOF MS. *Peptides*. 2006;27(4):841–849.
101. Soragni A, Zambelli B, Mukrasch MD, et al. Structural characterization of binding of Cu(II) to tau protein. *Biochemistry*. 2008;47(41):10841–10851.
102. Shin BK, Saxena S. Insight into potential Cu(II)-binding motifs in the four pseudorepeats of tau protein. *J Phys Chem*. 2011;115(50):15067–15078.
103. Zhou L-X, Du J-T, Zeng Z-Y, et al. Copper (II) modulates in vitro aggregation of a tau peptide. *Peptides*. 2007;28(11):2229–2234.
104. Su XY, Wu WH, Huang ZP, et al. Hydrogen peroxide can be generated by tau in the presence of Cu(II). *Biochem Biophys Res Commun*. 2007;358(2):661–665.
105. Larner F, Sampson B, Rehkamper M, et al. High precision isotope measurements reveal poor control of copper metabolism in Parkinsonism. *Metallomics*. 2013;5(2):125–132.
106. Pall HS, Blake DR, Gutteridge JM, et al. Raised cerebrospinal-fluid copper concentration in parkinson's disease. *Lancet*. 1987;330(8553):238–241.

107. Boll MC, Alcaraz-Zubeldia M, Montes S, Rios C. Free copper, ferroxidase and SOD1 activities, lipid peroxidation and NO(x) content in the CSF. A different marker profile in four neurodegenerative diseases. *Neurochem Res*. 2008;33(9):1717–1723.
108. Jimenez-Jimenez FJ, Molina JA, Aguilar MV, et al. Cerebrospinal fluid levels of transition metals in patients with Parkinson's disease. *J Neural Transm*. 1998;105(4-5):497–505.
109. Qureshi GA, Qureshi AA, Memon SA, Parvez SH. Impact of selenium, iron, copper and zinc in on/off Parkinson's patients on L-dopa therapy. *J Neural Transm Suppl*. 2006;(71):229–236.
110. Davies KM, Hare DJ, Cottam V, et al. Localization of copper and copper transporters in the human brain. *Metallomics*. 2013;5(1):43–51.
111. Choi BS, Zheng W. Copper transport to the brain by the blood-brain barrier and blood-CSF barrier. *Brain Res*. 2009;1248:14–21.
112. Ayton S, Lei P, Duce JA, et al. Ceruloplasmin dysfunction and therapeutic potential for Parkinson disease. *Ann Neurol*. 2013;73(4):554–559.
113. Davies KM, Bohic S, Carmona A, et al. Copper pathology in vulnerable brain regions in Parkinson's disease. *Neurobiol Aging*. 2014;35(4):858–866.
114. Wang X, Moualla D, Wright JA, Brown DR. Copper binding regulates intracellular alpha-synuclein localisation, aggregation and toxicity. *J Neurochem*. 2010;113(3):704–714.
115. Miotto MC, Rodriguez EE, Valiente-Gabioud AA, et al. Site-specific copper-catalyzed oxidation of alpha-synuclein: tightening the link between metal binding and protein oxidative damage in Parkinson's disease. *Inorg Chem*. 2014;53(9):4350–4358.
116. Miotto MC, Binolfi A, Zweckstetter M, Griesinger C, Fernandez CO. Bioinorganic chemistry of synucleinopathies: deciphering the binding features of Met motifs and His-50 in AS-Cu(I) interactions. *J Inorg Biochem*. 2014;141:208–211.
117. De Ricco R, Valensin D, Dell'Acqua S, et al. Remote His50 Acts as a coordination switch in the high-affinity N-terminal centered copper(II) site of alpha-synuclein. *Inorg Chem*. 2015;54(10):4744–4751.
118. Miotto MC, Valiente-Gabioud AA, Rossetti G, et al. Copper binding to the N-terminally acetylated, naturally occurring form of alpha-synuclein induces local helical folding. *J Am Chem Soc*. 2015;137(20):6444–6447.
119. De Ricco R, Valensin D, Dell'Acqua S, Casella L, Hureau C, Faller P. Copper(I/II), alpha/beta-synuclein and amyloid-beta: menage a trois?. *Chembiochem*. 2015;16(16):2319–2328.
120. Paik SR, Shin HJ, Lee JH. Metal-catalyzed oxidation of alpha-synuclein in the presence of Copper(II) and hydrogen peroxide. *Arch Biochem Biophys*. 2000;378(2):269–277.
121. Cole NB, Murphy DD, Lebowitz J, Di Noto L, Levine RL, Nussbaum RL. Metal-catalyzed Oxidation of α-Synuclein: helping to define the relationship between oligomers, protofibrils, and filaments. *J Biol Chem*. 2005;280(10):9678–9690.
122. Uversky VN, Li J, Fink AL. Metal-triggered Structural transformations, aggregation, and fibrillation of human α-synuclein: a possible molecular link between Parkinson's disease and heavy metal exposure. *J Biol Chem*. 2001;276(47):44284–44296.
123. Rodriguez JA, Ivanova MI, Sawaya MR, et al. Structure of the toxic core of alpha-synuclein from invisible crystals. *Nature*. 2015;525(7570):486–490.
124. Pauly PC, Harris DA. Copper stimulates endocytosis of the prion protein. *J Biol Chem*. 1998;273(50):33107–33110.
125. Toni M, Massimino ML, Griffoni C, Salvato B, Tomasi V, Spisni E. Extracellular copper ions regulate cellular prion protein (PrPC) expression and metabolism in neuronal cells. *FEBS Lett*. 2005;579(3):741–744.
126. Perera WSS, Hooper NM. Ablation of the metal ion-induced endocytosis of the prion protein by disease-associated mutation of the octarepeat region. *Curr Biol*. 2001;11(7):519–523.
127. Brown DR, Qin K, Herms JW, et al. The cellular prion protein binds copper in vivo. *Nature*. 1997;390(6661):684–687.
128. Stys PK, You H, Zamponi GW. Copper-dependent regulation of NMDA receptors by cellular prion protein: implications for neurodegenerative disorders. *J Physiol*. 2012;590(Pt 6):1357–1368.
129. Jobling MF, Huang X, Stewart LR, et al. Copper and zinc binding modulates the aggregation and neurotoxic properties of the prion peptide PrP106-126. *Biochemistry*. 2001;40(27):8073–8084.
130. Redecke L, von Bergen M, Clos J, et al. Structural characterization of beta-sheeted oligomers formed on the pathway of oxidative prion protein aggregation in vitro. *J Struct Biol*. 2007;157(2):308–320.
131. Arnesano F, Scintilla S, Calo V, et al. Copper-triggered aggregation of ubiquitin. *PloS one*. 2009;4(9):e7052.
132. Prakash A, Bharti K, Majeed ABA. Zinc: indications in brain disorders. *Fundam Clin Pharmacol*. 2015;29(2):131–149.

133. Szewczyk B. Zinc homeostasis and neurodegenerative disorders. *Front Aging Neurosci.* 2013;5:33.
134. Burnet FM. A possible role of zinc in the pathology of dementia. *Lancet.* 1981;1(8213):186–188.
135. Vural H, Demirin H, Kara Y, Eren I, Delibas N. Alterations of plasma magnesium, copper, zinc, iron and selenium concentrations and some related erythrocyte antioxidant enzyme activities in patients with Alzheimer's disease. *J Trace Ekem Med Biol.* 2010;24(3):169–173.
136. Plantin LO, Lying-Tunell U, Kristensson K. Trace elements in the human central nervous system studied with neutron activation analysis. *Biol Trace Elem Res.* 1987;13(1):69–75.
137. Ward NI, Mason JA. Neutron activation analysis techniques for identifying elemental status in Alzheimer's disease. *J Radioanalyt Nuc Chem.* 1987;113(2):515–526.
138. Corrigan FM, Reynolds GP, Ward NI. Hippocampal tin, aluminum and zinc in Alzheimer's disease. *Biometals.* 1993;6(3):149–154.
139. Deibel MA, Ehmann WD, Markesbery WR. Copper, iron, and zinc imbalances in severely degenerated brain regions in Alzheimer's disease: possible relation to oxidative stress. *J Neurol Sci.* 1996;143(1-2):137–142.
140. Religa D, Strozyk D, Cherny RA, et al. Elevated cortical zinc in Alzheimer disease. *Neurology.* 2006;67(1):69–75.
141. Suh SW, Jensen KB, Jensen MS, et al. Histochemically-reactive zinc in amyloid plaques, angiopathy, and degenerating neurons of Alzheimer's diseased brains. *Brain Res.* 2000;852(2):274–278.
142. Zhang LH, Wang X, Stoltenberg M, Danscher G, Huang L, Wang ZY. Abundant expression of zinc transporters in the amyloid plaques of Alzheimer's disease brain. *Brain Res Bull.* 2008;77(1):55–60.
143. Lee JY, Cole TB, Palmiter RD, Suh SW, Koh JY. Contribution by synaptic zinc to the gender-disparate plaque formation in human Swedish mutant APP transgenic mice. *Proc Natl Acad Sci USA.* 2002;99(11):7705–7710.
144. Sensi SL, Rapposelli IG, Frazzini V, Mascetra N. Altered oxidant-mediated intraneuronal zinc mobilization in a triple transgenic mouse model of Alzheimer's disease. *Exp Gerontol.* 2008;43(5):488–492.
145. Bush AI, Pettingell WH, Multhaup G, et al. Rapid induction of Alzheimer A beta amyloid formation by zinc. *Science.* 1994;265(5177):1464–1467.
146. Bush AI, Pettingell Jr WH, Paradis MD, Tanzi RE. Modulation of A beta adhesiveness and secretase site cleavage by zinc. *J Biol Chem.* 1994;269(16):12152–12158.
147. Faller P, Hureau C, Berthoumieu O. Role of metal ions in the self-assembly of the Alzheimer's amyloid-beta peptide. *Inorg Chem.* 2013;52(21):12193–12206.
148. Tõugu V, Palumaa P. Coordination of zinc ions to the key proteins of neurodegenerative diseases: Aβ, APP, α-synuclein and PrP. *Coord Chem Rev.* 2012;256(19-20):2219–2224.
149. Alies B, Hureau C, Faller P. The role of metal ions in amyloid formation: general principles from model peptides. *Metallomics.* 2013;5(3):183–192.
150. Hoernke M, Falenski JA, Schwieger C, Koksch B, Brezesinski G. Triggers for β-sheet formation at the hydrophobic–hydrophilic interface: high concentration, in-plane orientational order, and metal ion complexation. *Langmuir.* 2011;27(23):14218–14231.
151. Uversky VN, Li J, Fink AL. Metal-triggered structural transformations, aggregation, and fibrillation of human alpha-synuclein. A possible molecular NK between Parkinson's disease and heavy metal exposure. *J Biol Chem.* 2001;276(47):44284–44296.
152. Lowe R, Pountney DL, Jensen PH, Gai WP, Voelcker NH. Calcium(II) selectively induces alpha-synuclein annular oligomers via interaction with the C-terminal domain. *Prot Sci.* 2004;13(12):3245–3252.
153. Valiente-Gabioud AA, Torres-Monserrat V, Molina-Rubino L, Binolfi A, Griesinger C, Fernandez CO. Structural basis behind the interaction of Zn(2)(+) with the protein alpha-synuclein and the Abeta peptide: a comparative analysis. *J Inorg Biochem.* 2012;117:334–341.
154. Santner A, Uversky VN. Metalloproteomics and metal toxicology of α-synuclein. *Metallomics.* 2010;2(6):378–392.
155. Hokenson MJ, Uversky VN, Goers J, Yamin G, Munishkina LA, Fink AL. Role of individual methionines in the fibrillation of methionine-oxidized alpha-synuclein. *Biochemistry.* 2004;43(15):4621–4633.
156. Yamin G, Glaser CB, Uversky VN, Fink AL. Certain metals trigger fibrillation of methionine-oxidized α-synuclein. *J Biol Chem.* 2003;278(30):27630–27635.
157. Meloni G, Vašák M. Redox activity of α-synuclein–Cu is silenced by Zn7-metallothionein-3. *Free Radic Biol Med.* 2011;50(11):1471–1479.
158. Thomas MP, Chartrand K, Reynolds A, Vitvitsky V, Banerjee R, Gendelman HE. Ion channel blockade attenuates aggregated alpha synuclein induction of microglial reactive oxygen species: relevance for the pathogenesis of Parkinson's disease. *J Neurochem.* 2007;100(2):503–519.

159. Kong SM, Chan BK, Park JS, et al. Parkinson's disease-linked human PARK9/ATP13A2 maintains zinc homeostasis and promotes alpha-Synuclein externalization via exosomes. *Hum Mol Genet*. 2014;23(11):2816–2833.
160. Watt NT, Hooper NM. The prion protein and neuronal zinc homeostasis. *Trends Biochem Sci*. 2003;28(8):406–410.
161. Brown DR, Wong B-S, Hafiz F, Clive C, Haswell SJ, Jones IM. Normal prion protein has an activity like that of superoxide dismutase. *Biochem J*. 1999;344(1):1–5.
162. Klamt F, Dal-Pizzol F, Conte da Frota Jr ML, et al. Imbalance of antioxidant defense in mice lacking cellular prion protein. *Free Radic Biol Med*. 2001;30(10):1137–1144.
163. Choi CJ, Kanthasamy A, Anantharam V, Kanthasamy AG. Interaction of metals with prion protein: possible role of divalent cations in the pathogenesis of prion diseases. *Neurotoxicology*. 2006;27(5):777–787.
164. Brown LR, Harris DA. Copper and zinc cause delivery of the prion protein from the plasma membrane to a subset of early endosomes and the Golgi. *J Neurochem*. 2003;87(2):353–363.
165. Pandey KK, Snyder JP, Liotta DC, Musaev DG. Computational studies of transition metal selectivity of octapeptide repeat region of prion protein (PrP). *J Phys Chem*. 2010;114(2):1127–1135.
166. Chattopadhyay M, Walter ED, Newell DJ, et al. The octarepeat domain of the prion protein binds Cu(II) with three distinct coordination modes at pH 7.4. *J Am Chem Soc*. 2005;127(36):12647–12656.
167. Kenward AG, Bartolotti LJ, Burns CS. Copper and zinc promote interactions between membrane-anchored peptides of the metal binding domain of the prion protein. *Biochemistry*. 2007;46(14):4261–4271.
168. Pan K, Yi CW, Chen J, Liang Y. Zinc significantly changes the aggregation pathway and the conformation of aggregates of human prion protein. *Biochim Biophys Acta*. 2015;1854(8):907–918.
169. Jackson GS, Murray I, Hosszu LLP, et al. Location and properties of metal-binding sites on the human prion protein. *Proc Natl Acad Sci USA*. 2001;98(15):8531–8535.
170. Sensi SL, Paoletti P, Bush AI, Sekler I. Zinc in the physiology and pathology of the CNS. *Nat Rev Neurosci*. 2009;10(11):780–791.
171. Liddell JR. Targeting mitochondrial metal dyshomeostasis for the treatment of neurodegeneration. *Neurodegener Dis Manag*. 2015;5(4):345–364.
172. Mena NP, Urrutia PJ, Lourido F, Carrasco CM, Núñez MT. Mitochondrial iron homeostasis and its dysfunctions in neurodegenerative disorders. *Mitochondrion*. 2015;21:92–105.
173. Horowitz MP, Greenamyre JT. Mitochondrial iron metabolism and its role in neurodegeneration. *J Alzheimers Dis*. 2010;20(suppl 2):S551–568.
174. Santambrogio P, Biasiotto G, Sanvito F, Olivieri S, Arosio P, Levi S. Mitochondrial ferritin expression in adult mouse tissues. *J Histochem Cytochem*. 2007;55(11):1129–1137.
175. Shvartsman M, Kikkeri R, Shanzer A, Cabantchik ZI. Non-transferrin-bound iron reaches mitochondria by a chelator-inaccessible mechanism: biological and clinical implications. *Am J Physiolo Cell Physiol*. 2007;293(4):C1383–1394.
176. Wu WS, Zhao YS, Shi ZH, et al. Mitochondrial ferritin attenuates beta-amyloid-induced neurotoxicity: reduction in oxidative damage through the Erk/P38 mitogen-activated protein kinase pathways. *Antioxid Redox Signal*. 2013;18(2):158–169.
177. Gao G, Chang YZ. Mitochondrial ferritin in the regulation of brain iron homeostasis and neurodegenerative diseases. *Front Pharm*. 2014;5:19.
178. Sheftel AD, Zhang AS, Brown C, Shirihai OS, Ponka P. Direct interorganellar transfer of iron from endosome to mitochondrion. *Blood*. 2007;110(1):125–132.
179. Hadzhieva M, Kirches E, Wilisch-Neumann A, et al. Dysregulation of iron protein expression in the G93A model of amyotrophic lateral sclerosis. *Neuroscience*. 2013;230:94–101.
180. Sinha M, Bhowmick P, Banerjee A, Chakrabarti S. Antioxidant role of amyloid β protein in cell-free and biological systems: implication for the pathogenesis of Alzheimer disease. *Free Rad Biol Med*. 2013;56:184–192.
181. Paula-Lima AC, Adasme T, SanMartin C, et al. Amyloid beta-peptide oligomers stimulate RyR-mediated Ca2+ release inducing mitochondrial fragmentation in hippocampal neurons and prevent RyR-mediated dendritic spine remodeling produced by BDNF. *Antioxid Redox Signal*. 2011;14(7):1209–1223.
182. Sanmartin CD, Paula-Lima AC, Garcia A, et al. Ryanodine receptor-mediated Ca(2+) release underlies iron-induced mitochondrial fission and stimulates mitochondrial Ca(2+) uptake in primary hippocampal neurons. *Front Mol Neurosci*. 2014;7:13.
183. Devi L, Raghavendran V, Prabhu BM, Avadhani NG, Anandatheerthavarada HK. Mitochondrial import and accumulation of alpha-synuclein impair complex I in human dopaminergic neuronal cultures and Parkinson disease brain. *J Biol Chem*. 2008;283(14):9089–9100.

184. Chinta SJ, Mallajosyula JK, Rane A, Andersen JK. Mitochondrial alpha-synuclein accumulation impairs complex I function in dopaminergic neurons and results in increased mitophagy in vivo. *Neurosci Lett.* 2010;486(3):235–239.
185. Lee DW, Kaur D, Chinta SJ, Rajagopalan S, Andersen JK. A disruption in iron-sulfur center biogenesis via inhibition of mitochondrial dithiol glutaredoxin 2 may contribute to mitochondrial and cellular iron dysregulation in mammalian glutathione-depleted dopaminergic cells: implications for Parkinson's disease. *Antioxid Redox Signal.* 2009;11(9):2083–2094.
186. Mena NP, Bulteau AL, Salazar J, Hirsch EC, Nunez MT. Effect of mitochondrial complex I inhibition on Fe-S cluster protein activity. *Biochem Biophys Res Commun.* 2011;409(2):241–246.
187. Perfeito R, Lazaro DF, Outeiro TF, Rego AC. Linking alpha-synuclein phosphorylation to reactive oxygen species formation and mitochondrial dysfunction in SH-SY5Y cells. *Mol Cell Neurosci.* 2014;62:51–59.
188. Yuan F, Yang L, Zhang Z, et al. Cellular prion protein (PrPC) of the neuron cell transformed to a PK-resistant protein under oxidative stress, comprising main mitochondrial damage in prion diseases. *J Mol Neurosci.* 2013;51(1):219–224.
189. Xu W, Barrientos T, Andrews Nancy C. Iron and copper in mitochondrial diseases. *Cell Metab.* 2013;17(3):319–328.
190. Faes L, Callewaert G. Mitochondrial dysfunction in familial amyotrophic lateral sclerosis. *J Bioenerg Biomembr.* 2011;43(6):587–592.
191. Sensi SL, Ton-That D, Sullivan PG, et al. Modulation of mitochondrial function by endogenous Zn^{2+} pools. *Proc Natl Acad Sci USA.* 2003;100(10):6157–6162.

CHAPTER

16

Metal Transporters in Neurodegeneration

Hong Jiang[*,**]

[*]Medical College of Qingdao University, Qingdao, China

[**]Shandong Provincial Collaborative Innovation Center for Neurodegenerative Disorders, Qingdao University, Qingdao, China

OUTLINE

Biometals in Neurodegenerative Diseases. http://dx.doi.org/10.1016/B978-0-12-804562-6.00016-6

Metal transporters, including transporters for iron, zinc, copper, etc., play a key role in the pathogenesis of neurodegenerative diseases.[1–5] Elevated iron and zinc levels and decreased copper levels were found in the substantia nigra (SN) in patients with Parkinson's disease (PD),[6–11] suggesting the role of iron, zinc, and copper in PD.[12] Recent studies have also shown that iron accumulates in the hippocampus and cerebral cortex,[13–17] and higher zinc and copper levels are present in mature amyloid plaques in patients with Alzheimer's disease (AD).[18–20] Furthermore, an increased deposition of iron level is detectable in the basal ganglia of patients with early-stage of Huntington's disease (HD).[21] Besides these, the alterations of other biometals including manganese, magnesium and aluminum as well as their corresponding transporters in various brain regions are involved in the pathological process of neurodegeneration.[22–24] For instance, manganese accumulation in globus pallidus, striatum, and SN,[25,26] decreased magnesium in the hippocampus, cerebrospinal fluid, but not serum,[27,28] and increased aluminum in the gray matter of brain[29,30] that have been linked to the neurotoxicity in PD, the cognitive impairments in AD, and neurological dysfunctions in other diseases. In this chapter, we summarize the metal transporters, their function and role in different neurodegenerative diseases.

IRON TRANSPORTERS AND NEURODEGENERATION

There are two kinds of iron transporters, one is responsible for its import and another for its export. Iron importers include transferrin (Tf)-transferrin receptor (TfR), divalent metal transporter 1 (DMT1), lactoferrin (Lf)-lactoferrin receptor (LfR), melanotransferrin (MTf), etc.[31–33] However, up to now, the only known iron exporter is ferroportin (Fpn)[34–36] (Fig. 16.1). Here, we summarize these iron transporters and their relevance to neurodegeneration.

Tf-TfR

The major pathway for cellular iron uptake in the brain is the Tf-TfR pathway. There are two types of TfRs, namely TfR1 and TfR2. The Tf-TfR1 complexes are internalized into the cell and form an intracellular endosome via receptor-mediated endocytosis. When pH value decreases, Tf binds iron that is released and transported across the endosomal membrane by DMT1.[37,38] TfR1 is expressed throughout the brain and especially on neurons, suggesting that iron could be transported through the classic Tf-TfR1 pathway.[39] There are five iron responsive elements (IRE) in the 5′-untranslated region of its mRNA, therefore, it can be regulated by intracellular iron levels through iron response proteins (IRP).[40] Through binding to IREs,

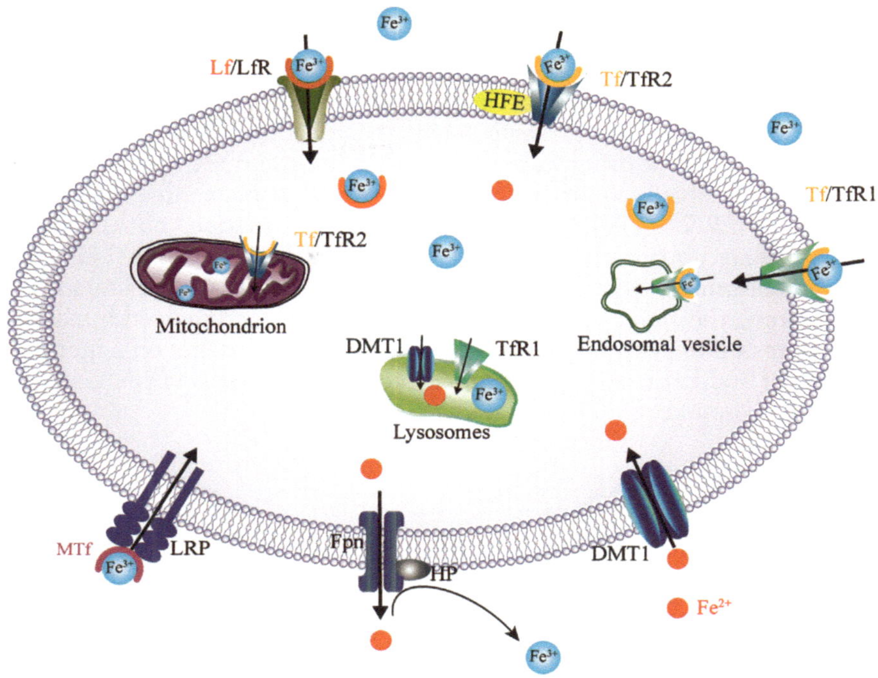

FIGURE 16.1 **Model of neuronal iron transport.** Iron is transported into the cell mainly by Tf-TfR1, DMT1, Lf-LfR, and MTf. Tf-TfR2 is also involved in the iron uptake in the presence of HFE. TfR2 is principally expressed within the mitochondria in the nigral dopaminergic neurons and mediates iron sequestration into mitochondria. The only way for iron transported out of the cell is by Fpn with the help of HP. *DMT1*, divalent metal transporter 1; *Fpn*, ferroportin; *HFE*, hemochromatosis protein; *HP* hephaestin; *Lf-LfR*, lactoferrin-lactoferrin receptor, *MTf*, melanotransferrin; *Tf-TfR*, transferrin-transferrin receptor. Schematic drawings are modified from previous study.[87]

IRPs are able to posttranscriptionally regulate the TfR1 mRNAs. IRPs are capable of maintaining cellular iron homeostasis by coordinating mRNA-encoding proteins, which are the critical components of a sensory and regulatory system. There are two distinct forms of IRPs, IRP1 and IRP2, in mammalian cells. IRP2 is the chief iron sensor and dominates posttranscriptional regulation of iron metabolism in the central nervous system (CNS). IRP1 is a bifunctional protein with the IRE binding activity and the enzymatic activity as cytosolic isoform of aconitase (c-acon). Unlike IRP1, IRP2 lacks enzyme activity and is without Fe-S clusters.

TfR2, is a homologue of TfR1 and shares about 45% homology with TfR1, identified in 1999.[41,42] Unlike TfR1, TfR2 mRNA does not contain the IRE, therefore it cannot be regulated by intracellular iron levels.[40] TfR2 is expressed mainly within the mitochondria in the nigral dopaminergic neurons.[43] Although TfR2 has a lower affinity for Tf binding than TfR1,[40] it is involved in Tf-TfR-dependent iron uptake, which is enhanced in the presence of hemochromatosis protein (HFE).[41] TfR2 can form a stable complex on the cell membrane with HFE.[41,44] This TfR2/HFE complex is the sensor of extracellular iron levels and could regulate the expression of hepcidin to maintain iron homeostasis.[45–48]

DMT1

DMT1, also known as nature resistance associated macrophage protein 2 (Nramp2) or divalent cation transporter 1 (DCT1), is believed to be responsible for initial uptake of iron from the duodenal lumen into the cells of the apical brush border membrane.[49–51] There are at least four distinct isoforms, which differ in both the C-terminus and the N-terminus. Of the two C-terminal spliced variants, one possesses a iron responsive element in the 3′-untranslated region (UTR) of its mRNA (DMT1 + IRE), whereas the other does not (DMT1−IRE).[49,52,53] DMT1 can be regulated posttranscriptionally through IRE and posttranslationally through the ubiquitin-proteasome system.[54] It is present in endothelial cells of the brain microvasculature, astrocytes lining the blood vessels, in the choroid plexus and in ependymal cells.[55] In rat SN, DMT1 is expressed on neurons, astrocytes, and microglia, but not on oligodendrocytes.[56] Decreased levels of brain iron in Belgrade rats, which have a defect in DMT1, suggest its critical role in brain iron uptake.[57]

Fpn

Fpn, also known as metal transport protein 1[58] or iron-regulated transporter 1 (IREG1),[59] is a transmembrane protein and expressed at the basolateral membrane of duodenal enterocytes, macrophages of the spleen and liver, placental syncytiotrophoblasts, as well as neurons and neuroglia.[35,55,58] Fpn transports ferrous iron across the basolateral membrane of enterocytes with the auxiliary ferroxidase activity of ceruloplasmin (CP) or hephaestin (HP).[59–61] In the brain, Fpn is found in the BBB endothelial cells, neurons, oligodendrocytes, astrocytes, the choroid plexus, and ependymal cells.[55,62,63] Fpn and HP are both expressed in neurons, astrocytes, oligodendrocytes and microglia, suggesting that HP could facilitate Fpn-mediated iron export from a variety of brain cells.[64]

Lf-LfR

Lf is an 80 kDa iron-binding cation glycoprotein, which exists widely in various secretory fluids. In the brain, Lf is synthesized by activated microglia and detected in dopaminergic neurons.[65] The structure of Lf is similar to Tf, which are both composed of two lobes with each possessing one iron-binding site for ferric ion.[66] Lf plays various physiological roles, such as enhancement in natural immunity, bone growth and wound healing. Furthermore, Lf is clarified to function as pathogen resistance including antiinflammatory, antifungal, antibacterial, antiviral, and anticancer activities.[67] Lf can transport various metal ions, such as iron, copper, zinc, and manganese, across BBB by the mediation of the LfR present at the endothelial cells of BBB.[68,69] In fact, in the AD or PD state, the expression of LfR is increased in the endothelial cells of the BBB. Moreover, Lf has a high affinity for iron that plays a role similar to that of Tf in iron transport in the brain, ensuring that an adequate amount of iron is present under normal circumstances.

MTf

MTf, also known as p97 protein, was first identified as a surface marker of melanoma cells and a member of iron-binding protein family.[70] MTf shares similar structural and functional aspects with serum Tf. Of these, there are many disulphide bonds including an almost identical N-terminal iron-binding site, which binds to trivalent iron and is hypothesized to have roles in cellular iron uptake.[71,72] Although MTf binds iron, it is not rapidly internalized into the cells as a soluble molecule but remains its own characterized function. Thus, it might play little role in iron uptake in vitro.[73,74] A number of studies reported that MTf could transport iron across the BBB through interacting with low-density lipoprotein receptor-related protein, and promote iron accumulation in the brain,[75,76] but the subsequent studies using transgenic mice demonstrated that MTf is not essential for iron transport in the brain, implicating it exerts an elusive role for iron homeostasis or metabolism.[77,78]

Iron Transporters and PD

Total iron levels are increased by 176% and levels of ferric iron are increased by 225% in the SN of PD patients relative to age-matched controls, suggesting the role of iron as an etiological factor for PD.[7] Other studies also showed increased iron levels in the SN of PD brains using a variety of methods, such as the spectrophotometric method and Perl's staining,[79] inductively coupled plasma spectroscopy,[10] magnetic resonance imaging,[80,81] laser microprobe mass analysis,[82] susceptibility-weighted imaging,[83,84] and enhanced T2 star weighted angiography.[85] However, there are no significant differences in the levels of total iron or ferric iron in other brain areas, such as cortex (Brodmann area 21), hippocampus, putamen, and globus pallidus.[7] In our previous study, we reported that the iron content was significantly lower in the temporal cortex of patients with PD when compared with age-matched healthy controls.[86,87] Unexpectedly, the levels of DMT1 + IRE, TfR1, FPN1, and IRP1 were shown to be decreased in the temporal cortex.[86]

The altered expression of iron transporters in the SN may be responsible for the nigral iron accumulation in PD. For example, a reduced density of transferrin binding sites is observed in the SN of PD patients.[88] More recent studies revealed that 1-methyl-4-phenylpyridinium (MPP^+) treatment enhanced the cell surface expression of TfR. Therefore, upregulation of TfR1-dependent iron influx could be involved in elevated iron levels in PD.[89,90] The selective localization of TfR2 in dopaminergic neurons and the accumulation of Tf in parallel with oxidative damage, suggests that the Tf/TfR2 system might lead to iron deposition in PD.[43,91]

A study on PD patients revealed that DMT1 + IRE levels in the SN are significantly increased in PD subjects compared with control subjects.[92] DMT1 is highly expressed in the nigral dopaminergic neurons in PD, which correlates with the abnormally deposited iron in the SN.[92] In addition, increased expression levels of DMT1 + IRE/DMT1-IRE[93] are prevalent in both animal and cell PD models.[64,94–96] These indicate that DMT1-dependent increases in iron levels play a prominent role in the degeneration of dopaminergic neurons in PD. As for the iron exporter, Fpn, decreased expression levels are observed in both animal and cell PD models.[64,94–96] Since both DMT1 + IRE and Fpn contain an IRE in their mRNA,[97] the upregulation of DMT1 + IRE and the concomitant downregulation of Fpn responsible for iron accumulation in the SN are due to an IRP-IRE-dependent pathway in 6-OHDA-induced PD models.[96,98] However, the upregulation of DMT1-IRE in MPTP-induced PD models is not an IRP/IRE-dependent pathway. A reactive oxygen species (ROS)-nuclear factor kappa B (NF-κB) activation pathway might also be involved in DMT1-IRE upregulation.[99,100]

LfR expression is increased in neurons and microvessels in PD patients, especially in those regions of the mesencephalon where the damage of dopaminergic neurons has occurred.[101] Moreover, dopamine content displays negative correlation with the intensity of neurons and microvessels where Lf is expressed, showing the more nigral dopamine loss the higher intensity of neurons and microvessels in the SN.[101,102] These studies imply that the increase in intracellular iron levels might be mediated through LfR on vulnerable neurons, which contribute to the degeneration of nigral dopaminergic neurons in PD.

Iron Transporters and AD

AD is a progressive neurodegenerative disorder, clinically characterized by a progressive loss of cognitive abilities and dementia, which is closely related to a degree of neuronal and synaptic loss.[103–105] The key features of the disease are the accumulation of extracellular amyloid-β (Aβ) plaques and neurofibrillary tangles inside neurons. It is the most common cause of dementia, affecting millions worldwide. Although genetic and nongenetic factors are involved in the etiology of AD, the exact mechanisms are largely unknown.

Increasing evidence suggests that iron might play an important role in the development or progression of AD.[106] The first evidence is that iron accumulates in the same brain regions that are characterized by Aβ deposition, such as hippocampus, parietal cortex, and motor cortex in AD patients.[16,17] High levels of iron have also been reported in the amyloid plaques in PS/APP (presenilin/amyloid precursor protein) and APP [V717I] transgenic mice,[107] resembling those seen in the brains of AD patients.

Another important link between iron and AD is based on the observation that APP expression is iron-regulated. APP is a single transmembrane metalloprotein that is cleaved to generate the 40–42-amino-acid Aβs by β-and γ-secretases.[15] The existence of a functional IRE in the 5′-UTR of APP mRNA makes it possible to be controlled at the level of mRNA translation by the action of IRE/IRP's response to iron.[108] This implies that high intracellular iron levels can cause increased APP translation and Aβ formation via this mechanism. In addition, iron can induce Aβ precipitation[109,110] and significantly enhance the toxicity of Aβ in cultured neuronal cells, whereas iron chelators protect the neurons from Aβ toxicity.[111] This provides a direct link between excessive iron and loss of neuronal function seen in AD patients.

The underlying mechanisms involved in the disturbance of iron homeostasis in AD brain remain unclear. It is reported that Aβ is a metalloprotein that binds transition metal ions through 3 histidine residues (His6, His13, and His14) located in the N-terminal domain.[15,112] Other proteins that accumulate in AD, such as tau protein also possesses metal-binding sites.[113] These might account for the iron accumulation in the affected brain regions in AD. DMT1 is colocalized with Aβ in the plaques of postmortem AD brain and the levels of DMT1 are significantly increased in the cortex and hippocampus in APP/PS1 transgenic mouse model when compared with that in wild type-control.[114] Another molecule for iron uptake, melanotransferrin (p97), is specifically localized on reactive microglial cells and associated with classic senile plaques of human AD brain tissues,[115] but it is not found to be associated with PD or HD.[115] The serum p97 concentration is elevated 3- to 4-fold in patients with AD as compared with non-AD dementia and normal controls.[116] In addition, heme oxygenase-1 (HO-1) is increased in neurofibrillary tangles, senile plaque neurites, granulovacuolar degeneration, and neuropil threads in human AD brains,[113,117] suggesting the redistribution of iron due to release from heme proteins in affected areas of the AD brain.

Iron and Other Neurodegenerative Disorders

HD is an autosomal dominant inherited neurological disorder characterized by progressive motor, psychiatric, and cognitive dysfunction, and is associated with selective neuronal loss and formation of intraneuronal protein aggregates in the striatum and the cortex. It is caused by abnormally expanded polyglutamine (polyQ) tracts in exon1 of huntingtin (Htt). Despite this genetic defect, the cause of the selective degeneration of neurons in the basal ganglia in HD remains unclear. Using X-ray fluorescence (XRF), iron oxide deposits are found in the basal ganglia of the HD transgenic mice. MRI studies have also found that iron accumulates in the basal ganglia early in the disease process in HD patients, even before the onset of symptoms.[21] It has been reported that deferoxamine alters the structure, localization, and oxidative potential of Htt exon1 polypeptide containing polyglutamine tracts of various sizes within inclusion bodies.[118] These results suggest that the accumulation of iron might play a causative role in the pathogenesis of the disease.[21,119] In addition, deferoxamine is reported to upregulate the expression of Htt, indicating that Htt is an iron-response protein.[120] Lumsden et al. reported that knockdown of Htt in Zebrafish led to microcytic, hypochromic anemia,[121] suggesting that the protein acts downstream of Tf-endocytosis involving the iron release from endocytic compartments into the cytosol to keep iron homeostasis.

Neurodegeneration with brain iron accumulation (NBIA) represents a group of rarely inherited neurological movement disorders with several causative gene mutations.[122] The common feature of NBIA is abnormal iron accumulation in the basal ganglia, primarily in the globuspallidus. NBIA includes pantothenate kinase–associated neurodegeneration (PKAN), infantile neuroaxonal dystrophy (INAD), neuroferritinopathy, and hereditary aceruloplasminemia.[38] The most frequent genetic form is PKAN, which is formerly known as Hallervorden-Spatz syndrome and caused by mutation in the pantothenate kinase 2 gene (PANK2).[123] INAD is a recessive disorder with psychomotor regression due to mutations in PLA2G6.[124] Neuroferritinopathy is a dominantly inherited, adult-onset disorder caused by mutations in the ferritin light chain (FTL1) gene[125] and hereditary aceruloplasminemia is an autosomal disorder of iron metabolism resulting from inherited mutations in CP and defective or absent CP function[126] as described earlier. Recently, mutations in the fatty acid hydroxylase gene FA2H are identified to lead to a novel form of NBIA with white matter degeneration.[122] These mutations in NBIA genes generate phenotypes that range from infantile and childhood to adult-onset iron accumulation disorders, indicating the importance of iron in the progress of this disease.[126–130]

ZINC TRANSPORTERS AND NEURODEGENERATION

In mammals, the concentration of zinc in the brain is around 150 μM which is higher than that in other organs.[131] The development of the CNS and maintenance of normal brain functions are highly dependent on zinc levels. Zinc exerts significant roles in catalyzing reactions or stabilizing protein structures and as a cofactor or key structural component of more than 300 metalloenzymes.[132] There are three distinct pools of zinc in the brain: a membrane bound metalloprotein pool, an ionic pool of free, or loosely bound ions and synaptic zinc which mostly exists at the glutamatergic terminals.[133] In both human and animals, high levels of zinc are involved in neurotoxicity and neurodegeneration relevant to various disorders.[134,135]

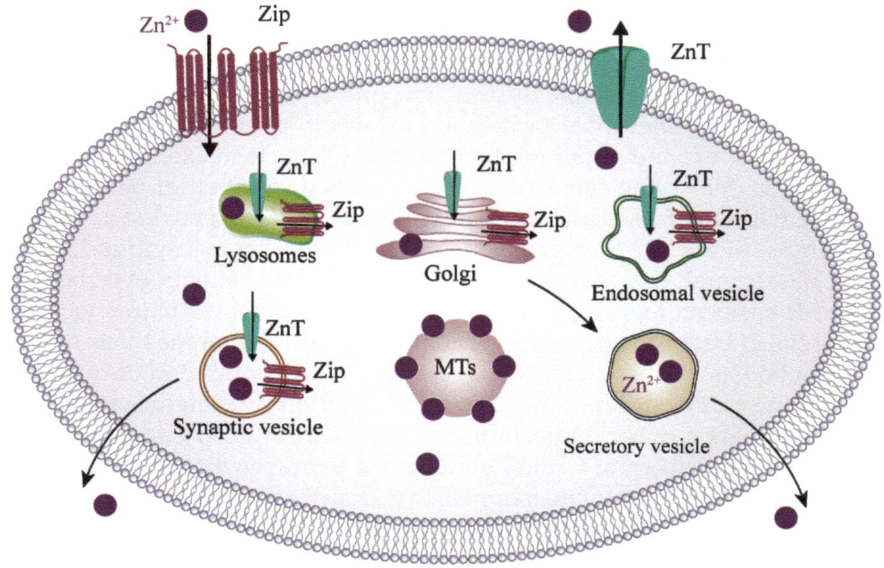

FIGURE 16.2 **Cellular localization of zinc transporters ZnT, ZIP, and MTs for zinc homeostasis.** Zinc is transported into the cytosol directly by ZIP family, and out of the cytosol directly by ZnT family. In the cytosol, MTs bind zinc to regulate its concentration at critical sites. *MTs*, metallothioneins; *ZIP*, iron-regulated transporter (Irt)-like proteins; *ZnT*, zinc transporter.

Zinc transporters contain three groups, including the zinc transporters (ZnTs), zinc-regulated transporter (Zrt) and iron-regulated transporter (Irt)-like proteins (ZIP) family, and metallothioneins (MTs). ZnTs mediate zinc efflux from cells or zinc influx into cellular compartments or organelles.[136,137] The ZIP family enhance zinc transport from the extracellular or from intracellular vesicles to the cytoplasm.[138] MTs are zinc homeostasis-regulating proteins.[139] In addition, DMT1, and ATP13A2 also regulate cellular zinc homeostasis[140] (Fig. 16.2).

ZnT

Most ZnT (SLC30A) members contain six predicted transmembrane (TM) domains with intracellular N-and C-terminals and a histidine/serine-rich loop between TM4 and TM5.[141,142] However, the recently reported human zinc transporters ZnT-like transporter 1 (hZTL1), a human apical intestinal zinc transporter, is predicted to have 12 TM domains with extracellular N- and C-terminals.[143] Ten ZnT family members are divided into four subtypes based on sequence, with ZnT5 and ZnT7 in subtype I, ZnT2, ZnT3, ZnT4, and ZnT8 in subtype II, ZnT1 and ZnT10 in subtype III, and ZnT6 and ZnT9 in subtype IV. All ZnT proteins are characterized by the cation diffusion facilitator proteins except for ZnT5 which contains additional TM domains at the N-terminal. The longest C-terminal tail of ZnTs is found in ZnT6 (203 amino acids) and the shortest one is found in ZnT7 (82 amino acids). The upstream of the first TM domain that contains subcellular targeting signals differs largely among ZnT proteins due to their length and the amino acid sequences. ZnT1 and two levels are directly regulated by intracellular zinc levels. ZnT1 in adult mouse brain[144] and ZnT3 in juvenile mouse brain[145] are generally found in areas where the immunoactive zinc is heavily stained.

ZIP

ZIPs (SLC39) are highly conserved in mice and humans where they share 93% amino acid similarity in sequence. The ZIP family is divided into four subfamilies: ZIP I, ZIP II, gufA, and LZT.[146] Most mammalian ZIP proteins, such as ZIP4, 5, 6, 7, 8, 10, 12, 13, and 14 belong to the LZT. ZIP1, 2 and 3 belong to the ZIP II; Zip9 belongs to the ZIP I; and ZIP11 clusters belong to the gufA.[138] Each ZIP contains eight putative TM domains and the fourth TM domain has conserved histidine, serine, and glycine residues.[142] In addition, a histidine-rich loop is present between the third and the fourth TM domains.[142,146] As the first member of ZIP, Irt1 was identified in *Arabidopsis*[147] and found to preferentially import iron, but can also transport manganese, calcium, and zinc.[147,148] ZIP1, 3, 4, 5, 6, 7, 10, 13, and 14 are expressed in the brain.[142,149–153] Among these, ZIP1 mRNA is highly expressed in hippocampus, thalamus, prefrontal cortex, commissural fiber tracts, ependymal cells lining the third and lateral ventricles, and epithelium cells in the choroid plexus, but little is found in the internal and external capsules and astrocytes.[149] ZIP3 mRNA is detected in all brain regions in embryos and adults of mice.[154] ZIP4 mRNA is found in the choroid plexus.[149] ZIP6 is expressed in most of the neurons which do not release hormones.[155] ZIP10 is predominantly expressed in the brain and spinal cord.[156]

MTs

MTs were discovered as unusual cadmium-binding proteins in horse kidney in 1957.[157] MTs are low-molecular-weight (6–7 kDa) metal-binding proteins that lack disulfides, aromatic amino acids or histidine, and contain one-third cysteine residues. All MTs are composed of a single polypeptide chain with 61–68 amino acids.[158–161] In humans, the MT genes are in the q13 region of chromosome 16, consisting of 11 functional isoforms that are sorted to four types, named MT1 (MT1A, B, E, F, G, H, M, and X), MT2 (MT2A), MT-3 (also named growth inhibitory factor, GIF), and MT4.[162–165] In cytoplasm, MTs bind zinc to reserve, buffer, and chelate.[166] MT1/2 is expressed in most tissues,[167,168] while MT3 and MT4 expression are restricted in the CNS and stratified squamous epithelia.[164,169–171] In the brain, MT1/2 is primarily expressed in the reactive astrocytes responding to neuronal injury[172,173] and to a lesser extent in activated microglia/macrophages.[174] In contrast, MT3 is expressed in astrocytes and neurons.[175–177] Expression of MT4 is thought to be restricted to epithelium.[178] The expressions of MTs are highly inducible by a range of stimuli, including metals, hormones, cytokines, oxidative agents, inflammation, and stress.[8,179–181]

Zinc Transporters and PD

Zinc transporters are implicated in neurodegenerative diseases and injuries, including PD,[182] AD,[183–185] amyotrophic lateral sclerosis (ALS),[186–188] and others.[189–196] The main functions of zinc transporters are not only related with metal chelation and free radical scavenging, but also have biological roles in the cell survival[197,198] and antiinflammation after brain injury.[199]

The strong increase in the expression of MT1/2A is found in both nigral reactive astrocytes and frontal cortex in PD patients.[173] Nevertheless, the content of MT1/2 is significantly reduced in the SN, striatum and myenteric plexus in PD models, whereas no changes in MT3 mRNA expression are observed.[182,200,201] MTs have been previously demonstrated that they have neuroprotective roles against DA neuronal damage in PD model. The nigral DA neurons in MT1/2 KO mice are more sensitive to 6-OHDA, rotenone, and DA quinone.[182,202,203] MT1/2 are suggested to play a role as scavengers in clearing ROS, including O_2^-, ·OH, $ONOO^-$, peroxy radicals, lipid peroxidation, and redox-active transition metals (copper, iron).[204–207] It has been reported that the MTs protect DA neurons and in vitro striatal astrocytes against DA quinone neurotoxicity by its quinone-quenching property.[203,207]

Zinc Transporters and AD

ZnTs (ZnT1, 3, 4, 5, 6, and 7) are detected in the Aβ-positive plaques in the cortex of human AD brains.[208] ZnT3 is also upregulated in APP/PS1 transgenic AD mice.[209,210] Moreover, the APP/ZnT3 double knockout mice do not develop Alzheimer's symptoms. However, it is also reported that ZnT3 levels are decreased in healthy older humans and particularly in AD, and in wild type mice with aging.[185] All these may indicate a critical role for ZnT3 in the pathogenesis of AD.[211,212] MT1/2 levels have been found to be consistently upregulated in AD patients.[184,213,214] MT1 alleviates AD by downregulating ROS levels, Aβ-induced downregulation of Bcl-2 and proinflammatory cytokine production, and inhibiting the activation of microglia.[184] However, contrary results showed that MT1/2-deficiency decreased the amyloid plaque burden, and partially rescued the hAPP-induced changes in mortality and body weight in a gender-dependent manner.[215] Data showed that protein levels of MT3 were reduced in AD patient brain and AD mice.[158,216,217] MT3 is related to the pathogenesis of AD and may connect with causing Aβ aggregation upon cysteine oxidation.[158,218–221] MT3 deficiency partially rescues the APP-induced mortality of females, and mildly affects APP-induced changes in behaviors.[221] The absence of MT3 results in actin disruption, and reduces Aβ uptake in astrocytes through an abnormality in actin polymerization.[222] On the contrary, in vitro studies on cultured cortical neurons demonstrated that MT3 alleviated the neurotoxic effects of Aβ probably by a metal swap between Zn_7MT3 and soluble and aggregated Cu(II)-Aβ1–40 leading to suppression of ·OHradical.[219,223,224] Therefore, the complex mechanisms of zinc transporters in AD need to be further investigated.

Zinc Transporters and Other Neurodegenerative Diseases

Although the expressions of MTs in Creutzfeldt–Jakob disease (CJD) brains differ from case to case, MT1/2 and MT3 in the astrocytes are significantly reduced.[225] It has also been revealed that MT1/2 accumulated upon a short disease duration, whereas MT3 was statistically reduced upon along disease duration in CJD brain.[225] In Gerstmann–Sträussler–Scheinker syndrome patients, MT1/2 expressions in the astrocytes are exclusively reduced, while the expression of MT3 is relatively well preserved.[225] PrP^C is evolutionarily related to the ZIP family. ZIP5, 6, and 10 have similar sequences to that of PrPC.[226] The cellular PrP^C facilitates the uptake of zinc into neuronal cells.[227] Thus, the ZIP proteins are also expected to open new ways of research to elucidate the biology of the prion disease.

MT1/2 and MT3 are detected mainly in the glia of sporadic ALS patients, and their expression levels are decreased in the spinal cords.[228,229] It has also been found that MT3-positive neurons are surrounded by definite MT3-positive glia in patients.[229] However, MT1/2 and MT3 expression within astrocytes are markedly upregulated in ALS (G93ASOD1 mutation) mice.[230,231] Without MT1/2 or MT3, ALS mice exhibited significant reductions in survival and motor dysfunction.[232] However, overexpression of MT1 or MT3 can prevent the loss of motor neurons, attenuate the pathological features, and prolong the life span of ALS mice.[186,233] Multiple sclerosis (MS) is a major chronic demyelinating and inflammatory disease of the CNS.[190,234] MT1/2 are mainly present in astrocytes and activated-monocytes/macrophages in MS patients and an MS model, and they are slightly increased in the inactive MS lesions.[190] Treatment with Zn-MT2 significantly decreases the expression of IL-6 and TNF-α in the CNS, reduces apoptosis of neurons and oligodendrocytes in MS model.[190,234] These results are consistent with the hypothesis that MTs may play an important protective function in ALS and MS.

COPPER TRANSPORTERS AND NEURODEGENERATION

Copper is an essential micronutrient and transition metal, which is necessary for different cellular functions, like cellular respiration, free radical defense, neurotransmitter synthesis, and neuronal myelination. However, copper is also toxic in excess of cellular requirements because of its participation in generation of free radicals.[235] A balance between absorption and excretion of copper is critical, in which transport proteins play a key role. Copper transporter 1 (CTR1),[236,237] as well as the copper transporting ATPases, ATP7A and ATP7B[238,239] are the major copper transport proteins, divalent metal transporter 1 (DMT1) may be also involved in the uptake of copper through the brain barriers.[240] Besides the transport proteins, there exists a subset of intracellular proteins regarded as copper chaperones delivering copper to specific intracellular targets which are also involved in the homeostasis of copper. These include antioxidant protein-1 (ATOX1), cytochrome oxidase enzyme complex (COX17), and copper chaperone for SOD[240,241] (Fig. 16.3).

Increasing evidence suggests that copper plays an important role in the pathogenesis of neurodegenerative diseases. For example, a high content of copper has been found in amyloid plaques from AD brains,[19,20] while a significant reduction in copper levels occurs in the dopaminergic neurons of the SN in the PD brains.[6] Since the SN contains twice more copper than that in other brain regions in normal conditions, it is feasible that a reduction of copper in this region may result from dysfunction of copper-dependent pathways which support neuronal function and survival, thus increasing the vulnerability of copper-deficient neurons during the pathogenesis of PD.[242] An imbalance in regulating extracellular and intracellular copper transport has been suggested to play a role in the etiology of these neurodegenerative diseases.

CTR1

CTR1 is a plasma membrane protein with three transmembrane domains that form a homotrimeric pore which is essential for copper uptake, as cuprous (Cu^{+}), in all cells. Before uptake by CTR1, cupric (Cu^{2+}) is thought to be reduced to Cu^{+} by different Steap proteins on the cell surface. The process of Cu^{+} uptake by CTR1 is energy dependent, acidic extracellular

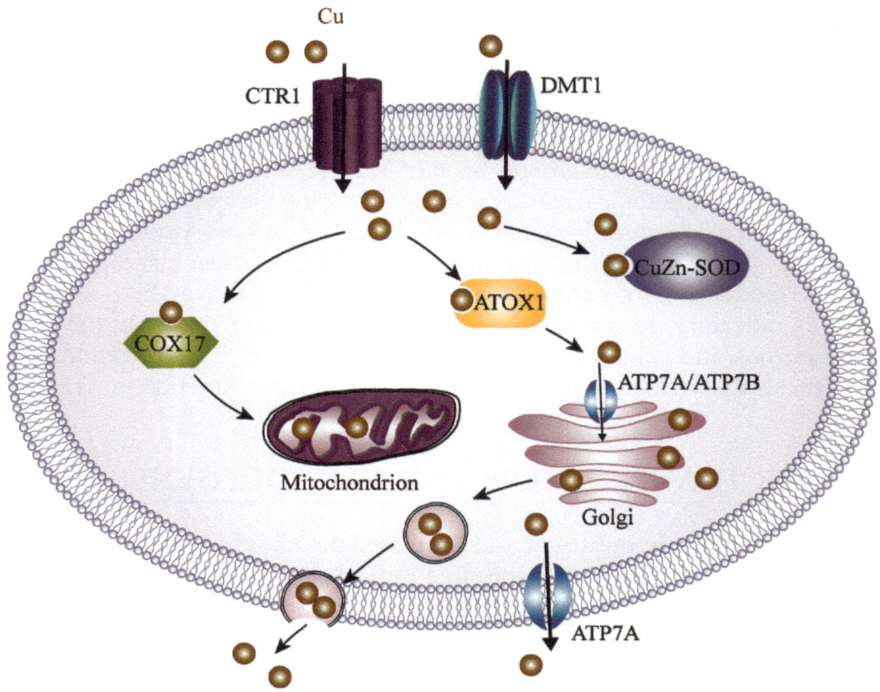

FIGURE 16.3 **A scheme for copper transport system in neuronal cells.** Copper is transported into the cell by CTR1. DMT1 may be also involved in the uptake of copper. After copper influx, they are distributed to different cellular locations by copper transport proteins, such as ATOX1, COX17, and CuZn-SOD. ATOX1 is suggested to transport copper to the ATPases, ATP7A, and ATP7B, which are normally located in the trans-Golgi network. When intracellular copper levels are elevated, ATP7A and ATP7B traffic from the trans-Golgi network to the cell periphery to export excess copper out of cells. *ATOX1*, antioxidant protein-1; *COX17*, cytochrome oxidase enzyme complex; *CTR1*, copper transporter 1; *DMT1*, divalent metal transporter 1.

pH sensitive, with high K^+ concentrations required, time-dependent and saturable.[243] CTR1 occurs as a pool of intracellular molecules which is quickly recruited to the plasma membrane when there is a copper shortage, then endocytosed according to high copper concentration in the medium.[244] Some research also suggested that the intracellular copper availability could regulate CTR1 posttranslationally.[243] CTR1 mRNA is ubiquitously expressed, but with the highest levels observed in the liver and lower levels detected in the brain and spleen. In the brain, CTR1 is expressed abundantly in the BBB, blood-cerebrospinal fluid barrier (BCB), and brain parenchyma, which plays an important role in cellular copper uptake.[240,245] The *Ctr1* family proteins are high affinity copper importers, which are conserved from yeast to humans.

The ATPases ATP7A/ATP7B

The copper-transporting P-type ATPases (copper-ATPases), ATP7A and ATP7B, are members of the P_{1B} subfamily of the P-type ATPases.[246–249] They have six copper-binding motifs within the cytoplasmic N-terminal domain, eight transmembrane domains, and highly conserved catalytic domains. Both ATP7A and ATP7B are widely expressed in cerebral cortex, hippocampus, cerebellum, olfactory bulb, SN, caudate putamen, and brainstem.[250,251] ATP7A and ATP7B possess dual functions, such as delivering copper into cell for the synthesis of copper-dependent enzymes, but on the other hand, is dependent on ATP hydrolysis to move excess copper across the cellular membranes. Under normal physiological conditions, ATP7A and ATP7B are localized at the trans-Golgi network (TGN). When intracellular copper levels are elevated, ATP7A and ATP7B traffic from the TGN to the cell periphery to export excess copper out of cells. When copper levels return to normal, ATP7A and ATP7B recycle back to the TGN. The trafficking and recycling of the copper-ATPases requires the specific signal sequences in the N- and C-terminal domains. Other processes also contribute to regulate copper-ATPase activity, such as posttranslational modifications, copper-stimulated phosphorylation by kinases, and protein interactions.[252]

Copper Transporters and PD

A growing body of evidence reports that disruption in copper homoeostasis and copper-associated pathways are linked to the neuronal death in PD. Studies have noted that occupational long-term exposure to copper increases the risk of PD.[253] Other environmentally based studies have also shown that the incidence of PD within urban populations is greater than that within suburban populations due to its severe emissions of copper.[254] Total copper levels in fresh-frozen and fixed SN in PD have been consistently reported to be decreased by 34%–51% compared with age-matched healthy controls.[6,11,255–257] Copper levels are also reduced in the striatum, being no longer available for the Cu-Zn-SOD, which is a major contributor to the antioxidant system in striatal neurons. In addition, decreased copper in striatal neurons would result in iron accumulation. A positive correlation has been observed between serum ceruloplasmin levels and the age of onset of PD, and a negative correlation between iron accumulation in the brain and the copper-dependent ferroxidase plasma activity has been demonstrated.[258,259] However, copper levels in the blood and CSF are controversial in PD patients.[9,260–262]

There is little information about the effect of copper transporters in the pathogenic process of PD. Moreover, there is no report about any mutation of CTR1 in PD until now, but only a marked reduction of CTR1 immunoreactivity in neurons and a correlation between CTR1 and copper levels in the SN of PD postmortem brains have been reported.[255] Neural tissue is especially sensitive to the dysfunction of CTR1, and the downregulation of CTR1 is a critical reason for cell death in the brain and spinal cord of zebrafish, implicating the copper depletion is probably caused by a disruption in CTR1 transport. More studies are needed to confirm the relevance of CTR1 in PD.[263] Sechi et al. found a nucleotide deletion at the 5′UTR region in a single allele of ATP7B gene in three sisters with a form of very-late-onset major depression and Parkinsonism, suggesting that a mutation in ATP7B could be associated with PD.[264]

Copper Transporters and AD

More and more evidence indicates that the formation of senile plaques is mediated by endogenous biometals, like copper, zinc, and iron.[265–267] In plaques isolated from the brains of AD patients, high concentrations of copper could be detected.[268] In addition, it was demonstrated that trace amounts of copper in water could induce β-amyloid plaques formation in a rabbit model of AD.[269] Though the total levels of copper are similar in healthy subjects and AD, the ratios of plasma/serum copper levels are significantly higher in AD.[270] And the correlation between free copper in blood and cognitive status in AD is negative.[271]

Genetic inhibition of human high affinity CTR1 orthologous, CTR1C, in an AD *Drosophila* model showed a prolonged life-span along with enhanced climbing ability, which prevented the role of increased copper accumulation from promoting brain neurodegeneration. After knock down of CTR1C, the flies were paraquat resistant, which suggests that the Aβ42 soluble fractions or the increased Aβ42 aggregates may have less toxicity in response to copper deficiency.[272]

Genetic analysis of AD patients and healthy controls uncovered ATP7B as a genetic risk factor for AD. A number of single nucleotide polymorphisms in ATP7B are associated with increased risk for AD.[273–276] These observations further support a crucial role for ATP7B in maintaining brain copper homeostasis and a potential role in AD pathogenesis.

MANGANESE TRANSPORTERS AND NEURODEGENERATION

Manganese Transporters

Multiple transporters are involved in manganese import, including DMT1, Tf/TfR, ZIP8 and ZIP14, and the dopamine transporter (DAT). Besides, many transporters are also involved in manganese export, such as ATPase 13A2 (ATP13A2), SLC30A10, Fpn, and the secretory pathway Ca^{2+}-ATPase 1 (SPCA1) (Fig. 16.4). Among these transporters, DMT1 was the first mammalian transporter identified for cellular uptake of manganese.[49] DMT1 has a robust ability for transporting manganese into the brain across the BBB, especially upon the condition of iron deficiency.[277,278] While DMT1 transports divalent manganese, the Tf/TfR unit is observed to transport trivalent manganese. The activated IREs in the Tf sense manganese levels in the cytoplasm so as to regulate the expression of TfR, which mediates the transport of trivalent manganese/Tf complex into the cells via ligand-receptor activity.[279] ZIP8 and ZIP14 were originally considered as zinc transporters, but subsequent studies showed that both ZIP8 and ZIP14 had high binding ability for manganese and they might participate in the regulation of body manganese level through its absorption from the liver and lung.[280] Moreover, manganese accumulation in the brain may be dependent on Ca^{2+} concentrations, showing that manganese uptake is inhibited by Ca^{2+} channel blocker,[281] and manganese enters cell membranes through store-operated Ca^{2+} channels in vitro.[282,283] In recent years, the main focus of studies on the role of efflux transporter in maintaining cellular manganese levels has just started to be appreciated. Genetic studies identified SLC30A10 as a cell surface-localized manganese efflux transporter. Patients who suffer from Parkinsonism harbor mutations in SLC30A10 resulting in manganese accumulation in brain.[284,285] Correspondingly, overexpression of SLC30A10 reduces cellular manganese levels and alleviates manganese-induced toxicity.[286] The iron exporter Fpn could also mediate cellular manganese export in a pH-dependent manner to attenuate manganese toxicity.[287] In addition to these cotransporters for multiple metal ions, a number of specific manganese importers and exporters are characterized to balance manganese levels for proper homeostasis.[288]

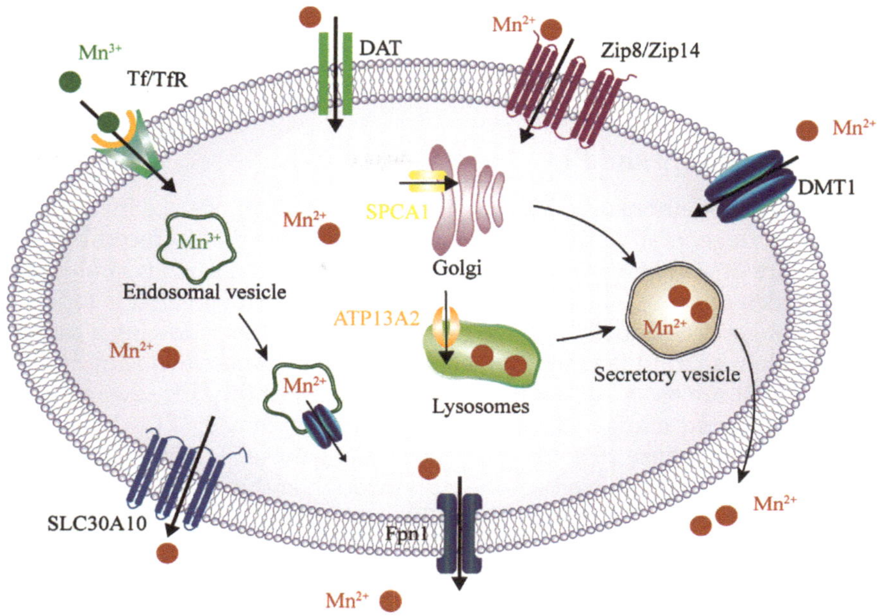

FIGURE 16.4 **The manganese homeostasis is tightly controlled by various transporters on the cell membrane and internal organelles surface.** Of these, DMT1, DAT, and ZIP8/ZIP14 are responsible for Mn^{2+} influx into the cytosol. Mn^{3+} is transported in cells through Tf/TfR. In addition, Mn^{3+} also enters cells through endocytosis and eventually released into cytoplasm as Mn^{2+} mediated by DMT1. When excess manganese crosses the membrane, SLC30A10 and Fpn1 will facilitate manganese efflux into the extracellular milieu. Furthermore, SPCA1 and ATP13A2 also transport extra manganese into the Golgi and lysosomes, which form vesicles containing manganese that secrete out of the cells. *DAT*, dopamine transporter; *DMT1*, divalent metal transporter 1; *Fpn*, ferroportin; *SLC30A10*, solute carrier family 30 member 10; *SPCA1*, secretory pathway calcium 1; *Tf/TfR*, transferrin-transferrin receptor; *ZIP*, iron-regulated transporter (Irt)-like proteins.

DAT is a membrane-spanning protein that induces the reuptake of neurotransmitter dopamine back into presynaptic vesicles for storage and later release. DAT expression is highly expressed in the ventral mesencephalon, medial forebrain bundle, globus pallidus, SNpc, and dorsal and ventral striatum.[289] Consistent with the studies on DAT inhibition, the experimental animals exposed to manganese chloride dramatically increased manganese accumulation in brain regions except in the striatum and globus pallidus where DAT are expressed,[277,290] implicating that DAT acts as a manganese transporter.

ATP13A2 (PARK9) is first characterized as a member of the mammalian P(5)-ATPase family,[291] which functions as a cation transporter and mutations in ATP13A2 are linked to Parkinsonism.[292,293] ATP13A2 plays a role in manganese and zinc metabolism.[292,294] Expression of ATP13A2 decreases intracellular manganese level and in turn protects the cells from manganese-induced lethality.[295]

SPCA1 is a P-type ion-transport ATPase that resembles the secretory pathway Ca^{2+} pump.[296] It primarily exists in the Golgi apparatus and is extensively expressed in keratinocytes, kidney, and brain tissues.[297,298] The SPCA1 homologue in yeast, PMR1, has been shown to mediate Ca^{2+} and manganese transport. Expression of SPCA1 in yeast fully rescues PMR1 phenotypes of high sensitivity to manganese toxicity. However, the roles of SPCA1 in the nervous system with high affinity manganese transport need to be well studied.[298]

Manganese Transporters and PD

Increasing evidence demonstrate that manganese accumulations are involved in the processes of the neurodegenerative disease. An animal model of PD induced by exposing the mice to the mixture of divalent and trivalent manganese displays behavioral and pathological alterations which are consistent with PD symptoms.[299,300] However, it is reported that the mechanism of manganese-induced pathologies in PD is complex, showing a severe neuronal cell death in the globus pallidus when challenged with manganese exposure.[301]

Changes in DMT1 are associated with increased susceptibility for several diseases, such as PD.[302] DMT1 mediated manganese accumulation occurs in a Tf/TfR-dependent manner. Tf binds trivalent manganese to form a trivalent manganese/Tf complex, which is transported by TfR in the endothelial cells of the BBB through endocytosis into the hippocampal and striatal neurons. After endosomes are acidified, trivalent manganese is released from the Tf/TfR complex.[303,304] Trivalent manganese is then reduced to divalent manganese by ferrireductase, and DMT1 transports divalent manganese into the cytosol for storage.[305,306] Patients with manganese-induced Parkinsonian syndrome carry one homozygous mutation in the SLC30A10 that result in increased manganese levels in brain, along with a severe neuronal loss in the basal ganglia and globus pallidus.[307,308] A latest study provides new views suggesting that SLC30A10 is a manganese exporter localized in cell membranes and that it mediates manganese neurotoxicity in PD via blockage of the efflux activity of the transporter.[286]

Manganese Transporters and AD

Manganese is a critical component of manganese superoxide dismutase (Mn-SOD). Mn-SOD plays an important role in maintaining mitochondria vitality in AD, and its disruption could lead to mitochondrial dysfunction, which explains the links between Aβ-induced oxidative stress and AD.[309] Recently, growing studies found that excess manganese level could lead to several cognitive impairments in AD, implicating a neurotoxic effect in brain.[25] Chronic manganese exposure changes the cellular response in the frontal cortex, showing diffused Aβ plaques and alpha-synuclein aggregation,[26] and a more recent study pointed out manganese could bind to the N-terminal part of the Aβ plaques,[310] these pathophysiological changes could explain the impairments in cognitive, learning, and memory observed in AD.

Manganese and Other Neurodegenerative Disorders

Numerous studies report that alterations in striatal manganese levels or deficiencies in manganese transporting contribute to the pathogenesis of HD. On the other hand, manganese accumulates in striatum and other basal ganglia leading to cytotoxicity via elevated oxidative stress or inhibited mitochondrial respiration.[311] In HD, the striatal medium spiny neurons display a decrease in manganese content and are resistant to manganese cytotoxicity.[312] It is reported that manganese-dependent phosphorylation of p53 is decreased, and ataxia telangiectasia mutated (ATM) kinase affects the process of p53 activation by manganese in HD cells, indicating manganese-dependent ATM-p53 signaling pathway is involved in the alteration of manganese in human and mouse striatal-like neuroprogenitor models of HD.[313] In other neurodegenerative disorders, the mutations in ATP13A2 are reported to lead to Kufor–Rakeb syndrome, which is a recessive disease different from PD.[314] ATP13A2 may exert inducible protective roles to cells; the evidence suggest that overexpression of ATP13A2 reduces intracellular manganese levels and prevents manganese neurotoxicity.[315]

MAGNESIUM TRANSPORTERS AND NEURODEGENERATION

Magnesium is an essential ion for sustaining health and life. It is involved in multiple enzymatic synthesis and cellular processes including nucleotide binding and energy metabolism.[316,317] Based on new technological detection, a number of magnesium transporters are identified, which include magnesium transporter 1 (MagT1), transporters transient receptor potential melastatin type 6 and 7 (TRPM6, TRPM7), solute carrier family 41 member 1 (SLC41A1), and cyclin M (CNNM) members (Fig. 16.5).

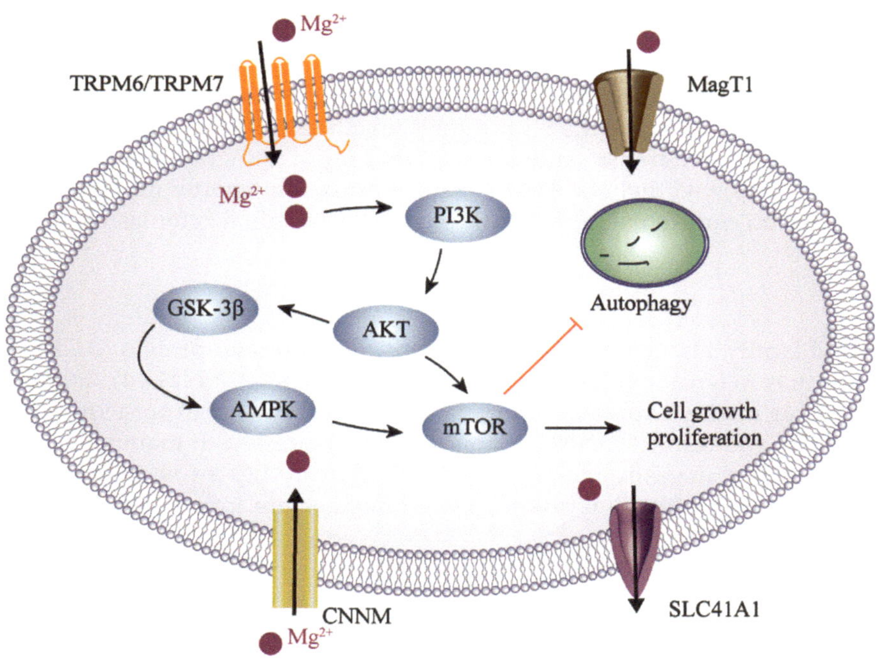

FIGURE 16.5 **Scheme of magnesium transport system and associated molecular pathway.** On the cell surface, TRPM6/TRPM7, MagT1, and CNNM family have been demonstrated to facilitate magnesium influx into the cell, while SLC41A1 mediates magnesium efflux. In cytoplasm, PI3K/Akt/mTOR is magnesium-sensitive. Activation of this signaling cascade by intracellular magnesium is essential for cell growth, proliferation as well as the inhibition of autophagy. *CNNM*, cyclin M; *MagT1*, magnesium transporter 1; *SLC41A1*, solute carrier family 41 member; *TRPM6/TRPM7*, transient receptor potential melastatin type 6 and 7.

MagT1

MagT1 is a protein of 335 amino acids that is ubiquitously expressed in tissues. It is composed of five putative transmembrane domains with a cleavage site, a N-glycosylation site, and numerous phosphorylation sites.[318] MagT1 mRNA and protein expression are significantly upregulated in epithelial cells cultured in low magnesium medium, and recent studies revealed that MagT1 could mediate magnesium influx transport into the cells through a ligand-receptor mechanism.[319,320]

TRPM6 and TRPM7

TRPM6 and TRPM7 are members of the long transient receptor potential channel subfamily that are identified respectively as ion channels and protein kinases.[321,322] TRPM6 is mainly expressed in epithelial cells, whereas TRPM7 is extensively expressed in body.[323] Both channels are considered as vital effectors in the maintenance of magnesium homeostasis. The epithelial TRPM6 channel is the magnesium entry pathway in the distal convoluted tubule of the kidney, and TRPM7 functions as part of an magnesium sensor and transducer in numerous neuronal cells.[324,325]

SLC41A1

Solute carrier family 41 member 1 (SLC41A1) functions as a sodium/magnesium exchanger, that consists of 513 amino acids with a molecular weight of 56 kDa. The protein structure possesses 11 putative transmembrane domains and it is highly expressed in heart and testis.[326,327] Studies showed that SLC41A1 is a magnesium transporter mediating magnesium efflux dependent on endosomal recycling through its N-terminal cytoplasmic domain.[328,329]

CNNM

The CNNM family, also known as ancient conserved domain protein (ACDP), has been identified to act as magnesium transporters.[330] Four proteins (CNNM1-4) share homolog to cyclin. CNNM1 is mainly expressed in brain and testis, CNNM2 expression is high in kidney, lung, spleen, and testis, CNNM3 is ubiquitously expressed in mammals, and CNNM4 is primarily expressed in gastrointestinal tract.[331] Recent studies are showing more evidence that the CNNM family plays important roles in magnesium influx to balance the cellular magnesium homeostasis.[332–334]

Magnesium Transporters and PD

Magnesium is essential for maintaining the physiological density of synapses in brain, magnesium deficiency results in memory impairment in numerous neurodegenerative disorders. The latest study pointed out that elevated magnesium level in brain could prevent the reduction in the number of dopamine neurons and increase the length of dopamine neurites in SN,[335] as well as inhibit cellular ROS generation and maintain ATP production, implicating the protective roles of magnesium against MPP^+ toxicity.[28]

As a sodium/magnesium exchanger, SLC41A1, is found to localize at locus PARK16 in PD and is a key component of cellular magnesium homeostasis. Mutations in SLC41A1 result in magnesium-efflux and thereby develop chronic intracellular magnesium deficiency in various brain regions of PD patients; and a decrease in magnesium level triggers processes inducing the neuronal damage.[336] In brain, TRPM7 is the most abundant TRPM channel in the CNS.[337] Knockdown of TRPM7 protects the neurons against H_2O_2 mediated injury.[338] In contrast, overexpression of TRPM7 channel has shown to increase the sensitivity of oxidative stress.[339]

Magnesium Transporters and AD

A number of studies demonstrated that magnesium levels were found to be significantly decreased in brain of AD patients. In the transgenic mouse model of AD, elevated magnesium level alleviates the pathological features of synapse loss, Aβ-plaque production and cognitive deficits.[340] In addition, treatment with magnesium sulfate improves insulin sensitivity, and also increases the inhibitory phosphorylation of GSK-3β, the activity of Akt and PI3K to reduce the hyperphosphorylated-tau,[341] indicating that magnesium functions as a synaptic protective factor in an animal model of AD.

In in vitro studies, knockdown of TRPM2 expression blocks the Aβ-mediated increase of the whole cell current magnitude, revealing that the interaction of TRPM2 channel activity and Aβ neuronal toxicity may advance the pathogenesis of AD.[342,343] Recently, TRPM7 has been found to coordinate the normal function of presenilin whose deficiency is associated with AD.[344] In addition, ALS and dementia are recognized to have low levels of Ca^{2+} and magnesium, which connect to the alteration of the functions of TRPM2 and TRPM7 channels.[345]

Magnesium and Other Neurodegenerative Disorders

Another progressive neurodegenerative disorder, HD, represents the polyglutamine expansions of huntingtin protein, which interacts with many synaptic vesicle proteins that are essential for exocytosis and endocytosis.[346,347] Huntingtin-interacting protein 14 (HIP14) and a related protein, HIP14-like (HIP14L), are identified to mediate magnesium transport and their transcripts are regulated by magnesium, suggesting the possibility that cellular magnesium alterations are associated with the pathology of HD.[348]

ALUMINUM TRANSPORTERS AND NEURODEGENERATION

Aluminum Transporters

Consistent with other trivalent metal ion transporters, aluminum transporters include Tf, DMT1, and others. Aluminum transport and uptake into cells are somewhat mixed-up with iron, showing that aluminum competed with iron in binding Tf, and the endothelial TfR helps aluminum to cross the BBB.[349] Aluminum could induce iron deregulation in neurons of AD via stabilization of IRP2, which achieves the oxidation and degradation of IRP2 in the ubiquitin-proteosomal pathway.[350] Moreover, a recent study reported that the metal ions transporter SMF-3/DMT1 involved in aluminum transport into the neurons and induced decreases in mitochondrial membrane potential and cellular ATP levels that resulted in dopaminergic neurons degeneration. The adverse effects of aluminum were mediated by SMF-3, a homologue to the human DMT1. Mutations in SMF-3 resulted in aluminum resistance showing reduced aluminum into an intracellular compartment.[351]

Aluminum Toxicity in PD and AD

A number of studies have identified the role of aluminum in involvement of neurodegenerative diseases including PD and AD. Chronic exposure to aluminum increases the prevalence of PD in the subjects.[352] Elevated aluminum concentration is found in the SN of PD patients, suggesting that aluminum contributes to the pathogenesis of idiopathic PD.[353] Aluminum is present in the lewy bodies and induces oxidative stress in the neurons and eventually cell death.[354,355] Recently, it was determined that alpha-synuclein is involved in aluminum-induced apoptosis and oxidative stress in PC12 cells.[356]

Since 1973, it was found that AD patients contain high aluminum levels in the gray matter of the brain, indicating that aluminum is regarded as a causative factor of AD.[29] Aluminum toxicity is characterized by three forms, termed as acute, subacute, and chronic. Acute aluminum neurotoxicity occurs when aluminum levels are more than 500 μg/L. This form of neurotoxicity could cause renal failure and a encephalopathy, which represent grand mal seizures, coma, and ultimately death.[357] Subacute aluminum neurotoxicity occurs when an intermediate amount of aluminum level occurs in blood or CSF, gradually leading to dialysis encephalopathy syndrome and dementia. In addition, when chronic aluminum neurotoxicity occurs this may lead to AD development in humans.

In vitro and in vivo studies showed that aluminum enhanced hyperphosphorylation and aggregation of tau protein through inhibiting PP2A activity.[358] Consistent with AD, the aggregation of hyperphosphorylated tau protein is also identified in dialysis patient brain with high level of aluminum.[359] A number of previous studies found that aluminum could influence the role of three important genes in AD, which are AβPP, presenilin-1, and presenilin-2.[360] In the cortical neurons of AD, high level of aluminum could increase the formation of Aβ plaque and enhance amyloidogenesis.[361] Moreover, aluminum also induces the formation of NRFs in the brain of AD patients.[362]

Aluminum and Other Neurodegenerative Disorders

ALS is induced by various environmental toxins including high levels of aluminum. Studies on mice injected with aluminum hydroxide showed a half decrease in muscular strength, an increase in anxiety and cell death in the spinal cord and motor cortex, along with long-term memory loss.[363,364] These severe locomotor deficits and motor nerve loss closely resemble the pathological processes obtained in human ALS.[365]

Dialysis encephalopathy is characterized by dementia, speech trouble, convulsions, and chronic renal dysfunction.[366,367] Bone biopsy showed that higher than normal aluminum levels are present, suggesting aluminum toxicity is a causal factor associated with this disease.[368]

CONCLUSIONS

Biometals play an important role in the pathophysiological processes of neurodegenerative diseases, but the molecular mechanisms for metal dyshomeostasis are not known accurately. A number of transporters and proteins are responsible for the metal homeostasis and balance, which is an issue that also deserves further research. This chapter mainly summarizes the information on the iron, zinc, copper, manganese, magnesium, and aluminum transporters, as well as the mechanistic aspects of their function and regulation in neurodegenerative diseases. Knowledge about these biometals in brain will help to establish promissory therapeutic strategies for neurodegeneration.

References

1. LaVaute T, Smith S, Cooperman S, Iwai K, Land W, Meyron-Holtz E, et al. Targeted deletion of the gene encoding iron regulatory protein-2 causes misregulation of iron metabolism and neurodegenerative disease in mice. *Nat Genet*. 2001;27(2):209–214.
2. Lieu PT, Heiskala M, Peterson PA, Yang Y. The roles of iron in health and disease. *Mol Aspects Med*. 2001;22(1-2):1–87.
3. Perez CA, Tong Y, Guo M. Iron chelators as potential therapeutic agents for Parkinson's Disease. *Curr Bioact Compd*. 2008;4(3):150–158.
4. Zhu WZ, Zhong WD, Wang W, Zhan CJ, Wang CY, Qi JP, et al. Quantitative MR phase-corrected imaging to investigate increased brain iron deposition of patients with Alzheimer disease. *Radiology*. 2009;253(2):497–504.
5. Sian-Hulsmann J, Mandel S, Youdim MB, Riederer P. The relevance of iron in the pathogenesis of Parkinson's disease. *J Neurochem*. 2011;118(6):939–957.
6. Dexter DT, Wells FR, Lees AJ, Agid F, Agid Y, Jenner P, et al. Increased nigral iron content and alterations in other metal ions occurring in brain in Parkinson's disease. *J Neurochem*. 1989;52(6):1830–1836.
7. Sofic E, Riederer P, Heinsen H, Beckmann H, Reynolds GP, Hebenstreit G, et al. Increased iron (III) and total iron content in post mortem substantia nigra of parkinsonian brain. *J Neural Transm*. 1988;74(3):199–205.
8. Mocchegiani E, Bertoni-Freddari C, Marcellini F, Malavolta M. Brain, aging and neurodegeneration: role of zinc ion availability. *Prog Neurobiol*. 2005;75(6):367–390.
9. Jimenez-Jimenez FJ, Molina JA, Aguilar MV, Meseguer I, Mateos-Vega CJ, Gonzalez-Munoz MJ, et al. Cerebrospinal fluid levels of transition metals in patients with Parkinson's disease. *J Neural Transm*. 1998;105(4–5):497–505.
10. Dexter DT, Carayon A, Javoy-Agid F, Agid Y, Wells FR, Daniel SE, et al. Alterations in the levels of iron, ferritin and other trace metals in Parkinson's disease and other neurodegenerative diseases affecting the basal ganglia. *Brain: J Neurol*. 1991;114(Pt 4):1953–1975.
11. Loeffler DA, LeWitt PA, Juneau PL, Sima AA, Nguyen HU, DeMaggio AJ, et al. Increased regional brain concentrations of ceruloplasmin in neurodegenerative disorders. *Brain Res*. 1996;738(2):265–274.
12. Jellinger K, Kienzl E, Rumpelmair G, Riederer P, Stachelberger H, Ben-Shachar D, et al. Iron-melanin complex in substantia nigra of parkinsonian brains: an X-ray microanalysis. *J Neurochem*. 1992;59(3):1168–1171.
13. Pinero DJ, Hu J, Connor JR. Alterations in the interaction between iron regulatory proteins and their iron responsive element in normal and Alzheimer's diseased brains. *Cell Mol Biol*. 2000;46(4):761–776.
14. Pinero DJ, Li N, Hu J, Beard JL, Connor JR. The intracellular location of iron regulatory proteins is altered as a function of iron status in cell cultures and rat brain. *J Nutr*. 2001;131(11):2831–2836.
15. Altamura S, Muckenthaler MU. Iron toxicity in diseases of aging: Alzheimer's disease, Parkinson's disease and atherosclerosis. *J Alzheimer's Dis*. 2009;16(4):879–895.
16. Dedman DJ, Treffry A, Candy JM, Taylor GA, Morris CM, Bloxham CA, et al. Iron and aluminium in relation to brain ferritin in normal individuals and Alzheimer's-disease and chronic renal-dialysis patients. *Biochem J*. 1992;287(Pt 2):509–514.
17. Good PF, Perl DP, Bierer LM, Schmeidler J. Selective accumulation of aluminum and iron in the neurofibrillary tangles of Alzheimer's disease: a laser microprobe (LAMMA) study. *Ann Neurol*. 1992;31(3):286–292.
18. Koh JY. Zinc and disease of the brain. *Mol Neurobiol*. 2001;24(1–3):99–106.

19. Lovell MA, Robertson JD, Teesdale WJ, Campbell JL, Markesbery WR. Copper, iron and zinc in Alzheimer's disease senile plaques. *J Neurol Sci*. 1998;158(1):47–52.
20. Rivera-Mancia S, Perez-Neri I, Rios C, Tristan-Lopez L, Rivera-Espinosa L, Montes S. The transition metals copper and iron in neurodegenerative diseases. *Chem-Biol Interact*. 2010;186(2):184–199.
21. Bartzokis G, Tishler TA. MRI evaluation of basal ganglia ferritin iron and neurotoxicity in Alzheimer's and Huntingon's disease. *Cell Mol Biol*. 2000;46(4):821–833.
22. Newland MC, Ceckler TL, Kordower JH, Weiss B. Visualizing manganese in the primate basal ganglia with magnetic resonance imaging. *Exp Neurol*. 1989;106(3):251–258.
23. McKinney AM, Filice RW, Teksam M, Casey S, Truwit C, Clark HB, et al. Diffusion abnormalities of the globi pallidi in manganese neurotoxicity. *Neuroradiology*. 2004;46(4):291–295.
24. Benedetto A, Au C, Avila DS, Milatovic D, Aschner M. Extracellular dopamine potentiates mn-induced oxidative stress, lifespan reduction, and dopaminergic neurodegeneration in a BLI-3-dependent manner in *Caenorhabditis elegans*. *PLoS Genet*. 2010;6(8):pii: e1001084. doi: 10.1371/journal.pgen.1001084.
25. Tong Y, Yang H, Tian X, Wang H, Zhou T, Zhang S, et al. High manganese, a risk for Alzheimer's disease: high manganese induces amyloid-beta related cognitive impairment. *J Alzheimers Dis*. 2014;42(3):865–878.
26. Guilarte TR. APLP1, Alzheimer's-like pathology and neurodegeneration in the frontal cortex of manganese-exposed non-human primates. *Neurotoxicology*. 2010;31(5):572–574.
27. Veronese N, Zurlo A, Solmi M, Luchini C, Trevisan C, Bano G, et al. Magnesium status in Alzheimer's disease: a systematic review. *Am J Alzheimer's Dis Other Demen*. 2016;31(3):208–213.
28. Shindo Y, Yamanaka R, Suzuki K, Hotta K, Oka K. Intracellular magnesium level determines cell viability in the MPP+ model of Parkinson's disease. *Bba-Mol Cell Res*. 2015;1853(12):3182–3191.
29. Crapper DR, Krishnan SS, Dalton AJ. Brain aluminum distribution in Alzheimer's disease and experimental neurofibrillary degeneration. *Science*. 1973;180(4085):511–513.
30. Bharathi, Shamasundar NM, Rao TSS, Naidu MD, Ravid R, Rao KSJ. A new insight on Al-maltolate-treated aged rabbit as Alzheimer's animal model. *Brain Res Rev*. 2006;52(2):275–292.
31. Lopez V, Suzuki YA, Lonnerdal B. Ontogenic changes in lactoferrin receptor and DMT1 in mouse small intestine: implications for iron absorption during early life. *Biochem Cell Biol*. 2006;84(3):337–344.
32. Mackenzie B, Takanaga H, Hubert N, Rolfs A, Hediger MA. Functional properties of multiple isoforms of human divalent metal-ion transporter 1 (DMT1). *Biochem J*. 2007;403(1):59–69.
33. Sekyere EO, Dunn LL, Rahmanto YS, Richardson DR. Role of melanotransferrin in iron metabolism: studies using targeted gene disruption in vivo. *Blood*. 2006;107(7):2599–2601.
34. Ganz T. Cellular iron: ferroportin is the only way out. *Cell Metab*. 2005;1(3):155–157.
35. Donovan A, Brownlie A, Zhou Y, Shepard J, Pratt SJ, Moynihan J, et al. Positional cloning of zebrafish ferroportin1 identifies a conserved vertebrate iron exporter. *Nature*. 2000;403(6771):776–781.
36. Nemeth E, Tuttle MS, Powelson J, Vaughn MB, Donovan A, Ward DM, et al. Hepcidin regulates cellular iron efflux by binding to ferroportin and inducing its internalization. *Science*. 2004;306(5704):2090–2093.
37. Baumann N, Pham-Dinh D. Biology of oligodendrocyte and myelin in the mammalian central nervous system. *Physiol Rev*. 2001;81(2):871–927.
38. Benarroch EE. Brain iron homeostasis and neurodegenerative disease. *Neurology*. 2009;72(16):1436–1440.
39. Moos T, Morgan EH. Transferrin and transferrin receptor function in brain barrier systems. *Cell Mol Neurobiol*. 2000;20(1):77–95.
40. Trinder D, Baker E. Transferrin receptor 2: a new molecule in iron metabolism. *Int J Biochem Cell Biol*. 2003;35(3):292–296.
41. Waheed A, Britton RS, Grubb JH, Sly WS, Fleming RE. HFE association with transferrin receptor 2 increases cellular uptake of transferrin-bound iron. *Arch Biochem Biophys*. 2008;474(1):193–197.
42. Kawabata H, Yang R, Hirama T, Vuong PT, Kawano S, Gombart AF, et al. Molecular cloning of transferrin receptor 2. A new member of the transferrin receptor-like family. *J Biol Chem*. 1999;274(30):20826–20832.
43. Lee DW, Andersen JK. Iron elevations in the aging Parkinsonian brain: a consequence of impaired iron homeostasis?. *J Neurochem*. 2010;112(2):332–339.
44. Fleming RE. Iron sensing as a partnership: HFE and transferrin receptor 2. *Cell Metab*. 2009;9(3):211–212.
45. Ganz T. Iron homeostasis: fitting the puzzle pieces together. *Cell Metab*. 2008;7(4):288–290.
46. Kielmanowicz MG, Laham N, Coligan JE, Lemonnier F, Ehrlich R. Mouse HFE inhibits Tf-uptake and iron accumulation but induces non-transferrin bound iron (NTBI)-uptake in transformed mouse fibroblasts. *J Cell Physiol*. 2005;202(1):105–114.

47. Lee PL, Beutler E. Regulation of hepcidin and iron-overload disease. *Annu Rev Pathol*. 2009;4:489–515.
48. Waheed A, Grubb JH, Zhou XY, Tomatsu S, Fleming RE, Costaldi ME, et al. Regulation of transferrin-mediated iron uptake by HFE, the protein defective in hereditary hemochromatosis. *Proc Natl Acad Sci USA*. 2002;99(5):3117–3122.
49. Gunshin H, Mackenzie B, Berger UV, Gunshin Y, Romero MF, Boron WF, et al. Cloning and characterization of a mammalian proton-coupled metal-ion transporter. *Nature*. 1997;388(6641):482–488.
50. Fleming MD, Trenor 3rd CC, Su MA, Foernzler D, Beier DR, Dietrich WF, et al. Microcytic anaemia mice have a mutation in Nramp2, a candidate iron transporter gene. *Nat Genet*. 1997;16(4):383–386.
51. Canonne-Hergaux F, Gruenheid S, Ponka P, Gros P. Cellular and subcellular localization of the Nramp2 iron transporter in the intestinal brush border and regulation by dietary iron. *Blood*. 1999;93(12):4406–4417.
52. Lee PL, Gelbart T, West C, Halloran C, Beutler E. The human Nramp2 gene: characterization of the gene structure, alternative splicing, promoter region and polymorphisms. *Blood Cells Mol Dis*. 1998;24(2):199–215.
53. Hubert N, Hentze MW. Previously uncharacterized isoforms of divalent metal transporter (DMT)-1: implications for regulation and cellular function. *Proc Natl Acad Sci USA*. 2002;99(19):12345–12350.
54. Howitt J, Putz U, Lackovic J, Doan A, Dorstyn L, Cheng H, et al. Divalent metal transporter 1 (DMT1) regulation by Ndfip1 prevents metal toxicity in human neurons. *Proc Natl Acad Sci USA*. 2009;106(36):15489–15494.
55. Burdo JR, Menzies SL, Simpson IA, Garrick LM, Garrick MD, Dolan KG, et al. Distribution of divalent metal transporter 1 and metal transport protein 1 in the normal and Belgrade rat. *J Neurosci Res*. 2001;66(6):1198–1207.
56. Song N, Jiang H, Wang J, Xie JX. Divalent metal transporter 1 up-regulation is involved in the 6-hydroxydopamine-induced ferrous iron influx. *J Neurosci Res*. 2007;85(14):3118–3126.
57. Burdo JR, Martin J, Menzies SL, Dolan KG, Romano MA, Fletcher RJ, et al. Cellular distribution of iron in the brain of the Belgrade rat. *Neuroscience*. 1999;93(3):1189–1196.
58. Abboud S, Haile DJ. A novel mammalian iron-regulated protein involved in intracellular iron metabolism. *J Biol Chem*. 2000;275(26):19906–19912.
59. McKie AT, Marciani P, Rolfs A, Brennan K, Wehr K, Barrow D, et al. A novel duodenal iron-regulated transporter, IREG1, implicated in the basolateral transfer of iron to the circulation. *Mol Cell*. 2000;5(2):299–309.
60. Kaplan J, Kushner JP. Mining the genome for iron. *Nature*. 2000;403(6771):711–713.
61. Le NT, Richardson DR. Ferroportin1: a new iron export molecule?. *Int J Biochem Cell Biol*. 2002;34(2):103–108.
62. Jiang DH, Ke Y, Cheng YZ, Ho KP, Qian ZM. Distribution of ferroportin1 protein in different regions of developing rat brain. *Dev Neurosci*. 2002;24(2–3):94–98.
63. Wu LJ, Leenders AG, Cooperman S, Meyron-Holtz E, Smith S, Land W, et al. Expression of the iron transporter ferroportin in synaptic vesicles and the blood-brain barrier. *Brain Res*. 2004;1001(1–2):108–117.
64. Wang J, Jiang H, Xie JX. Ferroportin1 and hephaestin are involved in the nigral iron accumulation of 6-OHDA-lesioned rats. *Eur J Neurosci*. 2007;25(9):2766–2772.
65. Fillebeen C, Ruchoux MM, Mitchell V, Vincent S, Benaissa M, Pierce A. Lactoferrin is synthesized by activated microglia in the human substantia nigra and its synthesis by the human microglial CHME cell line is upregulated by tumor necrosis factor alpha or 1-methyl-4-phenylpyridinium treatment. *Brain Res*. 2001;96(1–2):103–113.
66. Baker EN, Anderson BF, Baker HM, Day CL, Haridas M, Norris GE, et al. Three-dimensional structure of lactoferrin in various functional states. *Adv Exp Med Biol*. 1994;357:1–12.
67. Vogel HJ, Schibli DJ, Jing W, Lohmeier-Vogel EM, Epand RF, Epand RM. Towards a structure-function analysis of bovine lactoferricin and related tryptophan- and arginine-containing peptides. *Biochem Cell Biol*. 2002;80(1):49–63.
68. Qiao R, Jia Q, Huwel S, Xia R, Liu T, Gao F, et al. Receptor-mediated delivery of magnetic nanoparticles across the blood-brain barrier. *ACS Nano*. 2012;6(4):3304–3310.
69. Ye Y, Sun Y, Zhao H, Lan M, Gao F, Song C, et al. A novel lactoferrin-modified beta-cyclodextrin nanocarrier for brain-targeting drug delivery. *Int J Pharm*. 2013;458(1):110–117.
70. Brown JP, Hewick RM, Hellstrom I, Hellstrom KE, Doolittle RF, Dreyer WJ. Human melanoma-associated antigen p97 is structurally and functionally related to transferrin. *Nature*. 1982;296(5853):171–173.
71. Rose TM, Plowman GD, Teplow DB, Dreyer WJ, Hellstrom KE, Brown JP. Primary structure of the human melanoma-associated antigen p97 (melanotransferrin) deduced from the mRNA sequence. *Proc Natl Acad Sci USA*. 1986;83(5):1261–1265.
72. Richardson D, Baker E. The uptake of inorganic iron complexes by human melanoma cells. *Biochimica Biophysica Acta*. 1991;1093(1):20–28.
73. Kennard ML, Richardson DR, Gabathuler R, Ponka P, Jefferies WA. A novel iron uptake mechanism mediated by GPI-anchored human p97. *EMBO Jl*. 1995;14(17):4178–4186.

74. Richardson DR. The role of the membrane-bound tumour antigen, melanotransferrin (p97), in iron uptake by the human malignant melanoma cell. *Eur J Biochem/FEBS*. 2000;267(5):1290–1298.
75. Demeule M, Poirier J, Jodoin J, Bertrand Y, Desrosiers RR, Dagenais C, et al. High transcytosis of melanotransferrin (P97) across the blood-brain barrier. *J Neurochem*. 2002;83(4):924–933.
76. Moroo I, Ujiie M, Walker BL, Tiong JW, Vitalis TZ, Karkan D, et al. Identification of a novel route of iron transcytosis across the mammalian blood-brain barrier. *Microcirculation*. 2003;10(6):457–462.
77. Suryo Rahmanto Y, Richardson DR. Generation and characterization of transgenic mice hyper-expressing melanoma tumour antigen p97 (Melanotransferrin): no overt alteration in phenotype. *Biochimica Biophysica Acta*. 2009;1793(7):1210–1217.
78. Sekyere EO, Dunn LL, Suryo Rahmanto Y, Richardson DR. Role of melanotransferrin in iron metabolism: studies using targeted gene disruption in vivo. *Blood*. 2006;107(7):2599–2601.
79. Sofic E, Paulus W, Jellinger K, Riederer P, Youdim MB. Selective increase of iron in substantia nigra zona compacta of parkinsonian brains. *Journal Neurochem*. 1991;56(3):978–982.
80. Drayer BP, Olanow W, Burger P, Johnson GA, Herfkens R, Riederer S. Parkinson plus syndrome: diagnosis using high field MR imaging of brain iron. *Radiology*. 1986;159(2):493–498.
81. Ryvlin P, Broussolle E, Piollet H, Viallet F, Khalfallah Y, Chazot G. Magnetic resonance imaging evidence of decreased putamenal iron content in idiopathic Parkinson's disease. *Arch Neurol*. 1995;52(6):583–588.
82. Good PF, Olanow CW, Perl DP. Neuromelanin-containing neurons of the substantia nigra accumulate iron and aluminum in Parkinson's disease: a LAMMA study. *Brain Res*. 1992;593(2):343–346.
83. Bandyopadhyay S, Rogers JT. Alzheimer's disease therapeutics targeted to the control of amyloid precursor protein translation: maintenance of brain iron homeostasis. *Biochem Pharmacol*. 2014;88(4):486–494.
84. Rossi M, Ruottinen H, Soimakallio S, Elovaara I, Dastidar P. Clinical MRI for iron detection in Parkinson's disease. *Clin Imaging*. 2013;37(4):631–636.
85. Wang C, Fan G, Xu K, Wang S. Quantitative assessment of iron deposition in the midbrain using 3D-enhanced T2 star weighted angiography (ESWAN): a preliminary cross-sectional study of 20 Parkinson's disease patients. *Magn Reson Imaging*. 2013;31(7):1068–1073.
86. Yu X, Du T, Song N, He Q, Shen Y, Jiang H, et al. Decreased iron levels in the temporal cortex in postmortem human brains with Parkinson disease. *Neurology*. 2013;80(5):492–495.
87. Jiang H, Wang J, Rogers J, Xie J. Brain Iron Metabolism Dysfunction in Parkinson's Disease. *Mol Neurobiol*. 2016;:[Epub ahead of print].
88. Faucheux BA, Hauw JJ, Agid Y, Hirsch EC. The density of [125I]-transferrin binding sites on perikarya of melanized neurons of the substantia nigra is decreased in Parkinson's disease. *Brain Res*. 1997;749(1):170–174.
89. Kalivendi SV, Kotamraju S, Cunningham S, Shang T, Hillard CJ, Kalyanaraman B. 1-Methyl-4-phenylpyridinium (MPP+)-induced apoptosis and mitochondrial oxidant generation: role of transferrin-receptor-dependent iron and hydrogen peroxide. *Biochem J*. 2003;371(Pt 1):151–164.
90. Kaur D, Lee D, Ragapolan S, Andersen JK. Glutathione depletion in immortalized midbrain-derived dopaminergic neurons results in increases in the labile iron pool: implications for Parkinson's disease. *Free Radic Biol Med*. 2009;46(5):593–598.
91. Mastroberardino PG, Hoffman EK, Horowitz MP, Betarbet R, Taylor G, Cheng D, et al. A novel transferrin/TfR2-mediated mitochondrial iron transport system is disrupted in Parkinson's disease. *Neurobiol Dis*. 2009;34(3):417–431.
92. Salazar J, Mena N, Hunot S, Prigent A, Alvarez-Fischer D, Arredondo M, et al. Divalent metal transporter 1 (DMT1) contributes to neurodegeneration in animal models of Parkinson's disease. *Proc Natl Acad Sci USA*. 2008;105(47):18578–18583.
93. Gunshin H, Allerson CR, Polycarpou-Schwarz M, Rofts A, Rogers JT, Kishi F, et al. Iron-dependent regulation of the divalent metal ion transporter. *FEBS Lett*. 2001;509(2):309–316.
94. Jiang H, Qian ZM, Xie JX. [Increased DMT1 expression and iron content in MPTP-treated C57BL/6 mice]. *Sheng Li Xue Bao*. 2003;55(5):571–576.
95. Lee DW, Rajagopalan S, Siddiq A, Gwiazda R, Yang L, Beal MF, et al. Inhibition of prolyl hydroxylase protects against 1-methyl-4-phenyl-1,2,3,6-tetrahydropyridine-induced neurotoxicity: model for the potential involvement of the hypoxia-inducible factor pathway in Parkinson disease. *J Biol Chem*. 2009;284(42):29065–29076.
96. Song N, Wang J, Jiang H, Xie J. Ferroportin 1 but not hephaestin contributes to iron accumulation in a cell model of Parkinson's disease. *Free Radic Biol Med*. 2010;48(2):332–341.

97. Chung J, Wessling-Resnick M. Molecular mechanisms and regulation of iron transport. *Crit Rev Clin Lab Sci.* 2003;40(2):151–182.
98. Jiang H, Song N, Xu H, Zhang S, Wang J, Xie J. Up-regulation of divalent metal transporter 1 in 6-hydroxydopamine intoxication is IRE/IRP dependent. *Cell Res.* 2010;20(3):345–356.
99. Xu H, Jiang H, Wang J, Xie J. Rg1 protects the MPP(+)-treated MES23.5 cells via attenuating DMT1 up-regulation and cellular iron uptake. *Neuropharmacology.* 2010;58(2):488–494.
100. Zhang S, Wang J, Song N, Xie J, Jiang H. Up-regulation of divalent metal transporter 1 is involved in 1-methyl-4-phenylpyridinium (MPP(+))-induced apoptosis in MES23.5 cells. *Neurobiol Aging.* 2009;30(9):1466–1476.
101. Faucheux BA, Nillesse N, Damier P, Spik G, Mouatt-Prigent A, Pierce A, et al. Expression of lactoferrin receptors is increased in the mesencephalon of patients with Parkinson disease. *Proc Natl Acad Sci USA.* 1995;92(21): 9603–9607.
102. Leveugle B, Faucheux BA, Bouras C, Nillesse N, Spik G, Hirsch EC, et al. Cellular distribution of the iron-binding protein lactotransferrin in the mesencephalon of Parkinson's disease cases. *Acta Neuropathol.* 1996;91(6):566–572.
103. Selkoe DJ. Amyloid beta-protein and the genetics of Alzheimer's disease. *J Biol Chem.* 1996;271(31):18295–18298.
104. Hardy J. Amyloid, the presenilins and Alzheimer's disease. *Trends Neurosci.* 1997;20(4):154–159.
105. Mattson MP. Cellular actions of beta-amyloid precursor protein and its soluble and fibrillogenic derivatives. *Physiol Rev.* 1997;77(4):1081–1132.
106. Mandel S, Amit T, Bar-Am O, Youdim MB. Iron dysregulation in Alzheimer's disease: multimodal brain permeable iron chelating drugs, possessing neuroprotective-neurorescue and amyloid precursor protein-processing regulatory activities as therapeutic agents. *Prog Neurobiol.* 2007;82(6):348–360.
107. Falangola MF, Lee SP, Nixon RA, Duff K, Helpern JA. Histological co-localization of iron in Abeta plaques of PS/APP transgenic mice. *Neurochem Res.* 2005;30(2):201–205.
108. Rogers JT, Randall JD, Cahill CM, Eder PS, Huang X, Gunshin H, et al. An iron-responsive element type II in the 5′-untranslated region of the Alzheimer's amyloid precursor protein transcript. *J Biol Chem.* 2002;277(47): 45518–45528.
109. Huang X, Moir RD, Tanzi RE, Bush AI, Rogers JT. Redox-active metals, oxidative stress, and Alzheimer's disease pathology. *Ann NYAcad Sci.* 2004;1012:153–163.
110. Mantyh PW, Ghilardi JR, Rogers S, DeMaster E, Allen CJ, Stimson ER, et al. Aluminum, iron, and zinc ions promote aggregation of physiological concentrations of beta-amyloid peptide. *J Neurochem.* 1993;61(3):1171–1174.
111. Schubert D, Chevion M. The role of iron in beta amyloid toxicity. *Biochem Biophys Res Commun.* 1995;216(2): 702–707.
112. Nakamura M, Shishido N, Nunomura A, Smith MA, Perry G, Hayashi Y, et al. Three histidine residues of amyloid-beta peptide control the redox activity of copper and iron. *Biochemistry.* 2007;46(44):12737–12743.
113. Perry G, Taddeo MA, Petersen RB, Castellani RJ, Harris PL, Siedlak SL, et al. Adventiously-bound redox active iron and copper are at the center of oxidative damage in Alzheimer disease. *Biometals.* 2003;16(1):77–81.
114. Zheng W, Xin N, Chi ZH, Zhao BL, Zhang J, Li JY, et al. Divalent metal transporter 1 is involved in amyloid precursor protein processing and Abeta generation. *FASEB J.* 2009;23(12):4207–4217.
115. Jefferies WA, Food MR, Gabathuler R, Rothenberger S, Yamada T, Yasuhara O, et al. Reactive microglia specifically associated with amyloid plaques in Alzheimer's disease brain tissue express melanotransferrin. *Brain Res.* 1996;712(1):122–126.
116. Kim DK, Seo MY, Lim SW, Kim S, Kim JW, Carroll BJ, et al. Serum melanotransferrin, p97 as a biochemical marker of Alzheimer's disease. *Neuropsychopharmacology.* 2001;25(1):84–90.
117. Smith MA, Kutty RK, Richey PL, Yan SD, Stern D, Chader GJ, et al. Heme oxygenase-1 is associated with the neurofibrillary pathology of Alzheimer's disease. *Am J Pathol.* 1994;145(1):42–47.
118. Firdaus WJ, Wyttenbach A, Giuliano P, Kretz-Remy C, Currie RW, Arrigo AP. Huntingtin inclusion bodies are iron-dependent centers of oxidative events. *FEBS J.* 2006;273(23):5428–5441.
119. Bartzokis G, Cummings J, Perlman S, Hance DB, Mintz J. Increased basal ganglia iron levels in Huntington disease. *Arch Neurol.* 1999;56(5):569–574.
120. Hilditch-Maguire P, Trettel F, Passani LA, Auerbach A, Persichetti F, MacDonald ME. Huntingtin: an iron-regulated protein essential for normal nuclear and perinuclear organelles. *Hum Mol Genet.* 2000;9(19):2789–2797.
121. Lumsden AL, Henshall TL, Dayan S, Lardelli MT, Richards RI. Huntingtin-deficient zebrafish exhibit defects in iron utilization and development. *Hum Mol Genet.* 2007;16(16):1905–1920.
122. Kruer MC, Paisan-Ruiz C, Boddaert N, Yoon MY, Hama H, Gregory A, et al. Defective FA2H leads to a novel form of neurodegeneration with brain iron accumulation (NBIA). *Ann Neurol.* 2010;68(5):611–618.

123. Hayflick SJ, Westaway SK, Levinson B, Zhou B, Johnson MA, Ching KH, et al. Genetic, clinical, and radiographic delineation of Hallervorden-Spatz syndrome. *N Engl J Med*. 2003;348(1):33–40.
124. Morgan NV, Westaway SK, Morton JE, Gregory A, Gissen P, Sonek S, et al. PLA2G6, encoding a phospholipase A2, is mutated in neurodegenerative disorders with high brain iron. *Nat Genet*. 2006;38(7):752–754.
125. Curtis AR, Fey C, Morris CM, Bindoff LA, Ince PG, Chinnery PF, et al. Mutation in the gene encoding ferritin light polypeptide causes dominant adult-onset basal ganglia disease. *Nat Genet*. 2001;28(4):350–354.
126. Harris ZL, Takahashi Y, Miyajima H, Serizawa M, MacGillivray RT, Gitlin JD. Aceruloplasminemia: molecular characterization of this disorder of iron metabolism. *Proc Natl Acad Sci USA*. 1995;92(7):2539–2543.
127. Berg D, Youdim MB. Role of iron in neurodegenerative disorders. *Top MagnReson Imaging.*. 2006;17(1):5–17.
128. Gonzalez-Cuyar LF, Perry G, Miyajima H, Atwood CS, Riveros-Angel M, Lyons PF, et al. Redox active iron accumulation in aceruloplasminemia. *Neuropathology*. 2008;28(5):466–471.
129. Texel SJ, Xu X, Harris ZL. Ceruloplasmin in neurodegenerative diseases. *Biochem Soc Trans*. 2008;36(Pt 6): 1277–1281.
130. Yoshida K, Furihata K, Takeda S, Nakamura A, Yamamoto K, Morita H, et al. A mutation in the ceruloplasmin gene is associated with systemic hemosiderosis in humans. *Nat Genet*. 1995;9(3):267–272.
131. Wallwork JC. Zinc and the central nervous system. *Prog Food Nutr Sci*. 1987;11(2):203–247.
132. Takeda A. Movement of zinc and its functional significance in the brain. *Brain Res Brain Res Rev*. 2000;34(3): 137–148.
133. Sensi SL, Paoletti P, Koh JY, Aizenman E, Bush AI, Hershfinkel M. The neurophysiology and pathology of brain zinc. *J Neurosci*. 2011;31(45):16076–16085.
134. Weiss JH, Sensi SL, Koh JY. Zn(2+): a novel ionic mediator of neural injury in brain disease. *Trends Pharmacol Sci*. 2000;21(10):395–401.
135. Tonder N, Johansen FF, Frederickson CJ, Zimmer J, Diemer NH. Possible role of zinc in the selective degeneration of dentate hilar neurons after cerebral ischemia in the adult rat. *Neurosci Lett*. 1990;109(3):247–252.
136. Huang L, Tepaamorndech S. The SLC30 family of zinc transporters— a review of current understanding of their biological and pathophysiological roles. *Mol Aspects Med*. 2013;34(2-3):548–560.
137. Szewczyk B. Zinc homeostasis and neurodegenerative disorders. *Front Aging Neurosci*. 2013;5:33.
138. Cousins RJ, Liuzzi JP, Lichten LA. Mammalian zinc transport, trafficking, and signals. *J Biol Chem*. 2006;281(34):24085–24089.
139. Krezel A, Hao Q, Maret W. The zinc/thiolate redox biochemistry of metallothionein and the control of zinc ion fluctuations in cell signaling. *Arch Biochem Biophys*. 2007;463(2):188–200.
140. Park JS, Blair NF, Sue CM. The role of ATP13A2 in Parkinson's disease: clinical phenotypes and molecular mechanisms. *Mov Disord*. 2015;30(6):770–779.
141. Gaither LA, Eide DJ. Eukaryotic zinc transporters and their regulation. *Biometals*. 2001;14(3-4):251–270.
142. Dufner-Beattie J, Langmade SJ, Wang F, Eide D, Andrews GK. Structure, function, and regulation of a subfamily of mouse zinc transporter genes. *J Biol Chem*. 2003;278(50):50142–50150.
143. Cragg RA, Christie GR, Phillips SR, Russi RM, Kury S, Mathers JC, et al. A novel zinc-regulated human zinc transporter, hZTL1, is localized to the enterocyte apical membrane. *J Biol Chem*. 2002;277(25):22789–22797.
144. Sekler I, Moran A, Hershfinkel M, Dori A, Margulis A, Birenzweig N, et al. Distribution of the zinc transporter ZnT-1 in comparison with chelatable zinc in the mouse brain. *J Comp Neurol*. 2002;447(3):201–209.
145. Valente T, Auladell C. Developmental expression of ZnT3 in mouse brain: correlation between the vesicular zinc transporter protein and chelatable vesicular zinc (CVZ) cells. Glial and neuronal CVZ cells interact. *Mol Cell Neurosci*. 2002;21(2):189–204.
146. Taylor KM, Nicholson RI. The LZT proteins; the LIV-1 subfamily of zinc transporters. *Biochim Biophys Acta*. 2003;1611(1–2):16–30.
147. Eide D, Broderius M, Fett J, Guerinot ML. A novel iron-regulated metal transporter from plants identified by functional expression in yeast. *Proc Natl Acad Sci USA*. 1996;93(11):5624–5628.
148. Rogers EE, Eide DJ, Guerinot ML. Altered selectivity in an Arabidopsis metal transporter. *Proc Natl Acad Sci USA*. 2000;97(22):12356–12360.
149. Belloni-Olivi L, Marshall C, Laal B, Andrews GK, Bressler J. Localization of zip1 and zip4 mRNA in the adult rat brain. *J Neurosci Res*. 2009;87(14):3221–3230.
150. Emmetsberger J, Mirrione MM, Zhou C, Fernandez-Monreal M, Siddiq MM, Ji K, et al. Tissue plasminogen activator alters intracellular sequestration of zinc through interaction with the transporter ZIP4. *J Neurosci*. 2010;30(19):6538–6547.

151. Qian J, Xu K, Yoo J, Chen TT, Andrews G, Noebels JL. Knockout of Zn transporters Zip-1 and Zip-3 attenuates seizure-induced CA1 neurodegeneration. *J Neurosci*. 2011;31(1):97–104.
152. Girijashanker K, He L, Soleimani M, Reed JM, Li H, Liu Z, et al. Slc39a14 gene encodes ZIP14, a metal/bicarbonate symporter: similarities to the ZIP8 transporter. *Mol Pharmacol*. 2008;73(5):1413–1423.
153. Grubman A, Lidgerwood GE, Duncan C, Bica L, Tan JL, Parker SJ, et al. Deregulation of subcellular biometal homeostasis through loss of the metal transporter, Zip7, in a childhood neurodegenerative disorder. *Acta Neuropathol Commun*. 2014;2:25.
154. Dufner-Beattie J, Huang ZL, Geiser J, Xu W, Andrews GK. Generation and characterization of mice lacking the zinc uptake transporter ZIP3. *Mol Cell Biol*. 2005;25(13):5607–5615.
155. Taylor KM, Morgan HE, Johnson A, Hadley LJ, Nicholson RI. Structure-function analysis of LIV-1, the breast cancer-associated protein that belongs to a new subfamily of zinc transporters. *Biochem J*. 2003;375(Pt 1):51–59.
156. Taylor KM, Morgan HE, Smart K, Zahari NM, Pumford S, Ellis IO, et al. The emerging role of the LIV-1 subfamily of zinc transporters in breast cancer. *Mol Med*. 2007;13(7–8):396–406.
157. Kagi JH, Valee BL. Metallothionein: a cadmium- and zinc-containing protein from equine renal cortex. *J Biol Chem*. 1960;235:3460–3465.
158. Uchida Y, Takio K, Titani K, Ihara Y, Tomonaga M. The growth inhibitory factor that is deficient in the Alzheimer's disease brain is a 68 amino acid metallothionein-like protein. *Neuron*. 1991;7(2):337–347.
159. Vasak M. Metallothioneins: chemical and biological challenges. *J Biol Inorg Chem*. 2011;16(7):975–976.
160. Dziegiel P, Pula B, Kobierzycki C, Stasiolek M, Podhorska-Okolow M. Metallothioneins: structure and functions. *Adv Anat Embryol Cell Biol*. 2016;218:3–20.
161. Vasak M, Hasler DW. Metallothioneins: new functional and structural insights. *Curr Opin Chem Biol*. 2000;4(2):177–183.
162. Karin M, Eddy RL, Henry WM, Haley LL, Byers MG, Shows TB. Human metallothionein genes are clustered on chromosome 16. *Proc Natl Acad Sci USA*. 1984;81(17):5494–5498.
163. West AK, Stallings R, Hildebrand CE, Chiu R, Karin M, Richards RI. Human metallothionein genes: structure of the functional locus at 16q13. *Genomics*. 1990;8(3):513–518.
164. Palmiter RD. The elusive function of metallothioneins. *Proc Natl Acad Sci USA*. 1998;95(15):8428–8430.
165. West AK, Hidalgo J, Eddins D, Levin ED, Aschner M. Metallothionein in the central nervous system: roles in protection, regeneration and cognition. *Neurotoxicology*. 2008;29(3):489–503.
166. Kimura T, Kambe T. The functions of metallothionein and ZIP and ZnT transporters: an overview and perspective. *Int J Mol Sci*. 2016;17(3).
167. van Lookeren Campagne M, Thibodeaux H, van Bruggen N, Cairns B, Lowe DG. Increased binding activity at an antioxidant-responsive element in the metallothionein-1 promoter and rapid induction of metallothionein-1 and -2 in response to cerebral ischemia and reperfusion. *J Neurosci*. 2000;20(14):5200–5207.
168. Searle PF, Davison BL, Stuart GW, Wilkie TM, Norstedt G, Palmiter RD. Regulation, linkage, and sequence of mouse metallothionein I and II genes. *Mol Cell Biol*. 1984;4(7):1221–1230.
169. Mocchegiani E, Giacconi R, Cipriano C, Muzzioli M, Fattoretti P, Bertoni-Freddari C, et al. Zinc-bound metallothioneins as potential biological markers of ageing. *Brain Res Bull*. 2001;55(2):147–153.
170. Nordberg M. Metallothioneins: historical review and state of knowledge. *Talanta*. 1998;46(2):243–254.
171. Palmiter RD, Findley SD, Whitmore TE, Durnam DM. MT-III, a brain-specific member of the metallothionein gene family. *Proc Natl Acad Sci USA*. 1992;89(14):6333–6337.
172. Leung YK, Pankhurst M, Dunlop SA, Ray S, Dittmann J, Eaton ED, et al. Metallothionein induces a regenerative reactive astrocyte phenotype via JAK/STAT and RhoA signalling pathways. *Exp Neurol*. 2010;221(1):98–106.
173. Michael GJ, Esmailzadeh S, Moran LB, Christian L, Pearce RK, Graeber MB. Up-regulation of metallothionein gene expression in parkinsonian astrocytes. *Neurogenetics*. 2011;12(4):295–305.
174. Wunderlich KA, Leveillard T, Penkowa M, Zrenner E, Perez MT. Altered expression of metallothionein-I and -II and their receptor megalin in inherited photoreceptor degeneration. *Invest Ophthalmol Vis Sci*. 2010;51(9):4809–4820.
175. Penkowa M, Caceres M, Borup R, Nielsen FC, Poulsen CB, Quintana A, et al. Novel roles for metallothionein-I + II (MT-I + II) in defense responses, neurogenesis, and tissue restoration after traumatic brain injury: insights from global gene expression profiling in wild-type and MT-I + II knockout mice. *J Neurosci Res*. 2006;84(7):1452–1474.
176. Hozumi I, Inuzuka T, Tsuji S. Brain injury and growth inhibitory factor (GIF)—a minireview. *Neurochem Res*. 1998;23(3):319–328.

177. Inuzuka T, Hozumi I, Tamura A, Hiraiwa M, Tsuji S. Patterns of growth inhibitory factor (GIF) and glial fibrillary acidic protein relative level changes differ following left middle cerebral artery occlusion in rats. *Brain Res*. 1996;709(1):151–231.
178. Vasak M, Meloni G. Chemistry and biology of mammalian metallothioneins. *J Biol Inorg Chem*. 2011;16(7): 1067–1078.
179. Bremner I. Nutritional and physiological significance of metallothionein. *Experientia Suppl*. 1987;52:81–107.
180. Sato M, Bremner I. Oxygen free radicals and metallothionein. *Free Radic Biol Med*. 1993;14(3):325–337.
181. Juarez-Rebollar D, Manjarrez J, Nava-Ruiz C, Zaga-Clavellina V, Flores-Espinosa P, Heras-Romero Y, et al. Metallothionein expression in the rat brain following KA and PTZ treatment. *Environ Toxicol Pharmacol*. 2015;40(2):530–534.
182. Murakami S, Miyazaki I, Sogawa N, Miyoshi K, Asanuma M. Neuroprotective effects of metallothionein against rotenone-induced myenteric neurodegeneration in parkinsonian mice. *Neurotox Res*. 2014;26(3):285–298.
183. Yuan Y, Niu F, Liu Y, Lu N. Zinc and its effects on oxidative stress in Alzheimer's disease. *Neurol Sci*. 2014;35(6):923–928.
184. Kim JH, Nam YP, Jeon SM, Han HS, Suk K. Amyloid neurotoxicity is attenuated by metallothionein: dual mechanisms at work. *J Neurochem*. 2012;121(5):751–762.
185. Adlard PA, Parncutt JM, Finkelstein DI, Bush AI. Cognitive loss in zinc transporter-3 knock-out mice: a phenocopy for the synaptic and memory deficits of Alzheimer's disease?. *J Neurosci*. 2010;30(5):1631–1636.
186. Hashimoto K, Hayashi Y, Watabe K, Inuzuka T, Hozumi I. Metallothionein-III prevents neuronal death and prolongs life span in amyotrophic lateral sclerosis model mice. *Neuroscience*. 2011;189:293–298.
187. Morahan JM, Yu B, Trent RJ, Pamphlett R. Are metallothionein genes silenced in ALS?. *Toxicol Lett*. 2007;168(1):83–87.
188. Ono S, Endo Y, Tokuda E, Ishige K, Tabata K, Asami S, et al. Upregulation of metallothionein-I mRNA expression in a rodent model for amyotrophic lateral sclerosis. *Biol Trace Elem Res*. 2006;113(1):93–104.
189. Espejo C, Martinez-Caceres EM. The role of methallothioneins in experimental autoimmune encephalomyelitis and multiple sclerosis. *Ann NY Acad Sci*. 2005;1051:88–96.
190. Penkowa M, Espejo C, Ortega-Aznar A, Hidalgo J, Montalban X, Martinez Caceres EM. Metallothionein expression in the central nervous system of multiple sclerosis patients. *Cell Mol Life Sci*. 2003;60(6):1258–1266.
191. Adam P, Krizkova S, Heger Z, Babula P, Pekarik V, Vaculovicoa M, et al. Metallothioneins in prion- and amyloid-related diseases. *J Alzheimers Dis*. 2016;51(3):637–656.
192. Chung RS, Leung YK, Butler CW, Chen Y, Eaton ED, Pankhurst MW, et al. Metallothionein treatment attenuates microglial activation and expression of neurotoxic quinolinic acid following traumatic brain injury. *Neurotox Res*. 2009;15(4):381–389.
193. Pedersen MO, Larsen A, Stoltenberg M, Penkowa M. Cell death in the injured brain: roles of metallothioneins. *Prog Histochem Cytochem*. 2009;44(1):1–27.
194. Diaz-Ruiz A, Vacio-Adame P, Monroy-Noyola A, Mendez-Armenta M, Ortiz-Plata A, Montes S, et al. Metallothionein-II inhibits lipid peroxidation and improves functional recovery after transient brain ischemia and reperfusion in rats. *Oxid Med Cell Longev*. 2014;2014:436429.
195. Ito Y, Tanaka H, Hara H. The potential roles of metallothionein as a therapeutic target for cerebral ischemia and retinal diseases. *Curr Pharm Biotechnol*. 2013;14(4):400–407.
196. Sharma S, Ebadi M. Significance of metallothioneins in aging brain. *Neurochem Int*. 2014;65:40–48.
197. Ambjorn M, Asmussen JW, Lindstam M, Gotfryd K, Jacobsen C, Kiselyov VV, et al. Metallothionein and a peptide modeled after metallothionein, EmtinB, induce neuronal differentiation and survival through binding to receptors of the low-density lipoprotein receptor family. *J Neurochem*. 2008;104(1):21–37.
198. Inoue K, Takano H, Shimada A, Satoh M. Metallothionein as an anti-inflammatory mediator. *Mediators Inflamm*. 2009;2009:101659.
199. Penkowa M. Metallothionein I + II expression and roles during neuropathology in the CNS. *Dan Med Bull*. 2006;53(2):105–121.
200. Dhanasekaran M, Albano CB, Pellet L, Karuppagounder SS, Uthayathas S, Suppiramaniam V, et al. Role of lipoamide dehydrogenase and metallothionein on 1-methyl-4-phenyl-1,2,3,6- tetrahydropyridine-induced neurotoxicity. *Neurochem Res*. 2008;33(6):980–984.
201. Ono S, Hirai K, Tokuda E. Effects of pergolide mesilate on metallothionein mRNAs expression in a mouse model for Parkinson disease. *Biol Pharm Bull*. 2009;32(10):1813–1817.
202. Asanuma M, Miyazaki I, Higashi Y, Tanaka K, Haque ME, Fujita N, et al. Aggravation of 6-hydroxydopamine-induced dopaminergic lesions in metallothionein-I and -II knock-out mouse brain. *Neurosci Lett*. 2002;327(1):61–65.

203. Miyazaki I, Asanuma M, Hozumi H, Miyoshi K, Sogawa N. Protective effects of metallothionein against dopamine quinone-induced dopaminergic neurotoxicity. *FEBS Lett*. 2007;581(25):5003–5008.
204. Reinecke F, Levanets O, Olivier Y, Louw R, Semete B, Grobler A, et al. Metallothionein isoform 2A expression is inducible and protects against ROS-mediated cell death in rotenone-treated HeLa cells. *Biochem J*. 2006;395(2):405–415.
205. Jing L, Li L, Zhao J, Sun Z, Peng S. Zinc-induced metallothionein overexpression prevents doxorubicin toxicity in cardiomyocytes by regulating the peroxiredoxins. *Xenobiotica*. 2016;46(8):715–725.
206. Lim KS, Cha MJ, Kim JK, Park EJ, Chae JW, Rhim T, et al. Protective effects of protein transduction domain-metallothionein fusion proteins against hypoxia- and oxidative stress-induced apoptosis in an ischemia/reperfusion rat model. *J Control Release*. 2013;169(3):306–312.
207. Miyazaki I, Asanuma M, Kikkawa Y, Takeshima M, Murakami S, Miyoshi K, et al. Astrocyte-derived metallothionein protects dopaminergic neurons from dopamine quinone toxicity. *Glia*. 2011;59(3):435–451.
208. Zhang LH, Wang X, Stoltenberg M, Danscher G, Huang L, Wang ZY. Abundant expression of zinc transporters in the amyloid plaques of Alzheimer's disease brain. *Brain Res Bull*. 2008;77(1):55–60.
209. Zhang LH, Wang X, Zheng ZH, Ren H, Stoltenberg M, Danscher G, et al. Altered expression and distribution of zinc transporters in APP/PS1 transgenic mouse brain. *Neurobiol Aging*. 2010;31(1):74–87.
210. Zheng W, Wang T, Yu D, Feng WY, Nie YX, Stoltenberg M, et al. Elevation of zinc transporter ZnT3 protein in the cerebellar cortex of the AbetaPP/PS1 transgenic mouse. *J Alzheimers Dis*. 2010;20(1):323–331.
211. Lee JY, Cole TB, Palmiter RD, Suh SW, Koh JY. Contribution by synaptic zinc to the gender-disparate plaque formation in human Swedish mutant APP transgenic mice. *Proc Natl Acad Sci USA*. 2002;99(11):7705–7710.
212. Li LB, Wang ZY. Disruption of brain zinc homeostasis promotes the pathophysiological progress of Alzheimer's disease. *Histol Histopathol*. 2016;31(6):623–627.
213. Carrasco J, Adlard P, Cotman C, Quintana A, Penkowa M, Xu F, et al. Metallothionein-I and -III expression in animal models of Alzheimer disease. *Neuroscience*. 2006;143(4):911–922.
214. Martinho A, Goncalves I, Cardoso I, Almeida MR, Quintela T, Saraiva MJ, et al. Human metallothioneins 2 and 3 differentially affect amyloid-beta binding by transthyretin. *FEBS J*. 2010;277(16):3427–3436.
215. Manso Y, Carrasco J, Comes G, Adlard PA, Bush AI, Hidalgo J. Characterization of the role of the antioxidant proteins metallothioneins 1 and 2 in an animal model of Alzheimer's disease. *Cell Mol Life Sci*. 2012;69(21):3665–3681.
216. Meloni G, Sonois V, Delaine T, Guilloreau L, Gillet A, Teissie J, et al. Metal swap between Zn7-metallothionein-3 and amyloid-beta-Cu protects against amyloid-beta toxicity. *Nat Chem Biol*. 2008;4(6):366–372.
217. Martin BL, Tokheim AM, McCarthy PT, Doms BS, Davis AA, Armitage IM. Metallothionein-3 and neuronal nitric oxide synthase levels in brains from the Tg2576 mouse model of Alzheimer's disease. *Mol Cell Biochem*. 2006;283(1-2):129–137.
218. Uchida Y, Tomonaga M. Neurotrophic action of Alzheimer's disease brain extract is due to the loss of inhibitory factors for survival and neurite formation of cerebral cortical neurons. *Brain Res*. 1989;481(1):190–193.
219. Durand J, Meloni G, Talmard C, Vasak M, Faller P. Zinc release of Zn(7)-metallothionein-3 induces fibrillar type amyloid-beta aggregates. *Metallomics*. 2010;2(11):741–744.
220. Tougu V, Karafin A, Zovo K, Chung RS, Howells C, West AK, et al. Zn(II)- and Cu(II)-induced non-fibrillar aggregates of amyloid-beta (1-42) peptide are transformed to amyloid fibrils, both spontaneously and under the influence of metal chelators. *J Neurochem*. 2009;110(6):1784–1795.
221. Manso Y, Carrasco J, Comes G, Meloni G, Adlard PA, Bush AI, et al. Characterization of the role of metallothionein-3 in an animal model of Alzheimer's disease. *Cell Mol Life Sci*. 2012;69(21):3683–3700.
222. Lee SJ, Seo BR, Koh JY. Metallothionein-3 modulates the amyloid beta endocytosis of astrocytes through its effects on actin polymerization. *Mol Brain*. 2015;8(1):84.
223. Uchida Y, Gomi F, Masumizu T, Miura Y. Growth inhibitory factor prevents neurite extension and the death of cortical neurons caused by high oxygen exposure through hydroxyl radical scavenging. *J Biol Chem*. 2002;277(35):32353–32359.
224. Pedersen JT, Hureau C, Hemmingsen L, Heegaard NH, Ostergaard J, Vasak M, et al. Rapid exchange of metal between Zn(7)-metallothionein-3 and amyloid-beta peptide promotes amyloid-related structural changes. *Biochemistry*. 2012;51(8):1697–1706.
225. Kawashima T, Doh-ura K, Torisu M, Uchida Y, Furuta A, Iwaki T. Differential expression of metallothioneins in human prion diseases. *Dement Geriatr Cogn Disord*. 2000;11(5):251–262.
226. Zhou X, Yang C, Liu Y, Li P, Yang H, Dai J, et al. Lipid rafts participate in aberrant degradative autophagic-lysosomal pathway of amyloid-beta peptide in Alzheimer's disease. *Neural Regen Res*. 2014;9(1):92–100.

227. Watt NT, Taylor DR, Kerrigan TL, Griffiths HH, Rushworth JV, Whitehouse IJ, et al. Prion protein facilitates uptake of zinc into neuronal cells. *Nat Commun*. 2012;3:1134.
228. Ishigaki S, Niwa J, Ando Y, Yoshihara T, Sawada K, Doyu M, et al. Differentially expressed genes in sporadic amyotrophic lateral sclerosis spinal cords—screening by molecular indexing and subsequent cDNA microarray analysis. *FEBS Lett*. 2002;531(2):354–358.
229. Hozumi I, Yamada M, Uchida Y, Ozawa K, Takahashi H, Inuzuka T. The expression of metallothioneins is diminished in the spinal cords of patients with sporadic ALS. *Amyotroph Lateral Scler*. 2008;9(5):294–298.
230. Gong YH, Elliott JL. Metallothionein expression is altered in a transgenic murine model of familial amyotrophic lateral sclerosis. *Exp Neurol*. 2000;162(1):27–36.
231. Tokuda E, Ono S, Ishige K, Naganuma A, Ito Y, Suzuki T. Metallothionein proteins expression, copper and zinc concentrations, and lipid peroxidation level in a rodent model for amyotrophic lateral sclerosis. *Toxicology*. 2007;229(1-2):33–41.
232. Puttaparthi K, Gitomer WL, Krishnan U, Son M, Rajendran B, Elliott JL. Disease progression in a transgenic model of familial amyotrophic lateral sclerosis is dependent on both neuronal and non-neuronal zinc binding proteins. *J Neurosci*. 2002;22(20):8790–8796.
233. Tokuda E, Okawa E, Watanabe S, Ono S. Overexpression of metallothionein-I, a copper-regulating protein, attenuates intracellular copper dyshomeostasis and extends lifespan in a mouse model of amyotrophic lateral sclerosis caused by mutant superoxide dismutase-1. *Hum Mol Genet*. 2014;23(5):1271–1285.
234. Penkowa M, Hidalgo J. Metallothionein treatment reduces proinflammatory cytokines IL-6 and TNF-alpha and apoptotic cell death during experimental autoimmune encephalomyelitis (EAE). *Exp Neurol*. 2001;170(1):1–14.
235. Brewer GJ. The risks of free copper in the body and the development of useful anticopper drugs. *Curr Opin Clin Nutr Metab Care*. 2008;11(6):727–732.
236. Bauerly KA, Kelleher SL, Lonnerdal B. Functional and molecular responses of suckling rat pups and human intestinal Caco-2 cells to copper treatment. *J Nutr Biochem*. 2004;15(3):155–162.
237. Kuo YM, Gybina AA, Pyatskowit JW, Gitschier J, Prohaska JR. Copper transport protein (Ctr1) levels in mice are tissue specific and dependent on copper status. *J Nutr*. 2006;136(1):21–26.
238. Qian Y, Tiffany-Castiglioni E, Welsh J, Harris ED. Copper efflux from murine microvascular cells requires expression of the menkes disease Cu-ATPase. *J Nutr*. 1998;128(8):1276–1282.
239. Niciu MJ, Ma XM, El Meskini R, Pachter JS, Mains RE, Eipper BA. Altered ATP7A expression and other compensatory responses in a murine model of Menkes disease. *Neurobiol Dis*. 2007;27(3):278–291.
240. Zheng W, Monnot AD. Regulation of brain iron and copper homeostasis by brain barrier systems: implication in neurodegenerative diseases. *Pharmacol Ther*. 2012;133(2):177–188.
241. Harris ED. Copper homeostasis: the role of cellular transporters. *Nutr Rev*. 2001;59(9):281–285.
242. Davies KM, Hare DJ, Cottam V, Chen N, Hilgers L, Halliday G, et al. Localization of copper and copper transporters in the human brain. *Metallomics*. 2013;5(1):43–51.
243. Gaggelli E, Kozlowski H, Valensin D, Valensin G. Copper homeostasis and neurodegenerative disorders (Alzheimer's, prion, and Parkinson's diseases and amyotrophic lateral sclerosis). *Chem Rev*. 2006;106(6):1995–2044.
244. Klomp AE, Tops BB, Van Denberg IE, Berger R, Klomp LW. Biochemical characterization and subcellular localization of human copper transporter 1 (hCTR1). *Biochem J*. 2002;364(Pt 2):497–505.
245. Choi BS, Zheng W. Copper transport to the brain by the blood-brain barrier and blood-CSF barrier. *Brain Res*. 2009;1248:14–21.
246. Bull PC, Thomas GR, Rommens JM, Forbes JR, Cox DW. The Wilson disease gene is a putative copper transporting P-type ATPase similar to the Menkes gene. *Nat Genet*. 1993;5(4):327–337.
247. Chelly J, Tumer Z, Tonnesen T, Petterson A, Ishikawa-Brush Y, Tommerup N, et al. Isolation of a candidate gene for Menkes disease that encodes a potential heavy metal binding protein. *Nat Genet*. 1993;3(1):14–19.
248. Mercer JF, Livingston J, Hall B, Paynter JA, Begy C, Chandrasekharappa S, et al. Isolation of a partial candidate gene for Menkes disease by positional cloning. *Nat Genet*. 1993;3(1):20–25.
249. Vulpe C, Levinson B, Whitney S, Packman S, Gitschier J. Isolation of a candidate gene for Menkes disease and evidence that it encodes a copper-transporting ATPase. *Nat Genet*. 1993;3(1):7–13.
250. Iwase T, Nishimura M, Sugimura H, Igarashi H, Ozawa F, Shinmura K, et al. Localization of Menkes gene expression in the mouse brain; its association with neurological manifestations in Menkes model mice. *Acta Neuropathol*. 1996;91(5):482–488.
251. Saito T, Okabe M, Hosokawa T, Kurasaki M, Hata A, Endo F, et al. Immunohistochemical determination of the Wilson Copper-transporting P-type ATPase in the brain tissues of the rat. *Neurosci Lett*. 1999;266(1):13–16.

252. Telianidis J, Hung YH, Materia S, Fontaine SL. Role of the P-Type ATPases, ATP7A and ATP7B in brain copper homeostasis. *Front Aging Neurosci*. 2013;5:44.
253. Gorell JM, Johnson CC, Rybicki BA, Peterson EL, Kortsha GX, Brown GG, et al. Occupational exposure to manganese, copper, lead, iron, mercury and zinc and the risk of Parkinson's disease. *Neurotoxicology*. 1999;20(2-3):239–247.
254. Willis AW, Evanoff BA, Lian M, Galarza A, Wegrzyn A, Schootman M, et al. Metal emissions and urban incident Parkinson disease: a community health study of Medicare beneficiaries by using geographic information systems. *Am J Epidemiol*. 2010;172(12):1357–1363.
255. Davies KM, Bohic S, Carmona A, Ortega R, Cottam V, Hare DJ, et al. Copper pathology in vulnerable brain regions in Parkinson's disease. *Neurobiol Aging*. 2014;35(4):858–866.
256. Popescu BF, Robinson CA, Rajput A, Rajput AH, Harder SL, Nichol H. Iron, copper, and zinc distribution of the cerebellum. *Cerebellum*. 2009;8(2):74–79.
257. Ayton S, Lei P, Duce JA, Wong BX, Sedjahtera A, Adlard PA, et al. Ceruloplasmin dysfunction and therapeutic potential for Parkinson disease. *Ann Neurol*. 2013;73(4):554–559.
258. Martinez-Hernandez R, Montes S, Higuera-Calleja J, Yescas P, Boll MC, Diaz-Ruiz A, et al. Plasma ceruloplasmin ferroxidase activity correlates with the nigral sonographic area in Parkinson's disease patients: a pilot study. *Neurochem Res*. 2011;36(11):2111–2115.
259. Bharucha KJ, Friedman JK, Vincent AS, Ross ED. Lower serum ceruloplasmin levels correlate with younger age of onset in Parkinson's disease. *J Neurol*. 2008;255(12):1957–1962.
260. Jimenez-Jimenez FJ, Fernandez-Calle P, Martinez-Vanaclocha M, Herrero E, Molina JA, Vazquez A, et al. Serum levels of zinc and copper in patients with Parkinson's disease. *J Neurol Sci*. 1992;112(1-2):30–33.
261. Torsdottir G, Kristinsson J, Sveinbjornsdottir S, Snaedal J, Johannesson T. Copper, ceruloplasmin, superoxide dismutase and iron parameters in Parkinson's disease. *Pharmacol Toxicol*. 1999;85(5):239–243.
262. Mariani S, Ventriglia M, Simonelli I, Donno S, Bucossi S, Vernieri F, et al. Fe and Cu do not differ in Parkinson's disease: a replication study plus meta-analysis. *Neurobiol Aging*. 2013;34(2):632–633.
263. Mackenzie NC, Brito M, Reyes AE, Allende ML. Cloning, expression pattern and essentiality of the high-affinity copper transporter 1 (ctrl) gene in zebrafish. *Gene*. 2004;328:113–120.
264. Sechi G, Antonio Cocco G, Errigo A, Deiana L, Rosati G, Agnetti V, et al. Three sisters with very-late-onset major depression and parkinsonism. *Parkinsonism Relat Disord*. 2007;13(2):122–125.
265. Bush AI, Pettingell WH, Multhaup G, d Paradis M, Vonsattel JP, Gusella JF, et al. Rapid induction of Alzheimer A beta amyloid formation by zinc. *Science*. 1994;265(5177):1464–1467.
266. Cherny RA, Legg JT, McLean CA, Fairlie DP, Huang X, Atwood CS, et al. Aqueous dissolution of Alzheimer's disease Abeta amyloid deposits by biometal depletion. *J Biol Chem*. 1999;274(33):23223–23228.
267. Dong J, Atwood CS, Anderson VE, Siedlak SL, Smith MA, Perry G, et al. Metal binding and oxidation of amyloid-beta within isolated senile plaque cores: Raman microscopic evidence. *Biochemistry*. 2003;42(10):2768–2773.
268. Phinney AL, Horne P, Yang J, Janus C, Bergeron C, Westaway D. Mouse models of Alzheimer's disease: the long and filamentous road. *Neurolo Res*. 2003;25(6):590–600.
269. Sparks DL, Schreurs BG. Trace amounts of copper in water induce beta-amyloid plaques and learning deficits in a rabbit model of Alzheimer's disease. *Proc Natl Acad Sci USA*. 2003;100(19):11065–11069.
270. Ventriglia M, Bucossi S, Panetta V, Squitti R. Copper in Alzheimer's disease: a meta-analysis of serum, plasma, and cerebrospinal fluid studies. *J Alzheimers Dis*. 2012;30(4):981–984.
271. Arnal N, Morel GR, de Alaniz MJ, Castillo O, Marra CA. Role of copper and cholesterol association in the neurodegenerative process. *Int J Alzheimers Dis*. 2013;2013:414817.
272. Lang M, Fan Q, Wang L, Zheng Y, Xiao G, Wang X, et al. Inhibition of human high-affinity copper importer Ctr1 orthologous in the nervous system of Drosophila ameliorates Abeta42-induced Alzheimer's disease-like symptoms. *Neurobiol Aging*. 2013;34(11):2604–2612.
273. Bucossi S, Mariani S, Ventriglia M, Polimanti R, Gennarelli M, Bonvicini C, et al. Association between the c. 2495 A>G ATP7B Polymorphism and Sporadic Alzheimer's Disease. *Int J Alzheimers Dis*. 2011;2011:973692.
274. Bucossi S, Polimanti R, Mariani S, Ventriglia M, Bonvicini C, Migliore S, et al. Association of K832R and R952K SNPs of Wilson's disease gene with Alzheimer's disease. *J Alzheimers Dis*. 2012;29(4):913–919.
275. Squitti R, Polimanti R, Bucossi S, Ventriglia M, Mariani S, Manfellotto D, et al. Linkage disequilibrium and haplotype analysis of the ATP7B gene in Alzheimer's disease. *Rejuvenation Res*. 2013;16(1):3–10.
276. Bucossi S, Polimanti R, Ventriglia M, Mariani S, Siotto M, Ursini F, et al. Intronic rs2147363 variant in ATP7B transcription factor-binding site associated with Alzheimer's disease. *J Alzheimers Dis*. 2013;37(2):453–459.

277. Erikson KM, John CE, Jones SR, Aschner M. Manganese accumulation in striatum of mice exposed to toxic doses is dependent upon a functional dopamine transporter. *Environ Toxicol Pharmacol*. 2005;20(3):390–394.
278. Garrick MD, Singleton ST, Vargas F, Kuo HC, Zhao L, Knopfel M, et al. DMT1: which metals does it transport?. *Biol Res*. 2006;39(1):79–85.
279. Subramaniam VN, Summerville L, Wallace DF. Molecular and cellular characterization of transferrin receptor 2. *Cell Biochem Biophys*. 2002;36(2-3):235–239.
280. Genter MB, Kendig EL, Knutson MD. Uptake of materials from the nasal cavity into the blood and brain: are we finally beginning to understand these processes at the molecular level?. *Ann NY Acad Sci*. 2009;1170:623–628.
281. Lucaciu CM, Dragu C, Copaescu L, Morariu VV. Manganese transport through human erythrocyte membranes. An EPR study. *Biochimica Biophysica Acta*. 1997;1328(2):90–98.
282. Dobrydneva Y, Blackmore P. 2-Aminoethoxydiphenyl borate directly inhibits store-operated calcium entry channels in human platelets. *Mol Pharmacol*. 2001;60(3):541–552.
283. Baldi C, Vazquez G, Boland R. Characterization of a 1,25(OH)2-vitamin D3-responsive capacitative Ca2+ entry pathway in rat osteoblast-like cells. *J Cell Biochem*. 2002;86(4):678–687.
284. Quadri M, Federico A, Zhao T, Breedveld GJ, Battisti C, Delnooz C, et al. Mutations in SLC30A10 cause parkinsonism and dystonia with hypermanganesemia, polycythemia, and chronic liver disease. *Am J Hum Genet*. 2012;90(3):467–477.
285. Tuschl K, Clayton PT, Gospe Jr SM, Gulab S, Ibrahim S, Singhi P, et al. Syndrome of hepatic cirrhosis, dystonia, polycythemia, and hypermanganesemia caused by mutations in SLC30A10, a manganese transporter in man. *Am J Hum Genet*. 2012;90(3):457–466.
286. Leyva-Illades D, Chen P, Zogzas CE, Hutchens S, Mercado JM, Swaim CD, et al. SLC30A10 is a cell surface-localized manganese efflux transporter, and parkinsonism-causing mutations block its intracellular trafficking and efflux activity. *J Neurosc*. 2014;34(42):14079–14095.
287. Madejczyk MS, Ballatori N. The iron transporter ferroportin can also function as a manganese exporter. *Biochimica Biophysica Acta*. 2012;1818(3):651–657.
288. Chen P, Chakraborty S, Mukhopadhyay S, Lee E, Paoliello MM, Bowman AB, et al. Manganese homeostasis in the nervous system. *J Neurochem*. 2015;134(4):601–610.
289. Ciliax BJ, Heilman C, Demchyshyn LL, Pristupa ZB, Ince E, Hersch SM, et al. The dopamine transporter: immunochemical characterization and localization in brain. *J Neurosci*. 1995;15(3 Pt 1):1714–1723.
290. Anderson JG, Cooney PT, Erikson KM. Inhibition of DAT function attenuates manganese accumulation in the globus pallidus. *Environ Toxicol Pharmacol*. 2007;23(2):179–184.
291. Schultheis PJ, Hagen TT, O'Toole KK, Tachibana A, Burke CR, McGill DL, et al. Characterization of the P5 subfamily of P-type transport ATPases in mice. *Biochem Biophys Res Commun*. 2004;323(3):731–738.
292. Gitler AD, Chesi A, Geddie ML, Strathearn KE, Hamamichi S, Hill KJ, et al. Alpha-synuclein is part of a diverse and highly conserved interaction network that includes PARK9 and manganese toxicity. *Nat Genet*. 2009;41(3):308–315.
293. Di Fonzo A, Chien HF, Socal M, Giraudo S, Tassorelli C, Iliceto G, et al. ATP13A2 missense mutations in juvenile parkinsonism and young onset Parkinson disease. *Neurology*. 2007;68(19):1557–1562.
294. Kong SMY, Chan BKK, Park JS, Hill KJ, Aitken JB, Cottle L, et al. Parkinson's disease-linked human PARK9/ATP13A2 maintains zinc homeostasis and promotes alpha-Synuclein externalization via exosomes. *Hum Mol Genet*. 2014;23(11):2816–2833.
295. Tan J, Zhang T, Jiang L, Chi J, Hu D, Pan Q, et al. Regulation of intracellular manganese homeostasis by Kufor–Rakeb syndrome-associated ATP13A2 protein. *J Bioll Chem*. 2011;286(34):29654–29662.
296. Gunteski-Hamblin AM, Clarke DM, Shull GE. Molecular cloning and tissue distribution of alternatively spliced mRNAs encoding possible mammalian homologues of the yeast secretory pathway calcium pump. *Biochemistry*. 1992;31(33):7600–7608.
297. Hu Z, Bonifas JM, Beech J, Bench G, Shigihara T, Ogawa H, et al. Mutations in ATP2C1, encoding a calcium pump, cause Hailey-Hailey disease. *Nat Genet*. 2000;24(1):61–65.
298. Ton VK, Mandal D, Vahadji C, Rao R. Functional expression in yeast of the human secretory pathway Ca(2+), Mn(2+)-ATPase defective in Hailey-Hailey disease. *J Biol Chem*. 2002;277(8):6422–6427.
299. Ordonez-Librado JL, Anaya-Martinez V, Gutierrez-Valdez AL, Colin-Barenque L, Montiel-Flores E, Avila-Costa MR. Manganese inhalation as a Parkinson disease model. *Parkinson's Dis*. 2010;2011:612989.
300. Sanchez-Betancourt J, Anaya-Martinez V, Gutierrez-Valdez AL, Ordonez-Librado JL, Montiel-Flores E, Espinosa-Villanueva J, et al. Manganese mixture inhalation is a reliable Parkinson disease model in rats. *Neurotoxicology*. 2012;33(5):1346–1355.

301. Erikson KM, Shihabi ZK, Aschner JL, Aschner M. Manganese accumulates in iron-deficient rat brain regions in a heterogeneous fashion and is associated with neurochemical alterations. *Biol Trace Elem Res*. 2002;87(1–3):143–156.
302. He Q, Du T, Yu X, Xie A, Song N, Kang Q, et al. DMT1 polymorphism and risk of Parkinson's disease. *Neurosci Lett*. 2011;501(3):128–131.
303. Gunter TE, Gerstner B, Gunter KK, Malecki J, Gelein R, Valentine WM, et al. Manganese transport via the transferrin mechanism. *Neurotoxicology*. 2013;34:118–127.
304. Roth JA, Horbinski C, Higgins D, Lein P, Garrick MD. Mechanisms of manganese-induced rat pheochromocytoma (PC12) cell death and cell differentiation. *Neurotoxicology*. 2002;23(2):147–157.
305. Au C, Benedetto A, Aschner M. Manganese transport in eukaryotes: the role of DMT1. *Neurotoxicology*. 2008;29(4):569–576.
306. Tuschl K, Mills PB, Clayton PT. Manganese and the brain. *International review of neurobiology*. 2013;110:277–312.
307. Tuschl K, Mills PB, Parsons H, Malone M, Fowler D, Bitner-Glindzicz M, et al. Hepatic cirrhosis, dystonia, polycythaemia and hypermanganesaemia--a new metabolic disorder. *J Inherit Metab Dis*. 2008;31(2):151–163.
308. Lechpammer M, Clegg MS, Muzar Z, Huebner PA, Jin LW, Gospe Jr SM. Pathology of inherited manganese transporter deficiency. *Ann Neurol*. 2014;75(4):608–612.
309. Anantharaman M, Tangpong J, Keller JN, Murphy MP, Markesbery WR, Kiningham KK, et al. Beta-amyloid mediated nitration of manganese superoxide dismutase: implication for oxidative stress in a APPNLH/NLH X PS-1P264L/P264L double knock-in mouse model of Alzheimer's disease. *Am J Pathol*. 2006;168(5):1608–1618.
310. Wallin C, Kulkarni YS, Abelein A, Jarvet J, Liao Q, Strodel B, et al. Characterization of Mn(II) ion binding to the amyloid-beta peptide in Alzheimer's disease. *J Trace Elem Med Biol*. 2016;38:183–193.
311. Zhang S, Fu J, Zhou Z. In vitro effect of manganese chloride exposure on reactive oxygen species generation and respiratory chain complexes activities of mitochondria isolated from rat brain. *Toxicol In Vitro*. 2004;18(1):71–77.
312. Madison JL, Wegrzynowicz M, Aschner M, Bowman AB. Disease-toxicant interactions in manganese exposed Huntington disease mice: early changes in striatal neuron morphology and dopamine metabolism. *Plos One*. 2012;7(2):e31024.
313. Tidball AM, Bryan MR, Uhouse MA, Kumar KK, Aboud AA, Feist JE, et al. A novel manganese-dependent ATM-p53 signaling pathway is selectively impaired in patient-based neuroprogenitor and murine striatal models of Huntington's disease. *Hum Mol Genet*. 2015;24(7):1929–1944.
314. Eiberg H, Hansen L, Korbo L, Nielsen IM, Svenstrup K, Bech S, et al. Novel mutation in ATP13A2 widens the spectrum of Kufor–Rakeb syndrome (PARK9). *Clin Genet*. 2012;82(3):256–263.
315. Ramonet D, Podhajska A, Stafa K, Sonnay S, Trancikova A, Tsika E, et al. PARK9-associated ATP13A2 localizes to intracellular acidic vesicles and regulates cation homeostasis and neuronal integrity. *Hum Mol Genet*. 2012;21(8):1725–1743.
316. Misra VK, Draper DE. On the role of magnesium ions in RNA stability. *Biopolymers*. 1998;48(2–3):113–135.
317. Bairoch A. The ENZYME database in 2000. *Nucleic Acids Res*. 2000;28(1):304–305.
318. Goytain A, Quamme GA. Identification and characterization of a novel mammalian Mg^{2+} transporter with channel-like properties. *BMC Genomics*. 2005;6:48.
319. Li FY, Chaigne-Delalande B, Kanellopoulou C, Davis JC, Matthews HF, Douek DC, et al. Second messenger role for Mg^{2+} revealed by human T-cell immunodeficiency. *Nature*. 2011;475(7357):471–476.
320. Chaigne-Delalande B, Li FY, O'Connor GM, Lukacs MJ, Jiang P, Zheng L, et al. Mg^{2+} regulates cytotoxic functions of NK and CD8 T cells in chronic EBV infection through NKG2D. *Science*. 2013;341(6142):186–191.
321. Runnels LW, Yue L, Clapham DE. TRP-PLIK, a bifunctional protein with kinase and ion channel activities. *Science*. 2001;291(5506):1043–1047.
322. Schmitz C, Perraud AL, Johnson CO, Inabe K, Smith MK, Penner R, et al. Regulation of vertebrate cellular Mg^{2+} homeostasis by TRPM7. *Cell*. 2003;114(2):191–200.
323. Konrad M, Schlingmann KP, Gudermann T. Insights into the molecular nature of magnesium homeostasis. *Am J Physiol Renal Physiol*. 2004;286(4):F599–F605.
324. van der Wijst J, Bindels RJ, Hoenderop JG. Mg2+ homeostasis: the balancing act of TRPM6. *Curr Opin Nephrol Hypertens*. 2014;23(4):361–369.
325. Cabezas-Bratesco D, Brauchi S, Gonzalez-Teuber V, Steinberg X, Valencia I, Colenso C. The different roles of the channel-kinases TRPM6 and TRPM7. *Curr Med Chem*. 2015;22(25):2943–2953.
326. Wabakken T, Rian E, Kveine M, Aasheim HC. The human solute carrier SLC41A1 belongs to a novel eukaryotic subfamily with homology to prokaryotic MgtE Mg^{2+} transporters. *Biochem Biophys Res Commun*. 2003;306(3):718–724.
327. Goytain A, Quamme GA. Functional characterization of human SLC41A1, a Mg^{2+} transporter with similarity to prokaryotic MgtE Mg^{2+} transporters. *Physiol Genomics*. 2005;21(3):337–342.

328. Kolisek M, Launay P, Beck A, Sponder G, Serafini N, Brenkus M, et al. SLC41A1 is a novel mammalian Mg^{2+} carrier. *J Biol Chem*. 2008;283(23):16235–16247.
329. Mandt T, Song Y, Scharenberg AM, Sahni J. SLC41A1 Mg(2+) transport is regulated via Mg(2+)-dependent endosomal recycling through its N-terminal cytoplasmic domain. *Biochem J*. 2011;439(1):129–139.
330. Wang CY, Shi JD, Yang P, Kumar PG, Li QZ, Run QG, et al. Molecular cloning and characterization of a novel gene family of four ancient conserved domain proteins (ACDP). *Gene*. 2003;306:37–44.
331. de Baaij JH, Stuiver M, Meij IC, Lainez S, Kopplin K, Venselaar H, et al. Membrane topology and intracellular processing of cyclin M2 (CNNM2). *J Biol Chem*. 2012;287(17):13644–13655.
332. Hardy S, Uetani N, Wong N, Kostantin E, Labbe DP, Begin LR, et al. The protein tyrosine phosphatase PRL-2 interacts with the magnesium transporter CNNM3 to promote oncogenesis. *Oncogene*. 2015;34(8):986–995.
333. Stuiver M, Lainez S, Will C, Terryn S, Gunzel D, Debaix H, et al. CNNM2, encoding a basolateral protein required for renal Mg2+ handling, is mutated in dominant hypomagnesemia. *Am J Hum Genet*. 2011;88(3):333–343.
334. Yamazaki D, Funato Y, Miura J, Sato S, Toyosawa S, Furutani K, et al. Basolateral Mg2+ extrusion via CNNM4 mediates transcellular Mg2+ transport across epithelia: a mouse model. *PLoS genetics*. 2013;9(12):e1003983.
335. Hashimoto T, Nishi K, Nagasao J, Tsuji S, Oyanagi K. Magnesium exerts both preventive and ameliorating effects in an in vitro rat Parkinson disease model involving 1-methyl-4-phenylpyridinium (MPP+) toxicity in dopaminergic neurons. *Brain Res*. 2008;1197:143–151.
336. Kolisek M, Sponder G, Mastrototaro L, Smorodchenko A, Launay P, Vormann J, et al. Substitution p.A350V in Na(+)/Mg(2)(+) exchanger SLC41A1, potentially associated with Parkinson's disease, is a gain-of-function mutation. *Plos One*. 2013;8(8):e71096.
337. Kunert-Keil C, Bisping F, Kruger J, Brinkmeier H. Tissue-specific expression of TRP channel genes in the mouse and its variation in three different mouse strains. *BMC Genomics*. 2006;7:159.
338. Coombes E, Jiang J, Chu XP, Inoue K, Seeds J, Branigan D, et al. Pathophysiologically relevant levels of hydrogen peroxide induce glutamate-independent neurodegeneration that involves activation of transient receptor potential melastatin 7 channels. *Antioxid Redox Signal*. 2011;14(10):1815–1827.
339. Nadler MJ, Hermosura MC, Inabe K, Perraud AL, Zhu Q, Stokes AJ, et al. LTRPC7 is a Mg.ATP-regulated divalent cation channel required for cell viability. *Nature*. 2001;411(6837):590–595.
340. Li W, Yu J, Liu Y, Huang X, Abumaria N, Zhu Y, et al. Elevation of brain magnesium prevents synaptic loss and reverses cognitive deficits in Alzheimer's disease mouse model. *Mol brain*. 2014;7:65.
341. Xu ZP, Li L, Bao J, Wang ZH, Zeng J, Liu EJ, et al. Magnesium protects cognitive functions and synaptic plasticity in streptozotocin-induced sporadic Alzheimer's model. *Plos One*. 2014;9(9):e108645.
342. Braun AP. A novel disease connection for TRPM2 channels. *Channels*. 2014;8(6):475–476.
343. Ostapchenko VG, Chen M, Guzman MS, Xie YF, Lavine N, Fan J, et al. The transient receptor potential melastatin 2 (TRPM2) channel contributes to beta-amyloid oligomer-related neurotoxicity and memory impairment. *J Neurosci*. 2015;35(45):15157–15169.
344. Oh HG, Chun YS, Kim Y, Youn SH, Shin S, Park MK, et al. Modulation of transient receptor potential melastatin related 7 channel by presenilins. *Dev Neurobiol*. 2012;72(6):865–877.
345. Hermosura MC, Garruto RM. TRPM7 and TRPM2-Candidate susceptibility genes for Western Pacific ALS and PD?. *Biochimica Biophysica Acta*. 2007;1772(8):822–835.
346. Huang K, Yanai A, Kang R, Arstikaitis P, Singaraja RR, Metzler M, et al. Huntingtin-interacting protein HIP14 is a palmitoyl transferase involved in palmitoylation and trafficking of multiple neuronal proteins. *Neuron*. 2004;44(6):977–986.
347. Kegel KB, Sapp E, Yoder J, Cuiffo B, Sobin L, Kim YJ, et al. Huntingtin associates with acidic phospholipids at the plasma membrane. *J Biol Chem*. 2005;280(43):36464–36473.
348. Goytain A, Hines RM, Quamme GA. Huntingtin-interacting proteins, HIP14 and HIP14L, mediate dual functions, palmitoyl acyltransferase and Mg2+ transport. *J Biol Chem*. 2008;283(48):33365–33374.
349. Yokel RA. Blood-brain barrier flux of aluminum, manganese, iron and other metals suspected to contribute to metal-induced neurodegeneration. *J Alzheimers Dis*. 2006;10(2-3):223–253.
350. Yamanaka K, Minato N, Iwai K. Stabilization of iron regulatory protein 2, IRP2, by aluminum. *FEBS Lett*. 1999;462(1-2):216–220.
351. VanDuyn N, Settivari R, LeVora J, Zhou S, Unrine J, Nass R. The metal transporter SMF-3/DMT-1 mediates aluminum-induced dopamine neuron degeneration. *J Neurochem*. 2013;124(1):147–157.
352. Zayed J, Campanella G, Panisset JC, Ducic S, Andre P, Masson H, et al. [Parkinson disease and environmental factors]. *Rev Epidemiol Sante Publique*. 1990;38(2):159–160.

353. Altschuler E. Aluminum-containing antacids as a cause of idiopathic Parkinson's disease. *Med Hypotheses*. 1999;53(1):22–23.
354. Uversky VN, Li J, Fink AL. Metal-triggered structural transformations, aggregation, and fibrillation of human alpha-synuclein. A possible molecular NK between Parkinson's disease and heavy metal exposure. *J Biol Chem*. 2001;276(47):44284–44296.
355. Sanchez-Iglesias S, Mendez-Alvarez E, Iglesias-Gonzalez J, Munoz-Patino A, Sanchez-Sellero I, Labandeira-Garcia JL, et al. Brain oxidative stress and selective behaviour of aluminium in specific areas of rat brain: potential effects in a 6-OHDA-induced model of Parkinson's disease. *J Neurochem*. 2009;109(3):879–888.
356. Saberzadeh J, Arabsolghar R, Takhshid MA. Alpha synuclein protein is involved in Aluminum-induced cell death and oxidative stress in PC12 cells. *Brain Res*. 2016;1635:153–160.
357. Shoskes DA, Radzinski CA, Struthers NW, Honey RJ. Aluminum toxicity and death following intravesical alum irrigation in a patient with renal impairment. *J Urol*. 1992;147(3):697–699.
358. Yamamoto H, Saitoh Y, Yasugawa S, Miyamoto E. Dephosphorylation of tau factor by protein phosphatase 2A in synaptosomal cytosol fractions, and inhibition by aluminum. *J Neurochem*. 1990;55(2):683–690.
359. Shin RW, Iwaki T, Kitamoto T, Sato Y, Tateishi J. Massive accumulation of modified tau and severe depletion of normal tau characterize the cerebral cortex and white matter of Alzheimer's disease. Demonstration using the hydrated autoclaving method. *Am J Pathol*. 1992;140(4):937–945.
360. Sato N, Hori O, Yamaguchi A, Lambert JC, Chartier-Harlin MC, Robinson PA, et al. A novel presenilin-2 splice variant in human Alzheimer's disease brain tissue. *J Neurochem*. 1999;72(6):2498–2505.
361. Pratico D, Uryu K, Sung S, Tang S, Trojanowski JQ, Lee VM. Aluminum modulates brain amyloidosis through oxidative stress in APP transgenic mice. *Faseb J*. 2002;16(9):1138–1140.
362. Walton JR. Evidence for Participation of Aluminum in Neurofibrillary Tangle Formation and Growth in Alzheimer's Disease. *J Alzheimers Dis*. 2010;22(1):65–72.
363. Petrik MS, Wong MC, Tabata RC, Garry RF, Shaw CA. Aluminum adjuvant linked to Gulf War illness induces motor neuron death in mice. *Neuromol Med*. 2007;9(1):83–100.
364. Shaw CA, Petrik MS. Aluminum hydroxide injections lead to motor deficits and motor neuron degeneration. *J Inorg Biochem*. 2009;103(11):1555–1562.
365. Shaw CA, Hoglinger GU. Neurodegenerative diseases: neurotoxins as sufficient etiologic agents?. *Neuromol Med*. 2008;10(1):1–9.
366. Rozas VV, Port FK, Rutt WM. Progressive dialysis encephalopathy from dialysate aluminum. *Arch Intern Med*. 1978;138(9):1375–1377.
367. Zatta P, Zambenedetti P, Reusche E, Stellmacher F, Cester A, Albanese P, et al. A fatal case of aluminium encephalopathy in a patient with severe chronic renal failure not on dialysis. *Nephrol Dial Transplant*. 2004;19(11):2929–2931.
368. Andrade LG, Garcia FD, Silva VS, Gabriel DP, Rodrigues Jr AG, Nascimento GV, et al. Dialysis encephalopathy secondary to aluminum toxicity, diagnosed by bone biopsy. *Nephrol Dial Transplant*. 2005;20(11):2581–2582.

CHAPTER

17

Metal Imaging in the Brain

David C. Dorman

North Carolina State University, Raleigh, NC, United States

OUTLINE

INTRODUCTION

This chapter reviews current literature related to the assessment of metal accumulation using magnetic resonance imaging (MRI). The discussion primarily focuses on effects seen in humans with discussion of animal studies as appropriate. Associations between brain MRI changes and metal concentrations in affected brain regions are also discussed. Metals to be discussed include gadolinium, iron, copper, and manganese. No attempt has been made to provide an exhaustive review of each of the topics or metals addressed. Wherever possible, references to review articles are provided.

INTRODUCTION TO MRI PHYSICS

A simple review of MRI physics can assist the reader in understanding how paramagnetic metals are detected using this imaging modality.[1] Protons, found predominantly in tissue water, have an intrinsic nuclear spin that produces an extremely weak magnetic force (Fig. 17.1). Protons placed within an external magnetic field (Bø) will align with (lower energy state) or against (higher energy state) Bø which is measured in Teslas (T). Protons will precess (i.e., wobble) about the axis of Bø with a frequency proportional to the magnetic field strength.

Biometals in Neurodegenerative Diseases. http://dx.doi.org/10.1016/B978-0-12-804562-6.00017-8

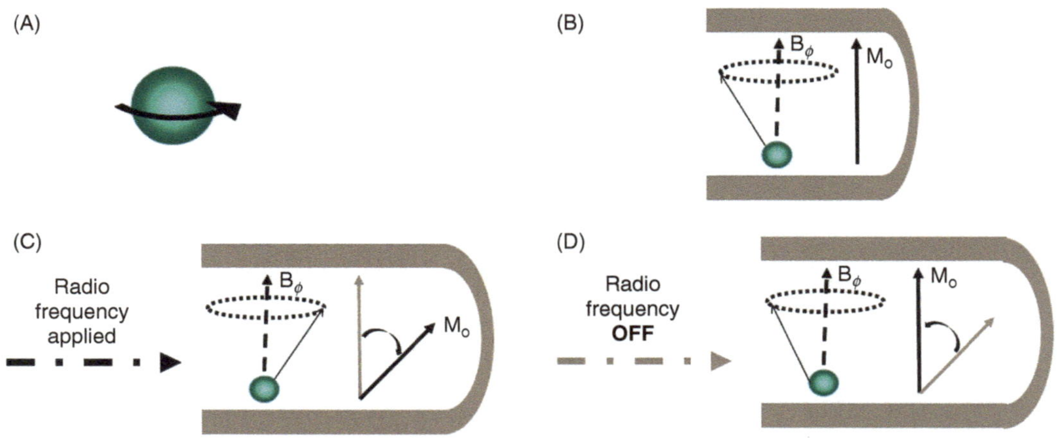

FIGURE 17.1 **Sequential steps involved during acquisition of a T1-weighted MRI.** (A) Spin of the proton causes the proton to act like a small magnet. (B) A hydrogen atom will precess (wobble) about an external magnetic field (Bø). The size of the magnetic field influences the amount the proton "wobbles." The net magnetization vector (i.e., summation of all the magnetic moments of the individual protons) is along the direction of the applied magnetic field Bø. this vector is called the equilibrium magnetization M_0 (C) The radio frequency causes a tipping of the longitudinal magnetization (result= transverse magnetization vector). (D) The time constant which describes how longitudinal magnetization returns to its equilibrium value is called the spin lattice relaxation time (T1).

The next step involves the application of an external radio frequency (RF) pulse. When the RF pulse is applied at the resonance frequency the protons absorb energy and "tilt" up to 180° from Bø. The resonance frequency of hydrogen is 64–85 MHz when the Bø is 1.5 and 2 T, respectively. When the RF pulse ends the absorbed RF energy is retransmitted at the resonance frequency and the excited proton's spin returns to its original orientation (i.e., longitudinal or spin-lattice relaxation). The time constant associated with this process is designated as T1. Recovery rates vary between different tissues (e.g., gray vs. white matter) resulting in the ability of MRI to identify different tissues. Simultaneously the excited protons begin to dephase due to spin–spin relaxation. The time constant associated with this relaxation process is referred to as T2. Such as T1, T2 varies among tissues and is influenced by the local chemical environment. Unlike T1, T2 values are less dependent on Bø. Transverse magnetization (T2) decay occurs faster than would be theoretically accounted for by atomic and molecular mechanisms associated with spin–spin relaxation. Another term, T2* relaxation, accounts for this difference and reflects what the coil receiver detects immediately after termination of the RF pulse. Irregularities in the homogeneity of Bø contribute to T2*. T2* occurs at a rate greater than T2.

MRI CONTRAST AGENTS

Paramagnetic ions including gadolinium, iron, and manganese are used as MRI contrast agents.[2] Protons in close (0.1–1 nm) proximity to these metals are affected by the paramagnetic metals' larger magnetic moment causing the protons to relax more quickly thus affecting the average relaxation times in a region of interest (Fig. 17.2).[2,3] Contrast agents signal

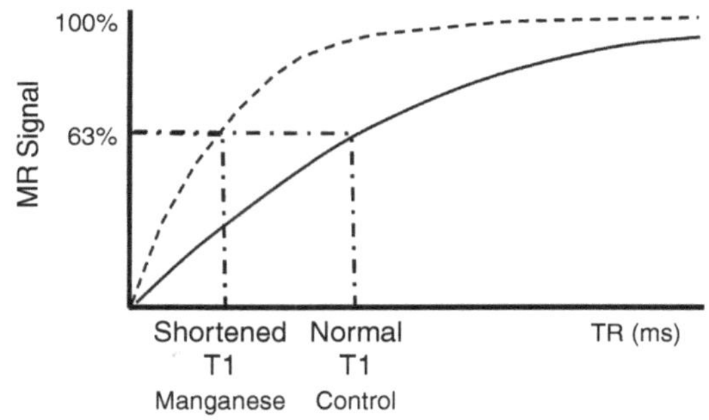

FIGURE 17.2 **Hypothetical curve illustrating the effect of manganese on longitudinal magnetization (T1) during the relaxation process.** The time after the excitation pulse to allow 63.2% of the magnetization to have recovered its alignment with Bø is termed the T1 time.

enhancement is defined by their relaxivity, which describes how solution relaxation rates change as a function of the contrast agent concentration. MRI contrast agents affect both relaxation rates (1/T1 and 1/T2) thus there are two relaxivities (r_1 and r_2) for these agents.[3,4] Contrast agents are categorized as T1 or T2 contrast agents depending on how they influence T1 or T2 relaxation times. Contrast agents lower the T1 and/or T2 at low (nM to mM) concentrations and doses are approximately 25–300 mmol/kg.[4]

GADOLINIUM

Several gadolinium-based contrast agents (GBCA) have been developed in which the gadolinium is chelated to reduce the availability of free gadolinium and thus its toxicity. Gadolinium chelates are broadly divided into linear and macrocyclic forms with further subdivision into ionic and nonionic subtypes.[3] Chelation increases the water solubility of the GBCA thereby reducing the ability of gadolinium to cross the blood brain barrier (BBB).[3] GBCAs are primarily used to enhance central nervous system (CNS) lesions with poor BBB integrity (e.g., brain tumors) and to enhance vessels during MR angiography.

The ionic radius of gadolinium (0.99 Å) is similar to that of calcium and gadolinium competitively inhibits voltage-gated calcium channels and interferes with calcium-dependent biological processes.[5] Zinc, copper, and calcium can displace gadolinium from the chelate resulting in toxicity.[6] The relative affinity of these cations for the chelates is copper > zinc > calcium. Because zinc has a relatively high serum concentration its ability to displace gadolinium is biologically most significant.[6]

Most GBCAs are given intravenously and these agents have favorable safety profiles. In mice the intravenous LD_{50} of free gadolinium (as $GdCl_3$) is approximately 100–200 mg/kg.[7] This salt form is approximately 20–100 times more toxic than the GBCAs.[6,8] Most GBCAs rapidly equilibrate with the intravascular and extracellular (interstitial) fluid compartments. Some GBCAs reach the extracellular fluid compartment while others target the liver or intravascular compartments. The fate of the GBCAs depends in part on their chemical structure. For example, cyclic gadolinium chelates generally undergo minimal biotransformation and are excreted unchanged by glomerular filtration.[8] Other GBCAs (e.g., gadoxetic acid) are taken up by hepatocytes and approximately 50% of the administered dose undergoes hepatobiliary/fecal elimination. The elimination half-life of cyclic gadolinium chelates in patients with normal renal function is approximately 1.5 h.[8] Individuals with compromised renal function can have delayed excretion and are at increased risk for gadolinium-induced renal toxicity.

An association exists between GBCA administration and the development of nephrogenic systemic fibrosis in humans with compromised renal function. Several GBCAs are contraindicated in patients with renal insufficiency, liver transplant patients, and infants.[9,10]

There is emerging evidence that gadolinium can be deposited in the brain following the repeated administration of certain GBCAs. Kanda and coworkers first described T1 signal hyperintensity in the globus pallidus (GP) and dentate nucleus (DN) in patients with normal renal function that had previously received a GBCA.[11] These findings have subsequently been corroborated by others[12–15] including studies demonstrating deposition of gadolinium in pediatric patients.[16] Increased signal intensity in the DN and GP on unenhanced T1-weighted images showed a positive correlation with previous exposure to linear chelate type GBCAs (e.g., gadopentetate dimeglumine or gadodiamide) whereas macrocyclic GBCAs did not.[17] Postmortem brain samples from affected patients have confirmed the presence of gadolinium in patients receiving GBCAs.[18–20] The mechanism of brain gadolinium deposition is poorly understood and is likely related to dechelation of gadolinium.[21] The neurotoxicological significance of gadolinium brain deposition is unknown and is being investigated by the United States Food and Drug Administration.[22,23]

IRON

Iron can change redox states and this property is critical for electron transport and other normal cellular functions. Free iron is highly reactive and readily produces cytotoxic reactive oxygen species. Numerous homeostatic mechanisms regulate the availability of iron in the CNS.[24] Extracellular iron is largely bound to transferrin and transported into the cell via transferrin receptor 1 (TFRC; TFR1) dependent endocytosis and via the divalent metal transporter 1 (DMT1; SLC11A2). Cytosolic iron is predominantly stored in ferritin or transferred to mitochondria and other iron rich organelles. Ferroportin 1 (FPN1; SLC40A1) transports iron out of the cell, and some studies have provided evidence that it is expressed in BBB endothelium.[24,25] Several mechanisms may be involved in increased deposition of iron in the CNS including changes in iron transport across the BBB, intracranial hemorrhage, and an influx of iron-containing macrophages from the bloodstream.[24,26]

Iron has a T1-shortening effect, and superparamagnetic iron oxides have been developed as MRI contrast agents.[27] Iron oxide nanoparticles (generally 10–3500 nm) used as MRI contrast agents are usually made of a crystalline core (e.g., magnetite [Fe_3O_4], maghemite [γ-Fe_2O_3], hematite [α-Fe_2O_3]) and a surface coating [e.g., dextran, starch, albumin, silicones, and poly(ethylene glycol)] for stabilizing the core.[28–30] Phantom studies using iron oxide have shown that iron concentrations in excess of 10 ppm can be detected using MRI.[31]

Brain MRI studies and tissue analyses show that iron (predominantly as ferritin iron) accumulates in the GP, red nucleus, DN, and substantia nigra (SN) during aging.[32,33] Mean iron concentrations found in the human GP, putamen, caudate nucleus, thalamus, and corpus callosum of 13 deceased subjects with no history of a neurological disorder or external evidence of brain trauma were 205, 160, 105, 50, and 29 ppm, respectively.[33]

Iron deposition in the GP and other iron rich brain regions is associated with a reduction in the T2 (T2*) relaxation time, leading to hypointensity on spin-echo and gradient-echo T2-weighted images.[34–36] A variety of MRI methods have been used to estimate brain iron content.[33,34,37] Some estimates are generated from the mathematical difference in transverse relaxivity (R2) measured at different field strengths (i.e., field-dependent R2 increase method) and these estimates have been validated with in vitro phantom studies.[34] Changes in the measured R2 values (R2*) attribute the relaxation enhancement at higher field strength to the presence of iron thus providing an estimate of tissue iron stores.[38] Imaging studies in rhesus monkeys show that R2 was correlated with total iron concentration and the relationship between R2 and tissue iron concentration appears to depend upon the iron concentration.[39] Brain iron concentrations in these monkeys ranged from 15 to 450 ppm, with the highest levels seen in the GP and the lowest levels in the cerebellum.[39] Other studies report a significant relationship between MRI findings evaluating tissue magnetic susceptibility, which is a dimensionless proportionality constant that indicates the degree of magnetization of a material in response to Bø, and iron concentration measured in human postmortem brain (grey matter) samples.[33] A complete description of these methods is beyond the scope of the present chapter and the reader is referred to recent reviews for additional information.[28,33,34]

Accumulation of iron in the brain in patients with essential tremor, Huntington's disease, Parkinson's disease, Alzheimer's disease, Wilson's disease, multiple sclerosis, chronic hemorrhage, and cerebral infarction is also inferred from MRI studies.[24,26,35,36,40–44] Brain iron and ferritin concentrations are elevated in people with Parkinson's or Huntington disease. Mean iron putamen concentrations found in normal patients (n = 6), patients with Parkinson disease (n = 10), and Huntington disease (n = 6) were 35, 52, and 116 ppm, respectively.[45] Although putamen iron concentrations were elevated in diseased patients they were not correlated with T2 shortening.[45] Several explanations have been postulated to account for this discordant finding including the observation that regional T2 signal intensity is affected by the water and myelin content of the tissue, iron transforms local chemistry causing different paramagnetic effects, and heterogeneous distribution of iron particles within the tissue.[35,46]

Additional neurologic syndromes have been classified as "neurodegeneration with brain iron overload accumulation" (NBIA) diseases.[47] Various NBIAs have been linked with mutations in genes that code for ceruloplasmin, ferritin light chain, pantothenate kinase 2 (PANK2), phospholipase A2 group 6 (PLA2G6), fatty acid hydroxylase 2, and coenzyme A synthase.[48] Some of the best studied NBIAs include pantothenate kinase associated neurodegeneration (PKAN, formerly known as Hallervorden-Spatz syndrome), PLA2G6-associated neurodegeneration (PLAN), and neuroferritinopathy–an adult onset autosomal dominant movement disorder.[49–51] NBIAs often present with progressive hypo- and/or hyperkinetic movement disorder and pathologically with excessive iron deposition in the brain, particularly affecting the GP and other portions of the basal ganglia.[51] Brain MRI can distinguish different NBIA subtypes.[52] For example, T2 imaging of patients with PKAN was associated with an abnormally low T2 signal in the GP and a longitudinal stripe of high signal due to gliosis and spongiosis (so called "eye of the tiger sign").[52]

The exact role that brain iron accumulation plays in NBIA and other neurodegenerative syndromes is poorly understood. It remains unknown whether iron accumulation contributes to disease progression or whether accumulation of iron occurs only after widespread neuronal death.[24] Despite the finding of inconsistent correlations between tissue iron concentration and brain MRI findings, MRI has proven valuable in the diagnosis of many iron storage diseases and has provided important insights into the role of this metal in neurodegenerative disease.

COPPER

As a component of cytochrome c oxidase, copper catalyzes electron transfer to oxygen during mitochondrial oxidative phosphorylation. Copper is also found in several antioxidants including superoxide dismutase and ceruloplasmin. Like iron, copper is also under tight homeostatic control. The major route of copper elimination is through hepatobiliary excretion. Two copper-transporting adenylpyrophosphatases (ATPases) play an essential role in copper homeostasis.[53] The gene for ATPase copper transporting alpha (ATP7A) encodes for a transmembrane copper transport protein that mediates copper uptake in the gastrointestinal tract and copper delivery to the brain. Mutations in this gene are associated with Menkes disease, X-linked distal spinal muscular atrophy, and occipital horn syndrome. ATPase copper transporting beta (ATP7B), exports copper out of the cells and mediates, hepatobiliary copper excretion.[53] Mutations in this gene are associated with Wilson disease (WD) and account for the gradual accumulation of copper that ultimately results in increased liver and brain copper concentrations and secondary hepatotoxicity and neurotoxicity.

Initial neurological symptoms seen during WD often emerge between 10 and 40 years of age. Patients often present with a parkinsonian syndrome characterized by difficulty swallowing, speech (dysarthria, apraxia) and writing disorders, as well as dystonia, kinetic tremor, or ataxia.[54] Many WD patients with neurological symptoms have liver disease at the time of detection.[54,55] Brain lesions are classically located in basal ganglia, midbrain, and DN and diffuse cerebral atrophy is frequently seen.[56] Cortical atrophy involving the frontal lobes and ventricular dilatation with flattening of the caudate nucleus and shrinkage of the thalamus and subcortical white matter have been reported.[54] Histologic changes in patients with WD include neuronal and oligodendroglia loss, spongy gliosis and astrocytosis, and rarefaction and cavitation of cerebral white matter with multifocal demyelination.[54] The presence or absence of lesions often vary since a spectrum of clinical presentations from pure hepatic, to pure neuropsychiatric, to essentially neurological, and mixed forms are reported. Neuronal injury is presumed to be predominantly due to direct copper toxicity, however glial abnormalities (e.g., Alzheimer type II glia) seen in WD suggest that hepatic encephalopathy may also contribute to the pathogenesis of neurologic disease in some patients.[57–59]

Brain MRI abnormalities in WD often reflect the neuropathologic findings.[60–62] Brain MRI findings also include intensity changes associated with the deposition of copper and other metals in the CNS. Individuals with WD often develop T1-weighted images with increased signal intensity in the GP, putamen, midbrain, and caudate nucleus and T2-weighted images with increased signal intensity in the putamen, caudate nucleus, GP, thalamus, midbrain, and pons.[46,57,59,62,63] Copper has a relatively small paramagnetic effect and copper accumulation in the brain may not directly account for the MR signal intensity changes seen in WD.[64,65]

Hypointensity of the SN, striatum, and GP on T2 weighted images in WD is thought to be due to increased accumulation of copper and iron.[35] The presence of T1 hyperintensity in the GP of WD patients has been attributed to the mixed paramagnetic effects of copper, iron, or manganese, and accumulation of Alzheimer's type II glial cells.[65–68] Direct support for these hypotheses however remains limited. Studies evaluating trace metal concentrations in the brain of patients with WD show that brain copper concentrations are often elevated (4- to 10-fold) when compared with normal reference ranges.[69,70] However, effects on other metal concentrations are more variable. For example, Faa and coworkers found decreased iron concentrations in the frontal cortex of a woman with WD and hepatic failure.[69] Litwin evaluated iron and manganese concentrations in the frontal cortex, putamen, pons, and DN of 12 WD patients.[70] Litwin reported that overall mean concentrations of iron, manganese, and zinc in these four brain regions were similar in WD and controls, but mean iron levels seen in the DN were higher in WD when compared with controls (56.8 vs. 32.6 μg/g).[70] Bruehlmeier and coworkers used positron emission tomography (PET) to evaluate brain uptake of radiolabeled iron (^{52}Fe-citrate) in 6 WD patients and 16 healthy volunteers.[71] They found that the rate of iron uptake into the WD brain was higher than that seen in healthy subjects.[71] Another line of evidence supporting a role for metal deposition accounting for the increased T1-weighted image signal intensity in the GP of WD patients comes from longitudinal studies that have evaluated MRI changes in patients receiving penicillamine and other chelation therapy.[63,72] For example, Kim and coworkers evaluated a cohort of children diagnosed with early WD.[63] They separated the cohort into three subtypes based on initial MRI findings: patients with normal MRI findings, patients with abnormally high signal intensity on T1-weighted images, and patients with abnormally high signal intensity on T2-weighted images. They found that children receiving penicillamine with normal initial findings had no appreciable change while patients with abnormally high signal intensity on their initial T1-weighted image had increased signal intensity in the involved area on T1-weighted images. In contrast, patients with high initial signal intensity on T2-weighted images showed improvement on their follow-up MRI.[63]

MANGANESE

Manganese is another essential nutrient under tight homeostatic regulation.[73] Manganese is incorporated into metalloproteins that play a critical role in normal cellular function. Manganese is an essential cofactor for arginase, glutamine synthetase, mitochondrial superoxide dismutase, and pyruvate carboxylase.[74] Manganese (Mn^{2+}) has a similar ionic radius to that of calcium (Ca^{2+}) and enters neurons through voltage-gated calcium channels.[75]

Manganese is paramagnetic and shortens the T1 of tissues where it has accumulated, resulting in positive contrast enhancement. Manganese undergoes anterograde axonal transport and demonstrates an ability to cross synapses.[76–79] These properties make manganese a very useful MRI contrast agent for anatomical and functional neuroimaging studies. Manganese-enhanced MRI (MEMRI) has emerged as an important means to evaluate neuronal function and networks.[80,81]

In addition to its use as a clinical and research tool, epidemiologic studies have established a causal association between chronic manganese inhalation and a parkinsonism syndrome

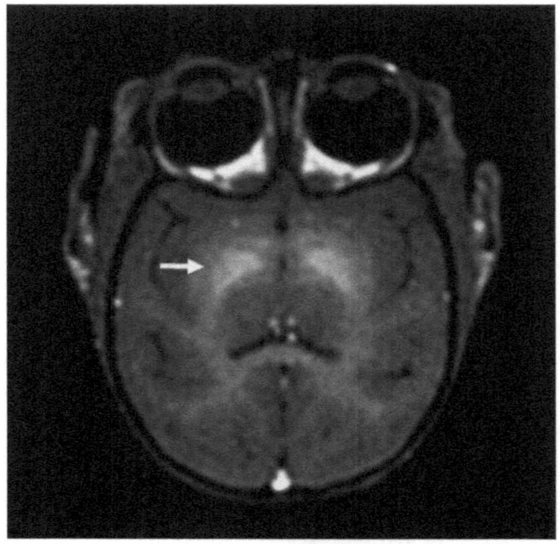

FIGURE 17.3 **T1 MRI image collected from a monkey exposed subchronically to a high dose of inhaled manganese.** The monkey demonstrates markedly increased signal intensity in the GP *(arrow)* which was consistent with manganese accumulation at this site.

known as manganism.[82,83] Manganese accumulates within the human striatum, GP, and SN.[82,83] Hallmarks of manganism include behavioral changes, extrapyramidal motor dysfunction, and neurochemical and neuropathologic changes in the basal ganglia and GP.[84] Cognitive deficits have also been reported in workers with exposure to manganese-based welding fumes.[84]

Brain MRI studies of highly exposed workers reveal signal changes in the GP, striatum, and midbrain consistent with manganese accumulation at these sites.[85,86] Changes in the pallidal index (i.e., ratio of the signal intensity in the GP over the intensity in the frontal white matter using T1-weighted MRI) has been used as a measure of manganese accumulation in the GP.[87–90] The pallidal index (PI) correlates with the pallidal manganese concentration seen in monkeys following subchronic exposure to inhaled manganese sulfate (Fig. 17.3).[91] However, increases in white matter manganese concentrations in manganese-exposed monkeys confound PI measurement and may lead to underestimation of pallidal manganese accumulation.[91] Changes in T1 relaxation rate (R1) in manganese-exposed monkeys is a better predictor of pallidal manganese concentration when compared with the PI.[94] Similar approaches to evaluate R1 in exposed welders have been used.[92–94] Lee and coworkers reported changes in the transverse relaxation rates (R2*) in the caudate nucleus of welders, a change which could be indicative of increased iron in this brain region.[93] Longitudinal changes in MRI signal intensity can be evaluated in workers to evaluate whether interventional approaches have been beneficial.[95]

Several MRI studies have been performed in children. Aschner and coworkers reported that infants with greater parenteral manganese exposure had shorter T1 relaxation times, consistent with manganese accumulation, in the basal ganglia when compared with infants with lower parenteral exposures.[96] Children with a defect in a putative manganese transporter protein encoded by the gene SLC39A14 also develop MRI changes consistent with manganese accumulation in the CNS (Tuschl et al., 2016).[97] Dion and coworkers, however were unable to detect increased MRI signal intensity in the GP of children exposed to high (145 μg/L) levels of manganese in drinking water when compared with children consuming a lower level (1 μg/L).[98]

The role of the olfactory route as a mechanism of brain delivery of manganese has also been studied with MRI.[99,100] Manganese-exposed monkeys demonstrate accumulation in the olfactory bulb following manganese inhalation.[94] Sen and coworkers used brain MRI to evaluate region-specific manganese accumulation in seven welders without obvious neurologic deficits.[101] When compared with age- and gender-matched controls, the manganese-exposed welders had significantly higher T1 relaxation rates in the olfactory bulb, as well as evidence of manganese accumulation in the frontal white matter, GP, and putamen.[101] Cross and coworkers used unilateral intranasal manganese instillation in rats and brain MRI to show significant transport of manganese in the olfactory bulb, lateral olfactory tract, and olfactory tubercle ipsilateral to the site of manganese administration.[102] Other MRI studies in mice have shown that parenterally administered manganese accumulates in the glomerular and mitral cell layers of the olfactory bulb, in the CA3 area of the hippocampus, and in the gray matter of the cerebellum.[103] The finding of olfactory bulb deposition of manganese following systemic delivery is consistent with other rodent studies examining manganese brain delivery after oral administration that show a propensity for this site to accumulate manganese.[104]

Patients with chronic hepatic failure often show a hyperintense GP, putamen, and red nucleus on T1 weighted images.[105,106] Similar MRI changes are seen in the lentiform nuclei of dogs with portosystemic shunts—and in one case a four-fold elevation in brain manganese concentration (vs. normal dogs) was associated with MRI hyperintensity.[107] Increased brain manganese concentrations are also seen in human patients with liver cirrhosis.[108] Manganese is considered to be the cause of MRI hyperintense GP in patients with chronic hepatic failure, however, copper and iron may also play a role.[35,109]

References

1. Pooley RA. Fundamental physics of MR imaging. *Radiographics*. 2005;25:1087–1099.
2. Lohrke J, Frenzel T, Endrikat J, Alves FC, Grist TM, Law M, Lee JM, Leiner T, Li KC, Nikolaou K, Prince MR, Schild HH, Weinreb JC, Yoshikawa K, Pietsch H. 25 years of contrast-enhanced MRI: developments, current challenges and future perspectives. *Adv Ther*. 2016;33:1–28.
3. Burtea C, Laurent S, Vander Elst L, Muller RN. Contrast agents: magnetic resonance. *Handb Exp Pharmacol*. 2008;185(Pt 1):135–165.
4. Hao D, Ai T, Goerner F, Hu X, Runge VM, Tweedle M. MRI contrast agents: basic chemistry and safety. *J Magn Reson Imaging*. 2012;36:1060–1071.
5. Rogosnitzky M, Branch S. Gadolinium-based contrast agent toxicity: a review of known and proposed mechanisms. *Biometals*. 2016;29:365–376.
6. Penfield JG, Reilly Jr RF. What nephrologists need to know about gadolinium. *Nat Clin Pract Nephrol*. 2007;3: 654–668.
7. Caillé JM, Lemanceau B, Bonnemain B. Gadolinium as a contrast agent for NMR. *AJNR Am J Neuroradiol*. 1983;4:1041–1042.
8. Aime S, Caravan P. Biodistribution of gadolinium-based contrast agents, including gadolinium deposition. *J Magn Reson Imaging*. 2009;30:1259–1267.
9. Grobner T. Gadolinium: a specific trigger for the development of nephrogenic fibrosing dermopathy and nephrogenic systemic fibrosis?. *Nephrol Dial Transpl*. 2006;21:1104–1108.
10. Forghani R. Adverse effects of gadolinium-based contrast agents: changes in practice patterns. *Top Magn Reson Imaging*. 2016;25:163–169.

11. Kanda T, Ishii K, Kawaguchi H, Kitajima K, Takenaka D. High signal intensity in the dentate nucleus and globus pallidus on unenhanced T1-weighted MR images: relationship with increasing cumulative dose of a gadolinium-based contrast material. *Radiology*. 2014;270:834–841.
12. Cao Y, Huang DQ, Shih G, Prince MR. Signal change in the dentate nucleus on T1-weighted MR images after multiple administrations of gadopentetate dimeglumine versus gadobutrol. *AJR Am J Roentgenol*. 2016;206: 414–419.
13. Errante Y, Cirimele V, Mallio CA, Di Lazzaro V, Zobel BB, Quattrocchi CC. Progressive increase of T1 signal intensity of the dentate nucleuson unenhanced magnetic resonance images is associated with cumulative doses of intravenously administered gadodiamide in patients with normal renal function, suggesting dechelation. *Invest Radiol*. 2014;49:685–690.
14. Murata N, Murata K, Gonzalez-Cuyar LF, Maravilla K. Gadolinium tissue deposition in brain and bone. *Magn Reson Imaging*. 2016;34(10):1359–1365.
15. Stojanov DA, Aracki-Trenkic A, Vojinovic S, Benedeto-Stojanov D, Ljubisavljevic S. Increasing signal intensity within the dentate nucleusand globus pallidus on unenhanced T1W magnetic resonance images in patients with relapsing-remitting multiple sclerosis: correlation with cumulative dose of a macrocyclic gadolinium-based contrast agent, gadobutrol. *Eur Radiol*. 2016;26:807–815.
16. Flood TF, Stence NV, Maloney JA, Mirsky DM. Pediatric brain: Repeated exposure to linear gadolinium-based contrast material is associated with increased signal intensity at unenhanced T1-weighted MR imaging. *Radiology*. 2017;282(1):160356.
17. Radbruch A, Weberling LD, Kieslich PJ, Hepp J, Kickingereder P, Wick W, Schlemmer HP, Bendszus M. Intraindividual analysis of signal intensity changes in the dentate nucleus after consecutive serial applications of linear and macrocyclic gadolinium-based contrast agents. *Invest Radiol*. 2016;51:683–690.
18. Kanda T, Fukusato T, Matsuda M, Toyoda K, Oba H, Kotoku J, Haruyama T, Kitajima K, Furui S. Gadolinium-based contrast agent accumulates in the brain even in subjects without severe renal dysfunction: Evaluation of autopsy brain specimens with inductively coupled plasma mass spectroscopy. *Radiology*. 2015;276: 228–232.
19. McDonald RJ, McDonald JS, Kallmes DF, Jentoft ME, Murray DL, Thielen KR, Williamson EE, Eckel LJ. Intracranial gadolinium deposition after contrast-enhanced MR imaging. *Radiology*. 2015;275:772–782.
20. Stojanov D, Aracki-Trenkic A, Benedeto-Stojanov D. Gadolinium deposition within the dentate nucleus and globus pallidus after repeated administrations of gadolinium-based contrast agents-current status. *Neuroradiology*. 2016;58:433–441.
21. Kanda T, Oba H, Toyoda K, Kitajima K, Furui S. Brain gadolinium deposition after administration of gadolinium-based contrast agents. *Jpn J Radiol*. 2016;34:3–9.
22. Ramalho J, Semelka RC, Ramalho M, Nunes RH, AlObaidy M, Castillo M. Gadolinium-based contrast agent accumulation and toxicity: an update. *AJNR Am J Neuroradiol*. 2016;37:1192–1198.
23. United States Food and Drug Administration, 2015. Gadolinium-based contrast agents for magnetic resonance imaging (MRI): Drug safety communication—FDA evaluating the risk of brain deposits with repeated use. Available from: http://www.fda.gov/Safety/MedWatch/SafetyInformation/SafetyAlertsforHumanMedicalProducts/ucm456012.htm
24. Rouault TA. Iron metabolism in the CNS: implications for neurodegenerative diseases. *Nat Rev Neurosci*. 2013;14:551–564.
25. Burkhart A, Skjørringe T, Johnsen KB, Siupka P, Thomsen LB, Nielsen MS, Thomsen LL, Moos T. Expression of iron-related proteins at the neurovascular unit supports reduction and reoxidation of iron for transport through the blood-brain barrier. *Mol Neurobiol*. 2016;53(10):7237–7253.
26. Dusek P, Bahn E, Litwin T, Jabłonka-Salach K, Łuciuk A, Huelnhagen T, Madai VI, Dieringer MA, Bulska E, Knauth M, Niendorf T, Sobesky J, Paul F, Schneider SA, Czlonkowska A, Brück W, Wegner C, Wuerfel J. Brain iron accumulation in Wilson disease: a post mortem 7 Tesla MRI—histopathological study. *Neuropathol Appl Neurobiol*. 2016;:(Epub ahead of print).
27. Wang Y-XJ. Superparamagnetic iron oxide based MRI contrast agents: current status of clinical application. *Quant Imaging Med Surg*. 2011;1:35–40.
28. Mao X, Xu J, Cui H. Functional nanoparticles for magnetic resonance imaging. *Wiley Interdiscip Rev Nanomed Nanobiotechnol*. 2016;8:814–841.
29. Shen Z, Wu A, Chen X. Iron oxide nanoparticles-based contrast agents for magnetic resonance imaging. *Mol Pharm*. 2016;:[Epub ahead of print].

30. Valdiglesias V, Fernández-Bertólez N, Kiliç G, Costa C, Costa S, Fraga S, Bessa MJ, Pásaro E, Teixeira JP, Laffon B. Are iron oxide nanoparticles safe? Current knowledge and future perspectives. *J Trace Elem Med Biol.* 2016;38:53–63.
31. Reimer P, Allkemper T, Schuierer G, Peters PE. Brain imaging: reduced sensitivity of RARE-derived techniques to susceptibility effects. *J Comput Assist Tomogr*. 1996;20:201–205.
32. Aoki S, Okada Y, Nishimura K, Nishimura K, Barkovich AJ, Kjos BO, Brasch RC, Norman D. Normal deposition of brain iron in childhood and adolescence: MR imaging at 1.5 T. *Radiology*. 1989;172:381–385.
33. Langkammer C, Schweser F, Krebs N, Deistung A, Goessler W, Scheurer E, Sommer K, Reishofer G, Yen K, Fazekas F, Ropele S, Reichenbach JR. Quantitative susceptibility mapping (QSM) as a means to measure brain iron? A post mortem validation study. *Neuroimage*. 2012;62:1593–1599.
34. Daugherty AM, Raz N. Appraising the role of iron in brain aging and cognition: promises and limitations of MRI methods. *Neuropsychol Rev*. 2015;25:272–287.
35. Kanda T, Nakai Y, Aoki S, Oba H, Toyoda K, Kitajima K, Furui S. Contribution of metals to brain MR signal intensity: review articles. *Jpn J Radiol*. 2016;34:258–266.
36. Novellino F, Cherubini A, Chiriaco C, Morelli M, Salsone M, Arabia G, Quattrone A. Brain iron deposition in essential tremor: a quantitative 3-Tesla magnetic resonance imaging study. *Mov Disord*. 2013;28:196–200.
37. Bilgic B, Pfefferbaum A, Rohlfing T, Sullivan EV, Adalsteinsson E. MRI estimates of brain iron concentration in normal aging using quantitative susceptibility mapping. *Neuroimage*. 2012;59:2625–2635.
38. Bartzokis G, Aravagiri M, Oldendorf WH, Mintz J, Marder SR. Field dependent transverse relaxation rate increase may be a specific measure of tissue iron stores. *Mag Res Med*. 1993;29:459–464.
39. Hardy PA, Gash D, Yokel R, Andersen A, Ai Y, Zhang Z. Correlation of R2 with total iron concentration in the brains of rhesus monkeys. *J Magn Reson Imaging*. 2005;21:118–127.
40. Berg D, Youdim MB. Role of iron in neurodegenerative disorders. *Top Magn Reson Imaging*. 2006;17:5–17.
41. Brass SD, Chen NK, Mulkern RV, Bakshi R. Magnetic resonance imaging of iron deposition in neurological disorders. *Top Magn Reson Imaging*. 2006;17:31–40.
42. Cherubini A, Péran P, Caltagirone C, Sabatini U, Spalletta G. Aging of subcortical nuclei: microstructural, mineralization and atrophy modifications measured in vivo using MRI. *Neuroimage*. 2009;48:29–36.
43. LeVine SM. Iron deposits in multiple sclerosis and Alzheimer's disease brains. *Brain Res*. 1997;760:298–303.
44. Shan DE, Pan HC, Ho DM, Teng MM, Chang C. Presence of activated microglia in a high-signal lesion on T1-weighted MR images: a biopsy sample re-examined. *AJNR Am J Neuroradiol*. 2007;28:602.
45. Chen JC, Hardy PA, Kucharczyk W, Clauberg M, Joshi JG, Vourlas A, Dhar M, Henkelman RM. MR of human postmortem brain tissue: correlative study between T2 and assays of iron and ferritin in Parkinson and Huntington disease. *AJNR Am J Neuroradiol*. 1993;14:275–281.
46. Dusek P, Dezortova M, Wuerfel J. Imaging of iron. *Int Rev Neurobiol*. 2013;110:195–239.
47. McNeill A, Chinnery PF. Neurodegeneration with brain iron accumulation. *Handb Clin Neurol*. 2011;100:161–172.
48. Arber CE, Li A, Houlden H, Wray S. Review: Insights into molecular mechanisms of disease in neurodegeneration with brain iron accumulation: unifying theories. *Neuropathol Appl Neurobiol*. 2016;42:220–241.
49. Kurian MA, Hayflick SJ. Pantothenate kinase-associated neurodegeneration (PKAN) and PLA2G6-associated neurodegeneration (PLAN): review of two major neurodegeneration with brain iron accumulation (NBIA) phenotypes. *Int Rev Neurobiol*. 2013;110:49–71.
50. Popławska-Domaszewicz K, Florczak-Wyspiańska J, Kozubski W. Update on neurodegeneration with brain iron accumulation. *Neurol Neurochir Pol*. 2014;48:206–213.
51. Schneider SA, Dusek P, Hardy J, Westenberger A, Jankovic J, Bhatia KP. Genetics and pathophysiology of neurodegeneration with brain iron accumulation (NBIA). *Curr Neuropharmacol*. 2013;11:59–79.
52. McNeill A, Birchall D, Hayflick SJ, Gregory A, Schenk JF, Zimmerman EA, Shang H, Miyajima H, Chinnery PF. T2* and FSE MRI distinguishes four subtypes of neurodegeneration with brain iron accumulation. *Neurology*. 2008;70:1614–1619.
53. Kaler SG. Inborn errors of copper metabolism. *Handb Clin Neurol*. 2013;113:1745–1754.
54. Patil M, Sheth KA, Krishnamurthy AC, Devarbhavi H. A review and current perspective on Wilson disease. *J Clin Exp Hepatol*. 2013;3:321–336.
55. Meenakshi-Sundaram S, Mahadevan A, Taly AB, Arunodaya GR, Swamy HS, Shankar SK. Wilson's disease: a clinico-neuropathological autopsy study. *J Clin Neurosci*. 2008;15:409–417.
56. Poujois A, Devedjian JC, Moreau C, Devos D, Chaine P, Woimant F, Duce JA. Bioavailable trace metals in neurological diseases. *Curr Treat Options Neurol*. 2016;18:46.

57. Hermann W. Morphological and functional imaging in neurological and non-neurological Wilson's patients. *Ann NY Acad Sci*. 2014;1315:24–29.
58. Norenberg MD. The role of astrocytes in hepatic encephalopathy. *Neurochem Pathol*. 1987;1:13–33.
59. van Wassenaer-van Hall HN, van den Heuvel AG, Algra A, Hoogenraad TU, Mali WP. Wilson disease: findings at MR imaging and CT of the brain with clinical correlation. *Radiology*. 1996;198:531–536.
60. Pulai S, Biswas A, Roy A, Guin DS, Pandit A, Gangopadhyay G, Ghorai PK, Sarkhel S, Senapati AK. Clinical features, MRI brain, and MRS abnormalities of drug-naïve neurologic Wilson's disease. *Neurol India*. 2014;62:153–158.
61. Trocello JM, Woimant F, El Balkhi S, Guichard JP, Poupon J, Chappuis P, Feillet F. Extensive striatal, cortical, and white matter brain MRI abnormalities in Wilson disease. *Neurology*. 2013;81:1557.
62. King AD, Walshe JM, Kendall BE, Chinn RJ, Paley MN, Wilkinson ID, Halligan S, Hall-Craggs MA. Cranial MR imaging in Wilson's disease. *AJR Am J Roentgenol*. 1996;167:1579–1584.
63. Kim TJ, Kim IO, Kim WS, Cheon JE, Moon SG, Kwon JW, Seo JK, Yeon KM. MR imaging of the brain in Wilson disease of childhood: findings before and after treatment with clinical correlation. *AJNR Am J Neuroradiol*. 2006;27:1373–1378.
64. Vymazal J, Bulte JW, Frank JA, Di Chiro G, Brooks RA. Frequency dependence of MR relaxation times. I. Paramagnetic ions. *J Magn Reson Imaging*. 1993;3:637–640.
65. Dusek P, Roos PM, Litwin T, Schneider SA, Flaten TP, Aaseth J. The neurotoxicity of iron, copper and manganese in Parkinson's and Wilson's diseases. *J Trace Elem Med Biol*. 2015;31:193–203.
66. Mochizuki H, Kamakura K, Masaki T, Okano M, Nagata N, Inui A, Fujisawa T, Kaji T. Atypical MRI features of Wilson's disease: high signal in globus pallidus on T1-weighted images. *Neuroradiology*. 1997;39:171–174.
67. Saatci I, Topcu M, Baltaoglu FF, Köse G, Yalaz K, Renda Y, Besim A. Cranial MR findings in Wilson's disease. *Acta Radiol*. 1997;38:250–258.
68. Sinha S, Taly AB, Ravishankar S, Prashanth LK, Venugopal KS, Arunodaya GR, Vasudev MK, Swamy HS. Wilson's disease: cranial MRI observations and clinical correlation. *Neuroradiology*. 2006;48:613–621.
69. Faa G, Lisci M, Caria MP, Ambu R, Sciot R, Nurchi VM, Silvagni R, Diaz A, Crisponi G. Brain copper, iron, magnesium, zinc, calcium, sulfur and phosphorus storage in Wilson's disease. *J Trace Elem Med Biol*. 2001;15:155–160.
70. Litwin T, Gromadzka G, Szpak GM, Jabłonka-Salach K, Bulska E, Członkowska A. Brain metal accumulation in Wilson's disease. *J Neurol Sci*. 2013;329:55–58.
71. Bruehlmeier M, Leenders KL, Vontobel P, Calonder C, Antonini A, Weindl A. Increased cerebral iron uptake in Wilson's disease: a ^{52}Fe-citrate PET study. *J Nucl Med*. 2000;41:781–787.
72. Sinha S, Taly AB, Prashanth LK, Ravishankar S, Arunodaya GR, Vasudev MK. Sequential MRI changes in Wilson's disease with de-coppering therapy: a study of 50 patients. *Br J Radiol*. 2007;80:744–749.
73. Chen P, Chakraborty S, Mukhopadhyay S, Lee E, Paoliello MM, Bowman AB, Aschner M. Manganese homeostasis in the nervous system. *J Neurochem*. 2015;134:601–610.
74. Horning KJ, Caito SW, Tipps KG, Bowman AB, Aschner M. Manganese is essential for neuronal health. *Annu Rev Nutr*. 2015;35:71–108.
75. Narita K, Kawasaki F, Kita H. Mn and Mg influxes through Ca channels of motor nerve terminals are prevented by verapamil in frogs. *Brain Res*. 1990;510:289–295.
76. Gallagher JJ, Zhang X, Ziomek GJ, Jacobs RE, Bearer EL. Deficits in axonal transport in hippocampal-based circuitry and the visual pathway in APP knock-out animals witnessed by manganese enhanced MRI. *Neuroimage*. 2012;60:1856–1866.
77. Ho LC, Wang B, Conner IP, van der Merwe Y, Bilonick RA, Kim SG, Wu EX, Sigal IA, Wollstein G, Schuman JS, Chan KC. In vivo evaluation of white matter integrity and anterograde transport in visual system after excitotoxic retinal injury with multimodal MRI and OCT. *Invest Ophthalmol Vis Sci*. 2015;56:3788–3800.
78. Jung DJ, Han M, Jin SU, Lee SH, Park I, Cho HJ, Kwon TJ, Lee HJ, Cho JH, Lee KY, Chang Y. Functional mapping of the auditory tract in rodent tinnitus model using manganese-enhanced magnetic resonance imaging. *Neuroimage*. 2014;100:642–649.
79. Thuen M, Berry M, Pedersen TB, Goa PE, Summerfield M, Haraldseth O, Sandvig A, Brekken C. Manganese-enhanced MRI of the rat visual pathway: acute neural toxicity, contrast enhancement, axon resolution, axonal transport, and clearance of Mn(2+). *J Magn Reson Imaging*. 2008;28:855–865.
80. Inoue T, Majid T, Pautler RG. Manganese enhanced MRI (MEMRI): neurophysiological applications. *Rev Neurosci*. 2011;22:675–694.
81. Malheiros JM, Paiva FF, Longo BM, Hamani C, Covolan L. Manganese-enhanced MRI: biological applications in neuroscience. *Front Neurol*. 2015;6:161.

82. Dorman DC. Extrapyramidal system neurotoxicity: animal models. *Handb Clin Neurol.* 2015;131:207–223.
83. Lucchini RG, Martin CJ, Doney BC. From manganism to manganese-induced parkinsonism: a conceptual model based on the evolution of exposure. *Neuromolecular Med.* 2009;11:311–321.
84. Roels HA, Bowler RM, Kim Y, Claus Henn B, Mergler D, Hoet P, Gocheva VV, Bellinger DC, Wright RO, Harris MG, Chang Y, Bouchard MF, Riojas-Rodriguez H, Menezes-Filho JA, Téllez-Rojo MM. Manganese exposure and cognitive deficits: a growing concern for manganese neurotoxicity. *Neurotoxicology.* 2012;33:872–880.
85. Fitsanakis VA, Zhang N, Avison MJ, Gore JC, Aschner JL, Aschner M. The use of magnetic resonance imaging (MRI) in the study of manganese neurotoxicity. *Neurotoxicology.* 2006;27:798–806.
86. Tuschl K, Mills PB, Clayton PT. Manganese and the brain. *Int Rev Neurobiol.* 2013;110:277–312.
87. Baker MG, Criswell SR, Racette BA, Simpson CD, Sheppard L, Checkoway H, Seixas NS. Neurological outcomes associated with low-level manganese exposure in an inception cohort of asymptomatic welding trainees. *Scand J Work Environ Health.* 2015;41:94–101.
88. Kim E, Kim Y, Cheong HK, Cho S, Shin YC, Sakong J, Kim KS, Yang JS, Jin YW, Kang SK. Pallidal index on MRI as a target organ dose of manganese: structural equation model analysis. *Neurotoxicology.* 2005;26:351–359.
89. Li SJ, Jiang L, Fu X, Huang S, Huang YN, Li XR, Chen JW, Li Y, Luo HL, Wang F, Ou SY, Jiang YM. Pallidal index as biomarker of manganese brain accumulation and associated with manganese levels in blood: a meta-analysis. *PLoS One.* 2014;9:e93900.
90. Shin YC, Kim E, Cheong HK, Cho S, Sakong J, Kim KS, Yang JS, Jin YW, Kang SK, Kim Y. High signal intensity on magnetic resonance imaging as a predictor of neurobehavioral performance of workers exposed to manganese. *Neurotoxicology.* 2007;28:257–262.
91. Dorman DC, Struve MF, Wong BA, Dye JA, Robertson ID. Correlation of brain magnetic resonance imaging changes with pallidal manganese concentrations in rhesus monkeys following subchronic manganese inhalation. *Toxicol Sci.* 2006;92:219–227.
92. Lee EY, Flynn MR, Du G, Lewis MM, Fry R, Herring AH, Van Buren E, Van Buren S, Smeester L, Kong L, Yang Q, Mailman RB, Huang X. T1 relaxation rate (R1) indicates nonlinear Mn accumulation in brain tissue of welders with low-level exposure. *Toxicol Sci.* 2015;146:281–289.
93. Lee EY, Flynn MR, Du G, Li Y, Lewis MM, Herring AH, Van Buren E, Van Buren S, Kong L, Fry RC, Snyder AM, Connor JR, Yang QX, Mailman RB, Huang X. Increased R2* in the caudate nucleus of asymptomatic welders. *Toxicol Sci.* 2016;150:369–377.
94. Lewis MM, Flynn MR, Lee EY, Van Buren S, Van Buren E, Du G, Fry RC, Herring AH, Kong L, Mailman RB, Huang X. Longitudinal T1 relaxation rate (R1) captures changes in short-term Mn exposure in welders. *Neurotoxicology.* 2016;57:39–44.
95. Han SH, Ahn SW, Youn YC, Shin HW. Reversal of pallidal magnetic resonance imaging T1 hyperintensity in a welder presenting as reversible parkinsonism. *Neurol India.* 2014;62:117–118.
96. Aschner JL, Anderson A, Slaughter JC, Aschner M, Steele S, Beller A, Mouvery A, Furlong HM, Maitre NL. Neuroimaging identifies increased manganese deposition in infants receiving parenteral nutrition. *Am J Clin Nutr.* 2015;102:1482–1489.
97. Dion LA, Bouchard MF, Sauvé S, Barbeau B, Tucholka A, Major P, Gilbert G, Mergler D, Saint-Amour D. MRI pallidal signal in children exposed to manganese in drinking water. *Neurotoxicology.* 2016;53:124–131.
98. Tuschl K, Meyer E, Valdivia LE, Zhao N, Dadswell C, Abdul-Sada A, Hung CY, Simpson MA, Chong WK, Jacques TS, Woltjer RL, Eaton S, Gregory A, Sanford L, Kara E, Houlden H, Cuno SM, Prokisch H, Valletta L, Tiranti V, Younis R, Maher ER, Spencer J, Straatman-Iwanowska A, Gissen P, Selim LA, Pintos-Morell G, Coroleu-Lletget W, Mohammad SS, Yoganathan S, Dale RC, Thomas M, Rihel J, Bodamer OA, Enns CA, Hayflick SJ, Clayton PT, Mills PB, Kurian MA, Wilson SW. Mutations in SLC39A14 disrupt manganese homeostasis and cause childhood-onset parkinsonism-dystonia. *Nat Commun.* 2016;7:11601.
99. Aschner M, Erikson KM, Dorman DC. Manganese dosimetry: species differences and implications for neurotoxicity. *Crit Rev Toxicol.* 2005;35:1–32.
100. Flynn MR, Susi P. Neurological risks associated with manganese exposure from welding operations—a literature review. *Int J Hyg Environ Health.* 2009;212:459–469.
101. Sen S, Flynn MR, Du G, Tröster AI, An H, Huang X. Manganese accumulation in the olfactory bulbs and other brain regions of "asymptomatic" welders. *Toxicol Sci.* 2011;121:160–167.
102. Cross DJ, Minoshima S, Anzai Y, Flexman JA, Keogh BP, Kim Y, Maravilla KR. Statistical mapping of functional olfactory connections of the rat brain in vivo. *Neuroimage.* 2004;23:1326–1335.

103. Sepúlveda MR, Dresselaers T, Vangheluwe P, Everaerts W, Himmelreich U, Mata AM, Wuytack F. Evaluation of manganese uptake and toxicity in mouse brain during continuous MnCl2 administration using osmotic pumps. *Contrast Media Mol Imaging*. 2012;7:426–434.
104. Foster ML, Bartnikas TB, Johnson LC, Herrera C, Pettiglio MA, Keene AM, Taylor MD, Dorman DC. Pharmacokinetic evaluation of the equivalency of gavage, dietary, and drinking water exposure to manganese in F344 rats. *Toxicol Sci*. 2015;145:244–251.
105. Das K, Singh P, Chawla Y, Duseja A, Dhiman RK, Suri S. Magnetic resonance imaging of brain in patients with cirrhotic and non-cirrhotic portal hypertension. *Dig Dis Sci*. 2008;53:2793–2798.
106. Rovira A, Alonso J, Córdoba J. MR imaging findings in hepatic encephalopathy. *AJNR Am J Neuroradiol*. 2008;29:1612–1621.
107. Torisu S, Washizu M, Hasegawa D, Orima H. Measurement of brain trace elements in a dog with a portosystemic shunt: relation between hyperintensity on T1-weighted magnetic resonance images in lentiform nuclei and brain trace elements. *J Vet Med Sci*. 2008;70:1391–1393.
108. Rose C, Butterworth RF, Zayed J, Normandin L, Todd K, Michalak A, Spahr L, Huet PM, Pomier-Layrargues G. Manganese deposition in basal ganglia structures results from both portal-systemic shunting and liver dysfunction. *Gastroenterology*. 1999;117:640–644.
109. Maeda H, Sato M, Yoshikawa A, Kimura M, Sonomura T, Terada M, Kishi K. Brain MR imaging in patients with hepatic cirrhosis: relationship between high intensity signal in basal ganglia on T1-weighted images and elemental concentrations in brain. *Neuroradiology*. 1997;39:546–550.

CHAPTER

18

Metalloregulation of Protein Clearance: New Therapeutic Avenues for Neurodegenerative Diseases

Alejandra Ramírez Muñoz, Mark A. Greenough, Ashley I. Bush, Carlos M. Opazo

The Florey Institute of Neuroscience and Mental Health, The University of Melbourne, Melbourne, VIC, Australia

OUTLINE

INTRODUCTION

Transition metals, such as copper, iron and zinc have an essential role in neuronal function. Several enzymes coordinate copper, iron, and zinc as cofactors for their activity, such as Zn/Cu superoxide dismutase.[1,2] These transition metals also regulate protein trafficking,

Biometals in Neurodegenerative Diseases. http://dx.doi.org/10.1016/B978-0-12-804562-6.00018-X

neurotransmission and synaptic plasticity in mature neurons.[1–4] Thus, there is an increase in the copper requirements at the secretory pathway for the synthesis of copper-dependent enzymes during neuronal differentiation.[1] Zinc blocks GABAA and *N*-methyl-D-aspartate (NMDA) receptors,[5] but copper has a biphasic effect on neurotransmission.[6] Iron is required for NMDA-induced ERK1/2 phosphorylation and further nuclear translocation, crucial for long-term potentiation (LTP).[2] Loss in metal homeostasis is also associated with neurodegeneration.[5,7–9]

Proteinopathy is a common feature of many neurodegenerative diseases including amyotrophic lateral sclerosis (ALS), Alzheimer's disease (AD), Parkinson's disease (PD), Huntington's and Prion diseases, which are characterized by the formation of protein aggregates in the Central Nervous System (Table 18.1). Extensive literature clearly indicates that transition metals interact with the proteins enriched in these structures promoting their aggregation, which are resistant to proteolysis and denaturation.[10–18] However, the role of these metals on the protein clearance mechanisms has received less attention, which is the major focus of this review.

Histopathological and biochemical studies indicate that ubiquitin proteasome system (UPS) dysfunction may be involved in the formation and accumulation of protein aggregates in the brains of patients with neurodegenerative diseases.[10–15] These aggregates are characterized by being enriched with ubiquitin, a feature that is commonly used to identify pathological lesions associated with these diseases.[10] Although how these aggregates are formed remains unknown, the presence of UPS and autophagy-lysosomal components in these aggregates suggest that these degradative pathways might be affected or involved in the onset

TABLE 18.1 Protein Aggregation is a Common Feature of Neurodegenerative Diseases

Neurodegenerative Disease	Brain localization	Protein aggregates/subcellular localization	References
Alzheimer's disease	Cerebral cortex, hippocampus	Neurofibrillary tangles; senile plaques, granulovacuolar inclusions and thread-like structures in the neuropil	[10–12]
Parkinson's disease	Cerebral cortex, midbrain (*substantia nigra*)	Intermediate filaments of Lewy bodies (cell body) and Lewy neurites (neuronal process)	[10,13]
Amyotrophic lateral sclerosis	Spinal cord, neostriatum	Cytoplasmic inclusions	[10,14,15]
Huntington's disease	Cerebral cortex and striatum	Intranuclear inclusions (INI) and dystrophic neurites (DNs)	[10,16]
Prion disease	Cerebral cortex, hippocampus, temporal cortex	Lysosome-related vesicles	[10,12]
Frontotemporal dementia	Frontal temporal lobes and neocortex	Cytoplasmic inclusions	[17]
Ischemia-reperfusion stroke	Hippocampus CAI region	Cytosol and juxtanuclear inclusions	[18]

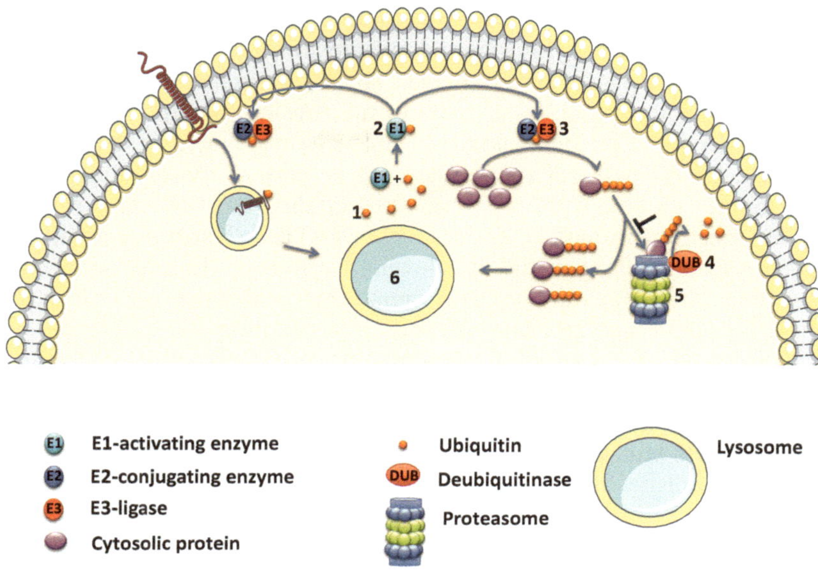

FIGURE 18.1 **Metalloregulation of protein clearance.** The figure depicts the general components of the ubiquitin proteasome system (UPS) and lysosomal pathways. The numbers in the figure indicate the intracellular components of the UPS and lysosomal pathways affected by copper, iron and zinc: (1) copper targets ubiquitin, (2) copper is delivered to E1 in the presence of copper-complexes, (3) copper and zinc bind E3 RING ligases, (4) zinc binds deubiquitinases (*DUB*), (5) copper (free or complexed to chelators), iron and zinc inhibit proteasome activity, and (6) copper, iron and zinc affect lysosome activity.

of these diseases.[10,19,20] Furthermore, disruption in ubiquitin homeostasis resulting in a decrease in free ubiquitin pools has been implicated in neurodegeneration.[21] Considering that the conjugation of free ubiquitin to proteins is a key step for the protein degradation driven by the UPS and the autophagy-lysosome system, the decrease of free ubiquitin is expected to adversely affect normal protein degradation[22,23] (Fig. 18.1). Both pathways have an important role in neuronal development, synaptic plasticity and neuronal survival,[24,25] and a disturbance in their function has been directly implicated in the pathogenesis and/or progression of several neurodegenerative diseases.[19,26,27]

The ALIGATOR and GSEA algorithms used in the International Genomics of Alzheimer's Project (IGAP) database, recently identified several genes that encodes components of the UPS to be involved in AD onset.[28] Also, it is well known that mutations in the *parkin* gene, a component of UPS, are particularly common in familial cases of PD that have an early age of onset.[29] Parkin has ubiquitin ligase activity, one of the key components of the ubiquitination machinery that regulates the degradation of mitochondrial and synaptic vesicle-associated proteins.[30,31]

Another AD hallmark is the presence of intracellular tau aggregates.[32] Evidence obtained from tau-expressing M1C cells suggest that the autophagy–lysosomal pathway is involved in the clearance of tau.[33] The perturbation of this pathway with chloroquine (CQ) decreases the activities of lysosomal proteases cathepsins D, B, and L, leading to the formation of tau oligomers and insoluble aggregates.[33] Furthermore, the molecular chaperone p62 mediates tau degradation by the autophagy–lysosomal system in a Presenilin 1 (PSEN1)-dependent manner, linking two of the major pathological proteins associated with AD.[34] Intriguingly, PSENs are required for normal cellular copper and zinc uptake and metalloenzyme function.[35,36] Together with the described role for PSEN1 in autophagy,[37,38] and the fact that lysosomes are enriched for copper and zinc, either one or both of these metals may play a key role in autolysosomal function. Certainly, calcium signaling has been linked to PSEN1's role in autophagy. The mechanism may be at the level of vATPase lysosomal acidification (which would also affect lysosomal copper and zinc levels),[39] although the precise mechanism is still debated.[40] The effect that PSEN may have on transition metal status and subsequent autophagy function is an area that our group is currently investigating.

Lysosomal dysfunction is a feature of many genetic mutations associated with PD.[20] These mutations lead to a failure in the lysosomal pathway, and have been associated with the accumulation of α-synuclein, Park2, and ubiquitinated proteins.[20] Furthermore, the TgCRND8 AD mice model exhibits enlarged cathepsin D-positive autolysosomes in the hippocampus, indicating a marked failure in the autophagy–lysosomal pathway.[41] This feature has also been observed in postmortem brains of AD patients.[19] The enlarged autolysosomes are specifically located within the neuronal soma and processes. Moreover, the autophagic vacuole and lysosome fractions contain abnormally high levels of LC3B-II, suggesting impairment in autophagic proteolysis.[41] In addition, these cathepsin D-positive autophagic-lysosomal compartments display immunoreactivity for ubiquitin and Aβ.[41] Furthermore, the deletion of cystatin B, a lysosomal cysteine protease inhibitor, stimulates autophagic-lysosomal proteolysis, promoting the clearance of ubiquitin and Aβ aggregates in TgCRND8 mice brains, which is correlated with a marked improvement in learning and memory functions.[41]

UPS components are sensitive to levels of metals, leading in some cases to inhibition of this pathway with concomitant protein accumulation.[42,43] While autophagy has been described as the initial cellular response to exposure to toxic metal concentrations,[44] a dysregulation of this pathway has also been associated with metal-dependent neurotoxicity.[45,46]

METALLOREGULATION OF THE UBIQUITIN PROTEASOME SYSTEM: IMPLICATION IN NEURODEGENERATIVE DISEASES

The UPS is one of the major intracellular protein degradative systems.[47] This pathway is highly selective and governed by the attachment of a Lys48-linked polyubiquitin chain to the protein target through a process called ubiquitination.[22] Ubiquitination is a posttranslational modification that forms a peptide bond between the lysine residue of the protein and the carboxy-terminal domain of ubiquitin. Ubiquitination is an ATP-dependent enzymatic process, whereby ubiquitin is first activated by the ubiquitin-activating enzymes (E1), then, transferred to a conjugating enzyme (E2), and finally covalently attached to lysine residues of the protein target in a process mediated by the ubiquitin-protein ligases (E3). The polyubiquitin chain is a signal for the 26S proteasome, a multienzymatic complex formed by a proteolytic core, the 20S proteasome, and the 19S complex with a regulatory function.[48,49] The protein is degraded, and the ubiquitin moieties are recycled by the deubiquitinating enzymes (DUBs) (Fig. 18.1).[27]

A growing body of evidence has demonstrated a regulatory role of metals in the function of components of the UPS. In the following section we will discuss the role of metals in the regulation of the different UPS components, and how a metal imbalance could have a direct impact on UPS failure.

Ubiquitin

Ubiquitin is a 76-amino acid globular protein that is highly conserved and stable.[22] Disruption in ubiquitin homeostasis resulting in a decrease in free ubiquitin pools has been implicated in neurodegeneration.[21] Depletion of ubiquitin has been associated to cycloheximide-induced toxicity in *Saccharomyces cerevisiae* cells.[50] Cycloheximide treatment reduces total levels of ubiquitin (free ubiquitin and conjugated ubiquitin), and its toxicity is reduced by ubiquitin overexpression. Moreover, cells with a deletion in the *UBP6* gene (Δ*ubp6* cells) that encodes Ubp6 deubiquitinating enzyme, are more sensitive to cycloheximide toxic effects than wild-type cells, which suggests a key role for free ubiquitin in cell viability. Ubiquitin overexpression also rescues Δubp6 cells from cycloheximide toxicity, in a less efficient rate than the wild-type cells, indicating an important role of the ubiquitin recycling system in the homeostasis of free ubiquitin pools.[50] Furthermore, evidence has shown that ubiquitin bioavailability is fundamental for neuronal survival. This was observed in a *Ubb*-null mice where the disruption of the *Ubb* gene, one of the two mammalian polyubiquitin genes, causes a decrease in free ubiquitin levels, inducing a progressive neurodegeneration in the hypothalamus.[21]

In vitro data has shown that Cu(II) interacts with ubiquitin at its N-terminus, leading to ubiquitin thermal destabilization and aggregation at the physiological pH range.[43,51] The ubiquitin aggregates promoted by Cu(II) are insoluble, SDS-stable, and resistant to trypsin proteolysis. The destabilization of ubiquitin is specific for Cu(II), since the incubation with other metals, such as Zn(II), Ni(II), Cd(II), or Al(III) does not alter ubiquitin structure nor induces its aggregation.[43] Ubiquitin has two Cu(II)-binding sites, the first one at the methionine 1 and the second one at the histidine 68, which is a preferred metal-binding site at the physiological pH.[52] Furthermore, Cu(II) reduction to Cu(I) prevents ubiquitin oligomerization. Therefore, this Cu(II)–ubiquitin interaction would be favored under oxidative stress conditions, a classical feature in neurodegenerative diseases.[53,54] The ubiquitin aggregation mediated by Cu(II) could lead to a decrease in free ubiquitin that has been associated with cellular toxicity and neurodegeneration.[50,55–57] In addition, ubiquitin Cu(II)-dependent aggregation significantly inhibits the formation of Lys48 and Lys63 polyubiquitin chains,[52] which is consistent with evidence that has shown an impairment in the UPS function due to protein aggregation.[58] Altogether, these studies suggest a pathological relevance for ubiquitin destabilization and aggregation promoted by its interaction with Cu(II).

E1 Ubiquitin-Activating Enzyme

The E1 ubiquitin-activating enzymes catalyze the first step of the ubiquitination cascade, which involves the formation of a thioester bond between the ubiquitin and the cysteine in the active site of E1 in an ATP-dependent reaction. Although it has not been described that the activity of this enzyme could be modulated by transition metals, a recent study showed that an increase in the intracellular levels of copper or zinc could inhibit its function.[59] HEK293 cells treated with dithiocarbamates Ziram or *N,N*-dimethyldithiocarbamate showed a significant decrease in E1 ubiquitin-activating enzyme activity, which correlated with an increase in copper and zinc intracellular levels. Moreover, the coincubation of dithiocarbamates with the copper chelator triethylenetetramine hydrochloride, prevented the inhibition of the E1-activating enzyme activity. The loss in the E1 ubiquitin-activating enzyme function could be associated to the oxidative stress promoted by these metals, as the presence of a cysteine residue in the active site of the enzyme makes its more susceptible to oxidative stress. Indeed, the cellular redox status of the ubiquitin-activating enzymes E1 is regulated by glutathione, the main antioxidant of the cells.[60] The factors that govern the activity of the E1-activating enzymes are relevant since loss in its function are related with apoptotic activation, motor impairment,[61] and also with the accumulation of mutant Huntingtin in the brain and peripheral tissues in a Huntington's disease mouse model.[62]

E3 Ubiquitin Ligases

Four main classes of E3 ubiquitin ligases have been described: homologous to E6-associated protein C-terminus (HECT), U-box, plant homeodomain (PHD) finger, and the really interesting novel gene (RING) finger.[63]

The RING fingers are characterized by the presence of an octet of cysteine and histidine residues organized in a conserved motif that coordinates two zinc ions. The coordination of the RING fingers with zinc ions is required for the domain folding, structure maintenance, and enzymatic function.[64,65]

For the E3 ubiquitin ligases, evidence suggests that the RING domains mediate the interaction between E2 ubiquitin conjugation enzymes with the E3 ubiquitin ligases, at the same time that the E3 ubiquitin ligase binds to the target protein for ubiquitination.[64–66]

Parkin has been described as a RING-type E3 ubiquitin ligase,[67] and failure in Parkin activity has been associated with an early-onset of PD.[29] It has been shown that *Drosophila* with a null *parkin* mutation are more vulnerable to 1-methyl-4-phenylpyridinium (MPP^+), rotenone, and paraquat toxicity, substances that have been associated with PD. *Drosophila parkin* mutant flies exposed to these agents suffered a significant decrease in their lifespan, that was prevented using copper and iron chelators.[68] Moreover, overexpression of the Ctr1B copper transporter in *Drosophila* lacking *parkin* exacerbated the rough eye phenotype associated to copper uptake.[68] Furthermore, it has been described a relevant role for Parkin in the clearance of damaged proteins by iron-induced oxidative stress.[69] These results indicate a protective role for the Parkin ubiquitin ligase activity against redox active metals implicated in PD pathogenesis.

X-linked inhibitor of apoptosis (XIAP) is another E3 Ligase that has been described to be regulated by metals.[70–72] It contains three amino-terminal baculovirus inhibitor of apoptosis protein repeat domain and a carboxy-terminal RING finger. These domains are capable of coordinating zinc by different combinations of cysteines and histidines.[71] XIAP plays an important role in copper homeostasis regulating the degradation of COMMD1, a protein that promotes the efflux of copper from the cell.[70–72] When cytosolic copper levels are low, XIAP efficiently degrades COMMD1, with a concomitant increase in the cytosolic copper levels. However, when cytosolic copper levels are elevated, XIAP binds copper resulting in a conformational change that is accompanied by a decrease in its half-life in cells. Under these conditions COMMD1 is not degraded, allowing the efflux of copper from the cytosol. Therefore,

XIAP is a cytosolic copper sensor that transduces the copper signal to UPS to regulate copper homeostasis.[70–72]

Furthermore, there is evidence that E3 ubiquitin ligase activity is necessary for the regulation of iron homeostasis. Cellular iron homeostasis is maintained by a balance between uptake and storage, and its bioavailability is regulated by the interaction between the iron-responsive elements (IREs) and iron regulatory proteins (IRPs).[73] It has been reported that the iron regulatory protein 2 (IRP2) turnover is regulated by the proteasome.[74,75] IRP2 is substrate of an E3 ubiquitin ligase complex, which contains a FBXL5 protein. Interestingly, FBXL5 has an iron- and oxygen-binding hemerythrin domain at the N-terminus (between the residues 1 and 161).[75] Moreover, the stability of FBXL5 is iron- and oxygen-dependent, and also it is degraded by the proteasome.[75] FBXL5 is accumulated under iron- and oxygen-replete conditions and degraded upon iron depletion. Therefore, this iron sensing mechanism regulates IRP2 degradation to maintain mammalian iron homeostasis.[75]

Deubiquitinases

Protein ubiquitination is a reversible process, mediated by the action of DUBs or deubiquitinases.[27] The deubiquitinases form part of the 19S regulatory complex of the 26S proteasome. The deubiquitinases are classified based on their enzymatic cleavage mechanism as zinc metalloproteases or cysteine proteases.[76]

POH1 or Rpn11 is a zinc metalloprotease[77] that contains a Jab1/MPN domain-associated metallopeptidase motif (JAMM) that is essential for the metal-dependent deubiquitinating activity of Rpn11.[78] Rpn11 has been described as a suppressor of the progressive neurodegeneration induced by expanded polyglutamine proteins associated with Huntington's disease and spinocerebellar ataxias.[79] Overexpression of Rpn11 protects against the toxicity produced by expanded polyglutamine and also abolishes the age-dependent decay in the proteasome activity, reducing the accumulation of ubiquitinated proteins and extending lifespan in a *Drosophila* model.[79]

The ubiquitin-specific peptidase 14 (Ups14), the mammalian ortholog for Ubp6 deubiquitinating enzyme, is a cysteine protease that is critical for the recycling of ubiquitin. It has been shown that the *ataxia* (*axJ*) mice exhibit neurological defects, as a result of a spontaneous recessive mutation that reduces the levels of Ups14.[57] In *axJ* mice, Ups14 expression is decreased in several tissues including the brain, which contains ~35% less free ubiquitin compared to wild-type mice.[55,56] The decrease in ubiquitin levels associated with the loss of Ups14 has a dramatic effect in neuromuscular junction activity.[56] Although there is not evidence that Usp14 activity is regulated by metals, it has been shown that copper complexes, such as copper (II) pyrithione can inhibit Ups14 activity,[80] suggesting that Ups14 has a specific metal-binding site.

Proteasome

The 26S proteasome is a multienzymatic complex (2000 kDa), composed by the 20S proteolytic core (750 kDa) and the 19S complex that contains the sites to recognize the K48-polyubiquinated proteins and the DUBs that remove the polyubiquitin chain, and translocate the proteins into the 20S core for their degradation.[49]

The accumulation of protein aggregates in neurodegenerative diseases has been associated to an impairment of the proteasome activity.[27] For example, in a mouse model of tauopathy there is a decrease in the chymotrypsin-like activity of the 26S proteasome.[26] Also, proteasomal inhibition has been used to develop a mouse model for PD.[81,82] Mice injected with lactacystin into the medial forebrain bundle have a decrease in motor activities related with dopaminergic neuron loss, mainly in the *substantia nigra*. Cellular changes include caspase-3 activation and early apoptotic changes, aberrant accumulation of ubiquitin positive and α-synuclein positive protein aggregates, and microglial activation.[82] Furthermore, iron levels are increased in this mouse model.[74,82] Treatments with iron-chelators, such as VK-28 [5-(4-(2-hydroxyethyl) piperazin-1-yl (methyl)-8-hydroxyquinoline], and its derivative M30 [5-(*N*-methyl-*N*-propargyaminomethyl)-8-hydroxyquinoline] have a neuroprotective effect against lactacystin-induced neurodegeneration by restoring proteasome activity, decreasing iron overload and microglial activation.[74] This evidence suggests that the proteasome activity could be modulated by iron.

The hydrolytic activity of the 20S proteasome can be inhibited by high concentration of Zn(II) and Cu(II), but not Fe(II) or Fe(III), which could suggest a role for Cu(II) and Zn(II) in protein aggregation due to inhibited proteasome activity.[42] However, the Cu(II) concentration (0.5 mM) needed to inhibit the proteasome activity exceeds the free copper levels expected under physiological conditions at the synaptic cleft and in the cytosol.[83,84]

METALS AS MEDIATORS OF AUTOPHAGY-LYSOSOMAL RESPONSE

The second main protein degradation system in eukaryotic cells occurs via autophagy–lysosomal system (Fig. 18.1). There are four specialized lysosomal proteolysis pathways. These pathways differ in the manner in which they deliver cargo into the lysosomes: macroautophagy, microautophagy, chaperone-mediated autophagy and the multivesicular body pathway.[23] Macroautophagy, or commonly called autophagy, is a multistep process, which includes the induction or cargo selection, isolation membrane nucleation, isolation membrane expansion, completion, fusion with the lysosome, breakdown, and finally export of the metabolites. Autophagy has a crucial role in the clearance of protein aggregates and dysfunctional organelles and is a source of amino acids for new protein synthesis.[23] During aging there is a decrease in lysosomal activity,[85] and also failures in the autophagy–lysosomal system have been associated with neurodegenerative diseases.[19,41] These changes in the autophagy–lysosomal system may be linked to the changes in metals associated to neurodegeneration and aging. It has been also reported that an increase in autophagy activity is associated with neuronal death under oxidative stress conditions, such as ischemia-reperfusion injury and metal neurotoxicity,[86–88] which could be directly related to neurodegenerative diseases pathogenesis as will be discussed in the following sections.

Copper

Copper imbalance plays a key role in neurodegenerative diseases.[5,8] In this context, it has been reported that Cu(II) forms a neurotoxic complex with dopamine.[89] The toxicity associated with the formation of this complex is prevented in the presence of the antioxidant ascorbic acid, indicating the importance of the redox state of the cell. Moreover, the cell death induced by the Cu–dopamine complexes is not related to activation of apoptotic pathways, but rather to an increase in autophagy.[88] Indeed, other studies have demonstrated that copper induces the accumulation of autophagosomes in a dose-dependent manner. The accumulation of copper-induced autophagosomes occurs with a concomitant increase in autophagy degradation activity,[90,91] which could be part of a homeostatic response that is activated by the generation of reactive oxygen species.[92] Also, evidence indicates that copper induces autophagy through the activation of adenosinemonophosphate (AMP)-activated protein kinase (AMPK), that in turn transiently activates Unc-51-like kinase 1 (Ulk1). Nonetheless, AMPK and Ulk1 knockout MEF cells are more sensitive to copper-induced toxicity, suggesting that activation of autophagy is a protective response of the cell against copper toxicity.[91]

Iron

Iron dyshomeostasis and accumulation has been linked with several neurodegenerative diseases, such as AD and PD.[81,93] Recent evidence has shown that iron homeostasis is regulated by autophagy–lysosomal proteolysis.[94]

The main intracellular iron storage is cytosolic ferritin.[95] Degradation of cytosolic ferritin, and further iron release, is mainly regulated by autophagic-lysosomal proteolysis.[94,96] Ferritin degradation is also carried by the proteasome degradation.[94] However, iron-mediated cell death in a cellular PD model results from excessive autophagy activity.[45] Furthermore, it has been reported that cells with increased autophagy activity are sensitive to oxidative stress associated with ferritin degradation and release of iron into the cytosol,[46] suggesting that iron could mainly affect protein degradation via the lysosomal pathway.

Zinc

Neuronal zinc homeostasis is mainly regulated by two types of transporters: Znt (zinc transporter) and Zip (Zrt/Irt-like protein) transporters.[97] Zinc dysregulation in the brain has been related with neurodegenerative diseases and neuronal damage associated with traumatic brain injury and seizure.[5,98]

There are reports that indicate that zinc acts as positive regulator of autophagy.[99,100] As mentioned earlier, autophagy has a crucial role in the degradation of intracellular protein aggregates (Fig. 18.1).[101] Thus, an increase in autophagy may have a protective effect against toxic protein aggregates characteristic of neurodegenerative diseases. In fact, clioquinol–zinc complexes induce autophagy and promote the accumulation of zinc entry in autophagic vacuoles.[100] The clioquinol-induced autophagy is blocked by *N,N,N′,N′*-tetrakis(2-pyridylmethyl) ethane-1,2-diamine (TPEN), a high affinity zinc chelator, corroborating the role of zinc as an autophagy inducer. Furthermore, clioquinol-induced autophagy increases the clearance of abnormal proteins in SH-SY5Y cells overexpressing a mutant Huntingtin protein, suggesting a protective role of zinc-mediated autophagy.[100]

In contrast, it has been shown that high levels of zinc induces toxicity and cell death via autophagy.[99] In addition, recurrent seizures in neonatal Sprague-Dawley rats induced an increase in the levels of autophagy-related proteins, Beclin-1 and LC3, in the cerebral cortex, indicating an increase in autophagy activity. Also, it has been shown that labile zinc accumulates in autophagic vacuoles under autophagy-induced conditions, leading to cell death. Furthermore, zinc chelation prevents autophagy-induced cell death.[102] Zinc-induced oxidative stress leads to autophagy-mediated cell death via lysosomal membrane permeabilization (LMP).[102] In addition, H_2O_2-induced oxidative stress induces the formation of zinc-containing enlarged lysosomes in hippocampal neurons, which are susceptible to disintegration as consequence of LMP.[87] Furthermore, neurons exposed to high zinc levels (500 μM) exhibited a dramatic focal swelling of neurites and an increase in zinc containing vesicles, which correlated with an increase in the lysosomal enzyme cathepsin D in the cytosol, a classical feature of LMP.[87] Altogether these studies suggest that zinc can modulate autophagy and therefore a dysregulation in zinc homeostasis could lead to autophagy–lysosomal dysfunction and ultimately to cell death.

CONCLUSIONS

The amount of evidence that supports a role of transition metals in neurodegenerative diseases has rapidly increased in the last decade. However, the mechanisms by which these metals are involved in these diseases are not fully elucidated. Understanding what role metals play in degradative pathways is a new area of investigation. Here, we describe the UPS components that are regulated by copper, iron and zinc. Moreover, we have discussed how these metals affect the autophagy–lysosomal system. In this case, specific lysosomal targets for transitional metals have not been identified yet. We propose that the UPS enzymes regulated by these transition metals are potential targets to generate new pharmacological treatment for these diseases. Further studies are required to identify the specific proteins in the autophagy–lysosomal system that sense transition metals.

Acknowledgments

The Florey Institute of Neuroscience and Mental Health acknowledges the strong support from the Victorian Government and in particular the funding from the Operational Infrastructure Support Grant. This work was supported by a NHMRC Dementia Research Fellowship (MAG), the Australian Research Council (AIB; CMO), the National Health and Medical Research Council, and the CRC for Mental Health (AIB); ARM is recipient of a BECA Chile Scholarship from the Chilean Government. Figures were produced using Servier Medical Art (http://www.servier.com).

References

1. Hatori Y, Yan Y, Schmidt K, et al. Neuronal differentiation is associated with a redox-regulated increase of copper flow to the secretory pathway. *Nat Commun*. 2016;7:10640.
2. Munoz P, Humeres A, Elgueta C, Kirkwood A, Hidalgo C, Nunez MT. Iron mediates *N*-methyl-D-aspartate receptor-dependent stimulation of calcium-induced pathways and hippocampal synaptic plasticity. *J Biol Chem*. 2011;15(286):13382–13392.
3. Greenough MA, RA, Bush AI, Opazo CM. Metallo-patways to Alzheimer's disease: lessons from genetic disorders of copper trafficking. *Metallomics*. 2016;8:831–839.
4. Castro PA, Ramirez A, Sepulveda FJ, et al. Copper-uptake is critical for the down regulation of synapsin and dynamin induced by neocuproine: modulation of synaptic activity in hippocampal neurons. *Front Aging Neurosci*. 2014;6:319.
5. Ayton S, Lei P, Bush AI. Metallostasis in Alzheimer's disease. *Free Radic Biol Med*. 2013;62:76–89.

6. Peters C, Munoz B, Sepulveda FJ, et al. Biphasic effects of copper on neurotransmission in rat hippocampal neurons. *J Neurochem*. 2011;119(1):78–88.
7. Bush AI. Metals and neuroscience. *Curr Opin Chem Biol*. 2000;4(2):184–191.
8. Bush AI. Copper, zinc, and the metallobiology of Alzheimer disease. *Alzheimer Dis Assoc Disord*. 2003;17(3): 147–150.
9. Bush AI, Masters CL, Tanzi RE. Copper, beta-amyloid, and Alzheimer's disease: tapping a sensitive connection. *Proc Natl Acad Sci USA*. 2003;100(20):11193–11194.
10. Lowe J, Hand N, Mayer RJ. Application of ubiquitin immunohistochemistry to the diagnosis of disease. *Methods Enzymol*. 2005;399:86–119.
11. Perry G, Friedman R, Shaw G, Chau V. Ubiquitin is detected in neurofibrillary tangles and senile plaque neurites of Alzheimer disease brains. *Proc Natl Acad Sci USA*. 1987;84(9):3033–3036.
12. Ironside JW, McCardle L, Hayward PA, Bell JE. Ubiquitin immunocytochemistry in human spongiform encephalopathies. *Neuropathol Appl Neurobiol*. 1993;19(2):134–140.
13. Lowe J, Blanchard A, Morrell K, et al. Ubiquitin is a common factor in intermediate filament inclusion bodies of diverse type in man, including those of Parkinson's disease, Pick's disease, and Alzheimer's disease, as well as Rosenthal fibres in cerebellar astrocytomas, cytoplasmic bodies in muscle, and mallory bodies in alcoholic liver disease. *J Pathol*. 1988;155(1):9–15.
14. Wakabayashi K, Piao YS, Hayashi S, Kakita A, Yamada M, Takahashi H. Ubiquitinated neuronal inclusions in the neostriatum in patients with amyotrophic lateral sclerosis with and without dementia—a study of 60 patients 31 to 87 years of age. *Clin Neuropathol*. 2001;20(2):47–52.
15. Leigh PN, Anderton BH, Dodson A, Gallo JM, Swash M, Power DM. Ubiquitin deposits in anterior horn cells in motor neurone disease. *Neurosci Lett*. 1988;93(2–3):197–203.
16. DiFiglia M, Sapp E, Chase KO, et al. Aggregation of huntingtin in neuronal intranuclear inclusions and dystrophic neurites in brain. *Science*. 1997;277(5334):1990–1993.
17. Neumann M, Rademakers R, Roeber S, Baker M, Kretzschmar HA, Mackenzie IR. A new subtype of frontotemporal lobar degeneration with FUS pathology. *Brain J Neurol*. 2009;132(Pt 11):2922–2931.
18. Liang J, Yao J, Wang G, Wang Y, Wang B, Ge P. Ischemic postconditioning protects neuronal death caused by cerebral ischemia and reperfusion via attenuating protein aggregation. *Int J Med Sci*. 2012;9(10):923–932.
19. Nixon RA, Wegiel J, Kumar A, et al. Extensive involvement of autophagy in Alzheimer disease: an immuno-electron microscopy study. *J Neuropathol Exp Neurol*. 2005;64(2):113–122.
20. Schneider L, Zhang J. Lysosomal function in macromolecular homeostasis and bioenergetics in Parkinson's disease. *Mol Neurodegener*. 2010;5:14.
21. Ryu KY, Garza JC, Lu XY, Barsh GS, Kopito RR. Hypothalamic neurodegeneration and adult-onset obesity in mice lacking the Ubb polyubiquitin gene. *Proc Natl Acad Sci USA*. 2008;105(10):4016–4021.
22. Haglund K, Dikic I. Ubiquitylation and cell signaling. *EMBO J*. 2005;24(19):3353–3359.
23. Huber LA, Teis D. Lysosomal signaling in control of degradation pathways. *Curr Opin Cell Biol*. 2016;39:8–14.
24. Jakawich SK, Neely RM, Djakovic SN, Patrick GN, Sutton MA. An essential postsynaptic role for the ubiquitin proteasome system in slow homeostatic synaptic plasticity in cultured hippocampal neurons. *Neuroscience*. 2010;171(4):1016–1031.
25. Tian X, Gala U, Zhang Y, et al. A voltage-gated calcium channel regulates lysosomal fusion with endosomes and autophagosomes and is required for neuronal homeostasis. *PLoS Biol*. 2015;13(3):e1002103.
26. Myeku N, Clelland CL, Emrani S, et al. Tau-driven 26S proteasome impairment and cognitive dysfunction can be prevented early in disease by activating cAMP-PKA signaling. *Nat Med*. 2016;22(1):46–53.
27. Ciechanover A, Brundin P. The ubiquitin proteasome system in neurodegenerative diseases: sometimes the chicken, sometimes the egg. *Neuron*. 2003;40(2):427–446.
28. International Genomics of Alzheimer's Disease Consortium (IGAP)Convergent genetic and expression data implicate immunity in Alzheimer's disease. *Alzheimers Dementia*. 2015;11(6):658–671.
29. Lucking CB, Durr A, Bonifati V, et al. Association between early-onset Parkinson's disease and mutations in the parkin gene. *N Engl J Med*. 2000;342(21):1560–1567.
30. Matheoud D, Sugiura A, Bellemare-Pelletier A, et al. Parkinson's disease-related proteins PINK1 and Parkin repress mitochondrial antigen presentation. *Cell*. 2016;166:314–327.
31. Zhang Y, Gao J, Chung KK, Huang H, Dawson VL, Dawson TM. Parkin functions as an E2-dependent ubiquitin-protein ligase and promotes the degradation of the synaptic vesicle-associated protein, CDCrel-1. *Proc Natl Acad Sci USA*. 2000;97(24):13354–13359.

32. Kosik KS, Joachim CL, Selkoe DJ. Microtubule-associated protein tau (tau) is a major antigenic component of paired helical filaments in Alzheimer disease. *Proc Natl Acad Sci USA*. 1986;83(11):4044–4048.
33. Hamano T, Gendron TF, Causevic E, et al. Autophagic-lysosomal perturbation enhances tau aggregation in transfectants with induced wild-type tau expression. *Eur J Neurosci*. 2008;27(5):1119–1130.
34. Tung YT, Wang BJ, Hsu WM, et al. Presenilin-1 regulates the expression of p62 to govern p62-dependent tau degradation. *Mol Neurobiol*. 2014;49(1):10–27.
35. Greenough MA, Volitakis I, Li QX, et al. Presenilins promote the cellular uptake of copper and zinc and maintain copper chaperone of SOD1-dependent copper/zinc superoxide dismutase activity. *J Biol Chem*. 2011;286(11):9776–9786.
36. Southon A, Greenough MA, Ganio G, Bush AI, Burke R, Camakaris J. Presenilin promotes dietary copper uptake. *PLoS One*. 2013;8(5):e62811.
37. Lee JH, Yu WH, Kumar A, et al. Lysosomal proteolysis and autophagy require presenilin 1 and are disrupted by Alzheimer-related PS1 mutations. *Cell*. 2010;141(7):1146–1158.
38. Neely KM, Green KN, LaFerla FM. Presenilin is necessary for efficient proteolysis through the autophagy-lysosome system in a gamma-secretase-independent manner. *J Neurosci*. 2011;31(8):2781–2791.
39. Lee JH, McBrayer MK, Wolfe DM, et al. Presenilin 1 maintains lysosomal Ca(2+) homeostasis via TRPML1 by regulating vATPase-mediated lysosome acidification. *Cell Rep*. 2015;12(9):1430–1444.
40. Bezprozvanny I. Presenilins: a novel link between intracellular calcium signaling and lysosomal function?. *J Cell Biol*. 2012;198(1):7–10.
41. Yang DS, Stavrides P, Mohan PS, et al. Reversal of autophagy dysfunction in the TgCRND8 mouse model of Alzheimer's disease ameliorates amyloid pathologies and memory deficits. *Brain J Neurol*. 2011;134(Pt 1):258–277.
42. Amici M, Forti K, Nobili C, et al. Effect of neurotoxic metal ions on the proteolytic activities of the 20S proteasome from bovine brain. *J Biol Inorg Chem*. 2002;7(7–8):750–756.
43. Arnesano F, Scintilla S, Calo V, et al. Copper-triggered aggregation of ubiquitin. *PLoS One*. 2009;4(9):e7052.
44. Chatterjee S, Sarkar S, Bhattacharya S. Toxic metals and autophagy. *Chem Res Toxicol*. 2014;27(11):1887–1900.
45. Chew KC, Ang ET, Tai YK, et al. Enhanced autophagy from chronic toxicity of iron and mutant A53T alpha-synuclein: implications for neuronal cell death in Parkinson disease. *J Biol Chem*. 2011;286(38):33380–33389.
46. Kurz T, Gustafsson B, Brunk UT. Cell sensitivity to oxidative stress is influenced by ferritin autophagy. *Free Radic Biol Med*. 2011;50(11):1647–1658.
47. Komander D, Rape M. The ubiquitin code. *Annu Rev Biochem*. 2012;81:203–229.
48. Liu CW, Millen L, Roman TB, et al. Conformational remodeling of proteasomal substrates by PA700, the 19 S regulatory complex of the 26 S proteasome. *J Biol Chem*. 2002;277(30):26815–26820.
49. Jung T, Catalgol B, Grune T. The proteasomal system. *Mol Aspects Med*. 2009;30(4):191–296.
50. Hanna J, Leggett DS, Finley D. Ubiquitin depletion as a key mediator of toxicity by translational inhibitors. *Mol Cell Biol*. 2003;23(24):9251–9261.
51. Milardi D, Arnesano F, Grasso G, et al. Ubiquitin stability and the Lys63-linked polyubiquitination site are compromised on copper binding. *Angew Chem Int Ed Engl*. 2007;46(42):7993–7995.
52. Arena G, Bellia F, Frasca G, et al. Inorganic stressors of ubiquitin. *Inorg Chem*. 2013;52(16):9567–9573.
53. Mandal PK, Saharan S, Tripathi M, Murari G. Brain glutathione levels—a novel biomarker for mild cognitive impairment and Alzheimer's disease. *Biol Psychiatry*. 2015;78.
54. Martin HL, Teismann P. Glutathione—a review on its role and significance in Parkinson's disease. *FASEB J*. 2009;23(10):3263–3272.
55. Anderson C, Crimmins S, Wilson JA, Korbel GA, Ploegh HL, Wilson SM. Loss of Usp14 results in reduced levels of ubiquitin in ataxia mice. *J Neurochem*. 2005;95(3):724–731.
56. Chen PC, Bhattacharyya BJ, Hanna J, et al. Ubiquitin homeostasis is critical for synaptic development and function. *J Neurosci*. 2011;31(48):17505–17513.
57. Wilson SM, Bhattacharyya B, Rachel RA, et al. Synaptic defects in ataxia mice result from a mutation in Usp14, encoding a ubiquitin-specific protease. *Nat Genet*. 2002;32(3):420–425.
58. Bence NF, Sampat RM, Kopito RR. Impairment of the ubiquitin-proteasome system by protein aggregation. *Science*. 2001;292(5521):1552–1555.
59. Dennis KE, Valentine WM. Ziram and sodium *N,N*-dimethyldithiocarbamate inhibit ubiquitin activation through intracellular metal transport and increased oxidative stress in HEK293 cells. *Chem Res Toxicol*. 2015;28(4):682–690.

60. Jahngen-Hodge J, Obin MS, Gong X, et al. Regulation of ubiquitin-conjugating enzymes by glutathione following oxidative stress. *J Biol Chem*. 1997;272(45):28218–28226.
61. Liu HY, Pfleger CM. Mutation in E1, the ubiquitin activating enzyme, reduces *Drosophila* lifespan and results in motor impairment. *PLoS One*. 2013;8(1):e32835.
62. Wade BE, Wang CE, Yan S, et al. Ubiquitin-activating enzyme activity contributes to differential accumulation of mutant huntingtin in brain and peripheral tissues. *J Neurosci*. 2014;34(25):8411–8422.
63. Upadhyay A, Amanullah A, Chhangani D, Mishra R, Mishra A. Selective multifaceted E3 ubiquitin ligases barricade extreme defense: potential therapeutic targets for neurodegeneration and ageing. *Ageing Res Rev*. 2015;24(Pt B):138–159.
64. Jackson PK, Eldridge AG, Freed E, et al. The lore of the RINGs: substrate recognition and catalysis by ubiquitin ligases. *Trends Cell Biol*. 2000;10(10):429–439.
65. Zhao JH, Yang CT, Wu JW, et al. RING domains functioning as E3 ligases reveal distinct structural features: a molecular dynamics simulation study. *J Biomol Struct Dyn*. 2008;26(1):65–74.
66. Zheng N, Wang P, Jeffrey PD, Pavletich NP. Structure of a c-Cbl-UbcH7 complex: RING domain function in ubiquitin-protein ligases. *Cell*. 2000;102(4):533–539.
67. Imai Y, Soda M, Takahashi R. Parkin suppresses unfolded protein stress-induced cell death through its E3 ubiquitin-protein ligase activity. *J Biol Chem*. 2000;275(46):35661–35664.
68. Saini N, Oelhafen S, Hua H, Georgiev O, Schaffner W, Bueler H. Extended lifespan of *Drosophila* parkin mutants through sequestration of redox-active metals and enhancement of anti-oxidative pathways. *Neurobiol Dis*. 2010;40(1):82–92.
69. Asano T, Koike M, Sakata S, et al. Possible involvement of iron-induced oxidative insults in neurodegeneration. *Neurosci Lett*. 2015;588:29–35.
70. Mufti AR, Burstein E, Csomos RA, et al. XIAP Is a copper binding protein deregulated in Wilson's disease and other copper toxicosis disorders. *Mol Cell*. 2006;21(6):775–785.
71. Mufti AR, Burstein E, Duckett CS. XIAP: cell death regulation meets copper homeostasis. *Arch Biochem Biophys*. 2007;463(2):168–174.
72. Burstein E, Ganesh L, Dick RD, et al. A novel role for XIAP in copper homeostasis through regulation of MURR1. *EMBO J*. 2004;23(1):244–254.
73. Rouault TA. The role of iron regulatory proteins in mammalian iron homeostasis and disease. *Nat Chem Biol*. 2006;2(8):406–414.
74. Zhu W, Li X, Xie W, et al. Genetic iron chelation protects against proteasome inhibition-induced dopamine neuron degeneration. *Neurobiol Dis*. 2010;37(2):307–313.
75. Salahudeen AA, Thompson JW, Ruiz JC, et al. An E3 ligase possessing an iron-responsive hemerythrin domain is a regulator of iron homeostasis. *Science*. 2009;326(5953):722–726.
76. Nijman SM, Luna-Vargas MP, Velds A, et al. A genomic and functional inventory of deubiquitinating enzymes. *Cell*. 2005;123(5):773–786.
77. Yao T, Cohen RE. A cryptic protease couples deubiquitination and degradation by the proteasome. *Nature*. 2002;419(6905):403–407.
78. Verma R, Aravind L, Oania R, et al. Role of Rpn11 metalloprotease in deubiquitination and degradation by the 26S proteasome. *Science*. 2002;298(5593):611–615.
79. Tonoki A, Kuranaga E, Tomioka T, et al. Genetic evidence linking age-dependent attenuation of the 26S proteasome with the aging process. *Mol Cell Biol*. 2009;29(4):1095–1106.
80. Liu N, Huang H, Dou QP, Liu J. Inhibition of 19S proteasome-associated deubiquitinases by metal-containing compounds. *Oncoscience*. 2015;2(5):457–466.
81. Smith MA, Harris PL, Sayre LM, Perry G. Iron accumulation in Alzheimer disease is a source of redox-generated free radicals. *Proc Natl Acad Sci USA*. 1997;94(18):9866–9868.
82. Xie W, Li X, Li C, Zhu W, Jankovic J, Le W. Proteasome inhibition modeling nigral neuron degeneration in Parkinson's disease. *J Neurochem*. 2010;115(1):188–199.
83. Kardos J, Kovacs I, Hajos F, Kalman M, Simonyi M. Nerve endings from rat brain tissue release copper upon depolarization. A possible role in regulating neuronal excitability. *Neurosci Lett*. 1989;103(2):139–144.
84. Rae TD, Schmidt PJ, Pufahl RA, Culotta VC, O'Halloran TV. Undetectable intracellular free copper: the requirement of a copper chaperone for superoxide dismutase. *Science*. 1999;284(5415):805–808.
85. Cuervo AM, Dice JF. When lysosomes get old. *Exp Gerontol*. 2000;35(2):119–131.

86. Cui D, Shang H, Zhang X, Jiang W, Jia X. Cardiac arrest triggers hippocampal neuronal death through autophagic and apoptotic pathways. *Sci Rep*. 2016;6:27642.
87. Hwang JJ, Lee SJ, Kim TY, Cho JH, Koh JY. Zinc and 4-hydroxy-2-nonenal mediate lysosomal membrane permeabilization induced by H_2O_2 in cultured hippocampal neurons. *J Neurosci*. 2008;28(12):3114–3122.
88. Paris I, Perez-Pastene C, Couve E, Caviedes P, Ledoux S, Segura-Aguilar J. Copper dopamine complex induces mitochondrial autophagy preceding caspase-independent apoptotic cell death. *J Biol Chem*. 2009;284(20): 13306–13315.
89. Paris I, Dagnino-Subiabre A, Marcelain K, et al. Copper neurotoxicity is dependent on dopamine-mediated copper uptake and one-electron reduction of aminochrome in a rat substantia nigra neuronal cell line. *J Neurochem*. 2001;77(2):519–529.
90. Zhang Z, Miah M, Culbreth M, Aschner M. Autophagy in neurodegenerative diseases and metal neurotoxicity. *Neurochem Res*. 2016;41(1–2):409–422.
91. Anandhan A, Rodriguez-Rocha H, Bohovych I, et al. Overexpression of alpha-synuclein at non-toxic levels increases dopaminergic cell death induced by copper exposure via modulation of protein degradation pathways. *Neurobiol Dis*. 2015;81:76–92.
92. Trejo-Solis C, Jimenez-Farfan D, Rodriguez-Enriquez S, et al. Copper compound induces autophagy and apoptosis of glioma cells by reactive oxygen species and JNK activation. *BMC Cancer*. 2012;12:156.
93. Takanashi M, Mochizuki H, Yokomizo K, et al. Iron accumulation in the substantia nigra of autosomal recessive juvenile parkinsonism (ARJP). *Parkinsonism Relat Disord*. 2001;7(4):311–314.
94. Zhang Y, Mikhael M, Xu D, et al. Lysosomal proteolysis is the primary degradation pathway for cytosolic ferritin and cytosolic ferritin degradation is necessary for iron exit. *Antioxid Redox Signal*. 2010;13(7):999–1009.
95. Arosio P, Ingrassia R, Cavadini P, Ferritins: a family of molecules for iron storage, antioxidation and more. *Biochim Biophys Acta*. 2009;1790(7):589–599.
96. Kidane TZ, Sauble E, Linder MC. Release of iron from ferritin requires lysosomal activity. *Am J Physiol Cell Physiol*. 2006;291(3):C445–C455.
97. Lichten LA, Cousins RJ. Mammalian zinc transporters: nutritional and physiologic regulation. *Annu Rev Nutr*. 2009;29:153–176.
98. Sun KJ, Zhu L, Wang HD, et al. Zinc as mediator of ubiquitin conjugation following traumatic brain injury. *Brain Res*. 2013;1506:132–141.
99. Lee SJ, Koh JY. Roles of zinc and metallothionein-3 in oxidative stress-induced lysosomal dysfunction, cell death, and autophagy in neurons and astrocytes. *Mol Brain*. 2010;3(1):30.
100. Park MH, Lee SJ, Byun HR, et al. Clioquinol induces autophagy in cultured astrocytes and neurons by acting as a zinc ionophore. *Neurobiol Dis*. 2011;42(3):242–251.
101. Redmann M, Darley-Usmar V, Zhang J. The role of autophagy, mitophagy and lysosomal functions in modulating bioenergetics and survival in the context of redox and proteotoxic damage: implications for neurodegenerative diseases. *Aging Dis*. 2016;7(2):150–162.
102. Hwang JJ, Kim HN, Kim J, et al. Zinc(II) ion mediates tamoxifen-induced autophagy and cell death in MCF-7 breast cancer cell line. *Biometals*. 2010;23(6):997–1013.

CHAPTER

19

Metals and Autophagy in Neurotoxicity

*Peng Su**, *Michael Aschner***, *Jingyuan Chen**, *Wenjing Luo**

*Fourth Military Medical University, Xi'an, China

**Albert Einstein College of Medicine, Bronx, NY, United States

OUTLINE

Biometals in Neurodegenerative Diseases. http://dx.doi.org/10.1016/B978-0-12-804562-6.00019-1

INTRODUCTION

We live in a metal-rich world and we can't live without metals. More than eighty metals have been found. Generally, according to their function in the human bodies, they are divided into two categories, essential metals [including sodium (Na), potassium (K), calcium (Ca), magnesium (Mg), iron (Fe), manganese (Mn), copper (Cu), etc.], and nonessential metals [including lead (Pb), cadmium (Cd), mercury (Hg), chromium (Cr), etc.]. Metals are one of the most dangerous pollutants because of their ubiquity, chemical versatility, and easiness of spreading.[1] Excessive exposure to essential and nonessential metals or lack of essential metals can give rise to a variety of adverse clinical conditions which leads to homeostasis disorders in different organs and cell types, particularly in neurodegenerative diseases. The conditions of clinical symptoms or diseases are highly dependent on exposure dose and duration time.

The concentration of Na, K, and Ca ions in neurons can directly affect their electrical activities, and the levels of Mg ions regulate ionotropic receptors, including γ-aminobutyric acid (GABA) and glutamate receptors. Zn and Cu are two essential trace metals for several enzymatic functions. Both hyper- and hypoconcentration of these metal ions can lead to neurological and psychotic syndromes, and other neural disorders. Several heavy metals, such as Pb, Hg, Cd, and Cr, have no biological function and their accumulation in brain parenchyma or spine is detrimental and toxic. In this review, we will summarize metal-related neurotoxicity and neurodegenerative diseases.

Autophagy, as an essential homeostatic process, is a general term for pathways by which cytoplasmic material, including soluble macromolecules and organelles, is delivered to lysosomes for degradation to adaptation to exogenous disruption.[2] There are three basic types of autophagy: macroautophagy, microautophagy, and chaperone-mediated autophagy (CMA).[3] Autophagy is essential for cell survival and the maintenance of homeostasis. The autophagy system is made up of autophagy-related proteins (Atgs), such as ULK1 (Atg1), Atg3-5, Beclin (Atg6), LC3 (Atg8), Atg12-14, Atg16L1, and FIP200 (Atg17). The coordinated action of Atgs mediates the membrane trafficking required for autophagosome formation.[4]

Autophagy plays a pivotal role in neuronal homeostasis. The function and survival of neurons are heavily dependent on the efficient removal of altered proteins and damaged organelles by autophagic degradation, because cytotoxic proteins cannot be diluted by cell division.[5] The importance of autophagy in the brain is highlighted by observations that genetic inactivation of essential autophagy genes (Atg5 or Atg7) in neurons causes accumulation of protein aggregates and spontaneous neurodegeneration,[6] suggesting that defective autophagy is implicated in the pathogenesis of neurodegenerative disorders. Neurodegenerative diseases share a common cellular and molecular pathogenic mechanism involving aggregated proteins that form inclusion bodies inside affected neurons, with a primary failure in autophagy being one possible cause of such scenarios.[7] Indeed, autophagic dysfunction has been implicated in numerous neurodegenerative diseases.

Many metal ions have crucial roles on autophagic pathway and proteins. Autophagy may regulate the beneficial and detrimental effects of metal ions. However, the interaction between autophagy and metals are much more complex. Herein, we will highlight recent advances on the emerging role of autophagy in central neural system (CNS), focusing on the regulation of autophagy during metal ion-induced neurotoxicity, and the possible mechanism involved.

PART 1 METAL-RELATED NEUROTOXICITY AND NEURODEGENERATIVE DISEASES

Alzheimer's Disease

Alzheimer's disease (AD) is a progressive neurodegenerative disorder characterized by the presence of extracellular senile plaques and intraneuronal fibrillary tangles. The plaques are mainly composed of β-amyloid (Aβ) peptides, which are generated by the proteolytic cleavage of amyloid precursor protein (APP) via β- and γ-secretases. Neurofibrillary tangles consist of highly phosphorylated forms of the microtubule-associated proteins tau.[8–10]

Metal ions play vital roles in the progress of AD. Age-related metal ion dysfunction may alter levels of neuronal metal ions in AD-affected areas, and the crosstalk between metal ions and AD pathological proteins indicates a close relationship between protein misfolding, aggregation, and metal ion homeostasis.[11] In AD patients, it has been proved that Cu^{2+}, Zn^{2+}, and Fe^{2+} are found in the core and rims of senile plaques and colocalize with Aβ.[12–14] Cu^{2+} and Fe^{2+} are increased in the neuropil of AD patients, and Zn^{2+} is decreased in AD patients' serum and blood, but increased in the cerebrospinal fluid, neuropil, and neocortical tissue.[15,16] In addition, a recent study shows that Mn^{2+} ions can also bind to the N-terminal part of Aβ peptide.[17] These data indicate that the role of metal ions in AD pathogenesis is more complex than previously considered before.

Pb can affect cognitive abilities, intelligence, and memory, although the direct association with AD development has yet to be revealed. Despite few epidemiological studies reporting the relationship between Pb and AD, a potential role of Pb in AD etiology is suggested in several experimental studies. Recent studies showed that Pb could increase APP mRNA expression after neonatal exposure, but not in the adult period.[18] A similar study performed in primates also showed that monkeys exposed to Pb in young age increased the number of amyloid plaques in late life.[19] An in vitro study also showed that Pb increased Aβ secretion and APP expression and decreased the expression of NEP (an Aβ IDE) in differentiated SH-SY5Y cells.[20]

Hg, as a heavy metal, can disrupt brain development and produces cognitive and motor disabilities.[21] Increased levels of Hg and decreased levels of Se and Zn have been noted in AD brains.[22] Plasma Mn and Hg concentrations were significantly higher in the CSF of AD patients.[23] Experimental data also showed that Hg could increase Aβ levels. Rat pheochromocytoma (PC12) cells exposed to both inorganic and organic (MeHg) Hg (10–1000 nM) showed a dose-dependent overproduction of Aβ40, probably by an increase in APP levels as well as a reduction in Aβ degradation by NEP.[24] Exposure to Hg also increased Aβ42 levels, but not APP expression in differentiated SH-SY5Y cells.

Aluminum (Al) is a neurotoxic element involved in the etiology of neurodegenerative disorders, such as AD. The incident of Al pollution in Cornwall provided evidence of Al's potential neurotoxicity, with analogous brain pathological characteristics noted in AD patients to subjects exposed to Al.[25] Recent research conducted in China reported a marginal positive association between Al levels in soil and the mortality caused by AD.[26] Chronic oral Al administration in rats increased Aβ production by raising the levels of APP in hippocampal and cortical tissues.[27] An in vitro study showed that exposure to Al increased the accumulation of Aβ and reduced the expression of NEP in cultured rat cortical neurons.[28] Another study showed that Al treatment reduced the Aβ degradation by decreasing the activity of cathepsin B, suggesting the activation of the amyloidogenic pathway and a reduction of the catabolism of Aβ.[29]

Parkinson's Disease

Parkinson's disease (PD) is a late-onset neurodegenerative disease characterized by progressive and extensive loss of dopaminergic (DAergic) neurons in the substantia nigra pars compacta (SNpc) and the presence of aggregated α-synuclein-containing intracellular inclusions known as Lewy bodies.[30] Similar to AD, some metals, such as Mn, Cu, and Fe, have been reported to affect the progress of PD. Although a large environmental survey showed that exposure to Fe or Cu alone had no effect on PD,[30] coexposure to Cu and Fe or Mn and Fe lasting for two to three decades have been reported to markedly increase the risk of PD.[31,32]

Excessive Mn intake leads to manganism, which represents a specific motor and cognitive dysfunction with many similarities to PD. Manganism has similar motor symptoms with PD, but there are some different features including dystonia and the lack of response to dopamine replacement therapy. In addition, neuropathological assessments showed that preferential cell loss in the globus pallidus (GP) with lesser cell loss in the putamen and subthalamic nucleus. Some epidemiological studies have shown that Mn exposure had an association with the risk of developing idiopathic PD,[33,34] however, others did not support the association.[35] Recent clinical studies suggest that lifetime exposure to lower level of Mn in some individuals may be a risk for typical PD.[36]

Mn and α-synuclein can combine to form deleterious effects on cell survival. Overexpressing α-synuclein in a neuronal cell line showed increased sensitivity to Mn challenge.[37] Mn has been shown to induce the expression of α-synuclein in cultured neuronal cells, and Mn accelerates the rate of α-synuclein fibrillization in vitro.[38]

Recent in vitro studies characterizing the kinase activity of LRRK2 have shown that that Mg^{2+} or Mn^{2+} can be used as ATP cofactors to support the kinase activity of wild-type LRRK2, but Mg^{2+} is a much better cofactor at promoting this activity.[39,40] However, both Mn^{2+} and Mg^{2+} are equally effective at promoting the activity of G2019S LRRK2. It was shown that the difference was a result of dramatic changes in the kinetic properties for the ATP-DMC substrate. While wild-type LRRK2 showed much slower catalytic rates in the presence of Mn^{2+} compared to Mg^{2+}, G2019S LRRK2 demonstrated similar ATP turnover rates in the presence of Mn^{2+} and Mg^{2+}. More importantly, both wild-type and G2019S LRRK2 demonstrated significantly higher affinities for Mn-ATP compared to Mg-ATP.[39,40] Consequently, relatively low concentration of Mn^{2+} could inhibit the kinase activity of wild-type LRRK2 driven by ATP-Mg^{2+}, but under similar conditions, the kinase activity of the G2019S mutant remained highly active.

Some in vitro studies showed that the expression of parkin (PARK2) can protect against Mn-induced toxicity in cultured cells.[41] Recessive mutations in the parkin/PARK2 gene are the most common cause for early onset Parkinsonism. Parkin is an E3 ligase that can modify proteins, such as DMT1.[42] DMT1 has broad substrate specificity and plays an important role in the transport of Mn. These studies suggest that parkin may play a significant role in maintaining the steady state levels of this transporter.[42]

Amyotrophic Lateral Sclerosis

Amyotrophic lateral sclerosis (ALS) is an idiopathic and fatal neuromuscular disease, which is characterized by degeneration of both cortical and spinal motor neurons.[43] Emerging evidence supports the notion that ALS is caused by gene–environment interactions, and exposure to excessive metals may interact with individual genetic susceptibility.[44] Several studies showed that Pb exposure was associated with the survival of ALS patients and human mutant SOD1 G93A transgenic mice. Interestingly, some studies showed that higher tibia and blood Pb levels were found to be associated with increased survival of ALS patients, indicating that Pb exposure may delay disease progression.[45] A preliminary case-control study on a population of 34 ALS patients from Italy showed that blood Pb levels were not significantly increased in patients compared with control and did not correlate with disease severity.[46] However, other studies showed significantly higher levels in cerebrospinal fluid and blood from ALS patients compared with controls, and the results were confirmed by SOD1 G93A transgenic mice.[47] It was hypothesized that Pb exposure could stimulate the increased expression of vascular endothelial growth factor (VEGF) in the spinal anterior horns of the transgenic mice, thereby inducing decreased activation of astrocytes with neuroprotective effects.[48]

Hg has been shown to have a potential role in ALS. Epidemiological and case-control studies have shown an association between Hg exposure and risk of developing ALS.[49] Schwarz et al. found clinical symptoms similar to those typical of ALS in a patient with long-term accidental Hg exposure.[50] Sienko et al. reported a population of ALS patients in a small Wisconsin community, which was characterized by large consumption of fresh-caught fish contaminated with high levels of Hg.[51] Barber et al.[52] noted neurological changes similar to ALS in some employees of a mercuric oxide manufacturing plant. However, Pamphlett and Waley[53] found no significant difference between inorganic Hg levels and upper or lower motor neurons of ALS patients compared with control. Animal and cell studies indicated that Hg exposure might affect the etiology of ALS. Administration of mercuric chloride ($HgCl_2$) in mice caused deposition of Hg in upper and lower motor neurons.[54] Long-term exposure to low level of MeHg, which is the most important organic mercury compound, showed an anticipation of the onset of ALS phenotype.[55] Low dose of MeHg could interfere the expression and release of proinflammatory cytokines interleukin-6 (IL-6) from microglial cells and impaired glial function, which may be involved in several neurodegenerative conditions.[56]

Selenium (Se) is a trace element with both toxicological and nutritional functions, and epidemiological investigations indicate a causal link between Se exposure and ALS risk. Kilness et al.[57] reported an increased risk of ALS in seleniferous areas, and Vinceti et al.[58] found that 5182 inhabitants who drank for at least 5 years the high-Se tap water, revealed an increased ALS risk in this municipality. Therefore, the association between the high Se environmental levels and the numerous ALS cases detected in this area might be causal. In addition, Yang et al.[59] identified clusters of patients with neurological signs and symptoms affecting motor function in seleniferous areas of China, although this study did not include a detailed report on the relation between risk of developing degeneration of the motor system and degree of Se exposure.

Animal and laboratory models also support the Se-ALS association. Se showed a specific toxicity to motor neurons in swine and cattle.[60] Se intoxication could selectively damage motor neurons in swine, provoking a bilateral focal poliomalacia of spinal cord ventral horns.[61]

Recently, Estevez et al. found another mechanism linking Se to ALS etiology. They found that Se-induced oxidative stress led to decreased cholinergic signaling and degeneration of cholinergic motor neurons through depletion of glutathione (GSH).[62] Maraldi et al.[63] examined the role of exposure to low Se levels in triggering oxidative damage and apoptosis in a human neuronal cell line. In particular, the oxidant properties of Se species might lead to a compensatory response in the cell, antagonizing the onset of apoptosis. Se exposure may also influence SOD1 accumulation in mitochondria, a somatic feature occurring in neurons during ALS pathogenesis.

Zn and Cu have been shown to contribute to oxidative neurotoxicity in spinal cord motor neurons. Treatment with high dose of Zn induced a strong increase in reactive oxygen species (ROS) generation and a significant decrease of spinal cord neuron survival in cultured neuronal cells.[64] In addition, exposure to sublethal concentrations of Zn has been found to enhance *N*-methyl-D-aspartate receptor (NMDAR)-mediated excitotoxicity in primary neurons from SOD1 G93A transgenic mice.[65] However, Zn and Cu supplementation prevented early death from Zn treatment alone. Ermilova et al.[66] found that moderate levels of dietary Zn could protect against the toxicity of ALS-associated SOD1 mutation.

Wilson's Disease

Wilson's disease (WD) is a genetic disorder caused by mutation of the ATP7B protein which is mostly expressed in the liver.[67,68] Dysfunction of ATP7B leads to disturbed Cu metabolism with a gradual accumulation of Cu in the body and reduced synthesis of various Cu proteins, in particular ceruloplasmin.[69] Cu leads to its spillage into plasma and CSF, leading to cellular uptake and oxidative damage in the CNS.[70] Increased Fe content has been reported in the striatum, gray matter, white matter, and dentate nucleus of the cerebellum in postmortem studies.[71] MRI studies indicate that metals, such as Fe and Mn may accumulate in the brain over the course of WD.[72] T1 hyperintensities in GP support the notion that Mn deposits in patients with the hepatic form of WD. Another MRI study reported that T2 hypointensities in GP and other brain regions in WD patients are suggestive of deposits with paramagnetic properties.[73] Some studies showed that GP changes might reflect Cu deposits, since Cu species are paramagnetic. A PET study with radioactively labeled Fe in human subjects showed increased brain Fe uptake in WD patients compared to healthy volunteers.[74]

Other Neurotoxicity and Neurodegenerative Diseases

Menkes disease (MD) is an X-linked multisystemic lethal disorder of impaired Cu metabolism characterized by neurodegenerative symptoms and connective tissue manifestation.[75,76] MD is a fatal neurodegenerative disorder characterized by symptoms like progressive cerebral atrophy, seizures, hypotonia, coarse hair, and connective tissue abnormalities.[77,78] Lacking Cu absorption, MD patients suffer a systemic Cu deficiency, leading to reduced Cu in brain, liver, and serum, but elevated level in kidney and small intestine.[79] The dysfunction of Cu gives rise to the disorder of Cu-dependent enzymes, such as cytochrome C oxidase, lysol oxidase, and tyrosinase. As neurodevelopment is relatively fast in the early life, the requirement of Cu seems particularly acute during the initial 12 months of life. Danks et al. firstly reported the involvement of Cu metabolism in MD, showing low serum levels and defective intestinal absorption of the metal.[80] At first, Cu malabsorption was thought to be the primary cause, but later investigation showed that Cu also accumulated in other tissues, such as liver and kidney, which suggested that the cause of MD may be multisystemic.[79]

PART 2 AUTOPHAGY IN METAL NEUROTOXICITY

Manganese

Manganese (Mn) is an essential trace element required for normal growth, development, and cellular homeostasis.[81] It serves as a cofactor of several key enzymes necessary for neuronal cell function, such as glutamine synthetase, mitochondrial superoxide dismutase (SOD), and pyruvate carboxylase.[82] The main route for physiological Mn absorption is through dietary intake.[83] Inhalation of Mn fumes and dusts has been identified as a health hazard in occupations, such as welding and mining.[84] Increased accumulation of Mn in DA-rich brain regions, such as GP, substantia nigra, and striatum, triggers neurotoxicity resulting in a neurological disorder referred to as manganism.[85] It is characterized by a set of extrapyramidal symptoms resembling idiopathic PD.[86] Exposure to Mn disrupts DA neurotransmission and induces DAergic neurodegeneration, thereby leading to motor deficits.[87,88] Mn toxicity is mediated by the autoxidation or turnover of intracellular catecholamines, induction of protein aggregation, production of ROS and toxic metabolites, depletion of cellular antioxidant defense mechanisms, and alterations of mitochondrial function and ATP production.[84] Mn has also been linked to the etiology of other neurodegenerative diseases. For example, chronic Mn exposure directly increases fibril formation by α-synuclein, which is a hallmark of PD.[89] Mn overload increases the risk for developing ALS.[81] Several Mn-dependent enzymes are altered in human HD brains and animal models of HD.[81]

Few studies have focused on the role and regulation of autophagy in Mn-exposed neuronal cells. Zhang et al. investigated the effects of Mn on autophagy in a rat model after a single intrastriatal injection of $MnCl_2$.[89] They found that Mn-induced compensatory autophagy activation in the early phase of exposure (4–12 h), but inhibited autophagy in the long term (1–28 days). The inhibition of autophagy correlated to the activation of the mTOR pathway. Pretreatment with the autophagy inhibitor wortmannin induced loss of DAergic neurons and worsened animal behavioral abnormalities, suggesting that autophagic induction may play a protective role against Mn-induced neurotoxicity at early time points, while dysregulation of autophagy at later phases may mediate DAergic neurodegeneration. Consistent with this study, another research group showed that enhanced autophagy in response to short-term Mn exposure protected in vitro glial cells against Mn cytotoxicity; while intrastriatal Mn injection-induced loss of astrocytic soma accompanied by disrupted autophagic activity in the long term.[90] We postulated that Mn persistence within the cell might continuously damage proteins and impair long-term autophagic efficiency. Mn-mediated autophagy is likely mediated through the activation of extracellular signal-regulated kinase (ERK1/2) and c-Jun N-terminal kinase (JNK), as well as suppression of the Akt signaling pathway. Although the aforementioned studies demonstrated that autophagy could be activated to counteract the harmful effects caused by Mn; the role of autophagy in Mn neurotoxicity has yet to be fully understood. Ngwa et al. reported that Mn nanoparticle-activated autophagic cell death in in vitro DAergic neurons.[91] Overall, given the conflicting results regarding the protective versus detrimental effects of autophagy in Mn-induced cytotoxicity, further research clarifying autophagic activity in animal models exposed to chronic Mn treatment will be required to determine whether autophagy modulation is a viable therapy for manganism.

Copper

Copper (Cu) is an essential but also toxic trace element. It functions as a cofactor and/or a structural component of several key enzymes required for normal development and function of the CNS, such as cytochrome c oxidase (energy metabolism), Zn/Cu-dependent SOD (antioxidative defense), ceruloplasmin (Fe metabolism), and DA-β-monoxygenase (neurotransmitter synthesis).[92] Impaired Cu homeostasis has been associated with neurological disorders, such as MD, WD, AD, and PD.[93] Mutations of the Cu transporting ATPase ATP7A and ATP7B are the molecular underpinnings of the fatal hereditary Menkes (deficient Cu) and Wilson's (excessive Cu) diseases, respectively.[93] In AD, high Cu content was found in senile plaques involved in precipitating Aβ oligomers.[94] On the other hand, there is an overall low Cu level in the AD brain, suggesting Cu is abnormally redistributed to senile plaques, leaving the tissue and cells deficient in Cu.[93] Cu has been implicated in the pathophysiology of PD since its levels in the substantia nigra of PD patients are substantially lower.[93] Studies have also demonstrated that Cu binds to α-synuclein and induces oligomerization of this protein.[95,96] Cu has also been found to promote the aggregation of htt, which is thought to be neurotoxic.[96]

Cu has been reported to induce autophagy in both neuronal and cancer cells. Cu-DA complexes induced excessive mitophagy and subsequent apoptotic cell death in a catecholaminergic cell line.[97] In addition, Cu enhanced autophagy flux in human DAergic cells in a dose-dependent manner. The induction of autophagy resulted from activation of AMP-activated protein kinase (AMPK)-ULK1 signaling pathway. Genetic inhibition of autophagy aggravated Cu-induced cell death, indicating a protective effect of autophagy against Cu-related apoptosis.[98] Numerous Cu-containing compounds have been developed and tested as new anticancer agents. Cu coordinated complex Cas III-ia was found to induce autophagy in C6 glioma cells,[99] which may be partially due to the production of ROS and ROS-activated JNK signaling. Inhibition of autophagy potentiated cell death induced by Cas III-ia, suggesting that autophagy antagonized cell apoptosis. Another anticancer copper complex, HYF127c/Cu, has also been reported to induce protective autophagy though activation of mitogen-activated protein kinase (MAPK) p38 pathway.[100] By contrast, Cu-based compound LCu mediated autophagic cell death by generating ROS in HeLa cells.[101] The discrepancies among the studies may stem from the different cell types, concentration and exposure times; nonetheless, all the studies suggest that Cu is an inducer of autophagy. In the present scenario, it is hard to speculate whether autophagy is beneficial or detrimental in Cu-related neurotoxicity based on the limited and conflicting evidence. A greater understanding of the cellular response to Cu and its relation to autophagy will yield insights to pathophysiological mechanisms underlying Cu toxicity in brain.

Cadmium

Cadmium (Cd) is a widespread industrial and environmental pollutant that is mainly released from smelting, burning of fossil fuels and municipal wastes, refining of metals, and cigarette smoking.[102] Human exposure to a Cd-contaminated environment or food chain causes accumulation of Cd in many organs, including lungs,[103] liver,[104,105] kidney,[104] testis,[106] bone,[107] and brain.[108] Cd can pass through the blood–brain barrier, causing the dysfunction of the CNS with symptoms including olfactory dysfunction, Parkinsonian like symptoms, slowing of vasomotor functioning, and neurological defects in attention, learning, and memory.[109] Cd toxicity is in part due to its disruption of intracellular Ca^{2+} homeostasis by compromising Ca^{2+}-dependent ATPases and inducing ER Ca^{2+} release. The subsequent elevation of free Ca^{2+} triggers various cascades that lead to apoptosis.[110] Moreover, Cd stimulates free radical production, resulting in oxidative damage of lipids, proteins, and DNA.[111,112] Cd also affects glutamatergic,[113] monoaminergic,[114] as well as the cholinergic systems.[115] Clinical investigations have pointed to Cd intoxication as a possible etiological factor for neurodegenerative diseases, such as AD.[116] Transgenic AD mice treated with Cd showed increased production of Aβ and senile plaque accumulation accompanied with more severe cognitive deficits compared with nontreated mice.[117] Cd may also accelerate tau aggregation.[118] In addition, it has been reported that Cd exposure causes ALS by reducing SOD activity.[119]

Cd-induced autophagy has been shown in various cell and animal models as demonstrated by an increase in autophagic vacuole formation and ATGs expression. The consequence of autophagy induction by Cd has remained unsettled due to contradictory results. Some studies found autophagy to be a prosurvival mechanism, with inhibition of autophagy exacerbating cell death. Liu and coworkers noted that Cd-induced cytoprotective autophagy in PC12 cells,[120] rat liver cells,[121] and primary rat neuron cultures,[122] since chloroquine (an autophagy inhibitor) further aggravated cell apoptosis, whereas rapamycin (an autophagy inhibitor) was able to decrease Cdinduced injury. These data are supported by two studies showing that Cd-mediated autophagy was protective against apoptotic cell death in both vascular[123] and pulmonary endothelial cells.[124] In addition, Lim et al. demonstrated that induction of autophagy interrupted apoptosis by counterbalancing ER stress after Cd exposure in lung epithelial fibroblasts.[125] A study using a rat model has also suggested that autophagy triggered by subtoxic Cd exposure suppressed apoptosis in the kidney.[126] On the other hand, a handful of studies showed programmed cell death as a direct consequence of autophagy induction. Cd cytotoxicity was attenuated by the autophagy inhibitor 3-MA in epidermal cells.[115] Cd induced autophagic cell death in mesangial cells through both Ca^{2+}-dependent activation of ERK[127] and ROS-dependent activation of glycogen synthase kinase (GSK)-3β.[128] Furthermore, Cd-mediated overactivation of mitophagy may contribute to cellular energy depletion and cell death.[129,130] The discrepancy in all these data may be explained by factors intrinsic to the different cell types. Further research is warranted to clarify the function of autophagy in Cd-mediated cytotoxicity.

Lead

Lead (Pb) is a ubiquitous environmental neurotoxicant that continues to be considered as a major global environmental health hazard.[131] The general population is primarily exposed to Pb through contaminated food and water, Pb-based paint in older housing, and from air pollution which is caused by industrial emissions and anthropogenic Pb contributions.[132] Exposure to Pb, especially during early development, causes a wide variety of deleterious effects on the CNS, such as behavioral disturbance, difficulties in learning and memory, and cognitive deficits.[132] The neurotoxicity of Pb is linked to its interference with several neurotransmission systems, such as the dopaminergic, cholinergic and glutamatergic systems.[133] Previous studies have demonstrated that Pb is a potent noncompetitive antagonist of the *N*-methyl-D-aspartate (NMDA) receptor.[134] Chronic Pb exposure inhibits hippocampal NMDA receptor-dependent long-term potentiation, alters the expression of NMDA receptor subunits and impairs synaptic plasticity, and decreases learning and memory.[134] Pb also disrupts Ca^{2+}-related cell signaling by substituting for Ca^{2+}.[135] Moreover, Pb induces oxidative stress and exerts some of its toxic effects through the disruption of prooxidant/antioxidant balance.[136] Experiments on animal models have shown that early postnatal Pb exposure augments Aβ plaques and phosphorylated tau later in life.[137] In addition, cumulative exposure to Pb increases risk for developing PD.[137]

Pb has been found to induce autophagy in both in vitro cell models and in vivo animal brain. Whether the autophagy induction is prosurvival or prodeath is controversial. In a rat model, Zhang et al. demonstrated that chronic exposure to Pb-containing drinking water significantly increased autophagosome formation and ATG proteins expression in CA1 neurons of hippocampus.[138] The enhanced autophagy was possibly due to suppression of the Akt/mTOR signaling pathway. The authors suggested that Pb-induced excess autophagy led to programmed cell death. In contrast, a study using cardiofibroblast culture showed that Pb-mediated autophagy alleviated cell stress and promoted survival.[139] Thus, very limited literature on the effect of autophagy on Pb neurotoxicity is available at the time of writing. This could open up a new area for the research of Pb field.

Methylmercury (MeHg)

Mercury (Hg) is an environmental pollutant that is of major public concern due to its ubiquitous nature. Hg that has been released into aquatic environments from anthropogenic sources becomes readily methylated by sulfate and iron-reducing bacteria giving rise to MeHg.[140] MeHg then bioaccumulates up the aquatic food chain. Consumption of large seafood, such as tuna or swordfish is the primary source of exposure to humans.[141] MeHg can readily cross the blood–brain barrier. This in part is due to its ability to bind thiol groups on proteins and amino acids. In particular, MeHg binds to cysteine, and therefore mimics the structure of methionine, thus enhancing its likelihood to be taken up by amino acid transporters.[142] MeHg can accumulate in human bodies with a biological half-life in the blood of 2–3 months.[143]

Exposure to MeHg is detrimental, particularly for the developing brain. MeHg has been reported to induce deformities and neurological impediments in the fetus, as well as cause stillbirths. In addition, it can cause visual, auditory, and speech impairment and ataxia.[144] MeHg-induced neurodegeneration has been examined in a variety of animal models including *Caenorhabditi elegans*, rats, and monkeys.[145–147]

While many studies have focused on the role of MeHg-induced oxidative stress, recent studies are focused on other mechanisms underlying its neurotoxicity, such as autophagy. In an in vitro study by Chang et al. (2013), human neural stem cells exposed to chronic doses of MeHg (0.01–1 μM) exhibited decreased mTOR protein levels in a dose-dependent manner.[148] As previously mentioned, mTOR is a negative regulator of autophagy. Therefore, loss of mTOR may suggest that MeHg-induces excessive autophagy, resulting in the conversion of the recycling nature of the autophagic system to a degenerative process. It has yet to be investigated how MeHg decreases mTOR expression. Increase in Atg6/Beclin-1 protein levels was also observed, suggesting a possible upregulation in autophagic activity. Finally, an increase in the microtubule-associated protein 1 light chain 3 (LC3)-II to LC3-I ratio was detected subsequent to exposure. The conversion of LC3-I (cytosolic form) to LC3-II (lipidated form that binds to the autophagosome membrane) is a widely used marker to assess the autophagy induction in mammalian cells.[149] The increased ratio of LC3-II to LC3-I in cells exposed to MeHg indicated higher autophagic activity. Transmission electron microscopy further verified that more autophagic vacuoles existed in the cells after MeHg exposure.[148]

Yuntao et al. (2014) examined autophagic biomarkers in rat astrocytes treated with MeHg.[150] They observed the presence of autophagosomes postexposure, increased LC3-II to LC3-I ratio, and an increase in Beclin-1 protein, indicating enhanced autophagy in astrocytes. Inducing autophagy with rapamycin led to cytoprotection, whereas suppression of autophagy with chloroquine exacerbated cytotoxicity post-MeHg exposure,[150] suggesting that autophagy is protective against MeHg-induced cytotoxicity. The study also showed that the protective effect of autophagy is possibly through attenuating cell apoptosis. To date, the mechanisms underlying MeHg-induced autophagy upregulation remain unclear. As mentioned previously, MeHg binds thiol groups on the proteins and may lead to protein destabilization and/or functional changes which possibly serve as an autophagy inducer. MeHg also triggers oxidative stress as indicated by ROS generation.[151] Oxidative stress has been shown to activate the autophagy-signaling pathway.

Due to the continued exposure of the general public to MeHg and the very limited literature on the role of autophagy in the mechanisms of its neurotoxicity, further investigation in this area is warranted.

Iron

Iron (Fe) is an essential metal required for survival, serving as a cofactor for a wide variety of metalloproteins, such as heme.[152] Its oxidative nature makes it useful in oxidation–reduction reactions, but potentially dangerous in an oxygen-rich environment. Cellular Fe content is regulated by ferritin which stores unused Fe to prevent haphazard reaction with oxygen.[153] Most Fe is taken up through the diet. Increased accumulation of Fe in the brain, possibly due to dyshomeostasis, can lead to neurodegeneration.[153] Indeed, increased Fe levels have been associated with neurological disorders including PD, AD, and HD, and are the hallmark of the inherited progressive neurological disorders known as neurodegeneration with brain Fe accumulation (NBIA).[152]

Two subgroups of NBIA patients exhibit mutations in genes that regulate the autophagic degradation process: WD repeat domain 45 (WDR45) and the previously mentioned ATP13A2. WDR45 mediates the fusion of autophagosomes with lysosomes and the subsequent formation of autolysosomes. ATP13A2, which typically locates on the lysosomal membrane, has been found to accumulate at ER, leading to ER stress and lysosomal dysfunction.[154–156] This suggests improper autophagic signaling as a result of enhanced Fe accumulation.

He et al. (2008) observed increased cathepsin D expression, a lysosome biomarker and a mediator of autophagy, and increased LC3-II to LC3-I ratio in the neuronal tissue of a rat model of intracranial hemorrhage (ICH) subsequent to Fe exposure. They further verified presence of autophagic vacuoles via electron microscopy. Fe chelation suppressed autophagy in this model, suggesting a significant role of Fe in autophagic cell death observed in ICH.[157]

Chen et al. (2012) proposed estradiol-mediated autophagic inhibition as an approach to Fe-induced autophagy after ICH, and provided evidence for sex differences as a result of this treatment.[158] In vitro studies also demonstrated increased Fe-associated autophagy and found that autophagic inhibition protected against Fe-induced cell death.[159–161]

There is some evidence that Fe accumulation may be the byproduct of neurodegenerative processes and not the cause.[162,163] Studies are conflicting on the dynamic between autophagy and Fe accumulation. In one instance, Fe accumulation downstream of oxidative stress, serves as a trigger for increased autophagy.[164] In another study, however, oxidative stress led to autophagy, which subsequently increased Fe accumulation.[165] In reality, cellular signaling pathways are rarely linear processes. Thus, Fe accumulation may be both the cause and the effect of cellular autophagy in response to oxidative stress.[165,166] Although much research has been devoted to Fe neurotoxicity and its aberrant accumulation, studies on its connections to autophagy are limited. Further investigation on autophagy regulation in Fe neurotoxicity is merited.

Zinc

Zinc (Zn) is an essential metal required for humans and many other living organisms. It is a cofactor for over 300 enzymes and metalloproteins, regulating gene transcription and the antioxidant response.[167] In childhood, Zn deficiency affects mental and physical development as well as learning abilities. Zn homeostasis has been associated with AD, brain trauma, epilepsy, etc. Increasing evidence show that Zn is a positive regulator of autophagy. Excessive Zn in medium has been shown to enhance autophagy induced by tamoxifen in MCF-7 breast cancer cells.[168] Zn can also increase autophagic protein expression in PC12 cells and cultured neurons. Zn promotes the formation of the autophagic signal, ROS, and increases autophagy in astrocytes after treatment with hypoxia and reoxygenation. On the other hand, Zn depletion by Zn chelation can suppress autophagy.

The detailed mechanisms of how Zn modulates autophagy still need to be defined. Studies showed that phosphorylation of ERK1/2 is necessary for the regulation of basal and induced autophagy by Zn.[168,169] ERK1/2 has been shown to activate autophagy through at least two pathways: ERK1/2 can activate the Beclin1-PI3K complex by phosphorylating the negative regulator of Beclin1, Bcl-2[170]; ERK1/2 activation was shown to activate autophagy by promoting disassembly of mTORC1 complex through a nonclassical pathway.[171] Metallothionein (MT), as a small molecular weight protein that binds Zn, has been reported to play an important role in Zn-induced autophagy activation during oxidative stress. Astrocytes from metallothionein 3 (MT3) knockout mice exhibited lower induction of autophagy by H_2O_2.[172] Zn can also potentially regulate autophagy by modulating the expression of genes involved in autophagy. Studies have shown that Zn induce the expression of genes through activation of the metal-responsive transcription factor (MTF1), which can regulate autophagic proteins, such as ATG7.[173] Bioinformatics analysis shows that the promoters of ATG7 and DFCP1 contain four binding sites for MTF1 within 2.0 kb upstream of the transcription start site.[174]

Zn may also regulate autophagy through regulation of microRNA expression[175] and modulation of methylation of genes.[176] In addition to regulating the initiation of autophagy (early autophagy), Zn takes effect in the degradation of the cargo in autolysosomes (late autophagy).

Julien et al. reported that Zn deficiency caused accumulation of lipofuscin, an indicator of incomplete lysosomal digestion, in retinal epithelium of rats.[177] Knock out of MT3 exhibited reduced acid phosphatase and neuraminidase activities, decreased expression of cathepsin D and L as well as increased lysosomal accumulation of cholesterol and lipofuscin in astrocytes.[172] Lysosome integrity was found to be disrupted in macrophages after treatment with TPEN, a zinc chelator.[178] Treatment with 4 μM TPEN for 72 h caused impaired degradation of LC3-II and p62/SQSTM in human hepatoma cells.[167,170]

Arsenic

Arsenic (As), as a wood preservative in the past, is a toxic metalloid and well-known carcinogen, which over 200 million people worldwide chronically suffer exposure to.[179,180] Research has shown that As exposure induces mitochondrial oxidative stress, imbalance of intracellular Ca^{2+}, disruption in ATP production, altered membrane potential, changes in cytoskeletal morphology, and neuronal cell death, among other effects.[180,181] Early-life exposure to As can cause lower brain weight and a reduction in glia and neurons,[182] which has been proved to be associated with AD and ALS.[137,181] Dimethylarsenic acid, a metabolite of As in humans, has been shown to increase β-amyloid levels.[183] Arsenic could inhibit the translocation of neurofilament (NF) and decreased NF content at peripheral nerves, which affect the etiology of ALS.[184]

Studies have shown that short-term As exposure triggers an autophagy response,[185,186] and the underlying mechanisms may be As-elevated ROS.[187,188] As-damaged organelles are the major source of ROS. Normally damaged organelles are removed by autophagy. Once the autophagy process disorders, ROS can leak from these damaged organelles, leading to the elevation of intracellular ROS levels.[189] Thus, ROS elevation induced by As activates autophagy, and activated autophagy in turn is able to remove damaged mitochondria and hence suppresses ROS induction. Zhang et al. reported that 16 weeks of low-dose As exposure induced BEAS-2B cell (human bronchial epithelial cells) transformation, which was accompanied with increased ROS generation and autophagy activation.[190] The same group further showed that enhancement of autophagy activity increased mitochondria turnover, decreased As-induced ROS generation and cell transformation, and inhibition of autophagy decreases mitochondria turnover, promotes ROS generation and cell transformation, which suggests that autophagy is actually a cellular self-defense mechanism against arsenic's action.

CONCLUSIONS

Neurodegenerative diseases and metal-induced neurotoxicity continue to pose a significant risk to human health and longevity. This review emphasizes the critical need to better understand the connection between autophagy and neurodegenerative disorders (Fig. 19.1). Furthermore, it highlights the probable association of metal-induced toxicity and autophagic processes. An enhanced research effort is paramount in order to effectively address the dynamic nature of autophagy, and potentially manipulate this process for therapeutic benefit.

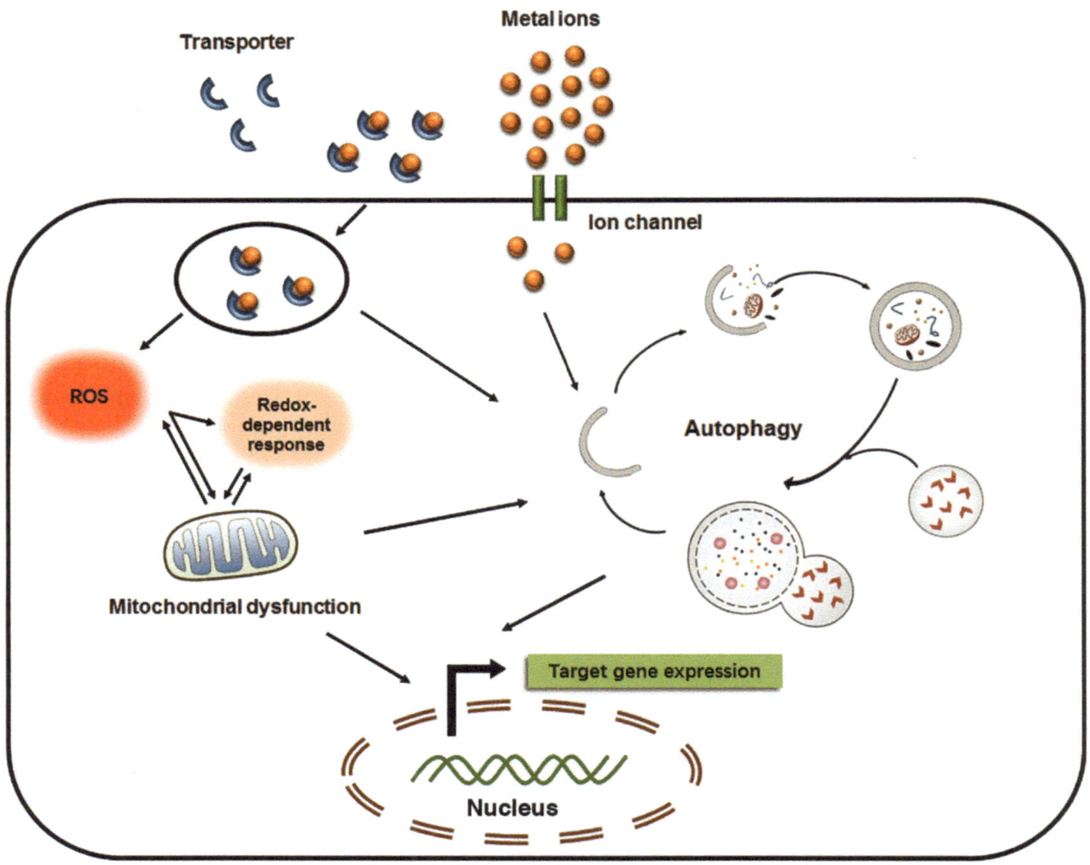

FIGURE 19.1 **Metal ions involved in autophagic function in cell homeostasis.** When exposure to hyper- and hypoconcentration of essential or heavy metals, metal ions can enter into cell plasm in ionic state or combined state. Metal ions affect redox balance and autophagic balance, leading to related target gene expression, and finally decide the survival or death of cells.

Acknowledgments

This work was supported in part by National Basic Research Program of China (973 Program, 2012CB525004), Key Project of Natural Science Foundation of China (30830087, 81230063), National Natural Science Foundation of China (30972499, 30771768, 30800898, 30901176, 81001256, 81001233), Program for Changjiang Scholars (T2011153), and Innovative Research Team in University (PCSIRT); MA was supported in part by NIEHS grants R01ES07331, R01ES10563, and R01ES020852.

References

1. Florea AM, Busselberg D. Occurrence, use and potential toxic effects of metals and metal compounds. *Biometals*. 2006;19(4):419–427.
2. Levine B, Mizushima N, Virgin HW. Autophagy in immunity and inflammation. *Nature*. 2011;469(7330):323–335.
3. Jiang P, Mizushima N. Autophagy and human diseases. *Cell Res*. 2014;24(1):69–79.

4. Saitoh T, Akira S. Regulation of innate immune responses by autophagy-related proteins. *J Cell Biol.* 2010;189(6):925–935.
5. Wong E, Cuervo AM. Autophagy gone awry in neurodegenerative diseases. *Nat Neurosci.* 2010;13(7):805–811.
6. Komatsu M, Waguri S, Chiba T, Murata S, Iwata J, Tanida I, et al. Loss of autophagy in the central nervous system causes neurodegeneration in mice. *Nature.* 2006;441(7095):880–884.
7. Martinez-Vicente M. Autophagy in neurodegenerative diseases: from pathogenic dysfunction to therapeutic modulation. *Semin Cell Dev Biol.* 2015;40:115–126.
8. Cheung ZH, Ip NY. Autophagy deregulation in neurodegenerative diseases—recent advances and future perspectives. *J Neurochem.* 2011;118(3):317–325.
9. Price DL, Tanzi RE, Borchelt DR, Sisodia SS. Alzheimer's disease: genetic studies and transgenic models. *Annu Rev Genet.* 1998;32:461–493.
10. Ju HL, Han KH, Lee JD, Ro SW. Transgenic mouse models generated by hydrodynamic transfection for genetic studies of liver cancer and preclinical testing of anti-cancer therapy. *Int J Cancer.* 2016;138(7):1601–1608.
11. Cristóvão JS, Santos R, Gomes CM. Metals and neuronal metal binding proteins implicated in Alzheimer's disease. *Oxid Med Cell Longev.* 2016;2016:1–13.
12. Ozcankaya R, Delibas N. Malondialdehyde, superoxide dismutase, melatonin, iron, copper, and zinc blood concentrations in patients with Alzheimer disease: cross-sectional study. *Croat Med J.* 2002;43(1):28–32.
13. Zatta P, Drago D, Bolognin S, Sensi SL. Alzheimer's disease, metal ions and metal homeostatic therapy. *Trends Pharmacol Sci.* 2009;30(7):346–355.
14. Roberts BR, Ryan TM, Bush AI, Masters CL, Duce JA. The role of metallobiology and amyloid-beta peptides in Alzheimer's disease. *J Neurochem.* 2012;120(suppl 1):149–166.
15. Religa D, Strozyk D, Cherny RA, Volitakis I, Haroutunian V, Winblad B, et al. Elevated cortical zinc in Alzheimer disease. *Neurology.* 2006;67(1):69–75.
16. Bishop GM, Robinson SR, Liu Q, Perry G, Atwood CS, Smith MA. Iron: a pathological mediator of Alzheimer disease?. *Dev Neurosci.* 2002;24(2–3):184–187.
17. Wallin C, Kulkarni YS, Abelein A, Jarvet J, Liao Q, Strodel B, et al. Characterization of Mn(II) ion binding to the amyloid-beta peptide in Alzheimer's disease. *J Trace Elem Med Biol.* 2016;38:183–193.
18. Basha MR, Wei W, Bakheet SA, Benitez N, Siddiqi HK, Ge YW, et al. The fetal basis of amyloidogenesis: exposure to lead and latent overexpression of amyloid precursor protein and beta-amyloid in the aging brain. *J Neurosci.* 2005;25(4):823–829.
19. Wu J, Basha MR, Brock B, Cox DP, Cardozo-Pelaez F, McPherson CA, et al. Alzheimer's disease (AD)-like pathology in aged monkeys after infantile exposure to environmental metal lead (Pb): evidence for a developmental origin and environmental link for AD. *J Neurosci.* 2008;28(1):3–9.
20. Huang H, Bihaqi SW, Cui L, Zawia NH. In vitro Pb exposure disturbs the balance between Abeta production and elimination: the role of AbetaPP and neprilysin. *Neurotoxicology.* 2011;32(3):300–306.
21. Johansson C, Castoldi AF, Onishchenko N, Manzo L, Vahter M, Ceccatelli S. Neurobehavioural and molecular changes induced by methylmercury exposure during development. *Neurotox Res.* 2007;11(3-4):241–260.
22. Wenstrup D, Ehmann WD, Markesbery WR. Trace element imbalances in isolated subcellular fractions of Alzheimer's disease brains. *Brain Res.* 1990;533(1):125–131.
23. Gerhardsson L, Lundh T, Minthon L, Londos E. Metal concentrations in plasma and cerebrospinal fluid in patients with Alzheimer's disease. *Dement Geriatr Cogn Disord.* 2008;25(6):508–515.
24. Song JW, Choi BS. Mercury induced the accumulation of amyloid beta (Abeta) in PC12 Cells: the role of production and degradation of Abeta. *Toxicol Res.* 2013;29(4):235–240.
25. Exley C, Esiri MM. Severe cerebral congophilic angiopathy coincident with increased brain aluminium in a resident of Camelford, Cornwall, UK. *J Neurol Neurosurg Psychiatry.* 2006;77(7):877–879.
26. Shen XL, Yu JH, Zhang DF, Xie JX, Jiang H. Positive relationship between mortality from Alzheimer's disease and soil metal concentration in mainland China. *J Alzheimers Dis.* 2014;42(3):893–900.
27. Walton JR, Wang MX. APP expression, distribution and accumulation are altered by aluminum in a rodent model for Alzheimer's disease. *J Inorg Biochem.* 2009;103(11):1548–1554.
28. Luo Y, Niu F, Sun Z, Cao W, Zhang X, Guan D, et al. Altered expression of Abeta metabolism-associated molecules from D-galactose/AlCl(3) induced mouse brain. *Mech Ageing Dev.* 2009;130(4):248–252.
29. Sakamoto T, Saito H, Ishii K, Takahashi H, Tanabe S, Ogasawara Y. Aluminum inhibits proteolytic degradation of amyloid beta peptide by cathepsin D: a potential link between aluminum accumulation and neuritic plaque deposition. *Febs Lett.* 2006;580(28–29):6543–6549.

30. Dick FD, De Palma G, Ahmadi A, Scott NW, Prescott GJ, Bennett J, et al. Environmental risk factors for Parkinson's disease and parkinsonism: the Geoparkinson study. *Occup Environ Med*. 2007;64(10):666–672.
31. Gorell JM, Johnson CC, Rybicki BA, Peterson EL, Kortsha GX, Brown GG, et al. Occupational exposures to metals as risk factors for Parkinson's disease. *Neurology*. 1997;48(3):650–658.
32. Zayed J, Ducic S, Campanella G, Panisset JC, Andre P, Masson H, et al. Environmental factors in the etiology of Parkinson's disease. *Can J Neurol Sci*. 1990;17(3):286–291.
33. Finkelstein MM, Jerrett M. A study of the relationships between Parkinson's disease and markers of traffic-derived and environmental manganese air pollution in two Canadian cities. *Environ Res*. 2007;104(3):420–432.
34. Willis AW, Evanoff BA, Lian M, Galarza A, Wegrzyn A, Schootman M, et al. Metal emissions and urban incident Parkinson disease: a community health study of Medicare beneficiaries by using geographic information systems. *Am J Epidemiol*. 2010;172(12):1357–1363.
35. Fored CM, Fryzek JP, Brandt L, Nise G, Sjogren B, McLaughlin JK, et al. Parkinson's disease and other basal ganglia or movement disorders in a large nationwide cohort of Swedish welders. *Occup Environ Med*. 2006;63(2):135–140.
36. Squitti R, Gorgone G, Panetta V, Lucchini R, Bucossi S, Albini E, et al. Implications of metal exposure and liver function in Parkinsonian patients resident in the vicinities of ferroalloy plants. *J Neural Transm (Vienna)*. 2009;116(10):1281–1287.
37. Covy JP, Giasson BI. α-Synuclein, leucine-rich repeat kinase-2, and manganese in the pathogenesis of parkinson disease. *Neurotoxicology*. 2011;32(5):622–629.
38. Bates CA, Fu S, Ysselstein D, Rochet JC, Zheng W. Expression and transport of alpha-Synuclein at the blood-cerebrospinal fluid barrier and effects of manganese exposure. *ADMET DMPK*. 2015;3(1):15–33.
39. Covy JP, Giasson BI. The G2019S pathogenic mutation disrupts sensitivity of leucine-rich repeat kinase 2 to manganese kinase inhibition. *J Neurochem*. 2010;115(1):36–46.
40. Lovitt B, Vanderporten EC, Sheng Z, Zhu H, Drummond J, Liu Y. Differential effects of divalent manganese and magnesium on the kinase activity of leucine-rich repeat kinase 2 (LRRK2). *Biochemistry*. 2010;49(14):3092–3100.
41. Zhang HT, Mi L, Wang T, Yuan L, Li XH, Dong LS, et al. PINK1/Parkin-mediated mitophagy play a protective role in manganese induced apoptosis in SH-SY5Y cells. *Toxicol In Vitro*. 2016;34:212–219.
42. Roth JA, Singleton S, Feng J, Garrick M, Paradkar PN. Parkin regulates metal transport via proteasomal degradation of the 1B isoforms of divalent metal transporter 1. *J Neurochem*. 2010;113(2):454–464.
43. Kiernan MC, Vucic S, Cheah BC, Turner MR, Eisen A, Hardiman O, et al. Amyotrophic lateral sclerosis. *Lancet*. 2011;377(9769):942–955.
44. Ludolph AC, Brettschneider J, Weishaupt JH. Amyotrophic lateral sclerosis. *Curr Opin Neurol*. 2012;25(5):530–535.
45. Kamel F, Umbach DM, Stallone L, Richards M, Hu H, Sandler DP. Association of lead exposure with survival in amyotrophic lateral sclerosis. *Environ Health Perspect*. 2008;116(7):943–947.
46. Das K, Nag C, Ghosh M. Familial, environmental, and occupational risk factors in development of amyotrophic lateral sclerosis. *N Am J Med Sci*. 2012;4(8):350–355.
47. Vinceti M, Guidetti D, Bergomi M, Caselgrandi E, Vivoli R, Olmi M, et al. Lead, cadmium, and selenium in the blood of patients with sporadic amyotrophic lateral sclerosis. *Ital J Neurol Sci*. 1997;18(2):87–92.
48. Barbeito AG, Martinez-Palma L, Vargas MR, Pehar M, Manay N, Beckman JS, et al. Lead exposure stimulates VEGF expression in the spinal cord and extends survival in a mouse model of ALS. *Neurobiol Dis*. 2010;37(3):574–580.
49. Praline J, Guennoc AM, Limousin N, Hallak H, de Toffol B, Corcia P. ALS and mercury intoxication: a relationship?. *Clin Neurol Neurosurg*. 2007;109(10):880–883.
50. Schwarz S, Husstedt I, Bertram HP, Kuchelmeister K. Amyotrophic lateral sclerosis after accidental injection of mercury. *J Neurol Neurosurg Psychiatry*. 1996;60(6):698.
51. Sienko DG, Davis JP, Taylor JA, Brooks BR. Amyotrophic lateral sclerosis. A case-control study following detection of a cluster in a small Wisconsin community. *Arch Neurol*. 1990;47(1):38–41.
52. Barber TE. Inorganic mercury intoxication reminiscent of amyotrophic lateral sclerosis. *J Occup Med*. 1978;20(10):667–669.
53. Pamphlett R, Waley P. Mercury in human spinal motor neurons. *ACTA Neuropathol*. 1998;96(5):515–519.
54. Chuu JJ, Liu SH, Lin-Shiau SY. Differential neurotoxic effects of methylmercury and mercuric sulfide in rats. *Toxicol Lett*. 2007;169(2):109–120.
55. Bassett T, Bach P, Chan HM. Effects of methylmercury on the secretion of pro-inflammatory cytokines from primary microglial cells and astrocytes. *Neurotoxicology*. 2012;33(2):229–234.

56. Philips T, Robberecht W. Neuroinflammation in amyotrophic lateral sclerosis: role of glial activation in motor neuron disease. *Lancet Neurol*. 2011;10(3):253–263.
57. Kilness AW, Hichberg FH. Amyotrophic lateral sclerosis in a high selenium environment. *JAMA*. 1977;237(26): 2843–2844.
58. Vinceti M, Guidetti D, Pinotti M, Rovesti S, Merlin M, Vescovi L, et al. Amyotrophic lateral sclerosis after long-term exposure to drinking water with high selenium content. *Epidemiology*. 1996;7(5):529–532.
59. Yang GQ, Wang SZ, Zhou RH, Sun SZ. Endemic selenium intoxication of humans in China. *Am J Clin Nutr*. 1983;37(5):872–881.
60. Davidson-York D, Galey FD, Blanchard P, Gardner IA. Selenium elimination in pigs after an outbreak of selenium toxicosis. *J Vet Diagn Invest*. 1999;11(4):352–357.
61. Vinceti M, Wei ET, Malagoli C, Bergomi M, Vivoli G. Adverse health effects of selenium in humans. *Rev Environ Health*. 2001;16(4):233–251.
62. Estevez AO, Mueller CL, Morgan KL, Szewczyk NJ, Teece L, Miranda-Vizuete A, et al. Selenium induces cholinergic motor neuron degeneration in *Caenorhabditis elegans*. *Neurotoxicology*. 2012;33(5):1021–1032.
63. Maraldi T, Riccio M, Zambonin L, Vinceti M, De Pol A, Hakim G. Low levels of selenium compounds are selectively toxic for a human neuron cell line through ROS/RNS increase and apoptotic process activation. *Neurotoxicology*. 2011;32(2):180–187.
64. Yao X. Effect of zinc exposure on HNE and GLT-1 in spinal cord culture. *Neurotoxicology*. 2009;30(1):121–126.
65. Nutini M, Frazzini V, Marini C, Spalloni A, Sensi SL, Longone P. Zinc pre-treatment enhances NMDAR-mediated excitotoxicity in cultured cortical neurons from SOD1(G93A) mouse, a model of amyotrophic lateral sclerosis. *Neuropharmacology*. 2011;60(7–8):1200–1208.
66. Ermilova IP, Ermilov VB, Levy M, Ho E, Pereira C, Beckman JS. Protection by dietary zinc in ALS mutant G93A SOD transgenic mice. *Neurosci Lett*. 2005;379(1):42–46.
67. Tanzi RE, Petrukhin K, Chernov I, Pellequer JL, Wasco W, Ross B, et al. The Wilson disease gene is a copper transporting ATPase with homology to the Menkes disease gene. *Nat Genet*. 1993;5(4):344–350.
68. Zischka H, Lichtmannegger J, Schmitt S, Jagemann N, Schulz S, Wartini D, et al. Liver mitochondrial membrane crosslinking and destruction in a rat model of Wilson disease. *J Clin Invest*. 2011;121(4):1508–1518.
69. Telianidis J, Hung YH, Materia S, Fontaine SL. Role of the P-type ATPases, ATP7A and ATP7B in brain copper homeostasis. *Front Aging Neurosci*. 2013;5:44.
70. Hayashi H, Yano M, Fujita Y, Wakusawa S. Compound overload of copper and iron in patients with Wilson's disease. *Med Mol Morphol*. 2006;39(3):121–126.
71. Horoupian DS, Sternlieb I, Scheinberg IH. Neuropathological findings in penicillamine-treated patients with Wilson's disease. *Clin Neuropathol*. 1988;7(2):62–67.
72. Sinha S, Taly AB, Prashanth LK, Ravishankar S, Arunodaya GR, Vasudev MK. Sequential MRI changes in Wilson's disease with de-coppering therapy: a study of 50 patients. *Br J Radiol*. 2007;80(957):744–749.
73. Sinha S, Taly AB, Ravishankar S, Prashanth LK, Venugopal KS, Arunodaya GR, et al. Wilson's disease: cranial MRI observations and clinical correlation. *Neuroradiology*. 2006;48(9):613–621.
74. Bruehlmeier M, Leenders KL, Vontobel P, Calonder C, Antonini A, Weindl A. Increased cerebral iron uptake in Wilson's disease: a 52Fe-citrate PET study. *J Nucl Med*. 2000;41(5):781–787.
75. Horn N, Tonnesen T, Tumer Z. Menkes disease: an X-linked neurological disorder of the copper metabolism. *Brain Pathol*. 1992;2(4):351–362.
76. Varadkar S. The biochemical basis of genetic epilepsies and the genetic basis of inherited metabolic disease. *Dev Med Child Neurol*. 2016;58:1001–1002.
77. Kaler SG. Menkes disease. *Adv Pediatr*. 1994;41:263–304.
78. Menkes JH, Alter M, Steigleder GK, Weakley DR, Sung JH. A sex-linked recessive disorder with retardation of growth, peculiar hair, and focal cerebral and cerebellar degeneration. *Pediatrics*. 1962;29:764–779.
79. Ahuja A, Dev K, Tanwar RS, Selwal KK, Tyagi PK. Copper mediated neurological disorder: visions into amyotrophic lateral sclerosis. Alzheimer and Menkes disease. *J Trace Elem Med Biol*. 2015;29:11–23.
80. Danks DM, Campbell PE, Walker-Smith J, Stevens BJ, Gillespie JM, Blomfield J, et al. Menkes' kinky-hair syndrome. *Lancet*. 1972;1(7760):1100–1102.
81. Bowman AB, Kwakye GF, Herrero HE, Aschner M. Role of manganese in neurodegenerative diseases. *J Trace Elem Med Biol*. 2011;25(4):191–203.
82. Sidoryk-Wegrzynowicz M, Aschner M. Manganese toxicity in the central nervous system: the glutamine/glutamate-gamma-aminobutyric acid cycle. *J Intern Med*. 2013;273(5):466–477.

83. Au C, Benedetto A, Aschner M. Manganese transport in eukaryotes: the role of DMT1. *Neurotoxicology*. 2008;29(4):569–576.
84. Martinez-Finley EJ, Gavin CE, Aschner M, Gunter TE. Manganese neurotoxicity and the role of reactive oxygen species. *Free Radic Biol Med*. 2013;62:65–75.
85. Aschner M, Guilarte TR, Schneider JS, Zheng W. Manganese: recent advances in understanding its transport and neurotoxicity. *Toxicol Appl Pharmacol*. 2007;221(2):131–147.
86. Finkelstein Y, Milatovic D, Aschner M. Modulation of cholinergic systems by manganese. *Neurotoxicology*. 2007;28(5):1003–1014.
87. Huang CC, Weng YH, Lu CS, Chu NS, Yen TC. Dopamine transporter binding in chronic manganese intoxication. *J Neurol*. 2003;250(11):1335–1339.
88. McDougall SA, Reichel CM, Farley CM, Flesher MM, Der-Ghazarian T, Cortez AM, et al. Postnatal manganese exposure alters dopamine transporter function in adult rats: Potential impact on nonassociative and associative processes. *Neuroscience*. 2008;154(2):848–860.
89. Zhang J, Cao R, Cai T, Aschner M, Zhao F, Yao T, et al. The role of autophagy dysregulation in manganese-induced dopaminergic neurodegeneration. *Neurotox Res*. 2013;24(4):478–490.
90. Gorojod RM, Alaimo A, Porte AS, Pomilio C, Saravia F, Kotler ML. The autophagic- lysosomal pathway determines the fate of glial cells under manganese-induced oxidative stress conditions. *Free Radic Biol Med*. 2015;87:237–251.
91. Afeseh NH, Kanthasamy A, Gu Y, Fang N, Anantharam V, Kanthasamy AG. Manganese nanoparticle activates mitochondrial dependent apoptotic signaling and autophagy in dopaminergic neuronal cells. *Toxicol Appl Pharmacol*. 2011;256(3):227–240.
92. Scheiber IF, Dringen R. Astrocyte functions in the copper homeostasis of the brain. *Neurochem Int*. 2013;62(5):556–565.
93. Scheiber IF, Mercer JF, Dringen R. Metabolism and functions of copper in brain. *Prog Neurobiol*. 2014;116:33–57.
94. Rivera-Mancia S, Perez-Neri I, Rios C, Tristan-Lopez L, Rivera-Espinosa L, Montes S. The transition metals copper and iron in neurodegenerative diseases. *Chem Biol Interact*. 2010;186(2):184–199.
95. Davies P, Wang X, Sarell CJ, Drewett A, Marken F, Viles JH, et al. The synucleins are a family of redox-active copper binding proteins. *Biochemistry*. 2011;50(1):37–47.
96. Dudzik CG, Walter ED, Abrams BS, Jurica MS, Millhauser GL. Coordination of copper to the membrane-bound form of alpha-synuclein. *Biochemistry*. 2013;52(1):53–60.
97. Paris I, Perez-Pastene C, Couve E, Caviedes P, Ledoux S, Segura-Aguilar J. Copper dopamine complex induces mitochondrial autophagy preceding caspase-independent apoptotic cell death. *J Biol Chem*. 2009;284(20):13306–13315.
98. Anandhan A, Rodriguez-Rocha H, Bohovych I, Griggs AM, Zavala-Flores L, Reyes-Reyes EM, et al. Overexpression of alpha-synuclein at non-toxic levels increases dopaminergic cell death induced by copper exposure via modulation of protein degradation pathways. *Neurobiol Dis*. 2015;81:76–92.
99. Trejo-Solis C, Jimenez-Farfan D, Rodriguez-Enriquez S, Fernandez-Valverde F, Cruz-Salgado A, Ruiz-Azuara L, et al. Copper compound induces autophagy and apoptosis of glioma cells by reactive oxygen species and JNK activation. *BMC CANCER*. 2012;12:156.
100. Zhong W, Zhu H, Sheng F, Tian Y, Zhou J, Chen Y, et al. Activation of the MAPK11/12/13/14 (p38 MAPK) pathway regulates the transcription of autophagy genes in response to oxidative stress induced by a novel copper complex in HeLa cells. *Autophagy*. 2014;10(7):1285–1300.
101. Guo WJ, Ye SS, Cao N, Huang J, Gao J, Chen QY. ROS-mediated autophagy was involved in cancer cell death induced by novel copper(II) complex. *Exp Toxicol Pathol*. 2010;62(5):577–582.
102. Chen L, Liu L, Huang S. Cadmium activates the mitogen-activated protein kinase (MAPK) pathway via induction of reactive oxygen species and inhibition of protein phosphatases 2A and 5. *Free Radic Biol Med*. 2008;45(7):1035–1044.
103. Manca D, Ricard AC, Tra HV, Chevalier G. Relation between lipid peroxidation and inflammation in the pulmonary toxicity of cadmium. *Arch Toxicol*. 1994;68(6):364–369.
104. Torra M, To-Figueras J, Rodamilans M, Brunet M, Corbella J. Cadmium and zinc relationships in the liver and kidney of humans exposed to environmental cadmium. *Sci Total Environ*. 1995;170(1–2):53–57.
105. Goering PL, Fisher BR, Kish CL. Stress protein synthesis induced in rat liver by cadmium precedes hepatotoxicity. *Toxicol Appl Pharmacol*. 1993;122(1):139–148.
106. Oliveira H, Lopes T, Almeida T, Pereira ML, Santos C. Cadmium-induced genetic instability in mice testis. *Hum Exp Toxicol*. 2012;31(12):1228–1236.

107. Akesson A, Bjellerup P, Lundh T, Lidfeldt J, Nerbrand C, Samsioe G, et al. Cadmium-induced effects on bone in a population-based study of women. *Environ Health Perspect*. 2006;114(6):830–834.
108. Baxter LC, Sparks DL, Johnson SC, Lenoski B, Lopez JE, Connor DJ, et al. Relationship of cognitive measures and gray and white matter in Alzheimer's disease. *J Alzheimers Dis*. 2006;9(3):253–260.
109. Wang B, Du Y. Cadmium and its neurotoxic effects. *Oxid Med Cell Longev*. 2013;2013:898034.
110. Chen S, Xu Y, Xu B, Guo M, Zhang Z, Liu L, et al. CaMKII is involved in cadmium activation of MAPK and mTOR pathways leading to neuronal cell death. *J Neurochem*. 2011;119(5):1108–1118.
111. Figueiredo-Pereira ME, Yakushin S, Cohen G. Disruption of the intracellular sulfhydryl homeostasis by cadmium-induced oxidative stress leads to protein thiolation and ubiquitination in neuronal cells. *J Biol Chem*. 1998;273(21):12703–21279.
112. Shukla GS, Hussain T, Chandra SV. Possible role of regional superoxide dismutase activity and lipid peroxide levels in cadmium neurotoxicity: in vivo and in vitro studies in growing rats. *Life Sci*. 1987;41(19): 2215–2221.
113. Borisova T, Krisanova N, Sivko R, Kasatkina L, Borysov A, Griffin S, et al. Presynaptic malfunction: the neurotoxic effects of cadmium and lead on the proton gradient of synaptic vesicles and glutamate transport. *Neurochem Int*. 2011;59(2):272–279.
114. Gutierrez-Reyes EY, Albores A, Rios C. Increase of striatal dopamine release by cadmium in nursing rats and its prevention by dexamethasone-induced metallothionein. *Toxicology*. 1998;131(2–3):145–154.
115. Del PJ, Zeballos G, Anadon MJ, Capo MA, Diaz MJ, Garcia J, et al. Higher sensitivity to cadmium induced cell death of basal forebrain cholinergic neurons: a cholinesterase dependent mechanism. *Toxicology*. 2014;325: 151–159.
116. Okuda B, Iwamoto Y, Tachibana H, Sugita M. Parkinsonism after acute cadmium poisoning. *Clin Neurol Neurosurg*. 1997;99(4):263–265.
117. Li X, Lv Y, Yu S, Zhao H, Yao L. The effect of cadmium on Abeta levels in APP/PS1 transgenic mice. *Exp Ther Med*. 2012;4(1):125–130.
118. Jiang LF, Yao TM, Zhu ZL, Wang C, Ji LN. Impacts of Cd(II) on the conformation and self-aggregation of Alzheimer's tau fragment corresponding to the third repeat of microtubule-binding domain. *Biochim Biophys Acta*. 2007;1774(11):1414–1421.
119. Bar-Sela S, Reingold S, Richter ED. Amyotrophic lateral sclerosis in a battery-factory worker exposed to cadmium. *Int J Occup Environ Health*. 2001;7(2):109–112.
120. Wang Q, Zhu J, Zhang K, Jiang C, Wang Y, Yuan Y, et al. Induction of cytoprotective autophagy in PC-12 cells by cadmium. *Biochem Biophys Res Commun*. 2013;438(1):186–192.
121. Zou H, Zhuo L, Han T, Hu D, Yang X, Wang Y, et al. Autophagy and gap junctional intercellular communication inhibition are involved in cadmium-induced apoptosis in rat liver cells. *Biochem Biophys Res Commun*. 2015;459(4):713–719.
122. Wang T, Wang Q, Song R, Zhang Y, Zhang K, Yuan Y, et al. Autophagy plays a cytoprotective role during cadmium-induced oxidative damage in primary neuronal cultures. *Biol Trace Elem Res*. 2015;168(2):481–489.
123. Dong Z, Wang L, Xu J, Li Y, Zhang Y, Zhang S, et al. Promotion of autophagy and inhibition of apoptosis by low concentrations of cadmium in vascular endothelial cells. *Toxicol In Vitro*. 2009;23(1):105–110.
124. Surolia R, Karki S, Kim H, Yu Z, Kulkarni T, Mirov SB, et al. Heme oxygenase-1-mediated autophagy protects against pulmonary endothelial cell death and development of emphysema in cadmium-treated mice. *Am J Physiol Lung Cell Mol Physiol*. 2015;309(3):L280–L292.
125. Lim SC, Hahm KS, Lee SH, Oh SH. Autophagy involvement in cadmium resistance through induction of multidrug resistance-associated protein and counterbalance of endoplasmic reticulum stress WI38 lung epithelial fibroblast cells. *Toxicology*. 2010;276(1):18–26.
126. Chargui A, Zekri S, Jacquillet G, Rubera I, Ilie M, Belaid A, et al. Cadmium-induced autophagy in rat kidney: an early biomarker of subtoxic exposure. *Toxicol Sci*. 2011;121(1):31–42.
127. Son YO, Wang X, Hitron JA, Zhang Z, Cheng S, Budhraja A, et al. Cadmium induces autophagy through ROS-dependent activation of the LKB1-AMPK signaling in skin epidermal cells. *Toxicol Appl Pharmacol*. 2011;255(3): 287–296.
128. Wang SH, Shih YL, Kuo TC, Ko WC, Shih CM. Cadmium toxicity toward autophagy through ROS-activated GSK-3beta in mesangial cells. *Toxicol Sci*. 2009;108(1):124–131.
129. Pi H, Xu S, Zhang L, Guo P, Li Y, Xie J, et al. Dynamin 1-like-dependent mitochondrial fission initiates overactive mitophagy in the hepatotoxicity of cadmium. *Autophagy*. 2013;9(11):1780–1800.

130. Wei X, Qi Y, Zhang X, Qiu Q, Gu X, Tao C, et al. Cadmium induces mitophagy through ROS-mediated PINK1/Parkin pathway. *Toxicol Mech Methods*. 2014;24(7):504–511.
131. Oteiza PI, Mackenzie GG, Verstraeten SV. Metals in neurodegeneration: involvement of oxidants and oxidant-sensitive transcription factors. *Mol Aspects Med*. 2004;25(1–2):103–115.
132. White LD, Cory-Slechta DA, Gilbert ME, Tiffany-Castiglioni E, Zawia NH, Virgolini M, et al. New and evolving concepts in the neurotoxicology of lead. *Toxicol Appl Pharmacol*. 2007;225(1):1–27.
133. Mason LH, Harp JP, Han DY. Pb neurotoxicity: neuropsychological effects of lead toxicity. *Biomed Res Int*. 2014;2014:840547.
134. Neal AP, Guilarte TR. Molecular neurobiology of lead (Pb(2+)): effects on synaptic function. *Mol Neurobiol*. 2010;42(3):151–160.
135. Marchetti C. Molecular targets of lead in brain neurotoxicity. *Neurotox Res*. 2003;5(3):221–236.
136. Nava-Ruiz C, Mendez-Armenta M, Rios C. Lead neurotoxicity: effects on brain nitric oxide synthase. *J Mol Histol*. 2012;43(5):553–563.
137. Chin-Chan M, Navarro-Yepes J, Quintanilla-Vega B. Environmental pollutants as risk factors for neurodegenerative disorders: Alzheimer and Parkinson diseases. *Front Cell Neurosci*. 2015;9:124.
138. Zhang J, Cai T, Zhao F, Yao T, Chen Y, Liu X, et al. The role of alpha-synuclein and tau hyperphosphorylation-mediated autophagy and apoptosis in lead-induced learning and memory injury. *Int J Biol Sci*. 2012;8(7):935–944.
139. Sui L, Zhang RH, Zhang P, Yun KL, Zhang HC, Liu L, et al. Lead toxicity induces autophagy to protect against cell death through mTORC1 pathway in cardiofibroblasts. *Biosci Rep*. 2015;35(2).
140. Parks JM, Johs A, Podar M, Bridou R, Hurt RJ, Smith SD, et al. The genetic basis for bacterial mercury methylation. *Science*. 2013;339(6125):1332–1335.
141. Sheehan MC, Burke TA, Navas-Acien A, Breysse PN, McGready J, Fox MA. Global methylmercury exposure from seafood consumption and risk of developmental neurotoxicity: a systematic review. *Bull World Health Organ*. 2014;92(4):254–269.
142. Kerper LE, Ballatori N, Clarkson TW. Methylmercury transport across the blood-brain barrier by an amino acid carrier. *Am J Physiol*. 1992;262(5 Pt 2):R761–R765.
143. Jo S, Woo HD, Kwon HJ, Oh SY, Park JD, Hong YS, et al. Estimation of the biological half-life of methylmercury using a population toxicokinetic model. *Int J Environ Res Public Health*. 2015;12(8):9054–9067.
144. Do NJ, Oliveira KR, Crespo-Lopez ME, Macchi BM, Maues LA, Pinheiro MC, et al. Methylmercury neurotoxicity and antioxidant defenses. *Indian J Med Res*. 2008;128(4):373–382.
145. Cao B, Lv W, Jin S, Tang J, Wang S, Zhao H, et al. Degeneration of peripheral nervous system in rats experimentally induced by methylmercury intoxication. *Neurol Sci*. 2013;34(5):663–669.
146. Martinez-Finley EJ, Caito S, Slaughter JC, Aschner M. The Role of skn-1 in methylmercury-induced latent dopaminergic neurodegeneration. *Neurochem Res*. 2013;38(12):2650–2660.
147. Shaw CM, Mottet NK, Body RL, Luschei ES. Variability of neuropathologic lesions in experimental methylmercurial encephalopathy in primates. *Am J Pathol*. 1975;80(3):451–470.
148. Chang SH, Lee HJ, Kang B, Yu KN, Minai-Tehrani A, Lee S, et al. Methylmercury induces caspase-dependent apoptosis and autophagy in human neural stem cells. *J Toxicol Sci*. 2013;38(6):823–831.
149. Gimenez-Xavier P, Francisco R, Platini F, Perez R, Ambrosio S. LC3-I conversion to LC3-II does not necessarily result in complete autophagy. *Int J Mol Med*. 2008;22(6):781–785.
150. Yuntao F, Chenjia G, Panpan Z, Wenjun Z, Suhua W, Guangwei X, et al. Role of autophagy in methylmercury-induced neurotoxicity in rat primary astrocytes. *Arch Toxicol*. 2016;90(2):333–345.
151. Farina M, Rocha JB, Aschner M. Mechanisms of methylmercury-induced neurotoxicity: evidence from experimental studies. *Life Sci*. 2011;89(15–16):555–563.
152. Batista-Nascimento L, Pimentel C, Menezes RA, Rodrigues-Pousada C. Iron and neurodegeneration: from cellular homeostasis to disease. *Oxid Med Cell Longev*. 2012;2012:128647.
153. Sheftel AD, Mason AB, Ponka P. The long history of iron in the Universe and in health and disease. *Biochim Biophys Acta*. 2012;1820(3):161–187.
154. Hayflick SJ, Kruer MC, Gregory A, Haack TB, Kurian MA, Houlden HH, et al. beta-Propeller protein-associated neurodegeneration: a new X-linked dominant disorder with brain iron accumulation. *Brain*. 2013;136(Pt 6):1708–1717.
155. Saitsu H, Nishimura T, Muramatsu K, Kodera H, Kumada S, Sugai K, et al. De novo mutations in the autophagy gene WDR45 cause static encephalopathy of childhood with neurodegeneration in adulthood. *Nat Genet*. 2013;45(4):445–449:441e-449e.

156. Meyer E, Kurian MA, Hayflick SJ. Neurodegeneration with brain iron accumulation: genetic diversity and pathophysiological mechanisms. *Annu Rev Genomics Hum Genet*. 2015;16:257–279.
157. He Y, Wan S, Hua Y, Keep RF, Xi G. Autophagy after experimental intracerebral hemorrhage. *J Cereb Blood Flow Metab*. 2008;28(5):897–905.
158. Chen CW, Chen TY, Tsai KL, Lin CL, Yokoyama KK, Lee WS, et al. Inhibition of autophagy as a therapeutic strategy of iron-induced brain injury after hemorrhage. *Autophagy*. 2012;8(10):1510–1520.
159. Zukor H, Song W, Liberman A, Mui J, Vali H, Fillebeen C, et al. HO-1-mediated macroautophagy: a mechanism for unregulated iron deposition in aging and degenerating neural tissues. *J Neurochem*. 2009;109(3): 776–791.
160. Chew KC, Ang ET, Tai YK, Tsang F, Lo SQ, Ong E, et al. Enhanced autophagy from chronic toxicity of iron and mutant A53T alpha-synuclein: implications for neuronal cell death in Parkinson disease. *J Biol Chem*. 2011;286(38):33380–33389.
161. Kamalinia G, Khodagholi F, Atyabi F, Amini M, Shaerzadeh F, Sharifzadeh M, et al. Enhanced brain delivery of deferasirox-lactoferrin conjugates for iron chelation therapy in neurodegenerative disorders: in vitro and in vivo studies. *Mol Pharm*. 2013;10(12):4418–4431.
162. Prohaska R, Sibon OC, Rudnicki DD, Danek A, Hayflick SJ, Verhaag EM, et al. Brain, blood, and iron: perspectives on the roles of erythrocytes and iron in neurodegeneration. *Neurobiol Dis*. 2012;46(3):607–624.
163. Colombelli C, Aoun M, Tiranti V. Defective lipid metabolism in neurodegeneration with brain iron accumulation (NBIA) syndromes: not only a matter of iron. *J Inherit Metab Dis*. 2015;38(1):123–136.
164. Sakaida I, Kyle ME, Farber JL. Autophagic degradation of protein generates a pool of ferric iron required for the killing of cultured hepatocytes by an oxidative stress. *Mol Pharmacol*. 1990;37(3):435–442.
165. Dixon SJ, Lemberg KM, Lamprecht MR, Skouta R, Zaitsev EM, Gleason CE, et al. Ferroptosis: an iron-dependent form of nonapoptotic cell death. *Cell*. 2012;149(5):1060–1072.
166. Fuchs Y, Steller H. Live to die another way: modes of programmed cell death and the signals emanating from dying cells. *Nat Rev Mol Cell Biol*. 2015;16(6):329–344.
167. Liuzzi JP, Guo L, Yoo C, Stewart TS. Zinc and autophagy. *Biometals*. 2014;27(6):1087–1096.
168. Hwang JJ, Kim HN, Kim J, Cho DH, Kim MJ, Kim YS, et al. Zinc(II) ion mediates tamoxifen-induced autophagy and cell death in MCF-7 breast cancer cell line. *Biometals*. 2010;23(6):997–1013.
169. Liuzzi JP, Yoo C. Role of zinc in the regulation of autophagy during ethanol exposure in human hepatoma cells. *Biol Trace Elem Res*. 2013;156(1-3):350–356.
170. Botti J, Djavaheri-Mergny M, Pilatte Y, Codogno P. Autophagy signaling and the cogwheels of cancer. *Autophagy*. 2006;2(2):67–73.
171. Wang J, Whiteman MW, Lian H, Wang G, Singh A, Huang D, et al. A non-canonical MEK/ERK signaling pathway regulates autophagy via regulating Beclin 1. *J Biol Chem*. 2009;284(32):21412–21424.
172. Lee SJ, Koh JY. Roles of zinc and metallothionein-3 in oxidative stress-induced lysosomal dysfunction, cell death, and autophagy in neurons and astrocytes. *Mol Brain*. 2010;3(1):30.
173. Lichtlen P, Schaffner W. The "metal transcription factor" MTF-1: biological facts and medical implications. *Swiss Med Wkly*. 2001;131(45–46):647–652.
174. Cartharius K, Frech K, Grote K, Klocke B, Haltmeier M, Klingenhoff A, et al. MatInspector and beyond: promoter analysis based on transcription factor binding sites. *Bioinformatics*. 2005;21(13):2933–2942.
175. Ryu MS, Langkamp-Henken B, Chang SM, Shankar MN, Cousins RJ. Genomic analysis, cytokine expression, and microRNA profiling reveal biomarkers of human dietary zinc depletion and homeostasis. *Proc Natl Acad Sci USA*. 2011;108(52):20970–20975.
176. Sharif R, Thomas P, Zalewski P, Fenech M. The role of zinc in genomic stability. *Mutat Res*. 2012;733(1-2):111–121.
177. Julien S, Biesemeier A, Kokkinou D, Eibl O, Schraermeyer U. Zinc deficiency leads to lipofuscin accumulation in the retinal pigment epithelium of pigmented rats. *PLoS One*. 2011;6(12):e29245.
178. Summersgill H, England H, Lopez-Castejon G, Lawrence CB, Luheshi NM, Pahle J, et al. Zinc depletion regulates the processing and secretion of IL-1beta. *Cell Death Dis*. 2014;5:e1040.
179. Prakash C, Soni M, Kumar V. Biochemical and molecular alterations following arsenic-induced oxidative stress and mitochondrial dysfunction in rat brain. *Biol Trace Elem Res*. 2015;167(1):121–129.
180. Prakash C, Soni M, Kumar V. Mitochondrial oxidative stress and dysfunction in arsenic neurotoxicity: a review. *J Appl Toxicol*. 2016;36(2):179–188.
181. Aung KH, Tsukahara S, Maekawa F, Nohara K, Nakamura K, Tanoue A. Role of environmental chemical insult in neuronal cell death and cytoskeleton damage. *Biol Pharm Bull*. 2015;38(8):1109–1112.

182. Tolins M, Ruchirawat M, Landrigan P. The developmental neurotoxicity of arsenic: cognitive and behavioral consequences of early life exposure. *Ann Glob Health*. 2014;80(4):303–314.
183. Zarazua S, Burger S, Delgado JM, Jimenez-Capdeville ME, Schliebs R. Arsenic affects expression and processing of amyloid precursor protein (APP) in primary neuronal cells overexpressing the Swedish mutation of human APP. *Int J Dev Neurosci*. 2011;29(4):389–396.
184. DeFuria J, Shea TB. Arsenic inhibits neurofilament transport and induces perikaryal accumulation of phosphorylated neurofilaments: roles of JNK and GSK-3beta. *Brain Res*. 2007;1181:74–82.
185. Qian W, Liu J, Jin J, Ni W, Xu W. Arsenic trioxide induces not only apoptosis but also autophagic cell death in leukemia cell lines via up-regulation of Beclin-1. *Leuk Res*. 2007;31(3):329–339.
186. Bolt AM, Byrd RM, Klimecki WT. Autophagy is the predominant process induced by arsenite in human lymphoblastoid cell lines. *Toxicol Appl Pharmacol*. 2010;244(3):366–373.
187. Azad MB, Chen Y, Gibson SB. Regulation of autophagy by reactive oxygen species (ROS): implications for cancer progression and treatment. *Antioxid Redox Signal*. 2009;11(4):777–790.
188. Scherz-Shouval R, Elazar Z. ROS, mitochondria and the regulation of autophagy. *Trends Cell Biol*. 2007;17(9):422–427.
189. Carames B, Taniguchi N, Otsuki S, Blanco FJ, Lotz M. Autophagy is a protective mechanism in normal cartilage, and its aging-related loss is linked with cell death and osteoarthritis. *Arthritis Rheum*. 2010;62(3):791–801.
190. Zhang T, Qi Y, Liao M, Xu M, Bower KA, Frank JA, et al. Autophagy is a cell self-protective mechanism against arsenic-induced cell transformation. *Toxicol Sci*. 2012;130(2):298–308.

CHAPTER

20

An Overview of Multifunctional Metal Chelators as Potential Treatments for Neurodegenerative Diseases

Frank W. Lewis, David Tétard

Northumbria University Newcastle, Newcastle, United Kingdom

OUTLINE

INTRODUCTION

The neurodegenerative diseases Alzheimer's disease (AD) and Parkinson's disease (PD) are currently the leading causes of dementia worldwide, with an ever-increasing health and economic burden as the global population ages. However, in comparison with other chronic diseases, such as heart disease, cancers, and stroke, research into the treatment and cure of dementia receives far less funding than other conditions.[1] As a result, new treatments are urgently needed as the burden of these chronic diseases continues to increase in the future.

The disease pathology of AD and PD is complex and multifactorial in nature. Postmortem brain tissue studies in AD patients reveal the presence of intracellular insoluble aggregates composed of misfolded amyloid β protein and extracellular hyperphosphorylated tau protein, while intracellular aggregates containing α-synuclein have been identified in PD

Biometals in Neurodegenerative Diseases. http://dx.doi.org/10.1016/B978-0-12-804562-6.00020-8

patients. In addition, metal ion dyshomeostasis is another characteristic feature of these conditions, and is believed to be an early event in the onset of AD and PD. Misplaced metals (iron, copper, and zinc) also exacerbate protein misfolding, deposition, and aggregation by forming insoluble metal–protein aggregates. When not tightly regulated and controlled, the redox-active metals iron and copper also have the potential to generate reactive oxygen species (ROS) that can cause oxidative damage to biomolecules in the neuron. In the case of PD, this can occur by the production of hydroxyl radicals through Fenton or Haber–Weiss chemistry. Another feature of these conditions is the depletion of the key neurotransmitters dopamine (in the substantia nigra of PD patients) and acetylcholine (throughout the brains of AD patients) that are essential for normal function. The exact order of events in AD and PD disease progression and their cause and effect relationships are still not clear and are the subject of intensive ongoing research.[2]

A simplified picture of iron regulation in a healthy neuron is presented in Fig. 20.1A. Iron levels in the neuron are tightly regulated and controlled by iron transport and storage proteins, particularly the iron import protein transferrin and the iron export protein ferroportin.[3,4] Once inside the cell, iron is usually stored in organelles by the iron storage protein ferritin. Within each cell there is also a small labile iron pool of weakly bound or unbound iron in the cytoplasm that acts as a temporary cellular iron store. With the exception of this iron pool, all iron in the cell is tightly bound by iron transport and storage proteins at all times, thus minimizing its ability to form metal–protein aggregates or to generate ROS.

A simplified picture of how neuronal iron regulation is disturbed in PD is shown in Fig. 20.1B. While iron import by transferrin continues, iron export by ferroportin and iron storage by ferritin both decrease due to reduced expression of these proteins, leading to a net build-up of iron in the labile iron pool. When weakly bound as in the labile iron pool, Fe(III) can be reduced by biological reductants (e.g., NADH) to Fe(II) which can then catalyze the Fenton/Haber–Weiss reactions to generate free radicals and other ROS. If unchecked, this

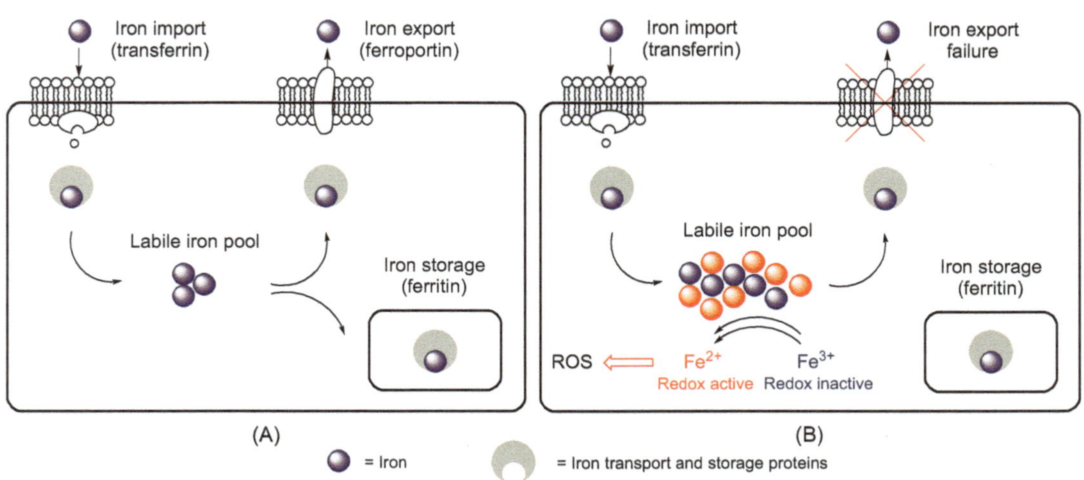

FIGURE 20.1 Simplified picture of (A) iron regulation in a healthy neuron, and (B) iron dysregulation in PD.

build-up of ROS can overwhelm cellular antioxidant defenses [e.g., glutathione, superoxide dismutase (SOD), catalase] and cause oxidative damage to biomolecules in the cell and, ultimately, to cell death.

The early involvement of misplaced metal ions (copper in AD, iron in PD) and their role in neurodegenerative disease progression (the metal hypothesis)[5] has opened up the possibility of developing metal chelators as potential disease modifying drug treatments for AD and PD.[6–12] The aim is to develop a chelator that can potentially resolubilize the metal–protein aggregates and redistribute the metals from regions of excess to regions of requirement. In addition, the chelator needs to passivate the redox-active metals iron and copper so that Fenton/Haber–Weiss chemistry and the associated build-up of ROS is prevented.

Strategies for drug development to combat AD and PD have to date mostly fallen under the "one drug, one target" paradigm. Classic examples are the development of acetylcholinesterase (AChE) inhibitors for AD treatment and monoamine oxidase (MAO) inhibitors for PD treatment. Both drug classes inhibit enzymes that catalytically break down the neurotransmitters acetylcholine and dopamine, and that are overexpressed in AD and PD, respectively. However, these types of drug treatments only offer temporary symptomatic relief and do not prevent further disease progression. Due to the complex multifactorial nature of AD and PD pathogenesis, the "one drug, multiple targets" approach to drug development has been gaining traction in recent years. In this approach, a drug with multiple modes of action against AD or PD is thought to have a greater chance of clinical success than a drug that has only one mode of action. This "multidrug action" approach to treating neurodegenerative diseases has been covered in several recent reviews.[13–20] In this chapter, we will provide a brief overview of the development of multifunctional metal chelators for AD and PD treatment, as well as the parent metal chelators on which these multifunctional drugs are based. For this review, we define multifunctional metal chelators as those having two or more therapeutic modes of action, as well as those having one mode of action and an additional structural feature that facilitates transport across the blood–brain barrier.

PARENT METAL CHELATORS

The metal chelators that have been studied as potential drug treatments against AD and PD are presented in Fig. 20.2. One of the first iron chelators to be studied as a potential treatment for PD was desferrioxamine **1** (Fig. 20.2), a hexadentate hydroxamate siderophore that is clinically used to treat iron overload diseases, such as β-thalassemia. Desferrioxamine **1** was previously found to be neuroprotective in the 6-hydroxydopamine toxin model of PD.[21,22] However, further development of **1** is unlikely due to its need for systemic administration and lack of oral bioavailability.

The clinically available 8-hydroxyquinoline clioquinol **2** (Fig. 20.2) is a bidentate chelator that shows good selectivity for Cu(II) and Zn(II), and was originally used as a topical antiseptic.[23] In early studies, **2** showed promising results as a potential drug treatment for AD. Oral administration of **2** to transgenic AD mice gave a nearly 50% decrease in amyloid β deposition compared to controls.[24] Compared to desferrioxamine **1**, clioquinol **2** also has the advantage of being able to cross the blood–brain barrier. However, despite promising results in clinical trials,[25] the drug was not further developed due to safety concerns over its

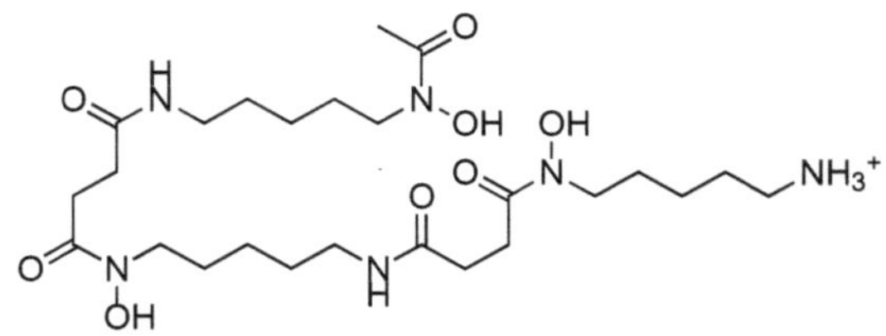

Desferrioxamine **1**

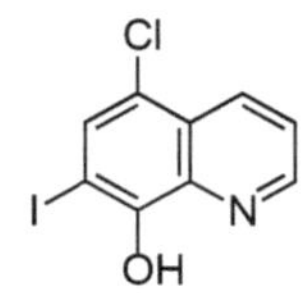

Clioquinol **2**

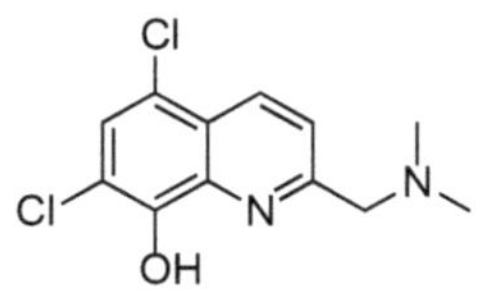

PBT2 **3**

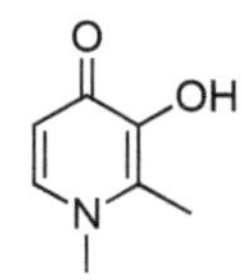

Deferiprone **4**

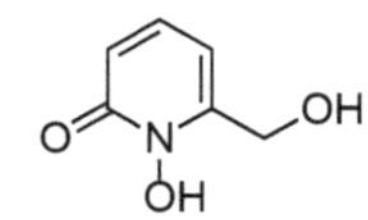

1,2-HOPO **5**

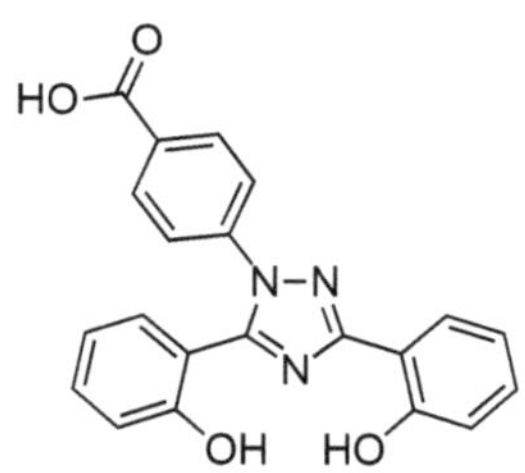

Deferasirox **6**

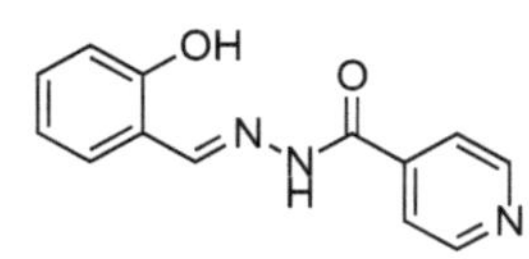

SIH **7**

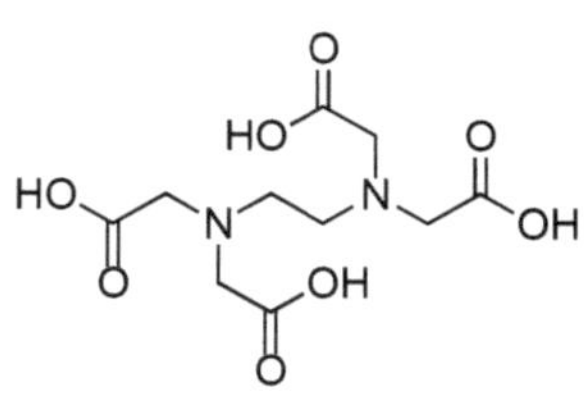

EDTA **8**

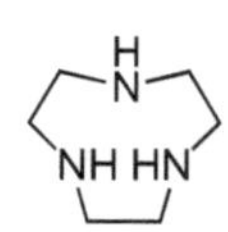

TACN **9**

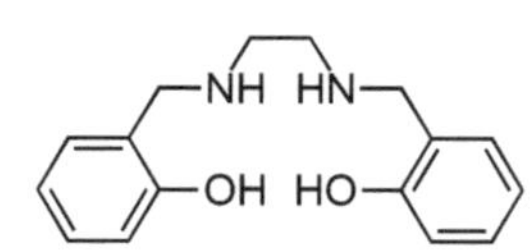

Tetrahydrosalen **10**

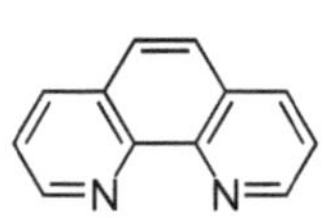

Phen **11**

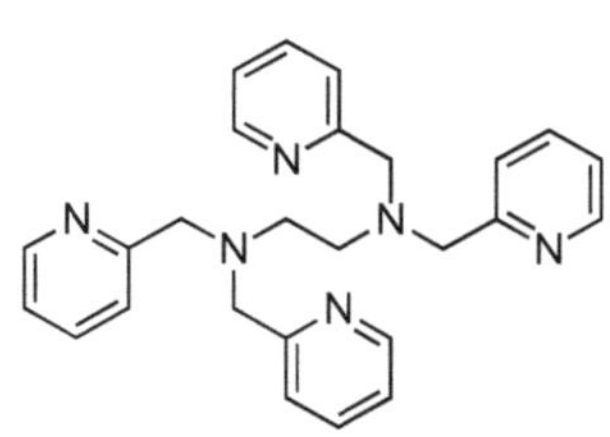

TPEN **12**

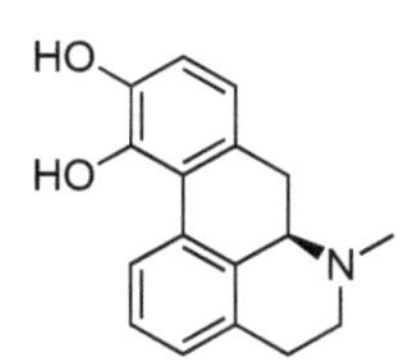

Apomorphine **13**

FIGURE 20.2 **Structures of parent metal chelators studied against neurodegenerative diseases.**

toxicity and issues with its synthesis. Subsequently, PBT2 **3** was developed as a successor to clioquinol **2** (Fig. 20.2), and is the most advanced drug in AD clinical trials. PBT2 **3** showed a reduction in amyloid β plaque formation and improved cognition when administered orally to mice.[26,27] In subsequent phase II clinical trials, PBT2 **3** significantly reduced cerebrospinal fluid levels of amyloid β and improved cognition at high doses.[28,29]

Hydroxypyridinones (HOPOs) have emerged as promising therapeutic candidates for a range of diseases where metal iron chelation is an essential therapeutic mode of action.[30,31] Deferiprone **4** (Fig. 20.2) is an orally available bidentate 3-hydroxypyridin-4-one (3,4-HOPO) iron chelator that is clinically used as a treatment for systemic iron overload diseases. Being a bidentate O-donor ligand, **4** is a hard Lewis base and thus highly selective for Fe(III) over Fe(II), Cu(II) and Zn(II).[32–36] Due to its high selectivity for Fe(III) over Fe(II), **4** is able to passivate Fe(III) and prevent its redox cycling to Fe(II), thereby preventing Fenton chemistry and ROS production.[37,38] Deferiprone **4** also has the ability to cross the blood–brain barrier and remove iron from the brain.[39] Due to these properties, deferiprone **4** was recently studied as a treatment for PD. Deferiprone **4** was neuroprotective in the 6-hydroxydopamine rat model of PD[22] and in a recent pilot clinical study, **4** showed a significant reduction in iron deposition in the substantia nigra in PD patients.[40] Further clinical studies with **4** are thus warranted.

In an effort to expand the range of bidentate O-donor ligands for the treatment of PD, some novel 1-hydroxypyridin-2-ones (1,2-HOPOs) were developed. From a preliminary drug screen, 1-hydroxypyridin-2-one **5** (Fig. 20.2) was identified as a promising lead candidate. This molecule was able to prevent neuronal loss in the 6-hydroxydopamine cell culture model of PD and its neuroprotective effects were comparable to that of the 3,4-HOPO deferiprone **4**.[41] Furthermore, both **5** and **4** normalized ferritin and transferrin expression levels to that in a healthy neuron when administered to either 6-hydroxydopamine or iron incubated neurons, indicating that both compounds act by reducing the labile iron pool.

The tridentate iron chelator deferasirox **6** (Fig. 20.2) is clinically used for the treatment of iron overload diseases. It has recently been studied as a potential treatment for AD. In a study on aged rats, administration of **6** significantly reduced age-related iron and amyloid β accumulation, oxidative damage and overexpression of ferritin and transferrin receptor 1 in rat brain, suggesting possible therapeutic potential in AD treatment.[42] In addition, deferasirox **6** showed promising neuroprotective effects against PD in 6-hydroxydopamine-lesioned rats.[22]

Other different metal chelators, such as EDTA **8**, chelators based on the 1,10-phenanthroline core **11** and TPEN **12** (Fig. 20.2) have been studied for the disaggregation of postmortem metal-amyloid β aggregates.[43,44] However, these chelators are unsuitable for further therapeutic development due to, among other reasons, poor blood–brain barrier permeability and poor metal ion specificity. The D1- and D2-receptor agonist apomorphine **13** (Fig. 20.2) showed iron chelating and antioxidant properties in both the 1-methyl-4-phenyl-1,2,3,6-tetrahydropyridine (MPTP), as well as in the 6-hydroxydopamine models of PD.[45] These were attributed to the drugs phenolic catechol moiety which can both chelate iron and scavenge free radical species. However, catechol groups are also known to be prooxidant compounds, giving rise to reactive *ortho*-quinones that are involved in neuronal damage.[46,47] The risk associated with the use of catechols as coordinating groups in chelators against neurodegenerative diseases will thus need to be assessed carefully.

MULTIFUNCTIONAL METAL CHELATORS

In this section, the multifunctional derivatives of the parent metal chelators shown in Fig. 20.2 will be reviewed. A number of multifunctional 8-hydroxyquinoline derivatives have been developed for the treatment of AD and PD (Fig. 20.3). Prochelator QBP **14** contains a boronate ester moiety that is designed to be unmasked in the presence of H_2O_2 to release the 8-hydroxyquinoline metal chelator. In the absence of H_2O_2, **14** does not prevent Cu-amyloid β aggregation but in the presence of H_2O_2, **14** is converted into the free metal chelator that passivates Cu, resolubilizes Cu-amyloid β aggregates, and prevents further Cu-amyloid β aggregation.[48] The strategy is a useful way to target prochelators to localized brain regions where metal–protein aggregation and ROS production occur simultaneously.

VK28 **19** (Fig. 20.3) was designed as a successor to clioquinol **2** and was chosen from a library of 8-hydroxyquinolines for further study due to its ability to inhibit lipid peroxidation. This chelator protected neurons from oxidative damage in the 6-hydroxydopamine model of PD both when directly injected into the brain, and when administered systemically, showing its ability to permeate the blood–brain barrier.[49] In a further improvement of this molecule, multifunctional chelators M30 **15** and HLA-20 **16** (Fig. 20.3) were developed. In addition to the metal binding 8-hydroxyquinoline motif, these molecules also contain the *N*-propargylamine moiety found in the monoamine oxidase B (MAO-B) inhibitors rasagiline and selegiline, which both irreversibly inhibit the breakdown of dopamine by the MAO-B enzyme. Thus **15** and **16** are designed to deliver two benefits in PD therapy; metal chelation/passivation and elevated dopamine levels through MAO-B inhibition. As well as showing good cell permeability and inhibition of MAO-B, both **15** and **16** showed neuroprotective effects in the 6-hydroxydopamine model of PD in vitro.[50,51] Studies in vivo showed that M30 **15** was also neuroprotective in the MPTP model, and M30 **15** selectively inhibited MAO-B in certain regions of the brain.[52]

Following these promising results, these molecules were further modified for AD therapy by the addition of a carbamate ester moiety to the coordinating hydroxyl group of **15** and **16**, giving rise to multifunctional prochelators M30D **17** and HLA-20A **18** (Fig. 20.3). The addition of the carbamate ester moiety is inspired by the active pharmacophore of the AChE inhibitor rivastigmine, which inhibits the breakdown of the neurotransmitter acetylcholine. Inhibition of AChE cleaves the carbamate ester thus releasing the free metal chelator. This endows **17** and **18** with three modes of action; metal chelation/passivation, elevated levels of acetylcholine (through AChE inhibition), and elevated levels of dopamine (through MAO-B inhibition). Both **17** and **18** were good AChE and MAO-B inhibitors similar to rivastigmine, and also showed neuroprotective effects in vitro by reducing metal-amyloid β aggregation.[53] These results illustrate the benefit of the "one drug, multiple targets" paradigm and further therapeutic development of these molecules is expected.[54]

Various other multifunctional 8-hydroxyquinolines were studied for their neuroprotective efficacy against AD and PD. Chelator M10 **21** (Fig. 20.3) contains a bound alanine residue and is designed to exploit the amino acid transporter system that carries neutral amino acids, including L-dopa, into the brain.[55] This molecule had neuroprotective effects comparable to rasagiline in the 6-hydroxydopamine model of PD in vitro as well as having good antioxidant and radical scavenging properties. Chelators M31 **22** and M32 **23** (Fig. 20.3) were good iron chelators and inhibitors of iron-induced lipid peroxidation. However, while M31 **22** was a

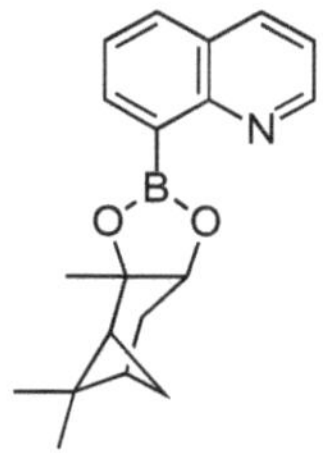

QBP **14**

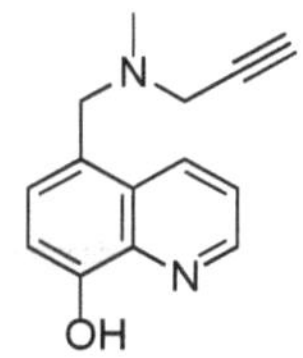

M30 **15**

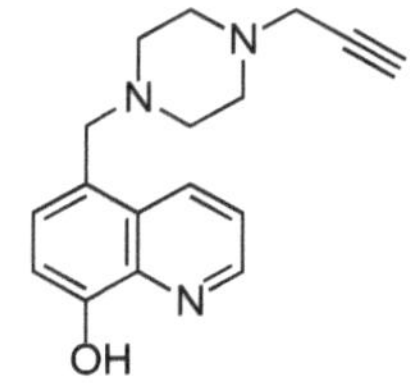

HLA-20 **16**

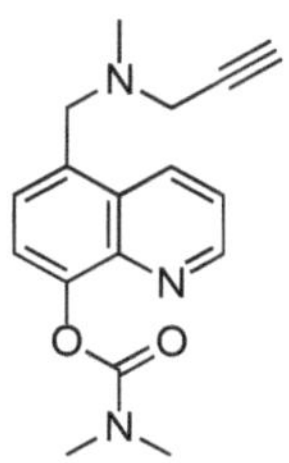

M30D **17**

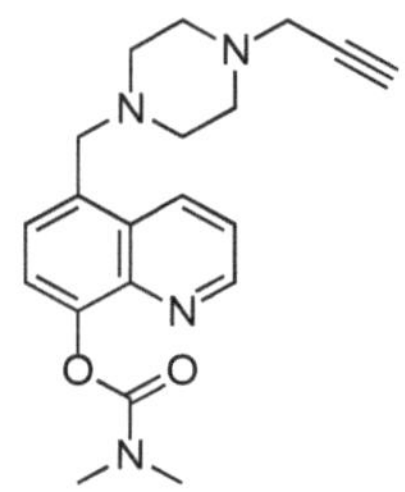

HLA-20A **18**

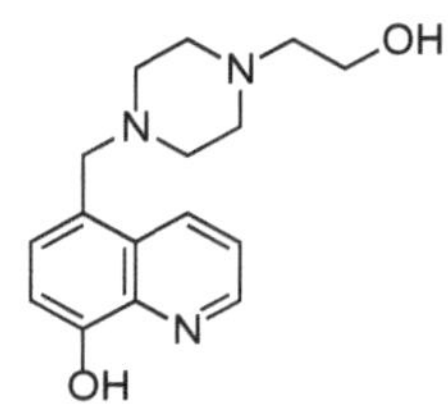

VK28 **19**

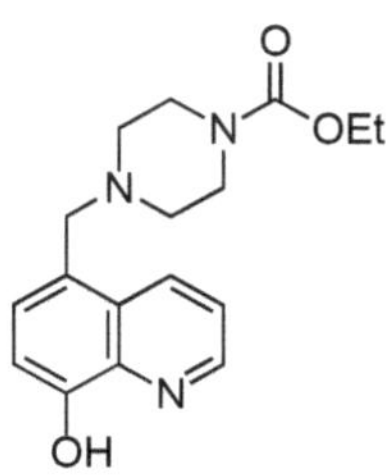

HLA16 **20**

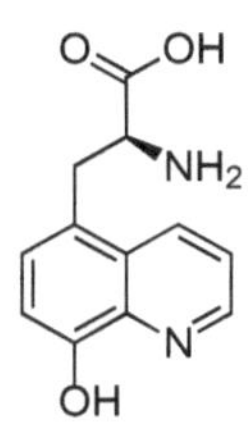

M10 **21**

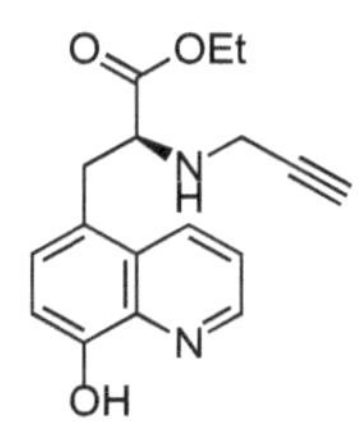

M31 **22**

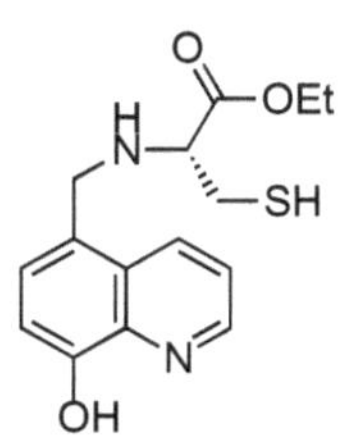

M32 **23**

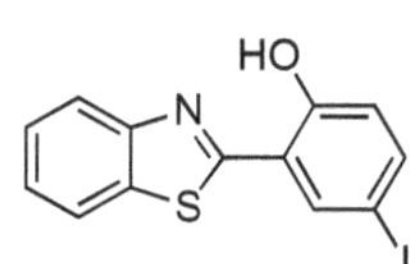

HBT1 **24**

FIGURE 20.3 **Structures of multifunctional 8-hydroxyquinoline derivatives studied against neurodegenerative diseases.**

selective MAO-B inhibitor (due to its *N*-propargylamine moiety), M32 **23** was not.[56] Due to the known concentration-dependent neurotoxicity of clioquinol **2**,[57] it remains to be seen if other derivatives of 8-hydroxyquinoline are suitable candidates for chelation therapy with a much improved safety profile. Chelator HBTI **24** (Fig. 20.3) has the same bidentate coordinating group as clioquinol **2** but is similar in structure to thioflavin-T, a dye used to detect amyloid deposits in brain tissue. Thus **24** contains both a metal chelating unit and an amyloid binding unit, and is designed to target brain regions containing amyloid aggregates. In a turbidity assay, this chelator was comparable to clioquinol **2** in its ability to dissolve amyloid β aggregates with Cu(II) and Zn(II), and fluorescence measurements in the presence of amyloid fibrils showed that **24** intercalated within these aggregates.[58]

Several multifunctional derivatives of deferiprone **4** have been developed for the treatment of AD and PD (Fig. 20.4). Due to the brain's high energy demand, the blood–brain barrier contains a number of glucose transporters (GLUT-1) that actively transport glucose into the brain. One strategy to target metal chelators to the brain is therefore glycoconjugation. A number of glycosylated derivatives of deferiprone **4** have been studied. Three such examples are shown in Fig. 20.4. Derivatives **25** and **26** are both prochelators where glycosylation on the chelating hydroxyl group has the added benefit of masking the chelating moiety, thus minimizing toxicity due to systemic metal chelation. Upon entering the brain, enzymatic cleavage of glucose releases the active chelator. Studies with **25** and **26** (Fig. 20.4) in vitro demonstrated the feasibility of this approach. Upon enzymatic removal of glucose from **25** and **26**, the hydroxyl group of the free chelators acted as an efficient radical scavenger, with **26** showing the best results.[59,60] In addition, the nonglycosylated analogs of **25** and **26** were able to reduce Cu(II)- and Zn(II)-induced amyloid β aggregation as measured by turbidity assay. Chelator **27** (Fig. 20.4) was able to penetrate the blood–brain barrier in rats when administered intravenously.[59] In contrast, glycosylated deferiprone **28** (Fig. 20.4) showed no ability to cross the blood–brain barrier in guinea pigs.[61]

Glycosylated prochelators **29** and **30** (Fig. 20.4) also contain an *N*-substituent which is structurally similar to the amyloid-selective dye thioflavin-T, and these derivatives are thus designed to target the prochelator to amyloid fibrils in the brain for the treatment of AD. Nonglycosylated derivatives of **29** and **30** showed an excellent ability to redissolve amyloid aggregates of Cu(II) and Zn(II) in vitro.[62] Chelator **31** (Fig. 20.4) is one of a number of amino acid-substituted derivatives that were developed as modified analogs of deferiprone **4**. Studies in vitro demonstrated the neuroprotective ability of these compounds to both amyloid β and iron-induced neurotoxicity.[63] In addition, in contrast to deferiprone **4**, **31** and related compounds did not inhibit the iron-containing enzyme tyrosine hydroxylase (an essential enzyme involved in the biosynthesis of dopamine), suggesting they could have applications as nontoxic alternatives to deferiprone **4**.

Chelators **32** and **33** (Fig. 20.4) are bifunctional chelators consisting of deferiprone **4** conjugated to the antioxidants butylated hydroxytoluene (BHT) and trolox, respectively. Thus **32** and **33** are designed to confer free radical trapping and antioxidant activity as well as metal chelation. These compounds showed superior neuroprotective activity in vitro than deferiprone, BHT, or trolox, as well as excellent antioxidant ability against lipid peroxidation in rat brain homogenate.[64,65] However, despite the authors mentioning potential applications against neurodegenerative diseases, the authors only report inhibition of lipid peroxidation and no studies with **32** and **33** have been reported yet in models of either AD or PD.

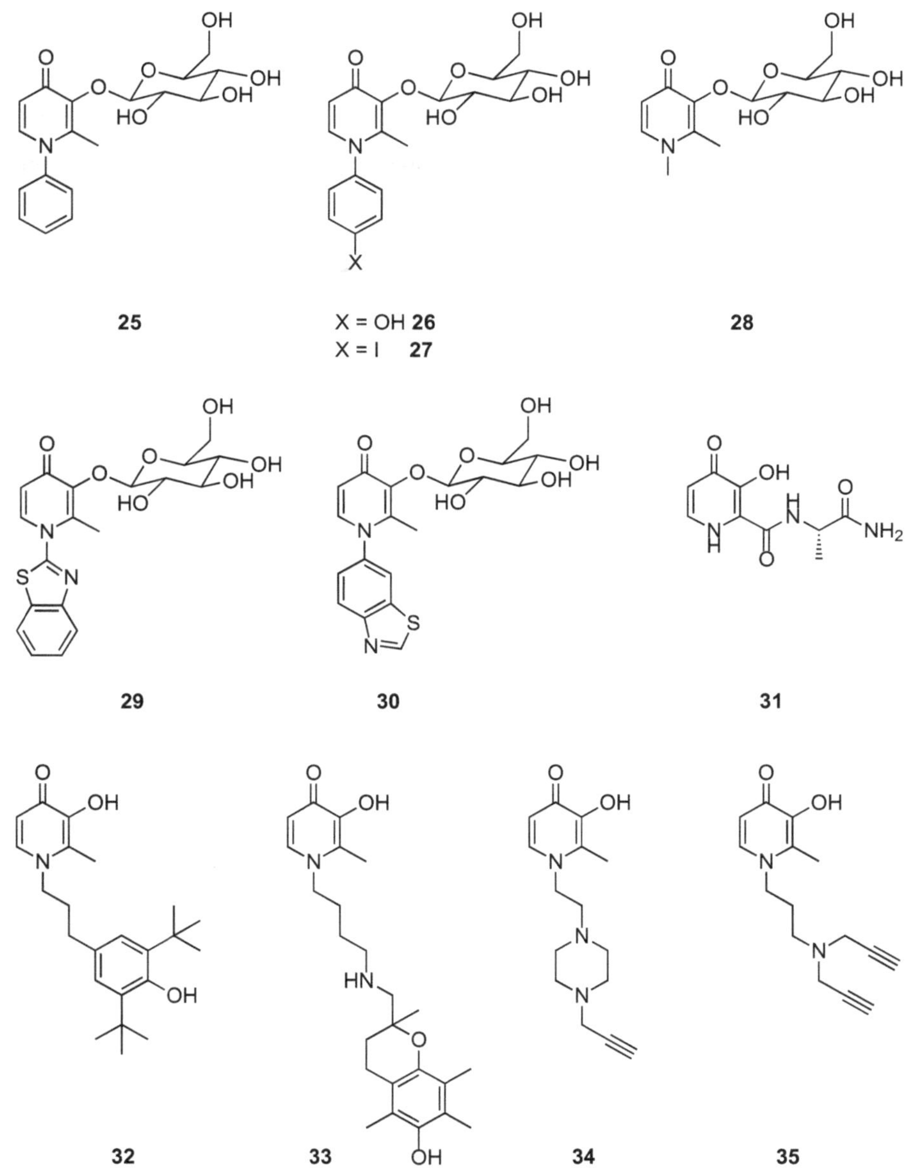

FIGURE 20.4 **Structures of multifunctional 3-hydroxypyridin-4-one derivatives studied against neurodegenerative diseases.**

Following the success of the bifunctional metal chelator/MAO-B inhibitor M30 **15** (Fig. 20.3), a similar bifunctional strategy was recently implemented with deferiprone **4**. Chelators **34** and **35** (Fig. 20.4) consist of deferiprone attached to one or more *N*-propargylamine moieties that are also found in M30 **15** and HLA-20 **16**, and are thus designed as dual action

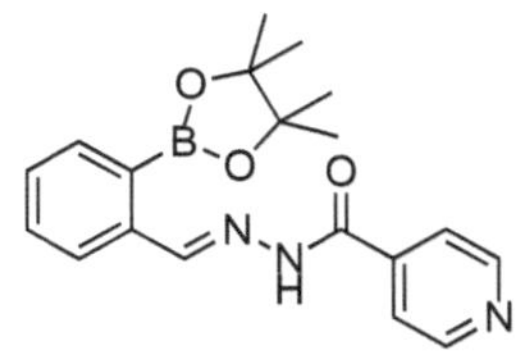

BSIH **36**

FIGURE 20.5 **Structure of a prochelator of salicylaldehyde isonicotinoyl hydrazone (SIH).**

metal chelators/MAO-B inhibitors. These compounds both displayed higher neuroprotective potencies than deferiprone **4** in models of both AD and PD in vitro, with **35** showing the most promising results.[66] Further studies are thus warranted on these promising molecules.

Boronic ester BSIH **36** (Fig. 20.5) is a prochelator of the tridentate iron chelator salicylaldehyde isonicotinoyl hydrazone **7** (Fig. 20.2) that is designed to unmask the chelator **7** in the presence of hydrogen peroxide.[67] This prochelator strategy is thus designed to take advantage of oxidative stress to release an active metal chelator in situ only in those brain regions where oxidative damage has occurred. Upon oxidation of **36** with hydrogen peroxide, chelator **7** will be released to chelate and passivate iron to prevent further oxidative damage. BSIH **36** protected retinal pigment epithelial cells from oxidative damage caused by hydrogen peroxide in vitro, and the use of **36** also avoided toxicity due to metal depletion (in contrast to desferrioxamine **1** or deferiprone **4**).[68]

Metal chelating agents that target amyloid fibrils have been proposed as promising potential treatments for AD. Following this strategy, the bifunctional chelator XH1 **37** (Fig. 20.6) was developed. This molecule consists of an EDTA-like metal chelator linked via two of its carboxylate groups to the amyloid-selective binding dye thioflavin-T. In studies on a model of AD in vitro, XH1 **37** significantly reduced Zn(II)-induced amyloid β deposition and the expression of amyloid precursor protein (APP), and in vivo studies in a transgenic mouse model also showed that **37** reduced amyloid β deposition in the mouse brain over a 4-week treatment period.[69]

Some multifunctional derivatives of the macrocyclic polyamines 1,4,7-triazacyclononane (tacn **9**, Fig. 20.2) and 1,4,7,10-tetraazacyclododecane (cyclen) have been studied as potential therapies for AD. These ligand backbones were selected due to the SOD activity of their Cu(II) and Zn(II) complexes. This enzyme catalyzes the breakdown of superoxide (O_2^-) and is

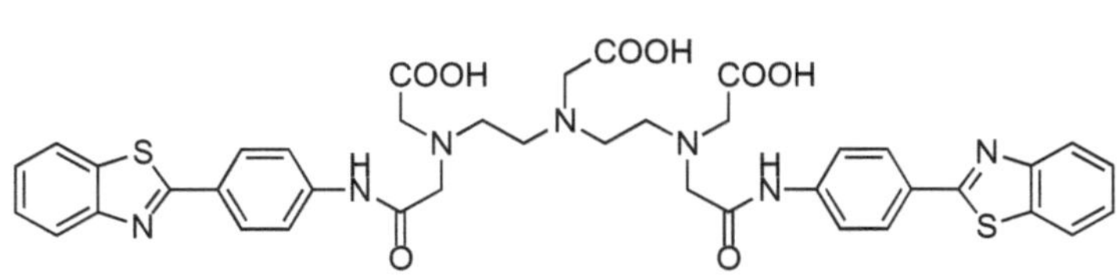

XH1 **37**

FIGURE 20.6 **Structure of a multifunctional EDTA derivative studied against neurodegenerative diseases.**

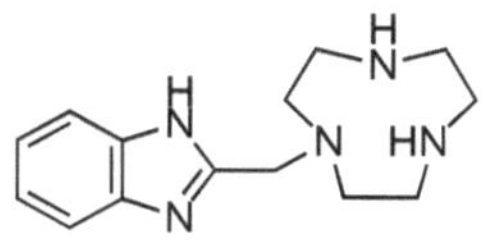

1-BYT **38**

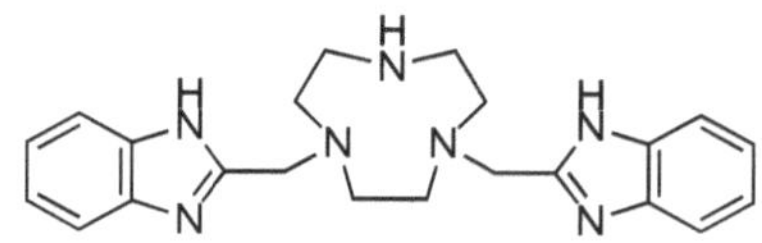

1,4-BYT **39**

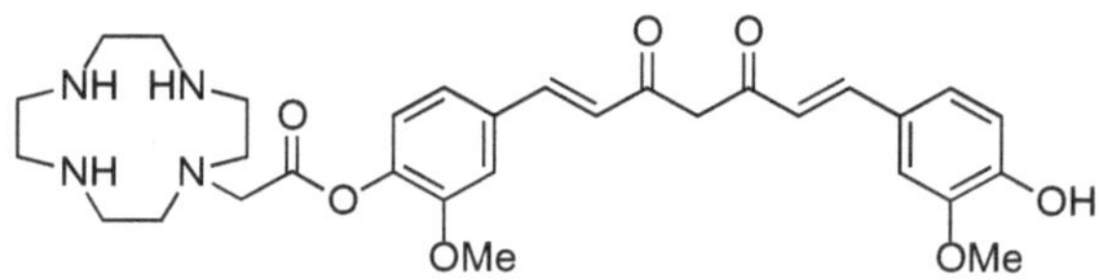

40

FIGURE 20.7 **Structures of multifunctional tacn and cyclen derivatives studied against neurodegenerative diseases.**

thus an important part of the cellular antioxidant defense. A computational study suggested 1-BYT **38** and 1,4-BYT **39** (Fig. 20.7), which both have additional benzimidazole metal binding groups, would show similar Cu(II) and Zn(II) chelating ability to clioquinol **2**.[70] Additionally, the Cu(II) complexes of **38** and especially **39** were predicted to have superior SOD activity to that of clioquinol **2**. These molecules therefore have two beneficial modes of action; metal chelation/passivation, and SOD activity. Bifunctional cyclen derivative **40** (Fig. 20.7) was inspired by a previous study on using Co(III)-cyclen complexes bound to amyloid recognition motifs for the proteolytic degradation of amyloid plaques. The idea was that the curcumin motif of **40** would direct the drug to amyloid deposits where the cyclen moiety would then chelate Cu(II) and form a complex that would hydrolyze the peptide bonds of the plaques. As predicted, **40** and other derivatives were able to bind Cu(II) and cleave amyloid oligomers in vitro, and protected the neurons from amyloid β-induced neurotoxicity.[71]

A number of glycosylated derivatives of the tetradentate ligand tetrahydrosalen have been developed. Two such examples are shown in Fig. 20.8. As mentioned previously, glycosylation of a parent ligand is designed to facilitate active transport of the ligand across the blood–brain barrier via the GLUT-1 transport protein. Ligand **41** (Fig. 20.8) is an active chelator with an additional masked hydroxyl group that can act as an antioxidant whereas ligand **42** is a prochelator that releases the active chelator upon enzymatic cleavage of glucose. Both compounds were able to efficiently chelate Cu(II) and Zn(II), disaggregate amyloid β oligomers, and act as antioxidants in vitro, while enzymatic cleavage of glucose from compound **42** by a bacterial β-glucosidase enzyme was also successfully demonstrated.[72,73] However, it is not yet known if these compounds are able to cross the blood–brain barrier.

Some dual-action metal chelators/ AChE inhibitors based on tacrine have been studied (Fig. 20.9). Tacrine was the first clinically approved AChE inhibitor for the treatment of AD, but its use was discontinued due to liver toxicity. Molecules **43–45** shown in Fig. 20.9 contain

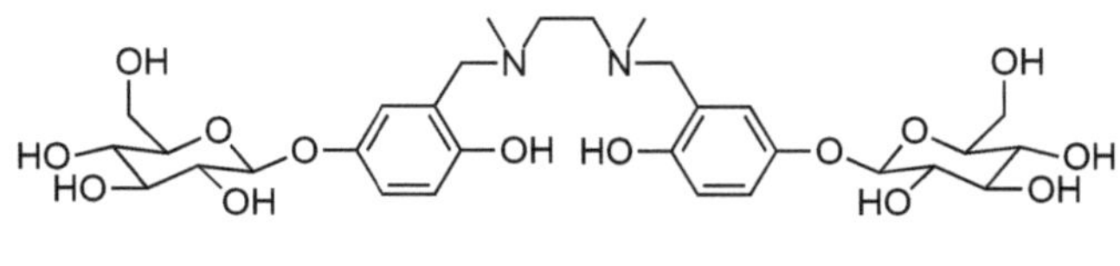

41

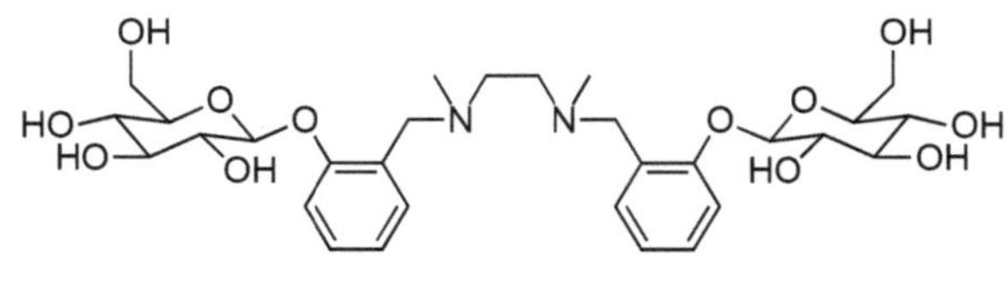

42

FIGURE 20.8 **Structures of multifunctional tetrahydrosalen derivatives studied against neurodegenerative diseases.**

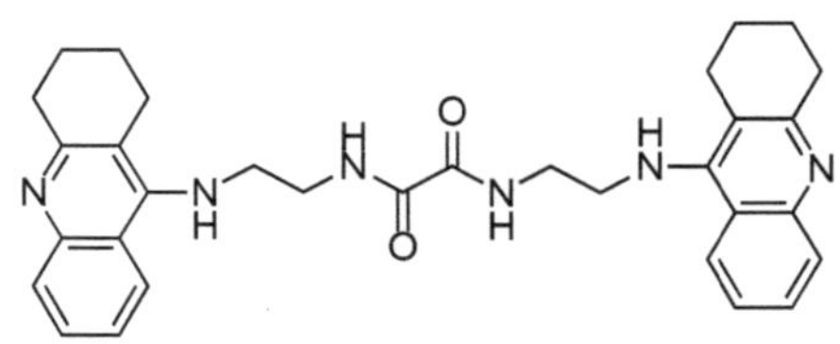

43

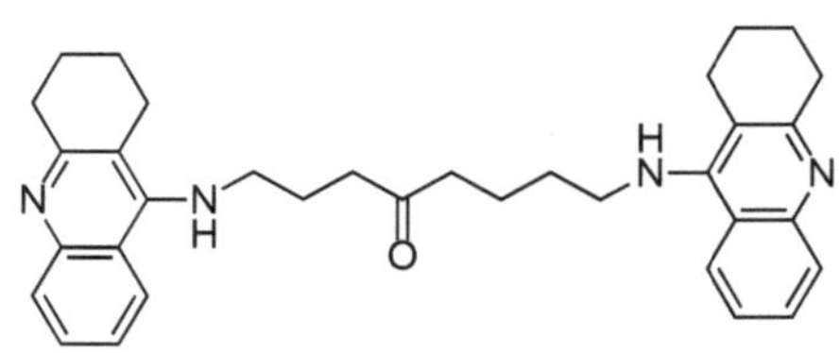

44

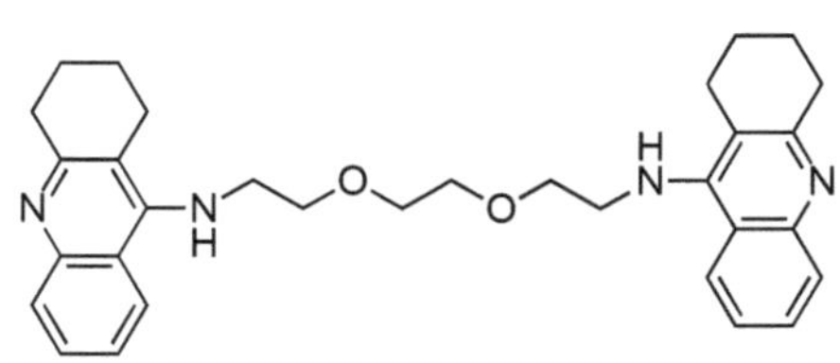

45

FIGURE 20.9 **Structures of multifunctional tacrine derivatives studied against neurodegenerative diseases.**

two tacrine moieties connected by a spacer containing one or more metal chelating O-donor atoms, and are based on a parent compound that contains a noncoordinating heptamethylene (C_7H_{14}) spacer. Molecules **43–45** retain the AChE inhibitory activity and reduction in

AChE-induced amyloid β aggregation of the parent compound and are also able to bind Fe(II) and Cu(II), albeit with low affinity for both metal ions.[74]

CONCLUSIONS

Since the advent of the "metal hypothesis" in neurodegenerative diseases, metal chelators have emerged as promising drug treatments for AD and PD due to their ability to restore metal ion homeostasis and passivate redox-active metals in neurons. More recently, multifunctional metal chelators have been proposed as superior treatments for these conditions, due to their ability to counteract multiple pathogenic disease pathways with more than one mode of action. The encouraging results obtained with some of these drugs both in animal studies and in human clinical trials bode well for the further development of these drugs as the first metal chelators to be used as disease-modifying drug treatments for these conditions.

References

1. Luengo-Fernandez R, Leal J, Gray A. Dementia 2010 The economic burden of dementia and associated research funding in the United Kingdom. A report produced by the Health Economics Research Centre, University of Oxford for the Alzheimer's Research Trust. www.alzheimersresearchuk.org/wp-content/uploads/2015/01/Dementia2010Full.pdf
2. Faller P, Hureau C. A bioinorganic view of Alzheimer's disease: when misplaced metal ions (re)direct the electrons to the wrong target. *Chem Eur J*. 2012;18:15910–15920.
3. Anderson CP, Shen M, Eisenstein RS, Leibold EA. Mammalian iron metabolism and its control by iron regulatory proteins. *Biochim Biophys Acta*. 2012;1823:1468–1483.
4. Zheng W, Monnot AD. Regulation of brain iron and copper homeostasis by brain barrier systems: implication in neurodegenerative diseases. *Pharmacol Ther*. 2012;133:177–188.
5. Ke Y, Qian ZM. Iron misregulation in the brain: a primary cause of neurodegenerative disorders. *Lancet Neurol*. 2003;2:246–253.
6. Kenche VB, Barnham KJ. Alzheimer's disease & metals: therapeutic opportunities. *Br J Pharmacol*. 2011;163:211–219.
7. Duce JA, Bush AI. Biological metals and Alzheimer's disease: implications for therapeutics and diagnostics. *Prog Neurobiol*. 2010;92:1–18.
8. Crouch PJ, Barnham KJ. Therapeutic redistribution of metal ions to treat Alzheimer's disease. *Acc Chem Res*. 2012;45:1604–1611.
9. Bush AI, Tanzi RE. Therapeutics for Alzheimer's disease based on the metal hypothesis. *Neurotherapeutics*. 2008;5:421–432.
10. Telpoukhovskaia MA, Orvig C. Werner coordination chemistry and neurodegeneration. *Chem Soc Rev*. 2013;42:1836–1846.
11. Crichton RR, Dexter DT, Ward RJ. Metal based neurodegenerative diseases–from molecular mechanisms to therapeutic strategies. *Coord Chem Rev*. 2008;252:1189–1199.
12. Ward RJ, Dexter DT, Crichton RR. Chelating agents for neurodegenerative diseases. *Curr Med Chem*. 2012;19:2760–2772.
13. Rodríguez- Rodríguez C, Telpoukhovskaia M, Orvig C. The art of building multifunctional metal-binding agents from basic molecular scaffolds for the potential application in neurodegenerative diseases. *Coord Chem Rev*. 2012;256:2308–2332.
14. Perez LR, Franz KJ. Minding metals: tailoring multifunctional chelating agents for neurodegenerative disease. *Dalton Trans*. 2010;39:2177–2187.

15. Cavalli A, Bolognesi ML, Minarini A, Rosini M, Tumiatti V, Recanatini M, Melchiorre C. Multi-target-directed ligands to combat neurodegenerative diseases. *J Med Chem*. 2008;51:347–372.
16. Geldenhuys WJ, Youdim MBH, Carroll RT, Van der Schyf CJ. The emergence of designed multiple ligands for neurodegenerative disorders. *Prog Neurobiol*. 2011;94:347–359.
17. Youdim MBH. Why do we need multifunctional neuroprotective and neurorestorative drugs for Parkinson's and Alzheimer's diseases as disease modifying agents. *Exp Neurobiol*. 2010;19:1–14.
18. Zheng H, Amit T, Bar-Am O, Fridkin M, Youdim MBH, Mandel SA. From anti-Parkinson's drug rasagiline to novel multitarget iron chelators with acetylcholinesterase and monoamine oxidase inhibitory and neuroprotective properties for Alzheimer's disease. *J Alzheimer's Dis*. 2012;30:1–16.
19. Youdim MBH, Kupershmidt L, Amit T, Weinreb O. Promises of novel multi-target neuroprotective and neurorestorative drugs for Parkinson's disease. *Parkinsonism Relat D*. 2014;20(S1):S132–S136.
20. Weinreb O, Amit T, Mandel S, Kupershmidt L, Youdim MBH. Neuroprotective multifunctional iron chelators: from redox-sensitive process to novel therapeutic opportunities. *Antioxid Redox Signal*. 2010;13:919–949.
21. Ben-Shachar D, Eshel G, Finberg JPM, Youdim MBH. The iron chelator desferrioxamine (desferal) retards 6-hydroxydopamine-induced degeneration of nigrostriatal dopamine neurons. *J Neurochem*. 1991;56:1441–1444.
22. Dexter DT, Statton SA, Whitmore C, Freinbichler W, Weinberger P, Tipton KF, Della Corte L, Ward RJ, Crichton RR. Clinically available iron chelators induce neuroprotection in the 6-OHDA model of Parkinson's disease after peripheral administration. *J Neural Trans (Vienna)*. 2011;118:223–231.
23. Bareggi SR, Cornelli U. Clioquinol: review of its mechanisms of action and clinical uses in neurodegenerative disorders. *CNS Neurosci Ther*. 2012;18:41–46.
24. Cherny RA, Atwood CS, Xilinas ME, Gray DN, Jones WD, McLean CA, Barnham KJ, Volitakis I, Fraser FW, Kim YS, Huang XD, Goldstein LE, Moir RD, Lim JT, Beyreuther K, Zheng H, Tanzi RE, Masters CL, Bush AI. Treatment with a copper-zinc chelator markedly and rapidly inhibits β-amyloid accumulation in Alzheimer's disease transgenic mice. *Neuron*. 2001;30:665–676.
25. Ritchie CW, Bush AI, Mackinnon A, Macfarlane S, Mastwyk M, MacGregor L, Kiers L, Cherny R, Li QX, Tammer A, Carrington D, Mavros C, Volitakis I, Xilinas M, Ames D, Davis S, Beyreuther K, Tanzi RE, Masters CL. Metal-protein attenuation with iodochlorhydroxyquin (clioquinol) targeting Aβ amyloid deposition and toxicity in Alzheimer disease: a pilot phase 2 clinical trial. *Arch Neurol*. 2003;60:1685–1691.
26. Adlard PA, Cherny RA, Finkelstein DI, Gautier E, Robb E, Cortes M, Volitakis I, Liu X, Smith JP, Pérez K, Laughton K, Li QX, Charman SA, Nicolazzo JA, Wilkins S, Deleva K, Lynch T, Kok G, Ritchie CW, Tanzi RE, Cappai R, Masters CL, Barnham KJ, Bush AI. Rapid restoration of cognition in Alzheimer's transgenic mice with 8-hydroxy quinoline analogs is associated with decreased interstitial Aβ. *Neuron*. 2008;59:43–55.
27. Crouch PJ, Savva MS, Hung LW, Donnelly PS, Mot AI, Parker SJ, Greenough MA, Volitakis I, Adlard PA, Cherny RA, Masters CL, Bush AI, Barnham KJ, White AR. The Alzheimer's therapeutic PBT2 promotes amyloid-β degradation and GSK3 phosphorylation via a metal chaperone activity. *J Neurochem*. 2011;119:220–230.
28. Lannfelt L, Blennow K, Zetterberg H, Batsman S, Ames D, Harrison J, Masters CL, Targum S, Bush AI, Murdoch R, Wilson J, Ritchie CW. Safety, efficacy, and biomarker findings of PBT2 in targeting Aβ as a modifying therapy for Alzheimer's disease: a phase IIa, double-blind, randomised, placebo-controlled trial. *Lancet Neurol*. 2008;7:779–786.
29. Faux NG, Ritchie CW, Gunn A, Rembach A, Tsatsanis A, Bedo J, Harrison J, Lannfelt L, Blennow K, Zetterberg H, Ingelsson M, Masters CL, Tanzi RE, Cummings JL, Herd CM, Bush AI. PBT2 rapidly improves cognition in Alzheimer's disease: additional phase II analyses. *J Alzheimer's Dis*. 2010;20:509–516.
30. Amélia Santos M, Marques SM, Chaves S. Hydroxypyridinones as "privileged" chelating structures for the design of medicinal drugs. *Coord Chem Rev*. 2012;256:240–259.
31. Amélia Santos M. Recent developments on 3-hydroxy-4-pyridinones with respect to their clinical applications mono and combined ligand approaches. *Coord Chem Rev*. 2008;252:1213–1224.
32. Liu ZD, Hider RC. Design of iron chelators with therapeutic application. *Coord Chem Rev*. 2002;232:151–171.
33. Liu ZD, Hider RC. Design of clinically useful iron(III)-selective chelators. *Med Res Rev*. 2002;22:26–64.
34. Hider RC, Zhou T. The design of orally active iron chelators. *Ann NY Acad Sci*. 2005;1054:141–154.
35. Hider RC, Roy S, Ma YM, Kong XL, Preston J. The potential application of iron chelators for the treatment of neurodegenerative diseases. *Metallomics*. 2011;3:239–249.
36. Zhou T, Ma Y, Kong X, Hider RC. Design of iron chelators with therapeutic application. *Dalton Trans*. 2012;41:6371–6389.
37. Timoshnikov VA, Kobzeva TV, Polyakov NE, Kontoghiorghes GJ. Inhibition of Fe^{2+}- and Fe^{3+}-induced hydroxyl radical production by the iron-chelating drug deferiprone. *Free Rad Biol Med*. 2015;78:118–122.

38. Chaves S, Canário S, Carrasco MP, Mira L, Santos MA. Hydroxy(thio)pyrone and hydroxy(thio)pyridinone iron chelators: physico-chemical properties and anti-oxidant activity. *J Inorg Biochem*. 2012;114:38–46.
39. Ward RJ, Dexter D, Florence A, Aouad F, Hider R, Jenner P, Crichton RR. Brain iron in the ferrocene-loaded rat: its chelation and influence on dopamine metabolism. *Biochem Pharmacol*. 1995;49:1821–1826.
40. Devos D, Moreau C, Devedjian JC, Kluza J, Petrault M, Laloux C, Jonneaux A, Ryckewaert G, Garçon G, Rouaix N, Duhamel A, Jissendi P, Dujardin K, Auger F, Ravasi L, Hopes L, Grolez G, Firdaus W, Sablonnière B, Strubi-Vuillaume I, Zahr N, Destée A, Corvol JC, Pöltl D, Leist M, Rose C, Defebvre L, Marchetti P, Cabantchik ZI, Bordet R. Targeting chelatable iron as a therapeutic modality in Parkinson's disease. *Antioxid Redox Signal*. 2014;21:195–210.
41. Workman DG, Tsatsanis A, Lewis FW, Boyle JP, Mousadoust M, Hettiarachchi NT, Hunter M, Peers CS, Tétard D, Duce JA. Protection from neurodegeneration in the 6-hydroxydopamine (6-OHDA) model of Parkinson's with novel 1-hydroxypyridin-2-one metal chelators. *Metallomics*. 2015;7:867–876.
42. Banerjee P, Sahoo A, Anand S, Bir A, Chakrabarti S. The oral iron chelator, deferasirox, reverses the age-dependent alterations in iron and amyloid-β homeostasis in rat brain: implications in the therapy of Alzheimer's disease. *J Alzheimer's Dis*. 2015;49:681–693.
43. Cherny RA, Legg JT, McLean CA, Fairlie DP, Huang X, Atwood CS, Beyreuther K, Tanzi RE, Masters CL, Bush AI. Aqueous dissolution of Alzheimer's disease Aβ amyloid deposits by biometal depletion. *J Biol Chem*. 1999;274:23223–23228.
44. Atwood CS, Perry G, Zeng H, Kato Y, Jones WD, Ling KQ, Huang XD, Moir RD, Wang DD, Sayre LM, Smith MA, Chen SG, Bush AI. Copper mediates dityrosine cross-linking of Alzheimer's amyloid-β. *Biochemistry*. 2004;43:560–568.
45. Grünblatt E, Mandel S, Gassen M, Youdim MBH. Potent neuroprotective and antioxidant activity of apomorphine in MPTP and 6-hydroxydopamine induced neurotoxicity. *J Neural Trans Suppl*. 1999;55:57–70.
46. Bisaglia M, Filograna R, Beltramini M, Bubacco L. Are dopamine derivatives implicated in the pathogenesis of Parkinson's disease?. *Ageing Res Rev*. 2014;13:107–114.
47. Segura-Aguilar J, Paris I, Muñoz P, Ferrari E, Zecca L, Zucca FA. Protective and toxic roles of dopamine in Parkinson's disease. *J Neurochem*. 2014;129:898–915.
48. Dickens MG, Franz KJ. A prochelator activated by hydrogen peroxide prevents metal-induced amyloid β aggregation. *ChemBioChem*. 2010;11:59–62.
49. Shachar DB, Kahana N, Kampel V, Warshawsky A, Youdim MBH. Neuroprotection by a novel brain permeable iron chelator, VK-28, against 6-hydroxydopamine lession in rats. *Neuropharmacol*. 2004;46:254–263.
50. Zheng H, Weiner LM, Bar-Am O, Epsztejn S, Cabantchik ZI, Warshawsky A, Youdim MBH, Fridkin M. Design, synthesis, and evaluation of novel bifunctional iron-chelators as potential agents for neuroprotection in Alzheimer's, Parkinson's, and other neurodegenerative diseases. *Bioorg Med Chem*. 2005;13:773–783.
51. Zheng H, Gal S, Weiner LM, Bar-Am O, Warshawsky A, Fridkin M, Youdim MBH. Novel multifunctional neuroprotective iron chelator-monoamine oxidase inhibitor drugs for neurodegenerative diseases: in vitro studies on antioxidant activity, prevention of lipid peroxide formation and monoamine oxidase inhibition. *J Neurochem*. 2005;95:68–78.
52. Gal S, Zheng H, Fridkin M, Youdim MBH. Novel multifunctional neuroprotective iron chelator-monoamine oxidase inhibitor drugs for neurodegenerative diseases. In vivo selective brain monoamine oxidase inhibition and prevention of MPTP-induced striatal dopamine depletion. *J Neurochem*. 2005;95:79–88.
53. Zheng H, Youdim MBH, Fridkin M. Site-activated chelators targeting acetylcholinesterase and monoamine oxidase for Alzheimer's therapy. *ACS Chem Biol*. 2010;5:603–610.
54. Zheng H, Fridkin M, Youdim MBH. From antioxidant chelators to site-activated multi-target chelators targeting hypoxia inducing factor, beta-amyloid, acetylcholinesterase and monoamine oxidase A/B. *Mini Rev Med Chem*. 2012;12:364–370.
55. Zheng H, Youdim MBH, Weiner LM, Fridkin M. Novel potential neuroprotective agents with both iron chelating and amino acid-based derivatives targeting central nervous system neurons. *Biochem Pharmacol*. 2005;70:1642–1652.
56. Youdim MBH, Fridkin M, Zheng H. Bifunctional drug derivatives of MAO-B inhibitor rasagiline and iron chelator VK-28 as a more effective approach to treatment of brain ageing and ageing neurodegenerative diseases. *Mech Ageing Dev*. 2005;126:317–326.
57. Mao X, Schimmer AD. The toxicology of clioquinol. *Toxicol Lett*. 2008;182:1–6.
58. Rodríguez-Rodríguez C, Sánchez de Groot N, Rimola A, Álvarez-Larena A, Lloveras V, Vidal-Gancedo J, Ventura S, Vendrell J, Sodupe M, González-Duarte P. Design, selection, and characterization of thioflavin-based intercalation compounds with metal chelating properties for application in Alzheimer's disease. *J Am Chem Soc*. 2009;131:1436–1451.

59. Schugar H, Green DE, Bowen ML, Scott LE, Storr T, Bohmerle K, Thomas F, Allen DD, Lockman PR, Merkel M, Patrick BO, Thompson KH, Orvig C. Combating Alzheimer's disease with multifunctional molecules designed for metal passivation. *Angew Chem Int Ed*. 2007;46:1716–1718.
60. Green DE, Bowen ML, Scott LE, Storr T, Merkel M, Böhmerle K, Thompson KH, Patrick BO, Schugar HJ, Orvig C. In vitro studies of 3-hydroxy-4-pyridinones and their glycosylated derivatives as potential agents for Alzheimer's disease. *Dalton Trans*. 2010;39:1604–1615.
61. Roy S, Preston JE, Hider RC, Ma YM. Glucosylated deferiprone and its brain uptake: implications for developing glucosylated hydroxypyridinone analogues intended to cross the blood–brain barrier. *J Med Chem*. 2010;53: 5886–5889.
62. Scott LE, Telpoukhovskaia M, Rodríguez-Rodríguez C, Merkel M, Bowen ML, Page BDG, Green DE, Storr T, Thomas F, Allen DD, Lockman PR, Patrick BO, Adam MJ, Orvig C. *N*-aryl-substituted 3-(β-D-glucopyranosyloxy)-2-methyl-4(1H)-pyridinones as agents for Alzheimer's therapy. *Chem Sci*. 2011;2:642–648.
63. Gaeta A, Molina-Holgado F, Kong XL, Salvage S, Fakih S, Francis PT, Williams RJ, Hider RC. Synthesis, physical–chemical characterisation and biological evaluation of novel 2-amido-3-hydroxypyridin-4(1H)-ones: Iron chelators with the potential for treating Alzheimer's disease. *Bioorg Med Chem*. 2011;19:1285–1297.
64. Bebbington D, Monck NJT, Gaur S, Palmer AM, Benwell K, Harvey V, Malcolm CS, Porter RHP. 3,5-Disubstituted-4-hydroxyphenyls linked to 3-hydroxy-2-methyl- 4(1H)-pyridinone: potent inhibitors of lipid peroxidation and cell toxicity. *J Med Chem*. 2000;43:2779–2782.
65. Bebbington D, Dawson CE, Gaur S, Spencer J. Prodrug and covalent linker strategies for the solubilization of dual-action antioxidants/iron chelators. *Bioorg Med Chem Lett*. 2002;12:3297–3300.
66. Arduino D, Silva D, Cardoso SM, Chaves S, Oliveira CR, Santos MA. New hydroxypyridinone iron-chelators as potential anti-neurodegenerative drugs. *Front Biosci*. 2008;13:6763–6774.
67. Charkoudian LK, Pham DM, Franz KJ. A pro-chelator triggered by hydrogen peroxide inhibits iron-promoted hydroxyl radical formation. *J Am Chem Soc*. 2006;128:12424–12425.
68. Charkoudian LK, Dentchev T, Lukinova N, Wolkow N, Dunaief JL, Franz KJ. Iron prochelator BSIH protects retinal pigment epithelial cells against cell death induced by hydrogen peroxide. *J Inorg Biochem*. 2008;102:2130–2135.
69. Dedeoglu A, Cormier K, Payton S, Tseitlin KA, Kremsky JN, Lai L, Li X, Moir RD, Tanzi RE, Bush AI, Kowall NW, Rogers JT, Huang X. Preliminary studies of a novel bifunctional metal chelator targeting Alzheimer's amyloidogenesis. *Exp Gerontol*. 2004;39:1641–1649.
70. Ji HF, Zhang HY. A new strategy to combat Alzheimer's disease. Combining radical-scavenging potential with metal-protein-attenuating ability in one molecule. *Bioorg Med Chem Lett*. 2005;15:21–24.
71. Wu W, Lei P, Liu Q, Hu J, Gunn AP, Chen M, Rui Y, Su X, Xie Z, Zhao Y, Bush AI, Li Y. Sequestration of copper from β-amyloid promotes selective lysis by cyclen-hybrid cleavage agents. *J Biol Chem*. 2008;283:31657–31664.
72. Storr T, Merkel M, Song-Zhao GX, Scott LE, Green DE, Bowen ML, Thompson KH, Patrick BO, Schugar H, Orvig C. Synthesis, characterization, and metal coordinating ability of multifunctional carbohydrate-containing compounds for Alzheimer's therapy. *J Am Chem Soc*. 2007;129:7453–7463.
73. Storr T, Scott LE, Bowen ML, Green DE, Thompson KH, Schugar HJ, Orvig C. Glycosylated tetrahydrosalens as multifunctional molecules for Alzheimer's therapy. *Dalton Trans*. 2009;:3034–3043.
74. Bolognesi ML, Cavalli A, Valgimigli L, Bartolini M, Rosini M, Andrisano V, Recanatini M, Melchiorre C. Multi-target-directed drug design strategy: from a dual binding site acetylcholinesterase inhibitor to a trifunctional compound against Alzheimer's disease. *J Med Chem*. 2007;50:6446–6449.

CHAPTER

21

Abnormal Function of Metalloproteins Underlies Most Neurodegenerative Diseases

Katja M. Kanninen, Anthony R. White***

*A.I. Virtanen Institute for Molecular Sciences, University of Eastern Finland, Kuopio, Finland
**QIMR Berghofer Medical Research Institute, Herston, QLD, Australia

OUTLINE

Biometals in Neurodegenerative Diseases. http://dx.doi.org/10.1016/B978-0-12-804562-6.00021-X

BACKGROUND

Neurodegenerative disease is a collective term covering a range of disorders that affect the brain, with the primary endpoint being loss of essential neuronal populations. These disorders include common diseases, such as Alzheimer's disease (AD) and Parkinson's disease (PD) and a range of less common disorders, such as frontotemporal dementia, motor neuron disease (MND), prion diseases, for example, Creutzfeldt–Jacob disease, lysosomal storage diseases, for example, Gaucher disease, and a group of diseases collectively known as "neurodegeneration with brain iron accumulation" (NBIA). The latter includes pantothenic kinase-associated neurodegeneration (PKAN), PLA2G6-associated neurodegeneration (PLAN), aceruloplasminemia (aCp), Kufor–Rakeb, and others.[1] While not being classically addressed as neurodegenerative diseases, additional neuropsychiatric conditions, such as autism spectrum disorders (ASDs) and schizophrenia are increasingly recognized to share a number of neuropathological characteristics with the conventional neurodegenerative diseases.[2]

As indicated, neurodegenerative diseases are characterized by loss of specific neuronal populations in the central nervous system (CNS). In each disease, the localization and pattern of loss is unique, for example, loss of hippocampal neurons in AD and loss of motor neurons in the spinal cord in MND,[3,4] although often there can be considerable overlap between different disorders, making definitive diagnosis difficult. Neuronal loss is rarely the only obvious pathological change in the CNS. Accompanying or preceding the loss of neurons is often accumulation of misfolded protein, for example, amyloid beta peptide and microtubule tau protein in AD, α-synuclein protein in PD, and prion protein in prion diseases.[5] In addition, activation of astrocytes and microglia, the brain's innate immune cell populations, is a common feature in neurodegeneration.[6,7] Other common changes include accumulation of oxidatively damaged proteins and lipids, epigenetic changes to DNA,[8,9] micro RNA abnormalities, demyelination, and changes to levels and/or localization of biological metals (biometals).

It is this last point (biometal abnormalities) that is perhaps the most overlooked and underappreciated event in neurodegeneration. Biometals include a range of metals that have important biological functions including iron (Fe), copper (Cu), and zinc (Zn) as major neurometals of importance. Each has a number of key roles in brain development and function, and these biometals show substantial changes in most forms of neurodegeneration. Changes to biometal levels and distribution alone does not prove their importance in driving neurodegenerative changes, as these may reflect secondary events caused by other changes, for example, protein aggregation; however, most neurodegenerative diseases are now known to be caused by, or involve major changes to, metalloproteins. These proteins have structural, enzymatic, transporter, transcription factor, and other key roles dependent on their interaction with biometals.[10] As this list of key metalloproteins underlying neurodegeneration continues to grow, the evidence is becoming overwhelming that neurodegenerative disorders are primarily metallopathies,[11] diseases cause by changes to metal homeostasis. This review will provide an overview of the metalloproteins that drive neurodegeneration, either directly or indirectly, with the hope that the biomedical field will start to view altered biometal stasis as a key neuropathological change and not simply "an inconvenient truth."

BIOMETALS

Biometals are essential cofactors in a range of biological functions in all cells, and have a number of specialized functions in the brain. Fe, in addition to its critical role in oxygen-carrying heme, is central to energy metabolism and DNA synthesis.[12] Fe is carefully coordinated due to its reactive state (transitioning readily between FeII and FeIII) and ability to generate reactive oxygen species (ROS) and reactive nitrogen species (RNS)[12] that damage lipids, proteins, and DNA. Proteins, such as transferrin and ferritin, as well as a range of other regulatory proteins carefully coordinate Fe levels.

Cu has essential roles in fundamental biochemical processes including mitochondrial energy production (cytochrome c oxidase), neurotransmitter synthesis (peptidylgycine α-amidating monooxygenase), melanin production (tyrosinase), antioxidant activity [Cu/Zn superoxide dismutase (SOD)], and antiinflammatory action (metallothionein).[13] Furthermore, Cu has been identified as a major regulator of synaptic activity[14] and has key roles in essential signaling processes.[13] As with Fe, Cu is highly redox active (CuI and CuII states predominate) and therefore can participate in generation of ROS and RNS if not carefully regulated. All cells, including neurons and glia have developed a highly complex and still largely unclear system of Cu transporters and chaperones to carefully shuttle and store Cu within the cell (Fig. 21.1). Cu largely enters cells via the copper transporter 1 (Ctr1), as CuI. It is then trafficked to various proteins for storage or utilization by several chaperones including copper chaperone to Cu/ZnSOD (CCS), cox17 to cytochrome c oxidase, Atox1 to Golgi and nucleus, or stored bound to metallothionein[13] (Fig. 21.1). Cu is loaded onto proteins by ATP7a in the Golgi and during excess Cu, the same protein traffics to the cell membrane and contributes to efflux of Cu (Fig. 21.1). Cu can also be loaded in vesicles at the synapse, most likely by ATP7a for release, where it controls the activity of NMDA-type glutamate receptors on the postsynaptic membrane.[13]

Zn is central to the action of a large number of structural, enzymatic, and transcription factor proteins. There are an estimated 3000 or more Zn proteins, and recently Zn has also become recognized as an essential second messenger taking its place alongside Ca^{2+}.[15] Zn has a critical structural role in zinc finger proteins that often act as transcription factors to drive gene transcription in nucleated cells.[16] Zn also has key modulatory roles in immunity, synaptic and eye function, bone development, and thyroid hormone production. An important role in neurotransmission is driven by Zn modulation of NMDA-type glutamate receptors by Zn released into the synapse. Although not as reactive as Cu and Fe, Zn must be carefully

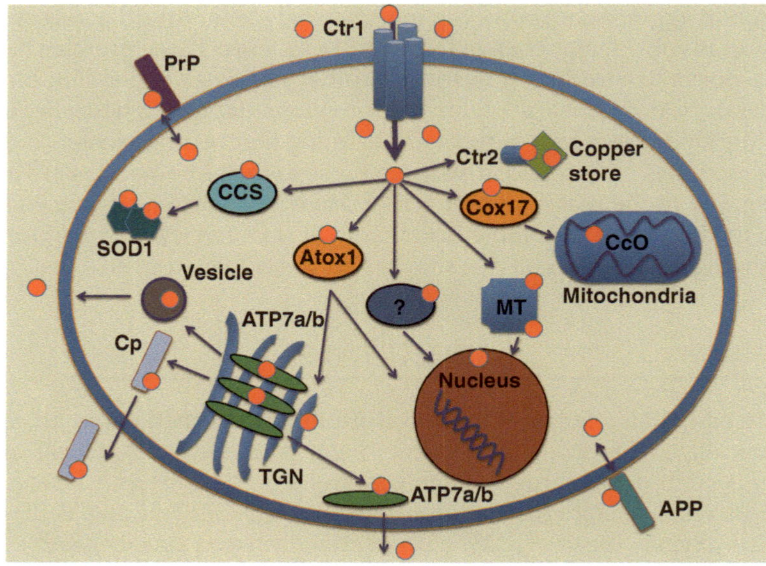

FIGURE 21.1 **Schematic representing cellular copper trafficking.** Copper enters the cell via the copper transporter 1 (*Ctr1*) and is directed to intracellular sites by copper chaperones. The copper chaperone for CCS transports copper to SOD1. Atox1 transports copper to the trans-Golgi network (*TGN*) where it is incorporated in proteins by ATP7a (or ATP7b in liver). Copper can also be transported into the nucleus by unknown chaperones or Atox1. Copper is transported to the mitochondria for incorporation into CcO by Cox17. Copper can also be sequestered by metallothionein (*MT*) or into intracellular stores by Ctr2. Export of copper from the cell is largely through secretion of copper-loaded proteins, such as Cp or via trafficking of ATP7a/b to the cell membrane. In neurons, copper is also released at the synapse in vesicles. Both prion protein (*PrP*) and amyloid precursor protein (*APP*) have additional, but as yet largely uncharacterized roles, in copper cycling between extra- and intracellular sites in neurons and potentially other cell types. *Source: Grubman A, White AR. Copper as a key regulator of cell signalling pathways.* Expert Rev Mol Med. *2014;16:e11. Published with permission from Cambridge University Press.*

regulated particularly due to its second messenger and kinase modulatory roles. Zn is stored by metallothionein or in vesicles. It is trafficked into cells and vesicles by Zn transporters (ZnT) and out of cells and vesicles by Zirt, Irt-like protein (Zip) transporters.[17]

ABNORMAL BIOMETAL LEVELS AND DISTRIBUTION UNDERLIE MOST FORMS OF NEURODEGENERATION

There is a large body of evidence supporting major changes to key biometal stasis in many neurodegenerative diseases[18] (Table 21.1). Unfortunately, much of the evidence is complex and often contradictory, which does not help the biomedical field engage in the importance of these biometals to the disease process. The main reasons for these issues are differences in postmortem time, animal models, tissue preparation, small numbers of tissue samples, lack of adequate control tissues, metal analysis techniques, and tissue regions

TABLE 21.1 Overview of Metallopathies and Associated Metal-Binding Proteins

Neurodegenerative diseases	Metal-associated protein	References
Neurodegenerative diseases caused by mutation in metalloproteins		
Wilson's disease	ATP7b	[24,25]
Menke's disease	ATP7a	[26]
Neurodegeneration with brain iron accumulation—neuroferritinopathy	Ferritin light (L)-chain	[27,28]
Neurodegeneration with brain iron accumulation—aceruloplasminemia	Ceruloplasmin	[29]
Neurodegeneration with brain iron accumulation—Kufor–Rakeb syndrome	ATP13a2/PARK9	[30]
Friedreich's ataxia	Frataxin	[31]
Motor neuron disease	Cu/Zn-superoxide dismutase	[32]
Alzheimer's disease	Amyloid precursor protein	[33]
Neurodegenerative diseases associated with abnormal metalloprotein function		
Autism	(ProSAP/Shank)	[34]
Schizophrenia	Dysbindin	[35]
CLN6 (variant late infantile) neuronal ceroid lipofuscinosis	Zip7	[22]
Parkinson's disease	α-Synuclein	[36]
Alzheimer's disease	Apolipoprotein E	[37]
Alzheimer's disease	Tau microtubule protein	[38]
Alzheimer's disease	Presenilin	[39]
Huntington's disease	Huntingtin	[40]
Motor neuron disease	TDP-43	[41]

examined. In addition, there will often be changes in many metals in the same tissues, which lead to the suspicion that we are simply observing a reaction to pathological tissue changes. While this may be true to some extent, our growing understanding of biometal stasis has revealed several important factors that support a critical contributory role for metal changes in neurodegeneration. Firstly, multiple metals are often changed in disease because they are intricately linked.[13,19] Metal handling pathways form a complex web in all cells (as shown for copper trafficking in Fig. 21.1). It is not surprising that a perturbation in one part of this network has major implications for the entire web. This is supported by our own research, which has shown that rectifying Zn homeostasis can restore altered Ca handling.[20] Second, studies are now showing substantial changes to biometal stasis as a very early event in the neurodegenerative disease process and not simply an end-stage change due to degenerating cells.[21–23] As discussed later in detail, the abnormalities seen in biometal stasis in neurodegeneration are likely to come from early changes caused by abnormal function of key metalloproteins.

ABNORMAL METALLOPROTEIN FUNCTION UNDERLYING NEURODEGENERATIVE DISEASES

As outlined earlier, there are many reports of altered biometals including Cu, Fe, and Zn in a range of neurodegenerative disorders, and many of these have been covered in other chapters. In this section, we will provide an insight into how abnormal expression, localization, and function of key metalloproteins drives a range of neurodegenerative diseases and examine what this means for those neurodegenerative diseases where the link to biometal abnormalities is less clear.

NEURODEGENERATIVE DISEASES CAUSED BY MUTATION IN METALLOPROTEINS

Wilson's Disease

Wilson's disease is an inherited disorder caused by mutation in the gene encoding for the Cu-transporting P-type ATPase, ATP7b.[24,25] Under basal Cu conditions, ATP7b is localized to the Golgi where it provides Cu for enzymes and proteins, including ceruloplasmin (Cp), which has a critical role in both Cu and Fe transport and storage in the body.[25] During excess Cu levels, ATP7b translocates to the cell membrane where it secretes excess Cu into the bile for removal.

More than 250 ATP7B gene mutations have been reported. Many of these are missense mutations. A common mutation H1069Q, occurs in nearly 40% of affected individuals with a Northern or Eastern European ancestry, while a third of Asians with Wilson's disease have an R778L mutation. These mutations generally affect protein structure, and subsequently its functional activity. Deletion and insertion mutations also occur and usually result in symptoms that are more severe than point mutations.[42,43]

The lack of ATP7b activity in the liver results in accumulation of Cu in liver and other organs, including the brain, due to failure of Cu excretion into the bile. Levels of Cu in the brain have been reported to reach 850% of normal levels.[25] Cu accumulation in Wilson's disease results in neurological and psychiatric symptoms. Symptoms include dysarthria, gait disturbance, *risus sardonicus*, dystonia, rigidity, tremor, and dysphagia. Less frequent manifestations include chorea and athetosis.[44]

ATP7b is also expressed in the brain, including choroid plexus, basal ganglia, cerebellum and cortex,[45] and its failure in Wilson's disease may lead to additional Cu-mediated neurological symptoms, possibly through abnormal astrocyte function. This may involve impairment of astrocyte production of Cp with associated consequences for Fe metabolism in the CNS.[25] Elevated Fe levels have been demonstrated in striatum, gray matter, white matter, and dentate nucleus (cerebellum) in postmortem Wilson's disease brain.[25] Additionally, failure of ATP7b in the choroid plexus may result in failure to eliminate excess Cu at the blood–CSF barrier. It remains uncertain whether the neurological symptoms observed in Wilson's disease are caused by Cu- or Fe-mediated oxidative damage or failure of metal-dependent enzyme activities (or both).

Menke's Disease

Menke's disease is a rare X-linked lethal inherited disorder caused by loss of Cu-transporting P-type ATPase, ATP7a activity. ATP7a has a similar function to ATP7b, however, the Cu-transporter is ubiquitously expressed (except liver).[26] ATP7a has an essential role in regulating dietary uptake of Cu in the intestinal epithelia.[26] In other organs, ATP7a resides in the Golgi providing Cu for cuproproteins and as with ATP7b, responds to elevated Cu by shuttling to the cell membrane to excrete excess Cu. Mutation in the ATP7A gene causes Menke's disease, with severe Cu deficiency in the brain, serum and liver, and Cu accumulation in duodenum, kidney, spleen, pancreas, and skeletal muscle. Abnormalities in Cu levels results in early childhood death if not diagnosed and treated.[26]

Menke's disease is caused by a large number of mutations in ATP7A including small deletions or insertions (22% of cases), nonsense mutations (18% of cases), splice junction mutations (18% of cases), large gene deletions (17% of cases), and missense mutations (17% of cases).[26]

Failure of intestinal Cu absorption leads to severe mental and developmental impairment due to loss of Cu-dependent enzyme activities in the brain.[45] In particular, impaired mitochondrial activity from loss of Cu-dependent cytochrome c oxidase function may have a major role in brain abnormalities in Menke's disease.[46] In addition, loss of activity of PAM results in impaired neurotransmitter synthesis (gastrin, cholecystokinin, vasoactive intestinal peptide, corticotrophin-releasing hormone, thyrotropin-releasing hormone, calcitonin, vasopressin, neuropeptide Y, and pituitary adenylyl cyclase-activating polypeptide) leading to severe developmental impairment in brain function together with seizures. Clinical neurological features include onset of seizures, diffuse atrophy, ventriculomegaly, tortuosity of cerebral blood vessels, and failure to thrive. Additional clinical features include connective tissue abnormalities, muscular hypotonia, and hypopigmentation of skin and hair.

Occipital horn syndrome (OHS) is a neurologically milder allelic variant of Menke's disease in which the neurological changes are milder (slight generalized muscle weakness and dysautonomia that includes syncope[26]). OHS is caused by exon skipping and a reduction in the level of correctly spliced ATP7A mRNA. The milder neurological phenotype of OHS likely reflects the fact that the mutant ATP7a is still able to traffic to the plasma membrane and secretes excess Cu.

Neurodegeneration With Brain Iron Accumulation

Modern brain imaging and genetics has led to the identification of a group of neurological disorders termed "neurodegeneration with brain iron accumulation" (NBIA). Collectively, these disorders share commonalities in extrapyramidal neurodegeneration and focal Fe accumulation, most often in the basal ganglia.[47] Symptoms include impairment in movement and cognition. NBIA includes a range of disorders with some caused by mutation in a well-recognized metalloprotein; neuroferritinopathy, aCp, and Kufor–Rakeb disease, and others caused by mutation in genes not previously recognized to be critical regulators of Fe homeostasis; pantothenate kinase-associated neurodegeneration (PKAN), phospholipase2, group VI-associated neurodegeneration (PLAN), mitochondrial membrane protein-associated neurodegeneration (MPAN), fatty acid hydroxylase-associated neurodegeneration (FAHN), and β-propeller protein-associated neurodegeneration (BPAN).[47,48] In the next section, we will initially discuss neuroferritinopathy and aCp and subsequently examine how mutations in diverse biochemical pathways also lead to abnormal Fe metabolism and impairment of brain function in the remaining disorders of NBIA.

NBIA—Neuroferritinopathy

Neuroferritinopathy (NBIA3)[27,28] is a rare monogenic autosomal-dominant (an exception in NBIA) neurodegenerative disorder caused by mutations in the ferritin light (L)-chain (FTL1) gene.

Ferritin is the ubiquitous, evolutionarily conserved Fe storage protein consisting of a near spherical shell with a cavity that can accommodate up to 4500 iron atoms.[49] The main role of ferritin is sequestration of free Fe to prevent formation of ROS.[50] Cytoplasmic ferritin is abundant in human cells,[49] but a mitochondrial form has also been identified.[51]

Disease onset in neuroferritinopathy normally occurs about age 40 and is characterized by chorea, dystonia, and mild cognitive decline. Cerebellar dysfunction can be seen in some cases. MRI reveals evidence of brain iron deposition on T2 MRI in globus pallidus, putamen, caudate nucleus, substantia nigra, and red nuclei.[52] Patients have low serum ferritin levels and severe neuronal loss in the basal ganglia, atrophy of cerebellum and cerebral cortex, abnormal iron accumulation, and the presence of ferritin inclusion bodies (IBs) in neurons and glia.[52] Additional extra-CNS pathology is also evident including ferritin IBs in hepatocytes, renal tubular epithelium, endothelial cells of capillaries, and skin fibroblasts.[52] Effective treatment still remains unknown.

The neuropathological features of neuroferritonopathy derive from ferritin and iron aggregates in neural tissue. In some cases, such as patients carrying the c.460dupA mutation,[27] granules, positive for Fe and ferritin staining are mainly extracellular but can also be colocalized in neurons, oligodendrocytes, and microglia. Alternatively, patients carrying c.442dupC and c.497_498dupTC mutations[53,54] reveal intracytoplasmic and intranuclear aggregates of ferritin in glial cells and in some neuronal subtypes, together with deposits of Fe, gliosis, and neuronal death.

Mutations in neuroferritinopathy are responsible for a frameshift at C-terminus of the L chain resulting in a partial or complete sequence change, although there is also one known case of a missense mutation (p.Ala69Thr). The mutations are thought to alter the L chain C-terminal region leading to a disorganization of the Fe channel, reduced stability of the ferritin complex, and formation of a wider and more permeable quaternary Fe channel. The resultant abnormalities in Fe storage are believed to induce Fe-mediated oxidative stress and neuronal degeneration.[52]

NBIA—Aceruloplasminemia

aCp is a neurodegenerative condition cause by mutations in the ceruloplasmin gene in an autosomal recessive manner.[29] In cases of aCp, neurological symptoms are caused by excessive Fe accumulation in affected brain regions (basal ganglia, nuclei, thalami, dentate nuclei, and cerebral and cerebellar cortices).[55] Other organs are also affected including liver and pancreas. Disease onset is usually around 50 years of age, and presents with classical extrapyramidal features, such as dystonia, dysarthria, chorea, and tremor, cognitive impairment, and often includes cerebellar ataxia.[56] Other presentations include retinal degeneration and diabetes mellitus. These changes coincide with undetectable serum Cp, low serum Cu and Fe together with increased serum ferritin (3–40 times normal).[57] T2-weighted brain MRI reveals hypointensity in the cerebral cortex, globus pallidus, putamen, caudate, thalamus, dentates, substantia nigra, and cerebellar cortex consistent with Fe deposition.[57]

Cp has a critical role in mobilizing Fe from tissues through its ferroxidase activity, a function that is dependent on Cu. Cp-bound Cu accounts for about 95% of all plasma Cu. Fe mobilization from intracellular stores is accompanied by ferroportin-dependent efflux. There are approximately 40 known mutations in Cp that cause aCp. The mutations alter the structural conformation of Cp leading to retention of Cp in the ER, abnormal Cu–Cp interactions, and impaired ferroxidase activity.[58] All these changes inhibit cellular (especially astrocyte) Fe export leading to Fe overload and toxicity. Autopsy studies reveal severe degeneration of the basal ganglia and dentate nucleus, together with substantial Fe deposits in both neuronal and glial cells.[59,60] In addition, Fe deposition is observed in glial cells but not neurons in the cerebral cortex. There is considerable evidence of elevated oxidative damage including lipid and protein oxidation, supporting a role for Fe-mediated oxidative stress in the neurodegeneration.

NBIA—Kufor–Rakeb and Neuronal Ceroid Lipofuscinosis (ATP13a2 Mediated)

Kufor–Rakeb syndrome (KRS) is a rare autosomal disorder caused by mutations in the gene for ATP13A2, which encodes a biometal (cation) transporter. It is also identified as a Parkinson's disease 9 (PARK9) gene. The disease is characterized by early-onset Parkinsonism, with pyramidal and extrapyramidal symptoms, altered eye movements, and dementia. Some cases reveal bilateral iron deposition in the basal ganglia by MRI, and are therefore included in the NBIA group.[61] Interestingly, different mutations in the same gene also cause a form of childhood neurodegeneration termed neuronal ceroid lipofuscinosis (NCL).[62]

ATP13A2 is a lysosomal type 5 P-type ATPase, a cation transporter, located in the late endosomes and lysosomes whose function is not well understood. Mutations lead to a truncation of the protein leading to accumulation in the ER and loss of function. The transporter has been reported to pump Zn and Mn ions across membranes in several organelles, however, recent studies reveal that ATP13A2 may have a specific role in autophagosomes and multivesicular bodies (MVBs).[30] ATP13A2 is closely associated with LC3, a marker of the autophagosomes. ATP13A2 is also localized to the outer limiting membrane of MVBs, a morphologically distinct late endosome compartment. MVBs can lead to the release of vesicles into the extracellular space as exosomes.[30] This process appears to be Zn mediated.

Analysis of ATP13A2 in patients' primary cells or knockdown of the protein in dopaminergic neuron cultures and in mouse models has demonstrated that impaired ATP13A2 function contributes to severe lysosomal and mitochondrial abnormities. These changes are also associated with decreased autophagosomal function.[63] It is believed that abnormal mitochondrial, lysosomal, and autophagic functions from mutant ATP13A2 are driven by altered Zn and/or Mn transport and/or homeostasis. Lysosomal Zn transport is impaired in patients' fibroblasts (Tsunemi, 2014) and this is associated with protein accumulation, increased ROS levels, ATP depletion, and mitochondrial dysfunction, leading to cell death. In addition, cells with ATP13A2 mutation are more susceptible to Mn-dependent toxicity.[64] It is uncertain how ATP12A2 handling of Zn and/or Mn is related to elevated Fe brain accumulation in some patients, but it may be related to the essential role the lysosome has in controlling cellular Fe homeostasis.

The previous discussion has considered the forms of NBIA that involve mutations in known metalloproteins [ferritin (Fe-storage protein), ceruloplasmin (ferroxidase), and ATP13a2 (biometal transporter)]. Other forms of NBIA involving proteins that affect biometal metabolism but without identified direct biometal modulation will be dealt with below.

NBIA—Other P-type ATPases in Neurological Disease

In addition to the neurological disorders associated with P1-type ATPases (ATP7a, Menke's disease and ATP7b, Wilson's disease) and P5-type ATPase (ATP13a2, Kufor–Rakeb disease, and NCL), P2-type ATPases are also linked to rare brain disease. Mutations in Na^+/K^+-ATPase underlies diseases, such as familial hemiplegic migraine type 2 (FHM2), alternating hemiplegia of childhood (AHC), and rapid-onset dystonia Parkinsonism (RDP).[65] The Na^+/K^+-ATPase is responsible for maintaining Na^+ and K^+ gradients across the cell membrane through exchange of Na^+ ions for K^+ ions, and is a critical process involved in control of cell volume and CNS function. In addition, mutations in ATP2B3, a Ca^{2+} pump maintaining cytosolic Ca^{2+} levels, are associated with early-onset X-linked spinocerebellar ataxia-1, a degenerative disease of the cerebellum.[66] It is not yet known what role these changes have, if any, on homeostasis of biometals, such as Fe, Cu or Zn.

Friedreich's Ataxia

Friedreich's ataxia (FRDA) is caused by a trinucleotide (GAA) repeat expansion in the first intron of the frataxin gene (FXN).[31] Most patients are homozygous for the expansion although in a small number of patients, one allele presents point mutations in the coding region. The repeat expansion results in inhibition of FXN expression by arrest of RNA polymerase II and heterochromatin-mediated gene silencing. This leads to diminished levels of the consequent protein, frataxin.[31,67]

The first symptoms of FRDA appear at puberty but onset of the disease can occur from infancy to after 60 years.[68] Symptoms of FRDA include progressive and unremitting ataxia,[69] including gait and limb ataxia, tendon areflexia, dysarthria, sensory loss, and pyramidal signs.[70] Additional disease features involve cardiomyopathy, skeletal and vision abnormalities, and diabetes.[70] FRDA involves neuropathological changes including degeneration of dorsal root ganglia, peripheral nerves, spinal cord, and the dentate nucleus in the cerebellum.[71] These are associated with axonal neuropathy with loss of large myelinated fibers.[72]

Frataxin is localized to the mitochondria of all cells and has an essential role in mitochondrial and cellular Fe homeostasis through a major role in iron–sulfur cluster biosynthesis, Fe sensing, and modulation of Fe redox actions.[73] High levels of frataxin are expressed in heart and CNS (major sites of pathological change in FRDA). During disease, large concentrations of Fe accumulate in mitochondria of affected cells. It is uncertain if these Fe aggregates directly participate in disease outcomes or whether the pathology is related to loss of Fe-related functions. Growing evidence indicates that microglial-mediated inflammatory responses in the affected areas of the CNS may be associated with altered Fe homeostasis and drive neurodegeneration in FRDA.

MND (SOD1)

MND is a group of disorders characterized by degeneration of upper and/or lower motor neurons in the CNS resulting in death, usually from respiratory failure. Amyotrophic lateral sclerosis (ALS), also known as Lou Gehrig's disease is the most common form and is associated with sporadic (sALS) or familial (fALS) forms. The latter comprise approximately 10% of all cases and caused by mutation in one of several causative genes including Cu/ZnSOD (SOD1), TDP-43, FUS, C9orf72, and several others.[74] While most cases of ALS are now thought to be associated with expansion of the nucleotide repeat region of C9orf72,[75] ALS brain and spinal cord commonly reveals neuropathological changes to TDP-43, an RNA-binding protein known to accumulate in the cytosol during disease.[76] The most common form of fALS is cause by mutation in SOD1, accounting for ~10% of fALS cases.[74] The mutations are autosomal dominant and approximately 150 mutations throughout the SOD1 gene have been identified. Much of our understanding of MND has come from animal models expressing mutant human SOD1.[74]

Motor neuron loss in ALS leads to muscle weakness and atrophy, fasciculations, spasticity and over time can include dysphagia and dysarthria.[74] In about 25% of cases, ALS can reveal brainstem symptoms (dysarthria, difficulty swallowing) followed by extremity weakness (progressive bulbar palsy). Neurons in the prefrontal and temporal cortex can also be affected in some patients associated with frontotemporal lobar degeneration, a disease closely related to ALS often with overlapping symptoms. The neuropathological changes in ALS include degeneration and loss of motor neurons in the anterior horns and motor nuclei of brain stem and also degeneration of upper motor neurons in the lateral corticospinal tracts. Neuronal degeneration is accompanied by presence of protein aggregates in remaining neurons and gliotic changes.[74]

While there are numerous reports of altered biometal homeostasis in ALS,[11,77] the main support is evidenced by the fact that mutations in SOD, a metalloantioxidant enzyme, are causative is a portion of fALS cases. SOD1 requires a single Cu and single Zn ion for antioxidant action.[32] Mutations in SOD1 most likely alter the interaction of these biometals with SOD1, leading to ROS production, possibly in a highly localized neuronal dysfunction. It is uncertain why motor neurons are preferentially affected, but may be due to the particularly high energy demands and oxygen consumption (and therefore ROS production) associated with the cell type. Studies with animal models have shown that loss of SOD1 activity alone is not sufficient to cause ALS, and therefore, the abnormal protein gains a toxic function through abnormal protein–metal association.[32]

Familial AD (APP)

AD is the most common form of adult-onset neurodegeneration, affecting ~36 million people worldwide. While the single most important factor in the disease is aging, AD is highly multifactorial with most cases being sporadic. A small number of cases are familial, involving mutation in the amyloid precursor protein (APP) gene, or in presenilin 1 or 2. Carriers of apolipoprotein E4 (ApoE4) have increased risk of disease over the general population. AD is primarily characterized by progressive cognitive failure (dementia) associated with hippocampal and cortical neuronal degeneration. The brain in AD patients normally reveals accumulation of extracellular amyloid plaques and intracellular neurofibrillary tangles (NFTs) comprised of hyperphosphorylated tau microtubule protein. Neurodegeneration is associated with neuroinflammatory changes including astrocytes and microglia.[78]

As would be expected for the most common form of neurodegeneration, AD has been the subject of many studies into the role of biometals. These studies have revealed accumulation of Cu, Zn, and Fe in amyloid deposits, concomitantly with loss of intracellular Cu in affected brain regions and in some cases Fe accumulation.[11] However, there still remains considerable debate on how accurate these studies are. Only a reduction in brain Cu levels has stood up to metaanalysis of reports on changes to brain biometals, reflecting the role of tissue preparation, analytical methods, and regions analyzed on outcome of measured biometal levels.[79] However, it has been clearly demonstrated that biometals do have a key role in the disease process. Both the full length precursor, APP, and the cleaved amyloid beta peptide (Aβ) fragment that accumulates in plaques are metalloproteins. APP is a large complex membrane protein with many observed cellular actions.[33] Cleavage of APP by secretase proteases results in formation of Aβ, which accumulates in the extracellular space. APP has N-terminal Cu (and Zn) binding domains, which likely has a key role in cellular Cu homeostasis and also regulation of Fe.[33] Altered APP function during ageing may be responsible for the loss of Cu in affected regions of the AD brain. In addition, Aβ itself also interacts directly with Cu, Zn, and Fe. The former two metals are known to potently drive aggregation of the peptide, leading to its accumulation into plaques. Neurotoxic accumulation of Aβ with consequent effects on tau metabolism is believed to underlie synaptic and subsequently neuronal degeneration in the AD brain. Whether this also involves biometal-mediated oxidative damage or additional biometal-driven changes is still uncertain.

NEURODEGENERATIVE DISEASES ASSOCIATED WITH ABNORMAL METALLOPROTEIN FUNCTION

Autism (ProSAP/Shank)

ASDs are lifelong developmental disabilities presenting from early life and affect human behaviors, such as social interaction, communication of feelings, imagination, and the relationships with others. ASDs include autistic disorder, Asperger syndrome, and several other developmental disabilities. They have multiple etiologies, including both genetic and environmental factors. Although ASDs are not classical neurodegenerative disorders, there is evidence of synaptic degeneration and there are important commonalities between ASDs and neurodegenerative diseases in relation to biometals. Significant changes to Zn and Cu have been reported in ASDs including serum Zn deficiency and elevated Cu in hair and nail samples in children with autism.[34,80] It is unknown how these changes relate to brain biometal stasis but recent studies have shown an important link between ASD-associated proteins and Zn/Cu.[34] In particular, the critical synaptic protein ProSAP2/Shank3 has been implicated in ASDs.[81,82] Mutations in ProSAP1/Shank2, ProSAP2/Shank3, and Shank1 have also been linked to autism.[83,84] The relationship to biometals exists through identification of a C-terminal Zn-binding domain in ProSAP/Shank proteins.[34] This domain has an important role in controlling synaptic localization of the ProSAP/Shank protein[85] and Zn binding controls the packing density of the proteins into macromolecular platforms.[86] ProSAP/Shank proteins also function as critical docking sites for a large number of interacting proteins in the postsynaptic density and therefore, may regulate the overall structure of the PSD.

Schizophrenia and Dysbindin

Schizophrenia is a neuropsychiatric disorder involving psychosis, apathy and social withdrawal, and cognitive impairment.[35] Due to a highly complex multifactorial disease process involving genetic and environmental influences, the causes of schizophrenia are still poorly understood. As with most forms of neurological disorder, studies have identified altered serum biometal levels in schizophrenia patients, although it has not been clear what this means to etiopathology. Recently, Gokhale et al. identified an important link between copper, dysbindin, and schizophrenia.[35] Dysbindin is encoded by the DTNBP1 gene, and polymorphisms have previously been linked to schizophrenia.[87] Dysbindin levels appear to be reduced in the brains of schizophrenia patients. Dysbindin is part of a larger protein complex (BLOC1), which is essential for regulating ATP7a localization. Alterations to dysbindin levels or function can lead to abnormal ATP7a activity and an increased susceptibility to Cu-mediated toxicity.[35]

CLN6 (Variant Late Infantile) Neuronal Ceroid Lipofuscinosis

The CLN6 form of NCL or Batten disease is mediated through mutation and loss of function of the CLN6 gene. CLN6 Batten disease is a form of lysosomal storage disorder and is characterized by accumulation of lipofuscin material in lysosome-derived fluorescent storage bodies[88] and progressive loss of neuronal function leading to loss of vision, motor dysfunction, and premature death.[88] As described earlier (Kufor–Rakeb) certain mutations in the gene of another biometal transporter (ATP13a2) results in a different form of Batten disease.[62] The function of the CLN6 gene product itself is unknown despite extensive studies. The protein is a multitransmembrane protein of the ER and mutations in CLN6 lead to loss of protein expression. Recently, we examined the affected brain regions of sheep that have a natural CLN6 mutation identical to that identified in some human patients.[22,89] The disease course in sheep is remarkably similar to humans in progression through different brain regions, neurological outcomes, and time frame. Our findings showed a striking loss of the Zn/Mn transporter Zip7 at very early stages of disease in affected brain regions.[19] The normal localization of Zip7 is the membrane of ER/Golgi, and we identified interaction between Zip7 and CLN6 protein in healthy cells. Subsequent studies revealed an important role for Zip7 in maintaining Zn and Ca homeostasis in neurons and this was altered in cells from CLN6 mice (harboring a natural CLN6 mutation). Together with ATP13a2, these studies are providing growing evidence for abnormal biometal regulation as a key factor in NCLs.

Parkinson's Disease and α-Synuclein

PD is the second most common neurodegenerative disorder in people over the age of 60. PD associates with clinical motor symptoms, rigidity, and bradykinesia, which result from progressive degeneration of dopaminergic neurons and loss of dopamine in the substantia nigra in the midbrain. Patients also present with a variety of nonmotor symptoms, such as cognitive decline, mood disorders, sleep disturbances, and difficulty in speaking.[90] Like with many other neurodegenerative diseases, the etiology of PD is largely unknown. The major pathological hallmark of both rare familial disease forms (less than 10% of cases) and sporadic PD is the accumulation of α-synuclein in intraneuronal Lewy bodies.[91] This cytosolic protein is abundantly expressed in the CNS and interestingly, while its physiological functions are not entirely understood, it has been shown to act as a cellular ferrireductase, using copper to reduce iron to its bioavailable form.[36] Overexpression of α-synuclein in dopaminergic neurons is sufficient to cause PD, thus demonstrating the importance of the protein in the disease pathogenesis.[92] Mutations in several other genes are also involved in the pathogenesis of PD (reviewed in[93]). These include autosomal-dominant mutations in ubiquitin-C-terminal hydrolase-L1 (UCH-L1) and leucine-rich repeat kinase (LRRK) 2[94] genes, and autosomal recessive mutations in Parkin,[95] PINK1,[96] DJ-1, and the ATP13A2[97] genes. As mentioned earlier, ATP13A2 mutations are also implicated in other diseases, including neuronal ceroid lipofuscinoses[62,98] and Kufor–Rakeb disease. Many of the proteins encoded by PD-associated genes function in diverse pathogenic pathways, such as altered autophagy, oxidative stress, and mitochondrial dysfunction, yet to date, a common pathway linking all the PD-related proteins has not been identified.

The involvement of biometals in PD stems from early epidemiological studies (reviewed in[99]) and postmortem analyses of PD patient brains.[100] Since then, the role of biometals in PD has attracted the interest of a growing number of researchers and the suggestion that dysregulation of intracellular metal homeostasis is a likely contributor to the disease pathogenesis has received significant support.[101] Out of the identified PD-related proteins, the interaction between α-synuclein and Fe and α-synuclein and Cu have received the most attention and will be discussed in the subsequent sections of this review.

While α-synuclein accumulation is considered by most to be an early event in the pathogenesis of PD, it has also been suggested that accumulation may occur secondary to other alterations, such as Fe mishandling. Various techniques have repeatedly demonstrated increased accumulation of Fe in specific brain areas of PD patients (reviewed in[102]) and perhaps even more importantly, Fe concentrations in the substantia nigra correlate with disease severity.[103,104] The fact that Fe accumulation occurs in patients with α-synuclein mutations, as well as in patients with mutations in the genes encoding LLRK2, parkin, PINK1 and DJ-1, as well as sporadic PD (summarized in[11]), suggests that Fe accumulation is a common feature in PD that is not necessarily related to α-synuclein alone. One of the main mechanisms through which Fe is proposed to mediate degeneration in PD is by increasing oxidative stress, and the other is through induction of a conformational change in α-synuclein that occurs during accumulation in Lewy bodies.[105] Fe is also enriched in Lewy bodies[106] The fact that the 5′ untranslated region of α-synuclein mRNA contains a predicted iron responsive element[107] suggests posttranscriptional regulation of α-synuclein protein production in response to Fe and provides further evidence for the importance of the Fe–α-synuclein interaction during

PD. Importantly, the finding that α-synuclein acts as a cellular ferrireductase implies that α-synuclein is a metalloprotein.[36]

Several studies support a link between brain Cu homeostasis, formation of complexes of Cu and α-synuclein, and PD. Although many studies have reported Cu alterations in CSF and blood of PD patients, a recent metaanalysis failed to demonstrate a difference between the Cu levels of PD patients and healthy controls.[108] Cu levels, however, are altered both in the degenerating PD brain[109] as well as in the surviving dopaminergic neurons of the substantia nigra.[110] As is the case with Fe, Cu in PD is related to increased oxidative stress, and α-synuclein aggregation that occurs during accumulation in Lewy bodies. It is becoming increasingly evident that that Cu binding enhances the aggregation of α-synuclein,[105,111] an interaction that leads to site-specific oxidation,[112] and cytotoxicity associated with neurodegeneration.[113] Cu may also have toxic effects independently of its α-synuclein aggregation-inducing activity, where Cu exposure and α-synuclein have a synergistic toxic effect on dopaminergic cells that is independent from α-synuclein aggregation.

AD and ApoE

Apolipoprotein E (ApoE) is expressed as three isoforms that differ by single amino acid substitutions. The APOE ε4 allele is the strongest risk factor for the development of late-onset AD[114,115] but the exact mode of ApoE function in AD remains unclear. The connection between ApoE and biometals in AD, especially Zn, has been the subject of intense research over the years, sparked by the finding that both ApoE and Zn are involved in the aggregation of Aβ and are found in amyloid plaques.[116] It is especially interesting that under physiological conditions the metal-induced aggregation of Aβ is highest for both Cu and Zn in the presence of the APOE ε4 allele when compared to the ε2 or ε3 alleles.[37] While some controversy exists over whether or not Zn levels are altered in the serum of AD patients,[117] the presence of the ApoE ε4 allele causes increased Zn concentrations in this subset of AD patients[118] thereby implying a connection between ApoE status and metal homeostasis.

It is known that the various ApoE isoforms interact with Zn and Cu via cysteine residues. As a consequence of an amino acid substitution for arginine (which is not a ligand for Zn),[119] the affinity of Zn is predicted to be lowest for the ApoE ε4 isoform. The ε2 and ε3 isoforms bind Zn with high affinity, which is suggested to be protective due to prevention of Zn binding to Aβ.[120] In contrast, due to the low affinity of Zn for the ApoE ε4 isoform it is more likely that Aβ readily interacts with surrounding metals and aggregates. In addition to binding to ApoE, Zn also affects the proteolytic stability of ApoE in an isoform-dependent manner, with the ε4 isoform being most susceptible for degradation. Therefore, mishandling of Zn in AD brains is suggested to affect ApoE ε4 degradation, leading to loss of functional full-length ApoE and increased fragments, which may be in part responsible for the higher risk of AD in ApoE ε4 carriers.[7]

Further evidence for the importance of the ApoE connection to Zn in AD comes from studies showing that Zn can modulate ApoE ε4-mediated phosphorylation of the tau protein, and that under ApoE deficiency the levels of synaptic Zn are reduced in parallel with reductions of the ZnT3 transporter.[120] Furthermore, increased dietary Zn impairs spatial memory in a mouse model of late-onset AD containing the ApoE ε4 allele.[121] Taken together, these studies suggest that ApoE, in addition to its well-described role in Aβ processing and clearance, may in fact be a metalloprotein that affects the cerebral pool of free Zn that contributes to multiple processes in AD pathology. These findings support an interaction between metals and ApoE that may be an important in the pathogenesis of AD.

AD and Tau

One of the defining features of AD pathology is the accumulation of abnormally phosphorylated tau protein in neurons. Tau is a microtubule-associated multifunctional protein that has well-described roles in stabilization and regulation of microtubule dynamics,[122] and in regulation of axonal transport of synaptic vesicles. Abnormal hyperphosphorylation of tau leads to its aggregation and accumulation in NFTs.[123,124]

It is known that tau codeposits in NFTs with several transition metals, including Cu[125] and Fe.[126] Several reports demonstrate that biometals bind to tau and influence its phosphorylation status and tendency to aggregate. For example, Cu has been shown to bind to tau,[38,127] enhance its phosphorylation,[128,129] and induce tau aggregation[130] at faster rates than in the absence of the metal.[38] Zn also induces tau hyperphosphorylation[131,132] and its direct binding to tau has been shown to modulate toxicity through two independent actions: phosphorylation and direct toxicity. Fe also interacts with hyperphosphorylated tau and increases the levels of tau phosphorylation at the typical AD-associated sites.[133,134] Interestingly, tau knockout mice develop parkinsonian symptoms caused by intracellular Fe accumulation that leads to dopaminergic cell degeneration.[135] Taken together, these reports provide evidence for the notion that tau is a metalloprotein, the function of which is affected by biometal status, as well as for the importance of biometals as key factors in tau regulation in AD.

AD and Presenilins

The presenilins function as the catalytic subunit of the γ-secretase protein complex. APP is cleaved by the γ-secretase complex at alternative sites to produce Aβ and the APP intracellular domain. Mutations in the *presenilin 1* (*PSEN1*) and *presenilin 2* (*PSEN2*) genes cause familial AD.[136]

There are relatively few studies describing the relationship between biometals and the presenilins. Deficiency of Cu and Zn has been demonstrated to occur in *PSEN1*-deficient mice, and mouse embryonic fibroblast cells derived from *PSEN1* and *PSEN2* knockout mice have reduced uptake of Cu and Zn.[39] Knockdown of *presenilin* in *Drosophila* is also associated with reduced Cu bioavailability.[137] These studies suggest that PS1 has a function in the cellular uptake of biometals. In addition, because Zn has been shown to modulate the synthesis of PS1,[138] it has been suggested that the high levels of Zn present in the amyloid plaques could enhance PS1 levels, thereby resulting in increased generation of Aβ. Recently, Fe was shown to increase the activity of the γ-secretase complex.[139] Although research on the metalloprotein role of the presenilins is sparse, the published reports support the idea that the presenilins have an important metalloprotein role in AD.

Finally, it should be noted that there are several important Aβ clearing enzymes, such as insulin degrading enzyme, neprilysin, and matrix metalloproteins, which are metalloproteins. Metals are also important for function of microglia that are essential for Aβ removal, providing additional links between metals and neurodegenerative processes.

NEURODEGENERATIVE DISEASES INVOLVING BIOMETAL CHANGES BUT WITHOUT A CLEARLY IDENTIFIED ROLE FOR METALLOPROTEIN ABNORMITIES

Huntington's Disease and Huntingtin

Huntington's disease (HD) is caused by dominant polyglutamine expansion within the N-terminus of the huntingtin protein, which leads to protein misfolding and intracellular aggregation in inclusions.[140] Degeneration occurs primarily in the cerebral cortex and striatum.[141] Clinically the disease is characterized by movement disturbances, cognitive dysfunction, and psychiatric symptoms.

Many studies report that biometal homeostasis is altered in HD. Biometals accumulate in the CNS of mouse models and human patients.[142] The huntingtin protein contains a domain that interacts with Cu and Fe and reduces them,[40] thus possibly contributing to oxidative stress. Toxic Fe accumulation appears to occur specifically in neurons. Cu has been shown to affect the fibrillation of huntingtin, thereby suggesting that HD could arise from a combinatory toxicity of Cu and polyglutamine.[143] The aggregation of wild-type huntingtin is promoted by Cu and inhibited by metal complexing compounds.[40] Furthermore, altering the levels of Cu has been reported to affect the aggregation and/or toxicity of an aggregation-prone N-terminal fragment of the huntingtin protein.[144] While it is clear that biometal changes occur and are an important feature of HD pathology, a precise metalloprotein role for huntingtin is yet to be discovered.

MND and TDP-43

As outlined earlier, mutations in SOD1 most likely alter the interaction of biometals with SOD1, leading to ROS production and neuronal dysfunction. Less is known about biometal changes and metalloprotein abnormalities in MND that is not caused by SOD1 mutations. However, a recent report by Dang et al. describes increased metal content in the TDP-43(A315T) transgenic mouse model of frontotemporal lobar degeneration and ALS.[41] While bulk metal levels in the brain were not affected by mutant TDP-43, Cu, Zn, and manganese concentrations were elevated in the spinal cords of A315T mutant mice. Further support for biometal association with TDP-43 comes from in vitro studies reporting that Zn is implicated in the aggregation of endogenous TDP-43[145] and that therapeutic targeting of biometal imbalance can prevent aberrant TDP-43 metabolism.[146] The mechanism through which TDP-43 alters metal levels remains to be determined, as does the exact metalloprotein function of TDP-43 in neurodegeneration.

NEURODEGENERATIVE DISEASES WHERE NO MAJOR ROLE FOR BIOMETALS OR METALLOPROTEINS HAS YET BEEN IDENTIFIED

In addition to the disorders discussed earlier in which a major role for biometals or metalloproteins has been demonstrated, a number of neurodegenerative diseases may be associated with metal imbalance, which is yet to be fully characterized. For example, it may well be that once metal changes are investigated in other recently described disease forms of MND (such as that caused by C9orf72 mutation), common metal homeostasis-related changes are discovered.

CONCLUSIONS

Biometal abnormalities are a central event in neurodegeneration that is often overlooked. It is now becoming more recognized that the majority of neurodegenerative disorders are caused by, or involve, changes to metalloproteins, which have critical, biometal-dependent functions in a wide variety of cellular processes.

In diseases where the contributing protein was discovered before its role in metallostasis was known, the latter fact is often ignored in favor of other protein actions (e.g., APP). Similarly, in cases where it is a known metalloprotein prior to its role in disease (e.g., Cu/ZnSOD in MND), the role of the metal is usually downplayed with the focus on nonmetal-related factors, such as protein aggregation. Even where its main function is to control metal stasis, the focus is frequently on the downstream effects, for example, ATP13a2 and its role in autophagy, rather than its primary role in ion stasis, which affects autophagy. Metal changes are usually seen as "peripheral" to the main neuropathology, not central. However, if oxidative stress and neuroinflammation are now seen as central components, metallostasis must also be included. It is hoped that in this review, we have presented a sound argument for why metalloprotein abnormalities are a central feature of many (most?) neurodegenerative diseases. Whether the disease is driven by mutations in known metalloproteins, such as SOD1 or ATP7a, or associated with changes to metalloprotein function (ApoE, tau, APP, etc.), many brain disorders involve metalloprotein changes and subsequent synaptic and neuronal dysfunction and death. It is highly plausible that for other forms of neurodegeneration, where no major metalloprotein function has yet been demonstrated, for example, TDP-43-associated MND, it may just be a matter of further investigation to demonstrate a critical role for these proteins in metal stasis. Continued understanding of these processes is essential if we are to develop new therapeutic approaches for neurodegeneration.

References

1. Schneider SA. Neurodegeneration with brain iron accumulation. *Curr Neurol Neurosci Rep*. 2016;16:9.
2. Chan AW, Kocerha J. The Path to microRNA therapeutics in psychiatric and neurodegenerative disorders. *Front Genet*. 2012;3:82.
3. Akhtar MW, Sanz-Blasco S, Dolatabadi N, Parker J, Chon K, Lee MS, Soussou W, McKercher SR, Ambasudhan R, Nakamura T, et al. Elevated glucose and oligomeric beta-amyloid disrupt synapses via a common pathway of aberrant protein S-nitrosylation. *Nat Commun*. 2016;7:10242.
4. Chen KS, Sakowski SA, Feldman EL. Intraspinal stem cell transplantation for amyotrophic lateral sclerosis. *Ann Neurol*. 2016;79:342–353.
5. Glabe CG. Common mechanisms of amyloid oligomer pathogenesis in degenerative disease. *Neurobiol Aging*. 2006;27:570–575.
6. Chung WS, Welsh CA, Barres BA, Stevens B. Do glia drive synaptic and cognitive impairment in disease? *Nat Neurosci*. 2015;18:1539–1545.
7. Xu H, Gupta VB, Martins IJ, Martins RN, Fowler CJ, Bush AI, Finkelstein DI, Adlard PA. Zinc affects the proteolytic stability of apolipoprotein E in an isoform-dependent way. *Neurobiol Dis*. 2015;81:38–48.

8. Dzamba D, Harantova L, Butenko O, Anderova M. Glial cells—the key elements of Alzheimer s disease. *Curr Alzheimer Res*. 2016;13:894–911.
9. Sanchez-Mut JV, Heyn H, Vidal E, Moran S, Sayols S, Delgado-Morales R, Schultz MD, Ansoleaga B, Garcia-Esparcia P, Pons-Espinal M, et al. Human DNA methylomes of neurodegenerative diseases show common epigenomic patterns. *Transl Psychiatry*. 2016;6:e718.
10. Zalups R, Koropatnick D. *Cellular and Molecular Biology of Metals*. New York, NY: CRC Press; 2010.
11. Barnham KJ, Bush AI. Biological metals and metal-targeting compounds in major neurodegenerative diseases. *Chem Soc Rev*. 2014;43:6727–6749.
12. Gozzelino R, Arosio P. Iron homeostasis in health and disease. *Int J Mol Sci*. 2016;17:130.
13. Grubman A, White AR. Copper as a key regulator of cell signalling pathways. *Expert Rev Mol Med*. 2014;16:e11.
14. D'Ambrosi N, Rossi L. Copper at synapse: release, binding and modulation of neurotransmission. *Neurochem Int*. 2015;90:36–45.
15. Bitanihirwe BK, Cunningham MG. Zinc: the brain's dark horse. *Synapse*. 2009;63:1029–1049.
16. Liu Y, Ma D, Ji C. Zinc fingers and homeoboxes family in human diseases. *Cancer Gene Ther*. 2015;22:223–226.
17. Prakash A, Bharti K, Majeed AB. Zinc: indications in brain disorders. *Fundam Clin Pharmacol*. 2015;29:131–149.
18. Aizenman E, Mastroberardino PG. Metals and neurodegeneration. *Neurobiol Dis*. 2015;81:1–3.
19. Grubman A, Pollari E, Duncan C, Caragounis A, Blom T, Volitakis I, Wong A, Cooper J, Crouch PJ, Koistinaho J, et al. Deregulation of biometal homeostasis: the missing link for neuronal ceroid lipofuscinoses? *Metallomics*. 2014;6:932–943.
20. Grubman A, James SA, James J, Duncan C, Volitakis I, Hickey JL, Crouch PJ, Donnelly PS, Kanninen KM, Liddell JR, et al. X-ray fluorescence imaging reveals subcellular biometal disturbances in a childhood neurodegenerative disorder. *Chem Sci*. 2014;5:2503–2516.
21. Rathnasamy G, Ling EA, Kaur C. Consequences of iron accumulation in microglia and its implications in neuropathological conditions. *CNS Neurol Disord Drug Targets*. 2013;12:785–798.
22. Grubman A, Lidgerwood GE, Duncan C, Bica L, Tan JL, Parker SJ, Caragounis A, Meyerowitz J, Volitakis I, Moujalled D, et al. Deregulation of subcellular biometal homeostasis through loss of the metal transporter, Zip7, in a childhood neurodegenerative disorder. *Acta Neuropathol Commun*. 2014;2:25.
23. Kumar KK, Lowe EWJ, Aboud AA, Neely MD, Redha R, Bauer JA, Odak M, Weaver CD, Meiler J, Aschner M, et al. Cellular manganese content is developmentally regulated in human dopaminergic neurons. *Sci Rep*. 2014;4:6801.
24. Bandmann O, Weiss KH, Kaler SG. Wilson's disease and other neurological copper disorders. *Lancet Neurol*. 2015;14:103–113.
25. Dusek P, Roos PM, Litwin T, Schneider SA, Flaten TP, Aaseth J. The neurotoxicity of iron, copper and manganese in Parkinson's and Wilson's diseases. *J Trace Elem Med Biol*. 2015;31:193–203.
26. Kaler SG. ATP7A-related copper transport diseases-emerging concepts and future trends. *Nat Rev Neurol*. 2011;7:15–29.
27. Curtis AR, Fey C, Morris CM, Bindoff LA, Ince PG, Chinnery PF, Coulthard A, Jackson MJ, Jackson AP, McHale DP, et al. Mutation in the gene encoding ferritin light polypeptide causes dominant adult-onset basal ganglia disease. *Nat Genet*. 2001;28:350–354.
28. Ohta E, Takiyama Y. MRI findings in neuroferritinopathy. *Neurol Res Int*. 2012;2012:197438.
29. Miyajima H, Nishimura Y, Mizoguchi K, Sakamoto M, Shimizu T, Honda N. Familial apoceruloplasmin deficiency associated with blepharospasm and retinal degeneration. *Neurology*. 1987;37:761–767.
30. Kong SM, Chan BK, Park JS, Hill KJ, Aitken JB, Cottle L, Farghaian H, Cole AR, Lay PA, Sue CM, et al. Parkinson's disease-linked human PARK9/ATP13A2 maintains zinc homeostasis and promotes α-Synuclein externalization via exosomes. *Hum Mol Genet*. 2014;23:2816–2833.
31. Campuzano V, Montermini L, Moltò MD, Pianese L, Cossée M, Cavalcanti F, Monros E, Rodius F, Duclos F, Monticelli A, et al. Friedreich's ataxia: autosomal recessive disease caused by an intronic GAA triplet repeat expansion. *Science*. 1996;271:1423–1427.
32. Hilton JB, White AR, Crouch PJ. Metal-deficient SOD1 in amyotrophic lateral sclerosis. *J Mol Med (Berl)*. 2015;93:481–487.
33. Bandyopadhyay S, Rogers JT. Alzheimer's disease therapeutics targeted to the control of amyloid precursor protein translation: maintenance of brain iron homeostasis. *Biochem Pharmacol*. 2014;88:486–494.
34. Bjorklund G. The role of zinc and copper in autism spectrum disorders. *Acta Neurobiol Exp (Wars)*. 2013;73:225–236.

35. Gokhale A, Vrailas-Mortimer A, Larimore J, Comstra HS, Zlatic SA, Werner E, Manvich DF, Iuvone PM, Weinshenker D, Faundez V. Neuronal copper homeostasis susceptibility by genetic defects in dysbindin, a schizophrenia susceptibility factor. *Hum Mol Genet*. 2015;24:5512–5523.
36. Davies P, Moualla D, Brown DR. Alpha-synuclein is a cellular ferrireductase. *PLoS One*. 2011;6:e15814.
37. Moir RD, Atwood CS, Romano DM, Laurans MH, Huang X, Bush AI, Smith JD, Tanzi RE. Differential effects of apolipoprotein E isoforms on metal-induced aggregation of A beta using physiological concentrations. *Biochemistry*. 1999;38:4595–4603.
38. Soragni A, Zambelli B, Mukrasch MD, Biernat J, Jeganathan S, Griesinger C, Ciurli S, Mandelkow E, Zweckstetter M. Structural characterization of binding of Cu(II) to tau protein. *Biochemistry*. 2008;47:10841–10851.
39. Greenough MA, Volitakis I, Li QX, Laughton K, Evin G, Ho M, Dalziel AH, Camakaris J, Bush AI. Presenilins promote the cellular uptake of copper and zinc and maintain copper chaperone of SOD1-dependent copper/zinc superoxide dismutase activity. *J Biol Chem*. 2011;286:9776–9786.
40. Fox JH, Kama JA, Lieberman G, Chopra R, Dorsey K, Chopra V, Volitakis I, Cherny RA, Bush AI, Hersch S. Mechanisms of copper ion mediated Huntington's disease progression. *PLoS One*. 2007;2:e334.
41. Dang TN, Lim NK, Grubman A, Li QX, Volitakis I, White AR, Crouch PJ. Increased metal content in the TDP-43(A315T) transgenic mouse model of frontotemporal lobar degeneration and amyotrophic lateral sclerosis. *Front Aging Neurosci*. 2014;6:15.
42. Lutsenko S. Modifying factors and phenotypic diversity in Wilson's disease. *Ann NY Acad Sci*. 2014;1315:56–63.
43. Wu F, Wang J, Pu C, Qiao L, Jiang C. Wilson's disease: a comprehensive review of the molecular mechanisms. *Int J Mol Sci*. 2015;16:6419–6431.
44. Ferenci P, Litwin T, Seniow J, Czlonkowska A. Encephalopathy in Wilson disease: copper toxicity or liver failure? *J Clin Exp Hepatol*. 2015;5:S88–S95.
45. La Fontaine S, Ackland ML, Mercer JF. Mammalian copper-transporting P-type ATPases, ATP7A and ATP7B: emerging roles. *Int J Biochem Cell Biol*. 2010;42:206–209.
46. Maehara M, Ogasawara N, Mizutani N, Watanabe K, Suzuki S. Cytochrome c oxidase deficiency in Menkes kinky hair disease. *Brain Dev*. 1983;5:533–540.
47. Poplawska-Domaszewicz K, Florczak-Wyspianska J, Kozubski W. Update on neurodegeneration with brain iron accumulation. *Neurol Neurochir Pol*. 2014;48:206–213.
48. Levi S, Finazzi D. Neurodegeneration with brain iron accumulation: update on pathogenic mechanisms. *Front Pharmacol*. 2014;5:99.
49. Arosio P, Levi S. Cytosolic and mitochondrial ferritins in the regulation of cellular iron homeostasis and oxidative damage. *Biochim Biophys Acta*. 2010;1800:783–792.
50. Graf E, Mahoney JR, Bryant RG, Eaton JW. Iron-catalyzed hydroxyl radical formation. Stringent requirement for free iron coordination site. *J Biol Chem*. 1984;259:3620–3624.
51. Levi S, Corsi B, Bosisio M, Invernizzi R, Volz A, Sanford D, Arosio P, Drysdale J. A human mitochondrial ferritin encoded by an intronless gene. *J Biol Chem*. 2001;276:24437–24440.
52. Levi S, Rovida E. Neuroferritinopathy: From ferritin structure modification to pathogenetic mechanism. *Neurobiol Dis*. 2015;81:134–143.
53. Vidal R, Ghetti B, Takao M, Brefel-Courbon C, Uro-Coste E, Glazier BS, Siani V, Benson MD, Calvas P, Miravalle L, et al. Intracellular ferritin accumulation in neural and extraneural tissue characterizes a neurodegenerative disease associated with a mutation in the ferritin light polypeptide gene. *J Neuropathol Exp Neurol*. 2004;63:363–380.
54. Mancuso M, Davidzon G, Kurlan RM, Tawil R, Bonilla E, Di Mauro S, Powers JM. Hereditary ferritinopathy: a novel mutation, its cellular pathology, and pathogenetic insights. *J Neuropathol Exp Neurol*. 2005;64:280–294.
55. Miyajima H, Takahashi Y, Kono S. Aceruloplasminemia, an inherited disorder of iron metabolism. *Biometals*. 2003;16:205–213.
56. McNeill A, Birchall D, Hayflick SJ, Gregory A, Schenk JF, Zimmerman EA, Shang H, Miyajima H, Chinnery PF. T2* and FSE MRI distinguishes four subtypes of neurodegeneration with brain iron accumulation. *Neurology*. 2008;70:1614–1619.
57. McNeill A, Pandolfo M, Kuhn J, Shang H, Miyajima H. The neurological presentation of ceruloplasmin gene mutations. *Eur Neurol*. 2008;60:200–205.
58. Hellman NE, Kono S, Miyajima H, Gitlin JD. Biochemical analysis of a missense mutation in aceruloplasminemia. *J Biol Chem*. 2002;277:1375–1380.

59. Morita H, Ikeda S, Yamamoto K, Morita S, Yoshida K, Nomoto S, Kato M, Yanagisawa N. Hereditary ceruloplasmin deficiency with hemosiderosis: a clinicopathological study of a Japanese family. *Ann Neurol.* 1995;37:646–656.
60. Yoshida K, Furihata K, Takeda S, Nakamura A, Yamamoto K, Morita H, Hiyamuta S, Ikeda S, Shimizu N, Yanagisawa N. A mutation in the ceruloplasmin gene is associated with systemic hemosiderosis in humans. *Nat Genet.* 1995;9:267–272.
61. Schneider SA, Paisan-Ruiz C, Quinn NP, Lees AJ, Houlden H, Hardy J, Bhatia KP. ATP13A2 mutations (PARK9) cause neurodegeneration with brain iron accumulation. *Mov Disord.* 2010;25:979–984.
62. Bras J, Verloes A, Schneider SA, Mole SE, Guerreiro RJ. Mutation of the parkinsonism gene ATP13A2 causes neuronal ceroid-lipofuscinosis. *Hum Mol Genet.* 2012;21:2646–2650.
63. Dehay B, Ramirez A, Martinez-Vicente M, Perier C, Canron MH, Doudnikoff E, Vital A, Vila M, Klein C, Bezard E. Loss of P-type ATPase ATP13A2/PARK9 function induces general lysosomal deficiency and leads to Parkinson disease neurodegeneration. *Proc Natl Acad Sci USA.* 2012;109:9611–9616.
64. Tan J, Zhang T, Jiang L, Chi J, Hu D, Pan Q, Wang D, Zhang Z. Regulation of intracellular manganese homeostasis by Kufor-Rakeb syndrome-associated ATP13A2 protein. *J Biol Chem.* 2011;286:29654–29662.
65. Retamales-Ortega R, Vio CP, Inestrosa NC. P2C-type ATPases and their regulation. *Mol Neurobiol.* 2016;53:1343–1354.
66. Zanni G, Calì T, Kalscheuer VM, Ottolini D, Barresi S, Lebrun N, Montecchi-Palazzi L, Hu H, Chelly J, Bertini E, et al. Mutation of plasma membrane Ca^{2+} ATPase isoform 3 in a family with X-linked congenital cerebellar ataxia impairs Ca^{2+} homeostasis. *Proc Natl Acad Sci USA.* 2012;109:14514–14519.
67. Gellera C, Castellotti B, Mariotti C, Mineri R, Seveso V, Didonato S, Taroni F. Frataxin gene point mutations in Italian Friedreich ataxia patients. *Neurogenetics.* 2007;8:289–299.
68. Santos R, Lefevre S, Sliwa D, Seguin A, Camadro JM, Lesuisse E. Friedreich ataxia: molecular mechanisms, redox considerations, and therapeutic opportunities. *Antioxid Redox Signal.* 2010;13:651–690.
69. Gomes CM, Santos R. Neurodegeneration in Friedreich's ataxia: from defective frataxin to oxidative stress. *Oxid Med Cell Longev.* 2013;2013:487534.
70. Harding AE. Friedreich's ataxia: a clinical and genetic study of 90 families with an analysis of early diagnostic criteria and intrafamilial clustering of clinical features. *Brain.* 1981;104:589–620.
71. Pandolfo M. Friedreich ataxia: the clinical picture. *J Neurol.* 2009;256(suppl 1):3–8.
72. Koeppen AH, Morral JA, Davis AN, Qian J, Petrocine SV, Knutson MD, Gibson WM, Cusack MJ, Li D. The dorsal root ganglion in Friedreich's ataxia. *Acta Neuropathol.* 2009;118:763–776.
73. Vaubel RA, Isaya G. Iron-sulfur cluster synthesis, iron homeostasis and oxidative stress in Friedreich ataxia. *Mol Cell Neurosci.* 2013;55:50–61.
74. Moujalled D, White AR. Advances in the development of disease-modifying treatments for amyotrophic lateral sclerosis. *CNS Drugs.* 2016;30:227–243.
75. Chew J, Gendron TF, Prudencio M, Sasaguri H, Zhang YJ, Castanedes-Casey M, Lee CW, Jansen-West K, Kurti A, Murray ME, et al. Neurodegeneration. C9ORF72 repeat expansions in mice cause TDP-43 pathology, neuronal loss, and behavioral deficits. *Science.* 2015;348:1151–1154.
76. Davidson Y, Robinson AC, Liu X, Wu D, Troakes C, Rollinson S, Masuda-Suzukake M, Suzuki G, Nonaka T, Shi J, et al. Neurodegeneration in frontotemporal lobar degeneration and motor neurone disease associated with expansions in C9orf72 is linked to TDP-43 pathology and not associated with aggregated forms of dipeptide repeat proteins. *Neuropathol Appl Neurobiol.* 2015;42:242–254.
77. Tokuda E, Watanabe S, Okawa E, Ono S. Regulation of intracellular copper by induction of endogenous metallothioneins improves the disease course in a mouse model of amyotrophic lateral sclerosis. *Neurotherapeutics.* 2015;12:461–476.
78. Ransohoff RM. How neuroinflammation contributes to neurodegeneration. *Science.* 2016;353:777–783.
79. Schrag M, Mueller C, Oyoyo U, Smith MA, Kirsch WM. Iron, zinc and copper in the Alzheimer's disease brain: a quantitative meta-analysis. Some insight on the influence of citation bias on scientific opinion. *Prog Neurobiol.* 2011;94:296–306.
80. Vela G, Stark P, Socha M, Sauer AK, Hagmeyer S, Grabrucker AM. Zinc in gut-brain interaction in autism and neurological disorders. *Neural Plast.* 2015;2015:972791.
81. Bonaglia MC, Giorda R, Borgatti R, Felisari G, Gagliardi C, Selicorni A, Zuffardi O. Disruption of the ProSAP2 gene in a t(12;22)(q24.1;q13.3) is associated with the 22q13.3 deletion syndrome. *Am J Hum Genet.* 2001;69:261–268.

82. Phelan MC, Rogers RC, Saul RA, Stapleton GA, Sweet K, McDermid H, Shaw SR, Claytor J, Willis J, Kelly DP. 22q13 deletion syndrome. *Am J Med Genet*. 2001;101:91–99.
83. Durand CM, Betancur C, Boeckers TM, Bockmann J, Chaste P, Fauchereau F, Nygren G, Rastam M, Gillberg IC, Anckarsäter H, et al. Mutations in the gene encoding the synaptic scaffolding protein SHANK3 are associated with autism spectrum disorders. *Nat Genet*. 2007;39:25–27.
84. Sato D, Lionel AC, Leblond CS, Prasad A, Pinto D, Walker S, O'Connor I, Russell C, Drmic IE, Hamdan FF, et al. SHANK1 deletions in males with autism spectrum disorder. *Am J Hum Genet*. 2012;90:879–887.
85. Boeckers TM, Liedtke T, Spilker C, Dresbach T, Bockmann J, Kreutz MR, Gundelfinger ED. C-terminal synaptic targeting elements for postsynaptic density proteins ProSAP1/Shank2 and ProSAP2/Shank3. *J Neurochem*. 2005;92:519–524.
86. Qiao F, Bowie JU. The many faces of SAM. *Sci STKE*. 2005;2005:re7.
87. Gornick MC, Addington AM, Sporn A, Gogtay N, Greenstein D, Lenane M, Gochman P, Ordonez A, Balkissoon R, Vakkalanka R, et al. Dysbindin (DTNBP1, 6p22.3) is associated with childhood-onset psychosis and endophenotypes measured by the Premorbid Adjustment Scale (PAS). *J Autism Dev Disord*. 2005;35:831–838.
88. Cárcel-Trullols J, Kovács AD, Pearce DA. Cell biology of the NCL proteins: what they do and don't do. *Biochim Biophys Acta*. 2015;1852:2242–2255.
89. McAllum EJ, Roberts BR, Hickey JL, Dang TN, Grubman A, Donnelly PS, Liddell JR, White AR, Crouch PJ. Zn II(atsm) is protective in amyotrophic lateral sclerosis model mice via a copper delivery mechanism. *Neurobiol Dis*. 2015;81:20–24.
90. Sung VW, Nicholas AP. Nonmotor symptoms in Parkinson's disease: expanding the view of Parkinson's disease beyond a pure motor, pure dopaminergic problem. *Neurol Clin*. 2013;31:S1–S16.
91. Spillantini MG, Schmidt ML, Lee VM, Trojanowski JQ, Jakes R, Goedert M. Alpha-synuclein in Lewy bodies. *Nature*. 1997;388:839–840.
92. Decressac M, Mattsson B, Lundblad M, Weikop P, Björklund A. Progressive neurodegenerative and behavioural changes induced by AAV-mediated overexpression of α-synuclein in midbrain dopamine neurons. *Neurobiol Dis*. 2012;45:939–953.
93. Houlden H, Singleton AB. The genetics and neuropathology of Parkinson's disease. *Acta Neuropathol*. 2012;124:325–338.
94. Zimprich A, Biskup S, Leitner P, Lichtner P, Farrer M, Lincoln S, Kachergus J, Hulihan M, Uitti RJ, Calne DB, et al. Mutations in LRRK2 cause autosomal-dominant parkinsonism with pleomorphic pathology. *Neuron*. 2004;44:601–607.
95. Kitada T, Asakawa S, Hattori N, Matsumine H, Yamamura Y, Minoshima S, Yokochi M, Mizuno Y, Shimizu N. Mutations in the parkin gene cause autosomal recessive juvenile parkinsonism. *Nature*. 1998;392:605–608.
96. Valente EM, Abou-Sleiman PM, Caputo V, Muqit MM, Harvey K, Gispert S, Ali Z, Del Turco D, Bentivoglio AR, Healy DG, et al. Hereditary early-onset Parkinson's disease caused by mutations in PINK1. *Science*. 2004;304:1158–1160.
97. Ramirez A, Heimbach A, Gründemann J, Stiller B, Hampshire D, Cid LP, Goebel I, Mubaidin AF, Wriekat AL, Roeper J, et al. Hereditary parkinsonism with dementia is caused by mutations in ATP13A2, encoding a lysosomal type 5 P-type ATPase. *Nat Genet*. 2006;38:1184–1191.
98. Farias FH, Zeng R, Johnson GS, Wininger FA, Taylor JF, Schnabel RD, McKay SD, Sanders DN, Lohi H, Seppälä EH, et al. A truncating mutation in ATP13A2 is responsible for adult-onset neuronal ceroid lipofuscinosis in Tibetan terriers. *Neurobiol Dis*. 2011;42:468–474.
99. Santner A, Uversky VN. Metalloproteomics and metal toxicology of α-synuclein. *Metallomics*. 2010;2:378–392.
100. Gerlach M, Ben-Shachar D, Riederer P, Youdim MB. Altered brain metabolism of iron as a cause of neurodegenerative diseases. *J Neurochem*. 1994;63:793–807.
101. Ayton S, Lei P, Bush AI. Metallostasis in Alzheimer's disease. *Free Radic Biol Med*. 2013;62:76–89.
102. Ayton S, Lei P. Nigral iron elevation is an invariable feature of Parkinson's disease and is a sufficient cause of neurodegeneration. *Biomed Res Int*. 2014;2014:581256.
103. Martin WR, Wieler M. Subthalamic nucleus stimulation in Parkinson disease: exciting or depressing. *Neurology*. 2008;71:704–705.
104. Pyatigorskaya N, Sharman M, Corvol JC, Valabregue R, Yahia-Cherif L, Poupon F, Cormier-Dequaire F, Siebner H, Klebe S, Vidailhet M, et al. High nigral iron deposition in LRRK2 and Parkin mutation carriers using R2* relaxometry. *Mov Disord*. 2015;30:1077–1084.

105. Uversky VN, Lee HJ, Li J, Fink AL, Lee SJ. Stabilization of partially folded conformation during alpha-synuclein oligomerization in both purified and cytosolic preparations. *J Biol Chem*. 2001;276:43495–43498.
106. Castellani RJ, Siedlak SL, Perry G, Smith MA. Sequestration of iron by Lewy bodies in Parkinson's disease. *Acta Neuropathol*. 2000;100:111–114.
107. Friedlich AL, Tanzi RE, Rogers JT. The 5'-untranslated region of Parkinson's disease alpha-synuclein messenger RNA contains a predicted iron responsive element. *Mol Psychiatry*. 2007;12:222–223.
108. Mariani S, Ventriglia M, Simonelli I, Donno S, Bucossi S, Vernieri F, Melgari JM, Pasqualetti P, Rossini PM, Squitti R. Fe and Cu do not differ in Parkinson's disease: a replication study plus meta-analysis. *Neurobiol Aging*. 2013;34:632–633.
109. Dexter DT, Wells FR, Lees AJ, Agid F, Agid Y, Jenner P, Marsden CD. Increased nigral iron content and alterations in other metal ions occurring in brain in Parkinson's disease. *J Neurochem*. 1989;52:1830–1836.
110. Davies KM, Bohic S, Carmona A, Ortega R, Cottam V, Hare DJ, Finberg JP, Reyes S, Halliday GM, Mercer JF, et al. Copper pathology in vulnerable brain regions in Parkinson's disease. *Neurobiol Aging*. 2014;35:858–866.
111. Tavassoly O, Nokhrin S, Dmitriev OY, Lee JS. Cu(II) and dopamine bind to α-synuclein and cause large conformational changes. *FEBS J*. 2014;281:2738–2753.
112. Miotto MC, Rodriguez EE, Valiente-Gabioud AA, Torres-Monserrat V, Binolfi A, Quintanar L, Zweckstetter M, Griesinger C, Fernández CO. Site-specific copper-catalyzed oxidation of α-synuclein: tightening the link between metal binding and protein oxidative damage in Parkinson's disease. *Inorg Chem*. 2014;53:4350–4358.
113. Wright JA, Wang X, Brown DR. Unique copper-induced oligomers mediate alpha-synuclein toxicity. *FASEB J*. 2009;23:2384–2393.
114. Corder EH, Saunders AM, Strittmatter WJ, Schmechel DE, Gaskell PC, Small GW, Roses AD, Haines JL, Pericak-Vance MA. Gene dose of apolipoprotein E type 4 allele and the risk of Alzheimer's disease in late onset families. *Science*. 1993;261:921–923.
115. Saunders AM, Schmader K, Breitner JC, Benson MD, Brown WT, Goldfarb L, Goldgaber D, Manwaring MG, Szymanski MH, McCown N. Apolipoprotein E epsilon 4 allele distributions in late-onset Alzheimer's disease and in other amyloid-forming diseases. *Lancet*. 1993;342:710–711.
116. Tanzi RE, Bertram L. New frontiers in Alzheimer's disease genetics. *Neuron*. 2001;32:181–184.
117. Rembach A, Hare DJ, Doecke JD, Burnham SC, Volitakis I, Fowler CJ, Cherny RA, McLean C, Grimm R, Martins R, et al. Decreased serum zinc is an effect of ageing and not Alzheimer's disease. *Metallomics*. 2014;6:1216–1219.
118. González C, Martín T, Cacho J, Breñas MT, Arroyo T, García-Berrocal B, Navajo JA, González-Buitrago JM. Serum zinc, copper, insulin and lipids in Alzheimer's disease epsilon 4 apolipoprotein E allele carriers. *Eur J Clin Invest*. 1999;29:637–642.
119. Karlin S, Zhu ZY. Classification of mononuclear zinc metal sites in protein structures. *Proc Natl Acad Sci USA*. 1997;94:14231–14236.
120. Lee JY, Cho E, Kim TY, Kim DK, Palmiter RD, Volitakis I, Kim JS, Bush AI, Koh JY. Apolipoprotein E ablation decreases synaptic vesicular zinc in the brain. *Biometals*. 2010;23:1085–1095.
121. Flinn JM, Bozzelli PL, Adlard PA, Railey AM. Spatial memory deficits in a mouse model of late-onset Alzheimer's disease are caused by zinc supplementation and correlate with amyloid-beta levels. *Front Aging Neurosci*. 2014;6:174.
122. Weingarten MD, Lockwood AH, Hwo SY, Kirschner MW. A protein factor essential for microtubule assembly. *Proc Natl Acad Sci USA*. 1975;72:1858–1862.
123. Grundke-Iqbal I, Iqbal K, Tung YC, Quinlan M, Wisniewski HM, Binder LI. Abnormal phosphorylation of the microtubule-associated protein tau (tau) in Alzheimer cytoskeletal pathology. *Proc Natl Acad Sci USA*. 1986;83:4913–4917.
124. Ihara Y, Nukina N, Miura R, Ogawara M. Phosphorylated tau protein is integrated into paired helical filaments in Alzheimer's disease. *J Biochem*. 1986;99:1807–1810.
125. Sayre LM, Perry G, Harris PL, Liu Y, Schubert KA, Smith MA. In situ oxidative catalysis by neurofibrillary tangles and senile plaques in Alzheimer's disease: a central role for bound transition metals. *J Neurochem*. 2000;74:270–279.
126. Good PF, Perl DP, Bierer LM, Schmeidler J. Selective accumulation of aluminum and iron in the neurofibrillary tangles of Alzheimer's disease: a laser microprobe (LAMMA) study. *Ann Neurol*. 1992;31:286–292.
127. Ma QF, Li YM, Du JT, Kanazawa K, Nemoto T, Nakanishi H, Zhao YF. Binding of copper (II) ion to an Alzheimer's tau peptide as revealed by MALDI-TOF MS, CD, and NMR. *Biopolymers*. 2005;79:74–85.

128. Kitazawa M, Cheng D, Laferla FM. Chronic copper exposure exacerbates both amyloid and tau pathology and selectively dysregulates cdk5 in a mouse model of AD. *J Neurochem*. 2009;108:1550–1560.
129. Voss K, Harris C, Ralle M, Duffy M, Murchison C, Quinn JF. Modulation of tau phosphorylation by environmental copper. *Transl Neurodegener*. 2014;3:24.
130. Zhou LX, Du JT, Zeng ZY, Wu WH, Zhao YF, Kanazawa K, Ishizuka Y, Nemoto T, Nakanishi H, Li YM. Copper (II) modulates in vitro aggregation of a tau peptide. *Peptides*. 2007;28:2229–2234.
131. Kim I, Park EJ, Seo J, Ko SJ, Lee J, Kim CH. Zinc stimulates tau S214 phosphorylation by the activation of Raf/mitogen-activated protein kinase-kinase/extracellular signal-regulated kinase pathway. *Neuroreport*. 2011;22:839–844.
132. Xiong Y, Jing XP, Zhou XW, Wang XL, Yang Y, Sun XY, Qiu M, Cao FY, Lu YM, Liu R, et al. Zinc induces protein phosphatase 2A inactivation and tau hyperphosphorylation through Src dependent PP2A (tyrosine 307) phosphorylation. *Neurobiol Aging*. 2013;34:745–756.
133. Guo C, Wang P, Zhong ML, Wang T, Huang XS, Li JY, Wang ZY. Deferoxamine inhibits iron induced hippocampal tau phosphorylation in the Alzheimer transgenic mouse brain. *Neurochem Int*. 2013;62:165–172.
134. Egaña JT, Zambrano C, Nuñez MT, Gonzalez-Billault C, Maccioni RB. Iron-induced oxidative stress modify tau phosphorylation patterns in hippocampal cell cultures. *Biometals*. 2003;16:215–223.
135. Lei P, Ayton S, Finkelstein DI, Spoerri L, Ciccotosto GD, Wright DK, Wong BX, Adlard PA, Cherny RA, Lam LQ, et al. Tau deficiency induces parkinsonism with dementia by impairing APP-mediated iron export. *Nat Med*. 2012;18:291–295.
136. Cruts M, Hendriks L, Van Broeckhoven C. The presenilin genes: a new gene family involved in Alzheimer disease pathology. *Hum Mol Genet*. 1996;5 Spec No:1449–1455.
137. Southon A, Greenough MA, Ganio G, Bush AI, Burke R, Camakaris J. Presenilin promotes dietary copper uptake. *PLoS One*. 2013;8:e62811.
138. Park IH, Jung MW, Mori H, Mook-Jung I. Zinc enhances synthesis of presenilin 1 in mouse primary cortical culture. *Biochem Biophys Res Commun*. 2001;285:680–688.
139. Li X, Liu Y, Zheng Q, Yao G, Cheng P, Bu G, Xu H, Zhang YW. Ferritin light chain interacts with PEN-2 and affects γ-secretase activity. *Neurosci Lett*. 2013;548:90–94.
140. DiFiglia M, Sapp E, Chase KO, Davies SW, Bates GP, Vonsattel JP, Aronin N. Aggregation of huntingtin in neuronal intranuclear inclusions and dystrophic neurites in brain. *Science*. 1997;277:1990–1993.
141. Vonsattel JP, Myers RH, Stevens TJ, Ferrante RJ, Bird ED, Richardson EP. Neuropathological classification of Huntington's disease. *J Neuropathol Exp Neurol*. 1985;44:559–577.
142. Rosas HD, Chen YI, Doros G, Salat DH, Chen NK, Kwong KK, Bush A, Fox J, Hersch SM. Alterations in brain transition metals in Huntington disease: an evolving and intricate story. *Arch Neurol*. 2012;69:887–893.
143. Xiao G, Fan Q, Wang X, Zhou B. Huntington disease arises from a combinatory toxicity of polyglutamine and copper binding. *Proc Natl Acad Sci USA*. 2013;110:14995–15000.
144. Hands SL, Mason R, Sajjad MU, Giorgini F, Wyttenbach A. Metallothioneins and copper metabolism are candidate therapeutic targets in Huntington's disease. *Biochem Soc Trans*. 2010;38:552–558.
145. Caragounis A, Price KA, Soon CP, Filiz G, Masters CL, Li QX, Crouch PJ, White AR. Zinc induces depletion and aggregation of endogenous TDP-43. *Free Radic Biol Med*. 2010;48:1152–1161.
146. Parker SJ, Meyerowitz J, James JL, Liddell JR, Nonaka T, Hasegawa M, Kanninen KM, Lim S, Paterson BM, Donnelly PS, et al. Inhibition of TDP-43 accumulation by Bis(thiosemicarbazonato)-copper complexes. *PLoS One*. 2012;7:e42277.

Further Reading

Steveson TC, Ciccotosto GD, Ma XM, Mueller GP, Mains RE, Eipper BA. Menkes protein contributes to the function of peptidylglycine alpha-amidating monooxygenase. *Endocrinology*. 2003;144:188–200.

Bousquet-Moore D, Mains RE, Eipper BA. Peptidylgycine alpha-amidating monooxygenase and copper: a gene-nutrient interaction critical to nervous system function. *J Neurosci Res*. 2010;88:2535–2545.

Kodama H, Fujisawa C, Bhadhprasit W. Pathology, clinical features and treatments of congenital copper metabolic disorders—focus on neurologic aspects. *Brain Dev*. 2011;33:243–251.

Index

I

N

O

P

R

U

V

W

X

Z

Kolibri 360 GmbH
Ferdinand-Jühlke-Straße 7
99095 Erfurt, Deutschland
produktsicherheit@kolibri360.de